D1154475

GENE EXPRESSION
AND ITS REGULATION

BASIC LIFE SCIENCES

Alexander Hollaender, General Editor
Biology Division
Oak Ridge National Laboratory
and The University of Tennessee

1973: VOLUME 1
  GENE EXPRESSION AND ITS REGULATION
  Edited by F. T. Kenney, B. A. Hamkalo, G. Favelukes, and J. T. August
  La Plata, Argentina, November 28 – December 3, 1971

In preparation:
  FUNDAMENTAL APPROACHES TO PLANT AND ANIMAL IMPROVEMENT
  Edited by A. Srb
  Cali, Colombia, November 27 – December 1, 1972

  REPRODUCTIVE PHYSIOLOGY AND GENETICS
  Edited by F. Fuchs and E. M. Coutinho
  Salvador, Bahia, Brazil, December, 1973

A Continuation Order Plan is available for this series. A continuation order will bring delivery of each new volume immediately upon publication. Volumes are billed only upon actual shipment. For further information please contact the publisher.

GENE EXPRESSION AND ITS REGULATION

Proceedings of the Eleventh International
Latin American Symposium, held at the University of
La Plata, Argentina, November 28–December 3, 1971

Edited by
Francis T. Kenney

and

Barbara A. Hamkalo

Biology Division
Oak Ridge National Laboratory
Oak Ridge, Tennessee

Gabriel Favelukes

Departamento de Bioquímica
Facultad de Ciencias Exactas
Universidad Nacional de La Plata
La Plata, Argentina

and

J. Thomas August

Department of Molecular Biology
Albert Einstein College of Medicine
Yeshiva University
Bronx, New York

International Symposium on
Gene Expression and Its Regulation

PLENUM PRESS • NEW YORK-LONDON • 1973

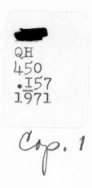
Library of Congress Catalog Card Number 72-90334
ISBN 0-306-36501-4

© 1973 Plenum Press, New York
A Division of Plenum Publishing Corporation
227 West 17th Street, New York, N. Y. 10011

United Kingdom edition published by Plenum Press, London
A Division of Plenum Publishing Company, Ltd.
Davis House (4th Floor), 8 Scrubs Lane, Harlesden, London,
NW10 6SE, England

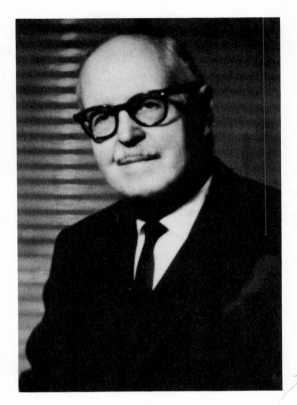

Bernardo Alberto Houssay (1887-1971)

This volume is dedicated to the memory of Dr. Bernardo Alberto Houssay, who was a member of the Organizing Committee for the La Plata symposium. Dr. Houssay, who passed on before the symposium actually took place, was a most outstanding physiologist. He was original in his approaches, and he did some of the most important pioneer work in endocrinology and related areas. Dr. Houssay played a vitally important role in the development of science in Latin America. Even under often adverse conditions, he insisted that new approaches in basic biology and biochemistry be encouraged. His influence was profoundly felt through his encouragement of younger men, and many of his own students now fill important positions in physiology. His leadership is now being reflected in the much broader view of science in general that is evidenced in Latin America. This present symposium demonstrates the high development that has taken place in basic biochemistry and biology.

Dr. Houssay will be very much missed not only by Latin Americans but by scientists all over the world.

ORGANIZING COMMITTEE

Honorary Presidents

Bernardo A. Houssay—Instituto de Biologia y Medicinia Experimental, Buenos Aires, Argentina.

Fritz Lipmann—Rockefeller University, New York, N.Y., U.S.A.

Severo Ochoa—Department of Biochemistry, New York University Medical Center, New York, N.Y., U.S.A.

Presidents

Alexander Hollaender—Biology Division, Oak Ridge National Laboratory, Oak Ridge, Tennessee, U.S.A., and University of Tennessee, Knoxville, Tennessee, U.S.A.

Luis F. Leloir—Instituto de Investigaciones Bioquímicas "Fundación Campomar" y Facultad de Ciencias Exactas y Naturales, Buenos Aires, Argentina.

Members

Israel D. Algranati—Instituto de Investigaciones Bioquímicas "Fundación Campomar" y Facultad de Ciencias Exactas y Naturales, Buenos Aires, Argentina.

Jorge E. Allende—Departmento de Biologia, Facultad de Ciencias, Universidad de Chile, Santiago, Chile.

J. Thomas August—Department of Molecular Biology, Albert Einstein College of Medicine, Yeshiva University, Bronx, New York, U.S.A.

Philip P. Cohen—Department of Physiological Chemistry, University of Wisconsin, Madison, Wisconsin, U.S.A.

Eduardo De Robertis—Instituto de Anatomía General y Embriología, Facultad de Medicina, Universidad de Buenos Aires, Argentina.

Héctor L. Fasano—Decano, Facultad de Ciencias Exactas, Universidad Nacional de La Plata, Argentina.

Oscar Grau—Departamento de Bioquímica, Facultad de Ciencias Exactas, Universidad Nacional de La Plata, Argentina.

Francis T. Kenney—Biology Division, Oak Ridge National Laboratory, Oak Ridge, Tennessee, U.S.A.

Francisco J. S. Lara—Departamento de Bioquímica, Instituto de Química, Universidade de São Paulo, Brasil.

Guillermo Soberón—Instituto de Investigaciones Biomédicas, Universidad Nacional Autónoma de México, México, D.F.

Andrés O. M. Stoppani—Instituto de Química Biológica, Facultad de Medicina, Universidad de Buenos Aires, Argentina.

General Secretary

Gabriel Favelukes—Departamento de Bioquímica, Facultad de Ciencias Exactas, Universidad Nacional de La Plata, Argentina.

SPONSORS

Facultad de Ciencias Exactas, Departamento de Bioquímica, Universidad Nacional de La Plata, Argentina.
Albert Einstein College of Medicine, Yeshiva University, Bronx, New York, U.S.A.
National Academy of Sciences of the United States, Washington, D.C., U.S.A.
Oak Ridge National Laboratory, Biology Division, Oak Ridge, Tennessee, U.S.A.

SUPPORTING INSTITUTIONS

Universidad Nacional de La Plata, Argentina.
Comisión de Investigaciones Científicas de la Provincia de Buenos Aires, Argentina.
Consejo Nacional de Investigaciones Científicas y Técnicas, Argentina.
Instituto Nacional de Farmacología y Bromatología, Argentina.
Organization of American States—Programa Regional de Desarrollo Científico y Tecnológico.
United States Atomic Energy Commission.
United States National Science Foundation.
Ford Foundation, U.S.A.

ACKNOWLEDGMENTS

The following Argentine institutions and firms have extended their generous collaboration and assistance:

Colegio de Abogados de La Plata.
Colegio de Escribanos de La Plata.
Consejo Profesional de Ciencias Económicas de la Provincia de Buenos Aires.
Colegio de Farmacéuticos de la Provincia de Buenos Aires.
Fundación Banco de Crédito Provincial, La Plata.
Laboratorios Bagó, La Plata.
Banco Río de la Plata.
Corporación Argentina de Productores de Carnes.
Olivetti Argentina, La Plata.
Philips Argentina.

Foreword

The Eleventh International Latin American Symposium is an important milestone reflecting the rapid development of basic biochemistry in Latin America. The topic "Gene Expression and Its Regulation" was received enthusiastically, and, thanks to the vision of our Argentine colleagues, the program developed rapidly under the leadership of Dr. Gabriel Favelukes as General Secretary of the Symposium. It is interesting to note the tremendous progress that has been made in basic and applied sciences in Latin America over the past few years. The increasing initiative and leadership being demonstrated by our Latin American colleagues in organizing these symposia is a most satisfying development that speaks well for the future of science in Latin America.

The early publication of this symposium has been made possible through the efforts of an editorial board consisting of Dr. F. T. Kenney (Oak Ridge National Laboratory), Dr. Gabriel Favelukes (University of La Plata), Dr. Barbara Hamkalo (Oak Ridge National Laboratory), and Dr. J. T. August (Albert Einstein College of Medicine).

As in previous symposia, excellent support has come from the Ford Foundation through a grant to the National Academy of Sciences, the United States Atomic Energy Commission, the National Science Foundation, OAS, and other groups.

Through the cooperation of the authorities at the University of La Plata, the Albert Einstein College of Medicine (the United States cosponsoring university), and other schools, this very successful symposium was made possible.

We were saddened by the loss of Dr. Bernardo Houssay, one of the Honorary Presidents of the Symposium. This volume is respectfully dedicated to Professor Houssay in recognition of his strong leadership in Latin American science.

A list of previous symposia in this series follows:

1961

International Symposium on Tissue Transplantation—Santiago, Viña del Mar, and Valparaiso, Chile. Published in 1962 by the University of Chile Press, Santiago; edited by A. P. Cristoffanini and Gustavo Hoecker; 269 pp.

1962

International Symposium on Mammalian Cytogenetics and Related Problems in Radiobio-
logy—São Paulo and Rio de Janeiro, Brazil. Published in 1964 by The Macmillan Company,
New York, under arrangement with Pergamon Press, Ltd., Oxford; edited by C. Pavan, C.
Chagas, O. Frota-Pessoa, and L. R. Caldas; 427 pp.

1963

International Symposium on Control of Cell Division and the Induction of Cancer—Lima,
Peru, and Cali, Colombia. Published in 1964 by the U.S. Department of Health, Education
and Welfare as *National Cancer Institute Monograph 14;* edited by C. C. Congdon and Pablo
Mori-Chavez; 403 pp.

1964

International Symposium on Genes and Chromosomes, Structure and Function—Buenos
Aires, Argentina. Published in 1965 by the U.S. Department of Health, Education and
Welfare as *National Cancer Institute Monograph 18;* edited by J. I. Valencia and Rhoda F.
Grell, with the cooperation of Ruby Marie Valencia; 354 pp.

1965

International Symposium on the Nucleolus—Its Structure and Function—Montevideo, Uruguay. Published in 1966 by the U.S. Department of Health, Education and Welfare as
National Cancer Institute Monograph 23; edited by W. S. Vincent and O. L. Miller, Jr.; 610
pp.

1966

International Symposium on Enzymatic Aspects of Metabolic Regulation—Mexico City,
Mexico. Published in 1967 by the U.S. Department of Health, Education and Welfare as
National Cancer Institute Monograph 27; edited by M. P. Stulberg; 343 pp.

1967

International Symposium on Basic Mechanisms in Photochemistry and Photobiology—
Caracas, Venezuela. Published in 1968 by Pergamon Press as *Photochemistry and Photobiology,* Vol. 7, No. 6; edited by J. W. Longworth; 326 pp.

1968

International Symposium on Nuclear Physiology and Differentiation—Belo Horizonte, Minas
Gerais, Brazil. Published in 1969 by The Genetics Society of America as a supplement to
Genetics, Vol. 61, No. 1; edited by R. P. Wagner; 469 pp.

1969

International Symposium on Fertility of the Sea—São Paulo, Brazil. Published in 1971 by
Gordon and Breach Science Publishers, New York; edited by J. D. Costlow; 2 vol., 622 pp.

1970

International Symposium on Visual Processes in Vertebrates—Santiago, Chile. Published in 1971 by Pergamon Press as Suppl. No. 3 to *Vision Research*, Vol. 11; edited by Thorne Shipley and J. E. Dowling; 477 pp.

Alexander Hollaender
Biology Division
Oak Ridge National Laboratory
Oak Ridge, Tennessee
and
University of Tennessee
Knoxville, Tennessee

Introduction

This volume contains the proceedings of the Eleventh Latin American Symposium—an International Symposium on Gene Expression and Its Regulation—which took place at the University of La Plata, Argentina, from November 28 to December 3, 1971. It is one of a series of symposia founded and conducted by Dr. Alexander Hollaender which are held annually in different Latin American universities to consider diverse areas of modern biology.

This symposium arose from a proposal made during the 1968 symposium in Belo Horizonte, to hold a meeting in which the current status of protein synthesis would be evaluated. This pointed not only to a need felt in this area after a decade of most intensive research but also to the growing interest and involvement of Latin American scientists in molecular biology.

The subject has been dealt with in its various classical as well as more recent aspects: transcription, tRNA and ribosome structure and origin, translation, and mitochondrial protein synthesis, treated from the mechanistic and regulatory points of view. Emphasis was placed on studies with eukaryotic systems. The results, a collection of two score papers and discussions at an impressive level, provide a picture of the field and reveal its present trends. They also show its remarkable progress in Latin America, reflected in the quality and number of contributions of this origin.

An important consequence of this symposium—as with preceding ones—has been the stimulating effect on Latin American participants, especially young scientists and students, of having personal contact and discussion with colleagues from abroad.

All these benefits have been attained thanks to the enthusiastic response and good will of the distinguished participants from far away and nearby countries, who created an atmosphere of active and fruitful exchange and left ties of friendship and cooperation. No less important have been the generous efforts and the sponsorship, support, and contributions of many individuals, institutions, and agencies toward the organization of the meeting. This recognition, and our thanks to all of them, should be especially directed to the members of the Organizing Committee, and to colleagues, students, and collaborators at the University of La Plata.

This symposium is a tribute to all those who have made possible the existence of science in Latin America. Three such men have been associated with our symposium: the late Bernardo A. Houssay, founder of physiology in Argentina, who largely influenced the growth of biological sciences in Latin America and to whose memory this volume is very fittingly dedicated; Luis F. Leloir, who has inspired and led the development and progress of biochemistry in our countries; and Alexander Hollaender, who with his vision, spirit, and energy has created effective means of communication and has stimulated and supported our scientific efforts and growth. Let this volume convey our indebtedness and gratitude to them.

The editing of this book has been in the charge of Dr. F. T. Kenney, Dr. Barbara Hamkalo, and Dr. J. T. August, besides myself. To them our grateful recognition for their efforts and their effective counselling, which helped in many ways to the realization of the symposium.

The Spanish translations of the summaries have been prepared by my wife, Dr. Susana S. de Favelukes, and the strenuous task of transcribing the recorded discussions was done untiringly by our secretaries, Mrs. Margarita Estrella de Fabre and Miss Clelia Volponi, with the collaboration of my colleagues and students. I wish to express to them my hearty thanks.

Gabriel Favelukes
General Secretary of the Symposium
University of La Plata
La Plata, Argentina

Symposium Participants

Alaniz, Jorge R.—Instituto de Fisiología Vegetal, Facultad de Agronomía, Universidad Nacional de La Plata, C.C. 31, La Plata, Argentina.

Alegria, Alvaro—Departamento de Ciencias Fisiológicas, Facultad de Medicina, Universidad del Valle, Apartado Aéreo 2188-Nacional 439, Cali, Colombia.

Algranati, Israel D.—Instituto de Investigaciones Bioquímicas "Fundación Campomar" y Facultad de Ciencias Exactas y Naturales, Obligado 2490, Buenos Aires, Argentina.

Algranati, Sara Goldenberg de—Instituto de Investigaciones Bioquímicas, "Fundación Campomar" y Facultad de Ciencias Exactas y Naturales, Obligado 2490, Buenos Aires, Argentina.

Allende, Jorge E.—Departamento de Química y Bioquímica, Facultad de Medicina, Universisidad de Chile, Casilla 6671, Santiago 4, Chile.

Añon, Maria Cristina—Departamento de Bioquímica, Facultad de Ciencias Exactas, Universidad Nacional de La Plata, Calles 47 y 115, La Plata, Argentina.

Anton, Dora—Departamento de Radiobiología, Comisión Nacional de Energía Atómica, Av. del Libertador 8250, Buenos Aires, Argentina.

August, J. Thomas—Department of Molecular Biology, Albert Einstein College of Medicine, Yeshiva University, 1300 Morris Park Avenue, Bronx, New York 10461, U.S.A.

Avila, Raquel—Departamento de Química Biológica, Facultad de Ciencias Exactas y Naturales, Universidad de Buenos Aires, Perú 222, Buenos Aires, Argentina.

Azzam, Manzur—Instituto de Investigaciones Bioquímicas "Fundación Campomar" y Facultad de Ciencias Exactas y Naturales, Obligado 2490, Buenos Aires, Argentina.

Bade, Ernesto G.—Cold Spring Harbor Laboratory, P.O. Box 100, Cold Spring Harbor, Long Island, New York 11724, U.S.A.

Bálsamo, Janne—Departamento de Bioquímica, Instituto de Química, Universidade de São Paulo, Caixa Postal 20780, São Paulo, Brasil.

Bard, Enzo—Departamento de Bioquímica, Facultad de Ciencias Exactas, Universidad Nacional de La Plata, Calles 47 y 115, La Plata, Argentina.

Barra, Hector S.—Departamento de Química Biológica, Facultad de Ciencias Químicas, Universidad Nacional de Córdoba, Córdoba, Argentina.

Basilio, Carlos—Departamento de Química y Bioquímica, Facultad de Medicina, Universidad de Chile, Casilla 6671, Santiago 4, Chile.

Bedetti, Carlos—Instituto de Química Biológica, Facultad de Medicina, Universidad de Buenos Aires, Paraguay 2155, Buenos Aires, Argentina.

Beorlegui, Norma—Departamento de Farmacología, Instituto Nacional de Farmacología y Bromatología, Caseros 2161, Buenos Aires, Argentina.

Bernard, Elena—Instituto de Biología y Medicina Experimental, Obligado 2490, Buenos Aires, Argentina.

Bertini, Francisco—Instituto de Histología y Embriología, Facultad de Ciencias Médicas, Universidad Nacional de Cuyo, Casilla de Correo 56, Mendoza, Argentina.

Bianchi, Nestor O.—Instituto Fitotecnico "Santa Catalina," Santa Catalina, Llavallol, Pcia Bs. As., Argentina.

Blaquier, Jorge—Instituto de Biología y Medicina Experimental, Obligado 2490, Buenos Aires, Argentina.

Bock, Robert M.—Laboratory of Molecular Biology, University of Wisconsin, Madison, Wisconsin 53706, U.S.A.

Borrajo, Celina Martone de—Departamento de Bioquímica, Facultad de Ciencias Exactas, Universidad Nacional de La Plata, Calles 47 y 115, La Plata, Argentina.

Bozzini, Pablo—Instituto Nacional de Microbiología "Carlos E. Malbrán," Av. Vélez Sarsfield 563, Buenos Aires, Argentina.

Bravo, Rodrigo—Departamento de Biología, Facultad de Ciencias, Universidad de Chile, Casilla 6671, Santiago 4, Chile.

Brenner, Rodolfo—Instituto de Fisiología, Facultad de Ciencias Médicas, Universidad Nacional de La Plata, Calles 60 y 120, La Plata, Argentina.

Brentani, Ricardo—Departamento de Bioquímica, Instituto de Química, Universidade de São Paulo, Cidade Universitaria, São Paulo, Brasil.

Burachik, Moises—Departamento de Bioquímica, Facultad de Ciencias Exactas, Universidad Nacional de La Plata, Calles 47 y 115, La Plata, Argentina.

Burdman, Jose A.—Orientación Química Biológica IV, Departamento de Química Biológica, Facultad de Farmacia y Bioquímica, Universidad de Buenos Aires, Junín 956, Buenos Aires, Argentina.

Burgos, Mario—Instituto de Histología y Embriología, Facultad de Ciencias Médicas, Universidad Nacional de Cuyo, Casilla de Correo 56, Mendoza, Argentina.

Buschiazzo, Hector—Instituto de Fisiología, Facultad de Ciencias Médicas, Universidad Nacional de La Plata, Calles 60 y 120, La Plata, Argentina.

Buschiazzo, Perla—Instituto de Fisiología, Facultad de Ciencias Médicas, Universidad Nacional de La Plata, Calles 60 y 120, La Plata, Argentina.

Bustamante Donayre, Ernesto—Departamento de Ciencias Fisiológicas, Universidad Peruana Cayetano Heredia, Km 3,5 Panamericana Norte, Apartado 5045, Lima, Perú.

Bustamante Monteverde, Carlos J.—Departamento de Bioquímica, Universidad Nacional Mayor de San Marcos, Apartado Postal 1546, Lima, Perú.

Cabada, Marcelo O.—Instituto de Biología, Facultad de Bioquímica, Química y Farmacia, Universidad Nacional de Tucumán, Ayacucho 482, San Miguel de Tucumán, Argentina.

Calandra, Roberto S.—Instituto de Biología y Medicina Experimental, Obligado 2490, Buenos Aires, Argentina.

Canessa J, Silvia—Departamento de Bioquímica, Universidad Católica, Casilla 114-D, Santiago, Chile.

Caputto, Ranwel—Departamento de Química Biológica, Facultad de Ciencias Químicas, Universidad Nacional de Córdoba, Ciudad Universitaria, Córdoba, Argentina.

Cárdenas, Marilu—Departamento de Biología, Facultad de Ciencias, Universidad de Chile, Casilla 6671, Santiago 4, Chile.

Castañeda, Mario—Departamento de Biología Molecular, Instituto de Investigaciones Biomédicas, Universidad Nacional Autónoma, Ciudad Universitaria 20, D.F., México.

Castro, Jacy Faro de—Instituto de Biofísica, Universidade Federal de Río de Janeiro, Av. Pasteur 458, Río de Janeiro, Brasil.

Castro, Roberto—Orientación Biología, Departamento de Ciencias Biológicas, Facultad de Farmacia y Bioquímica, Universidad de Buenos Aires, Junín 956, Buenos Aires, Argentina.

Cazorla T, Alberto—Departamento de Ciencias Fisiológicas, Universidad Peruana Cayetano Heredia, Km 3,5 Panamericana Norte, Apartado 5045, Lima, Perú.

Ceron, Gabriel—Instituto Nacional para Programas Especiales de Salud (IMPES), Av. El Dorado-Carrera SO, Apartado Aéreo 3951, Bogotá, D.E., Colombia.

Chambon, Pierre—Institut de Chimie Biologique, Faculté de Médecine de Strasbourg, 11, Rue Humann, Strasbourg, France.

Charreau, Eduardo—Instituto de Biología y Medicina Experimental, Obligado 2490, Buenos Aires, Argentina.

Cohen, Philip P.—Department of Physiological Chemistry, University of Wisconsin, Madison, Wisconsin 53706, U.S.A.

Colli, Walter—Departamento de Bioquímica, Instituto de Química, Universidade de São Paulo, Caixa Postal 20780, São Paulo, Brasil.

Contreras, Guillermo—Unidad de Virología, Universidad de Chile, Zañartu 1042, Santiago, Chile.

Corredor, Carlos—Departamento de Ciencias Fisiológicas, Facultad de Medicina, Universidad del Valle, Apartado Aéreo 2188, Cali, Colombia.

Costa Maia, Jose C. da—Departamento de Química, Instituto de Química, Universidade de São Paulo, Caixa Postal 20780, São Paulo, Brasil.

Coto, Celia—Departamento de Química Biológica, Facultad de Ciencias Exactas y Naturales, Universidad de Buenos Aires, Perú 222, Buenos Aires, Argentina.

Crosa, Jorge—Departamento de Química Biológica, Facultad de Ciencias Exactas y Naturales, Universidad de Buenos Aires, Perú 222, Buenos Aires, Argentina.

De Nicola, Alejandro F.—Instituto de Biología y Medicina Experimental, Obligado 2490, Buenos Aires, Argentina.

De Robertis, Eduardo—Instituto de Anatomía General y Embriología, Facultad de Medicina, Universidad de Buenos Aires, Paraguay 2155, Buenos Aires, Argentina.

De Robertis, Eduardo (h)—Instituto de Investigaciones Bioquímicas "Fundación Campomar" y Facultad de Ciencias Exactas y Naturales, Obligado 2490, Buenos Aires, Argentina.

Duvilanski, Beatriz—Orientación Química Biológica IV, Departamento de Química Biológica, Facultad de Farmacia y Bioquímica, Universidad de Buenos Aires, Junín 956, Buenos Aires, Argentina.

Echave Llanos, Julian—Instituto de Biología, Histología y Embriología, Facultad de Ciencias Médicas, Universidad Nacional de La Plata, Calles 60 y 120, La Plata, Argentina.

Escalante, Manuel—Departamento de Ciencias Biológicas, Facultad de Ciencias Exactas, Universidad Nacional de La Plata, Calles 47 y 115, La Plata, Argentina.

Ezcurra, Pedro—Instituto de Investigaciones Bioquímicas "Fundación Campomar" y Facultad de Ciencias Exactas y Naturales, Obligado 2490, Buenos Aires, Argentina.

Fasano, Hector L.—Facultad de Ciencias Exactas, Universidad Nacional de La Plata, Calles 47 y 115, La Plata, Argentina.

Favelukes, Gabriel—Departamento de Bioquímica, Facultad de Ciencias Exactas, Universidad Nacional de La Plata, Calles 47 y 115, La Plata, Argentina.

Favelukes, Susana S. de—Instituto de Química Biológica, Facultad de Medicina, Universidad de Buenos Aires, Paraguay 2155, Buenos Aires, Argentina.

Feix, Günter—Institut für Biologie III (Genetik und Molekular Biologie), Universität Freiburg, 78 Freiburg I Br., Germany.

Fernández, Maria T. Franze de—Departamento de Química Biológica, Facultad de Farmacia y Bioquímica, Universidad de Buenos Aires, Junín 956, Buenos Aires, Argentina.

Figini, Ruben V.—INIFTA, Facultad de Ciencias Exactas, Universidad Nacional de La Plata, Calles 47 y 115, La Plata, Argentina.

Fischer-Ferraro, Catalina—Instituto de Investigaciones Médicas, Hospital Tornú, Donato Alvarez 3000, Buenos Aires, Argentina.

Flawia, Mirtha—Instituto de Investigaciones Bioquímicas "Fundación Campomar" y Facultad de Ciencias Exactas y Naturales, Obligado 2490, Buenos Aires, Argentina.

Fontanive, Veronica—Departamento de Química Biológica, Facultad de Farmacia y Bioquímica, Universidad de Buenos Aires, Junín 956, Buenos Aires, Argentina.

Fossati, Alberto—Departamento de Bioquímica, Facultad de Ciencias Exactas, Universidad Nacional de La Plata, Calles 47 y 115, La Plata, Argentina.

Franchi, Carlos M.—Laboratorio de Biofísica, Instituto de Investigación de Ciencias Biológicas, Av. Italia 3318, Montevideo, Uruguay.

Gaede, Karl—Instituto Venezolano de Investigaciones Científicas, Apartado 1827, Caracas, Venezuela.

Gagliardino, Juan J.—Instituto de Fisiología, Facultad de Ciencias Médicas, Universidad Nacional de La Plata, Calles 60 y 120, La Plata, Argentina.

Galanti, Norbel—Departamento de Biología, Escuela de Medicina, Universidad de Chile, Zañartu 1042, Santiago, Chile.

Gambarini, Angelo G.—Departamento de Bioquímica, Instituto de Química, Universidade de São Paulo, Caixa Postal 20780, São Paulo, Brasil.

Garcia, Roberto—Departamento de Ultraestructura Celular, Instituto de Investigación de Ciencias Biológicas, Av. Italia 3318, Montevideo, Uruguay.

Garcia Oyola, Eliseo—Departamento de Ciencias Fisiológicas, Universidad Peruana Cayetano Heredia, Km 3,5 Panamericana Norte, Apartado 5045, Lima, Perú.

Garland, Peter B.—Medical Sciences Institute, Department of Biochemistry, The University Dundee DD1 4HN, Scotland.

Gatica, Marta—Departamento de Química y Bioquímica, Facultad de Medicina, Universidad de Chile, Casilla 6671, Santiago 4, Chile.

Gattoni, Renata C.—Universidad Nacional de Córdoba, Boulevard Las Heras 960, Córdoba, Argentina.

Geiduschek, E. Peter—Department of Biology, University of California at San Diego, P.O. Box 109, La Jolla, California 92037, USA.

Ghysen, Alain—Departamento de Biología, Facultad de Ciencias, Universidad de Chile, Casilla 6671, Santiago 4, Chile.

Goldstein, Daniel—Instituto de Investigaciones Médicas, Hospital Tornú, Donato Alvarez 3000, Buenos Aires, Argentina.

Gomez, Carlos J.—Orientación Química Biológica IV, Departamento de Química Biológica, Facultad de Farmacia y Bioquímica, Universidad de Buenos Aires, Junín 956, Buenos Aires, Argentina.

Gonzalez, Carmen—Departamento de Química y Bioquímica, Facultad de Medicina, Universidad de Chile, Casilla 6671, Santiago 4, Chile.

Gonzalez, Nelida—Instituto de Investigaciones Bioquímicas, Fundación Campomar y Facultad de Ciencias Exactas y Naturales, Obligado 2490, Buenos Aires, Argentina.

González Cadavid, Nestor F.—Departamento de Biología Celular, Facultad de Ciencias, Universidad Central de Venezuela, Apartado 10098, Caracas, Venezuela.

Grado, Carmen—Unidad de Virología, Universidad de Chile, Independencia 939, Santiago, Chile.

Grau, Oscar—Departamento de Bioquímica, Facultad de Ciencias Exactas, Universidad Nacional de La Plata, Calles 47 y 115, La Plata, Argentina.

Guglielmone, Alicia Ramirez de—Orientación Química Biológica IV, Departamento de Química Biológica, Facultad de Farmacia y Bioquímica, Universidad de Buenos Aires, Junín 956, Buenos Aires, Argentina.

Hamkalo, Barbara A.—Oak Ridge National Laboratory, Biology Division, P.O. Box Y, Oak Ridge, Tennessee 37830, U.S.A.

Hardesty, Boyd–Department of Chemistry, Clayton Foundation Biochemical Institute, University of Texas at Austin, Austin, Texas 78712, U.S.A.

Heredia, Claudio F.–Instituto de Enzimología, Centro de Investigaciones Biológicas, Velázquez 144, Madrid 6, España.

Hierro Quintana, Jose–Departamento de Bioquímica, Instituto de Química, Universidade de São Paulo, Caixa Postal 20780, São Paulo, Brasil.

Hoecker, Gustavo–Departamento de Biología, Escuela de Medicina, Universidad de Chile, Zañartu 1042, Santiago, Chile.

Hollaender, Alexander–Oak Ridge National Laboratory, Biology Division, P.O. Box Y, Oak Ridge, Tennessee 37830, U.S.A., and University of Tennessee at Knoxville, Tennessee, U.S.A.

Huberman, Alberto–Departamento de Bioquímica, Instituto Nacional de la Nutrición, México, D.F., México.

Hunau, Raquel Cohen de–Cátedra de Fisiología Vegetal, Facultad de Ciencias Agrarias, Universidad Nacional de Cuyo, Chacras de Coria, Mendoza, Argentina.

Iñon, Maria T. Tellez de–Instituto de Investigaciones Bioquímicas "Fundación Campomar" y Facultad de Ciencias Exactas y Naturales, Obligado 2490, Buenos Aires, Argentina.

Issaly, Abel–Laboratorio de Biología Molecular, Instituto Nacional de Microbiología "Carlos E. Malbrán," Av. Vélez Sarsfield 563, Buenos Aires, Argentina.

Issaly, Inda–Laboratorio de Biología Molecular, Instituto Nacional de Microbiología "Carlos E. Malbrán," Av. Vélez Sarsfield 563, Buenos Aires, Argentina.

Jiménez, Estela Sánchez de–Departamento de Bioquímica, Facultad de Química, Universidad Nacional Autónoma, Ciudad Universitaria 20, D.F., México.

Jiménez de Asua, Luis–Instituto de Investigaciones Bioquímicas "Fundación Campomar" y Facultad de Ciencias Exactas y Naturales, Obligado 2490, Buenos Aires, Argentina.

Jobbagy, Andres J.–Orientación Biología, Departamento de Ciencias Biológicas, Facultad de Farmacia y Bioquímica, Universidad de Buenos Aires, Junín 956, Buenos Aires, Argentina.

Jobbagy, Zulema Gampel de–Orientación Biología, Departamento de Ciencias Biológicas, Facultad de Farmacia y Bioquímica, Universidad de Buenos Aires, Junín 956, Buenos Aires, Argentina.

Judewicz, Norberto–Instituto de Investigaciones Bioquímicas "Fundación Campomar" y Facultad de Ciencias Exactas y Naturales, Obligado 2490, Buenos Aires, Argentina.

Kenney, Francis T.–Oak Ridge National Laboratory, Biology Division, P.O. Box Y, Oak Ridge, Tennessee 37830, U.S.A.

Kohan, Silvia Segre de–Instituto de Oncología "Angel H. Roffo," Facultad de Medicina, Universidad de Buenos Aires, Av. San Martín 5481, Buenos Aires, Argentina.

Krawiec, Leon–Orientación Química Biológica IV, Departamento de Química Biológica, Facultad de Farmacia y Bioquímica, Universidad de Buenos Aires, Junín 956, Buenos Aires, Argentina.

Lara, Francisco J. S.–Departamento de Bioquímica, Instituto de Química, Universidade de São Paulo, Caixa Postal 20780, São Paulo, Brasil.

Lejsek, Angela Vendola de–Departamento de Bioquímica, Facultad de Ciencias Exactas, Universidad Nacional de La Plata, Calles 47 y 115, La Plata, Argentina.

Leloir, Luis F.–Instituto de Investigaciones Bioquímicas "Fundación Campomar" y Facultad de Ciencias Exactas y Naturales, Obligado 2490, Buenos Aires, Argentina.

Lengyel, Peter–Department of Molecular Biophysics and Biochemistry, Yale University, New Haven, Connecticut 06520, U.S.A.

Lipmann, Fritz–Rockefeller University, New York, N.Y. 10021, U.S.A.

Lisanti, Norberto N.–Instituto de Oncología "Angel H. Roffo," Facultad de Medicina, Universidad de Buenos Aires, Av. San Martín 5481, Buenos Aires, Argentina.

Lizarraga, Beatriz—Departamento de Bioquímica, Universidad Nacional Mayor de San Marcos, Apartado Postal 1546, Lima, Perú.

Lombardo, Jorge—Departamento de Radiobiología, Comisión Nacional de Energía Atómica, Av. del Libertador 8250, Buenos Aires, Argentina.

Lucca, Fernando L. de—Departamento de Bioquímica, Faculdade de Medicina de Ribeirao Preto, da USP, Ribeirao Preto, S.P., Brasil.

Mahler, Henry R.—Department of Chemistry, Indiana University, Bloomington, Indiana 47401, U.S.A.

Manchester, Keith L.—Department of Biochemistry, University of the West Indies, Mona, Kingston 7, Jamaica.

Mariano, Marta—Facultad de Bioquímica, Química y Farmacia, Universidad Nacional de Tucumán, Ayacucho 482, San Miguel de Tucumán, Argentina.

Martinez, Estela Nora—Departamento de Bioquímica, Facultad de Ciencias Exactas, Universidad Nacional de La Plata, Calles 47 y 115, La Plata, Argentina.

Martinez Segovia, Zulema M. de—Laboratorio de Virus, Instituto Nacional de Microbiología "Carlos E. Malbrán," Av. Vélez Sarsfield 563, Buenos Aires, Argentina.

Martuscelli, Jaime—Departamento de Biología Molecular, Instituto de Investigaciones Biomédicas, Ciudad Universitaria 20, D.F., México.

Mazar Barnett, Beatriz Klein de—Departamento de Radiobiología, Comisión Nacional de Energía Atómica, Av. del Libertador 8250, Buenos Aires, Argentina.

Melgar, Ernesto—Departamento de Bioquímica, Universidad Nacional Mayor de San Marcos, Apartado Postal 1546, Lima, Perú.

Meneghini, Rogerio—Departamento de Bioquímica, Instituto de Química, Universidade de São Paulo, Caixa Postal 20780, São Paulo, Brasil.

Mersich, Susana—Departamento de Química Biológica, Facultad de Ciencias Exactas y Naturales, Universidad de Buenos Aires, Perú 222, Buenos Aires, Argentina.

Moldave, Kivie—California College of Medicine, University of California at Irvine, Irvine, California 92664, U.S.A.

Monasterio, Octavio—Departamento de Biológia, Facultad de Ciencias, Universidad de Chile, Casilla 6671, Santiago 4, Chile.

Mordoh, Jose—Instituto de Investigaciones Bioquímicas "Fundación Campomar" y Facultad de Ciencias Exactas y Naturales, Obligado 2490, Buenos Aires, Argentina.

Moussatche, Nissim—Laboratorio de Metabolismo Macromolecular, Instituto de Biofísica, Universidade Federal de Río de Janeiro, Av. Pasteur 458, Río de Janeiro, GB, Brasil.

Muñoz, Enzo—Departamento de Radiobiología, Comisión Nacional de Energía Atómica, Av. del Libertador 8250, Buenos Aires, Argentina.

Nethol, Victor—Departamento de Farmacología, Facultad de Ciencias Exactas, Universidad Nacional de La Plata, Calles 47 y 115, La Plata, Argentina.

Nomura, Masayasu—Institute for Enzyme Research, University of Wisconsin, Madison, Wisconsin 53706, U.S.A.

Novelli, G. David—Oak Ridge National Laboratory, Biology Division, P.O. Box Y, Oak Ridge, Tennessee 37830, U.S.A.

Oliver, Guillermo—Facultad de Bioquímica, Química y Farmacia, Universidad Nacional de Tucumán, Ayacucho 482, Tucumán, Argentina.

Orce, Luis F.—Departamento de Radiobiología, Comisión Nacional de Energía Atómica, Av. del Libertador 8250, Buenos Aires, Argentina.

Palatnik, Marcos—Departamento de Ciencias Biológicas, Facultad de Ciencias Exactas, Universidad Nacional de La Plata, Calles 47 y 115, La Plata, Argentina.

Palermo, Ana Maria—Departamento de Radiobiología, Comisión Nacional de Energía Atómica, Av. del Libertador 8250, Buenos Aires, Argentina.

Parada, Luis—Departamento de Investigación-Microbiología, Laboratorios Pfizer, SACI, Av. John McKeen 3501, Moreno, Pcia. de Buenos Aires, Argentina.

Parada, Nelda M. de—Cátedra de Bromatología, Facultad de Farmacia y Bioquímica, Universidad de Buenos Aires, Junín 956, Buenos Aires, Argentina.

Passeron, Susana—Instituto de Investigaciones Bioquímicas "Fundación Campomar" y Facultad de Ciencias Exactas y Naturales, Obligado 2490, Buenos Aires, Argentina.

Paz Aliaga, Benjamin—Departamento de Bioquímica, Universidad de San Agustín, Arequipa, Perú.

Peñaranda, Jose—Departamento de Química y Bioquímica, Facultad de Medicina, Universidad de Chile, Casilla 6671, Santiago 4, Chile.

Perazzolo, Clovis A.—Instituto de Biociencias-Bioquímica, Universidade de Río Grande do Sul, Porto Alegre, Brasil.

Peres, Clarita—Departamento de Bioquímica, Instituto de Química, Universidade de São Paulo, Cidade Universitaria, São Paulo, Brasil.

Perez Esandi, Miguela Vajlis de—Centro Panamericano de Zoonosis, Casilla de Correo 73, Ramos Mejía, Pcia, de Buenos Aires, Argentina.

Perretta, Marco—Laboratorio de Bioquímica, Departamento de Ciencias Fisiológicas, Facultad de Ciencias Pecuarias y Medicina Veterinaria, Universidad de Chile, Casilla 5539, Santiago, Chile.

Perry, Robert P.—The Institute for Cancer Research, Fox Chase, Philadelphia, Pennsylvania 19111, U.S.A.

Peso, Osvaldo A.—Centro de Investigaciones Microbiológicas, Facultad de Ciencias Exactas y Naturales, Universidad de Buenos Aires, Perú 222, Buenos Aires, Argentina.

Pirosky, Rosita R. de—Instituto de Oncología "Angel H. Roffo," Av. San Martín 5481, Buenos Aires, Argentina.

Pizarro, Olga—Departamento de Biología, Escuela de Medicina, Universidad de Chile, Zañartu 1042, Santiago, Chile.

Plata, Cecilia Aguilar de—Departamento de Ciencias Fisiológicas, Facultad de Medicina, Universidad del Valle, Apartado Aéreo 2188-Nacional 439, Cali, Colombia.

Quintans, Carlos J.—Departamento de Radiobiología, Comisión Nacional de Energía Atómica, Av. del Libertador 8250, Buenos Aires, Argentina.

Quinteros, Indalecio R.—Cátedra de Genética Microbiana, Facultad de Ciencias Veterinarias, Universidad Nacional de La Plata, Calles 60 y 119, La Plata, Argentina.

Ramirez, Jose L—Departamento de Biología Celular, Facultad de Ciencias, Universidad Central de Venezuela, Apartado 10098, Caracas, Venezuela.

Reyes, Oscar—Departamento de Bioquímica, Facultad de Ciencias, Universidad de Chile, Casilla 6671, Santiago 4, Chile.

Rivas, Carmen—Centro de Investigaciones Microbiológicas, Facultad de Ciencias Exactas y Naturales, Universidad de Buenos Aires, Perú 222, Buenos Aires, Argentina.

Rivas, Emilio—Centro de Investigaciones Microbiológicas, Facultad de Ciencias Exactas y Naturales, Universidad de Buenos Aires, Perú 222, Buenos Aires, Argentina.

Rho, Elena—Departamento de Bioquímica, Universidad Católica, Casilla 114-D, Santiago, Chile.

Rodriguez, Julio A.—Departamento de Química Biológica, Facultad de Ciencias Químicas, Universidad Nacional de Córdoba, Córdoba, Argentina.

Ruiz Holgado, Aida Pesce de—Instituto de Microbiología "Dr. Luis C. Verna," Facultad de Bioquímica, Química y Farmacia, Universidad Nacional de Tucumán, Ayacucho 482, Tucumán, Argentina.

Sacerdote, Fabio L.—Instituto de Histología y Embriología, Facultad de Ciencias Médicas, Universidad Nacional de Cuyo, Casilla de Correo 56, Mendoza, Argentina.

Sadnik, L. Isaac—Departamento de Bioquímica, Facultad de Ciencias Exactas, Universidad Nacional de La Plata, Calles 47 y 115, La Plata, Argentina.

Salum, Sonia Brieux de—Instituto de Investigaciones Hematológicas, Academia Nacional de Medicina, Andrés Pacheco de Melo 3081, Buenos Aires, Argentina.

Santelli, Glaucia M.—Departamento de Biología, Instituto de Biología, Universidade de São Paulo, São Paulo, Brasil.

Santelli, Roberto V.—Departamento de Bioquímica, Instituto de Química, Universidade de São Paulo, Caixa Postal 20780, São Paulo, Brasil.

Santiago, Ricardo—Departamento de Biología Molecular, Instituto de Investigaciones Biomédicas, Universidad Nacional Autónoma, Ciudad Universitaria 20, D.F., México.

Sarachu, Alberto N.—Departamento de Bioquímica, Facultad de Ciencias Exactas, Universidad Nacional de La Plata, Calles 47 y 115, La Plata, Argentina.

Schimke, Robert T.—Stanford University Medical Center, Department of Pharmacology, Stanford, California 94305, U.S.A.

Schuttenberg, Rita Fernandez de—Departamento de Bioquímica, Facultad de Ciencias Exactas, Universidad Nacional de La Plata, Calles 47 y 115, La Plata, Argentina.

Smith, John D.—MRC Laboratory of Molecular Biology, University Postgraduate Medical School, Hills Road, Cambridge CB2 2QH, England.

Soeiro, Ruy—Department of Medicine, Albert Einstein College of Medicine, 1300 Morris Park Avenue, Bronx, N.Y. 10461, U.S.A.

Sorarrain, Oscar—Departamento de Física, Facultad de Ciencias Exactas, Universidad Nacional de La Plata, Calles 47 y 115, La Plata, Argentina.

Sorgentini, Delia A.—Departamento de Bioquímica, Facultad de Ciencias Exactas, Universidad Nacional de La Plata, Calles 47 y 115, La Plata, Argentina.

Soto, Ana M.—Orientación Química Biológica IV, Departamento de Química Biológica, Facultad de Farmacia y Bioquímica, Universidad de Buenos Aires, Junín 956, Buenos Aires, Argentina.

Spirin, Alexander S.—Institute of Protein Research, Academy of Sciences of the U.S.S.R., Poustchino, Moscow Region, U.S.S.R.

Spitz, Moises—Departamento de Bioquímica, Facultad de Ciencias Exactas, Universidad Nacional de La Plata, Calles 47 y 115, La Plata, Argentina.

Stockert, Juan C.—Centro de Investigaciones en Reproducción, Facultad de Medicina, Universidad de Buenos Aires, Paraguay 2155, Buenos Aires, Argentina.

Stoppani, Andres O. M.—Instituto de Química Biológica, Facultad de Medicina, Universidad de Buenos Aires, Paraguay 2155, Buenos Aires, Argentina.

Tarlovsky, Martha Schwarcz de—Instituto de Química Biológica, Facultad de Medicina, Universidad de Buenos Aires, Paraguay 2155, Buenos Aires, Argentina.

Terenzi, Hector—Orientación Biología, Departamento de Ciencias Biológicas, Facultad de Farmacia y Bioquímica, Universidad de Buenos Aires, Junín 956, Buenos Aires, Argentina.

Terra, Walter—Departamento de Bioquímica, Instituto de Química, Universidade de São Paulo, São Paulo, Brasil.

Torres, Hector N.—Instituto de Investigaciones Bioquímicas "Fundación Campomar" y Facultad de Ciencias Exactas y Naturales, Obligado 2490, Buenos Aires, Argentina.

Torres, Ramon de—Cátedra de Microbiología, Facultad de Farmacia y Bioquímica, Universidad de Buenos Aires, Junín 956, Buenos Aires, Argentina.

Torres de Castro, Firmino—Instituto de Biofísica, Universidade Federal de Río de Janeiro, Av. Pasteur 458, Río de Janeiro, Brasil.

Travers, Andrew A.—MRC Laboratory of Molecular Biology, University Postgraduate Medical School, Hills Road, Cambridge CB2 2QH, England.

Tres, Laura—Centro de Investigaciones en Reproducción, Facultad de Medicina, Universidad de Buenos Aires, Paraguay 2155, Buenos Aires, Argentina.

Trione, Sinibaldo O.—Cátedra de Fisiología Vegetal, Facultad de Ciencias Agrarias, Universidad Nacional de Cuyo, Chacras de Coria, Mendoza, Argentina.

Ureta, Tito—Departamento de Química y Bioquímica, Facultad de Medicina, Universidad de Chile, Casilla 6671, Santiago 4, Chile.

Valencia, Helida Dopchiz de—Departamento de Bioquímica, Facultad de Ciencias Exactas, Universidad Nacional de La Plata, Calles 47 y 115, La Plata, Argentina.

Valenzuela, Alfonso—Laboratorio de Bioquímica, Departamento de Ciencias Fisiológicas, Facultad de Ciencias Pecuarias y Medicina Veterinaria, Universidad de Chile, Casilla 5539, Santiago, Chile.

Valenzuela, Pablo—Laboratorio de Bioquímica, Instituto de Ciencias Biológicas, Universidad Católica, Casilla 114-D, Santiago, Chile.

Vargas Linares, Clara E. Roig de—Instituto de Histología y Embriología, Facultad de Ciencias Médicas, Universidad Nacional de Cuyo, Casilla de Correo 56, Mendoza, Argentina.

Vasquez, Cesar—Instituto de Anatomía General y Embriología, Facultad de Medicina, Universidad de Buenos Aires, Paraguay 2155, Buenos Aires, Argentina.

Vazquez, David—Instituto de Biología Celular, Centro de Investigaciones Biológicas, Velázquez, 144, Madrid-6, España.

Verona, Carlos A.—Instituto de Biología Marina, Mar del Plata, Argentina.

Vilchez, Carlos—Instituto de Patología General y Experimental, Facultad de Ciencias Médicas, Universidad Nacional de Cuyo, Avenida Libertador 80, Mendoza, Argentina.

Weissmann, Charles—Institut für Molekularbiologie, Universität Zürich, Hönggerberg, CH-8049 Zürich, Switzerland.

Wettstein, Rodolfo—Departamento de Ultraestructura Celular, Instituto de Investigación de Ciencias Biológicas, Av. Italia 3318, Montevideo, Uruguay.

Yudelevich, Arturo—Laboratorio de Bioquímica, Departamento de Biología Celular, Universidad Católica, Casilla 114-D, Santiago, Chile.

Zachau, Hans G.—Institut für Physiologische Chemie und Physikalische Biochemie, Universität München, 8000 München 15, Germany.

Zingalles Oller do Nascimento, Bianca—Departamento de Bioquímica, Instituto de Química, Universidade de São Paulo, Cidade Universitaria, São Paulo, Brasil.

Zorzopulos, Jorge—Orientación Biología, Departamento de Ciencias Biológicas, Facultad de Farmacia y Bioquímica, Universidad de Buenos Aires, Junín 956, Buenos Aires, Argentina.

Contents

GENE EXPRESSION AND ITS REGULATION

1

What Do We Know
About Protein Synthesis?

Fritz Lipmann

Rockefeller University
New York, New York, U.S.A.

Of the three polymerizations that produce the tapes for the replication of genetic information, the framework of the biosynthetic process for protein synthesis is probably the one best understood. And yet close inspection shows our understanding to be still rather superficial. I will attempt here to summarize briefly what we know and to single out a few phases where we now hope to gain a deeper knowledge.

Genetic replication is performed by the master method of negative-positive image formation through hydrogen bonding between two pairs of purine and pyrimidine bases. The sequence of information transfer shown in Fig. 1 is one of two nucleic acid transcriptions: DNA to image DNA, and DNA to image RNA, the messenger RNA (mRNA). These transcriptions yield ribonucleotide sequences that are then translated into amino acid sequences through hydrogen bonding between triplet nucleotide codons of mRNA and anticodon triplets of aminoacyl-tRNA. This translation is the expression of the code and yields the proteins which are the principal ingredients that compound a new organism directly or by catalytic action.

Although this translation of the four-base shorthand tape into the 20 amino acid sequence is more complex than the preceding transcriptions, its mechanism was the earliest to be recognized in greater detail (1). It led us to find common features in the three consecutive stages of information transfer. This has become particularly clear recently in the transcription of chromosomal DNA to mRNA and its succeeding translation into amino acid sequence; in these two processes,

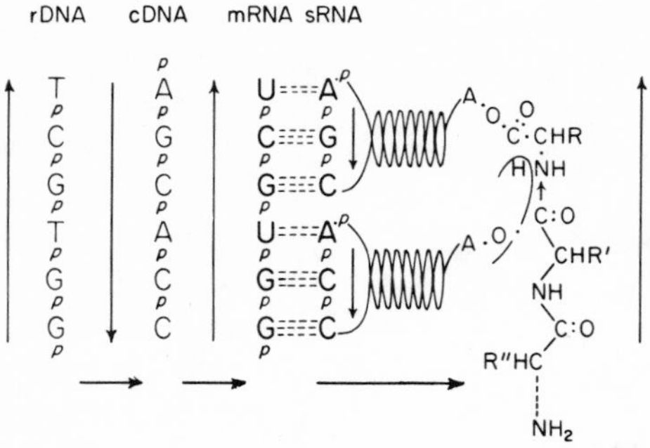

rDNA   cDNA   mRNA sRNA

Fig. 1. Transcription and expression of the code.

only limited parts of the nucleotide sequence are transcribed or translated. This implies that the replication mechanism has to be directed to start and terminate at specified places in the overall sequence.

The thus required division of the process into three stages, initiation, elongation, and termination, was first clearly recognized in protein synthesis (2). In this process, it appeared that the ribosome, which serves as the reactor for assembling the parts of the machinery, is complemented by a variety of cytoplasmic proteins—commonly called supernatant factors—which include special sets for the three phases, i.e., initiation factors, elongation factors, and termination factors. Clearly, initiation and termination are singular events, whereas elongation, framed within the two, is a repetitive addition of many units that form the new polymer. Only recently have the analogous factors been discovered in DNA-mRNA transcription, revealing, as expected, an analogous three-phase sequence for breaking up the large sequences in the chromosome into smaller messages for translation into a few proteins at a time. In this case, the factors are called sigma (σ) for initiation (3) and rho (ρ) for termination and release (4).

The scheme in Fig. 1 does not include the enzymatic machinery but merely summarizes chain elongation. Most emphasis is placed on the final process of assembling the 20 amino acids, showing more explicitly the reading of mRNA by the codon-anticodon interaction which yields the orderly arrangement of the amino acids in the protein chain. The dynamics of this polypeptide chain elongation is illustrated in Fig. 2. The ribosome is pictured moving on mRNA, which glides along the smaller ribosomal subunit. On the upper part of the ribosome, two tRNAs are pictured bound side-by-side to the larger subunit; the left one carries the elongating chain, the right one brings in the newly adding amino acid, and both are codon-anticodon linked to the message. The addition progresses from left to right. On the left, an empty tRNA, having added its amino acid to the elongating chain, is leaving, and the peptidyl-tRNA sitting on the donor site is in the process of transacting the transfer of its peptidyl to the new aminoacyl-tRNA on the acceptor site. Then the freshly elongated peptidyl-tRNA has to move from acceptor site to donor site to continue the next round of transfer to a new aminoacyl-tRNA. For this reason, transpeptidation is followed by a translocation of the elongated peptidyl-tRNA. On the right side of the scheme, a new aminoacyl-tRNA is already aiming to join its anticodon triplet to continue the process.

The events during every elongation step, which we call the elongation cycle (2,6), are elaborated in Fig. 3, using as an example poly U-linked polyphenyl-alanine synthesis. At the upper left, a ribosome is shown right after translocation. It carries a peptidyl-tRNA, and the triplet beside it is free. It is filled in stage 2 by an aminoacyl-tRNA, and immediately after its addition the ribosomal trans-peptidase located in the larger subunit transacts peptidyl transfer. This is followed in stage 3 by translocation of the newly elongated peptidyl-tRNA from acceptor to donor site, thereby expelling the empty tRNA. At the close of the cycle (stage 4) after translocation, the newly elongated peptidyl-tRNA has returned to stage 1 and is ready to repeat the cycle. The activities of the various supernatant factors are listed and explained in Table I.

INITIATION (1)

Initiation requires three factors, F1, F2, and F3 (7), which interact and appear to connect termination and initiation. After release of a protein by the termination process, the ribosome dissociates (8) where F3 seems to be involved

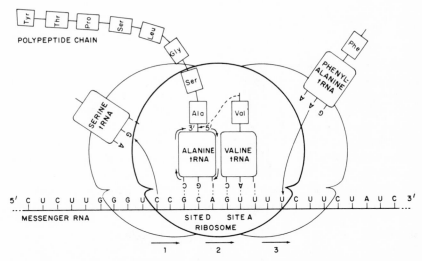

Fig. 2. Survey of sequential addition of amino acids, adapted from Crick (5). Site D, donor site; site A, acceptor site.

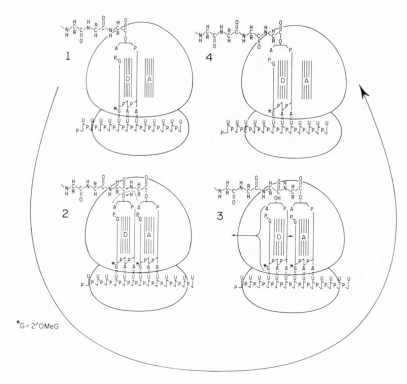

Fig. 3. Peptide elongation cycle. Details are discussed in the text.

(9). The initiation factors then connect the small subunit with a specially located AUG triplet on mRNA and a special initiation $tRNA_f^{Met}$ (10). In bacterial and mitochondrial systems, the Met on this tRNA is formylatable and carries formylmethionine (1, p. 411). Likewise, a special $tRNA_i^{Met}$ initiates in the eukaryote cytoplasm (1, p. 420) but is not formylated, carrying only methionine. A different $tRNA^{Met}$ is specific for the internal placement of methionine, which also connects with the methionine-coding AUG triplet. After formation, the initiation complex of the small subunit joins the large subunit and elongation begins. The initiating formylmethionine in bacteria or the methionine in eukaryotes are generally split off from the finished protein.

TERMINATION-RELEASE

In mapping out the coordination between triplets and amino acids, it appeared that three codons were singled out as nonsense codons since they did not connect with any of the aminoacyl-tRNAs (11). They are UAA, UAG, and UGA, and they turned out to be termination codons. There is no tRNA involved in termination, but instead the termination codon complexes with a protein, one of the two release factors: R1 for UAA and UAG, R2 for UAA and UGA (11). This complex in some manner induces the peptidyl transferase to catalyze transfer to water rather than to an amino group and thereby releases the protein from the tRNA of the terminally added amino acid.

COMPOSITION AND SHAPE OF THE RIBOSOME

The most important part in the protein synthesis machinery is surely the ribosome. A number of groups (12) have studied its composition. It was long known to contain nearly equal amounts of RNA and protein. But, in contrast to each subunit containing one larger RNA each, the larger in addition having a small 5S RNA, subunits were found to have an amazingly large number of proteins. The most studied subunits of the *Escherichia coli* ribosome contain 21 proteins for the 30S subunit and 30-35 for the 50S subunit. The functional coordination of these proteins, with a few exceptions, is not well understood.

Table I. Bacterial Complementary Factors[a]

Phase	Factor	Origin	Function
1. Initiation	F3	High salt ribosomal wash	Dissociation of ribosomal subunits
	$\left.\begin{array}{l}\text{F1}\\\text{F2}\\\text{F3}\end{array}\right\}$ +GTP		Binding of mRNA and initiator tRNA to 30S subunits
2. Elongation cycles	$\left.\begin{array}{l}T_u\\T_s\end{array}\right\}$ T + GTP	Supernatant fraction	Binding of aminoacyl-tRNA-T_u-GTP complex to ribosome
	Peptidyl transferase	50S Ribosomal subunit	Peptidyl transfer from peptidyl-tRNA to aminoacyl-tRNA
	G + GTP	Supernatant fraction	Translocation of elongated peptidyl-tRNA; release of empty tRNA
3. Termination	R1 R2	Supernatant fraction	Release of protein before UAA, UAG or UAA, UGA

[a] For details, compare text and Fig. 2 and 3.

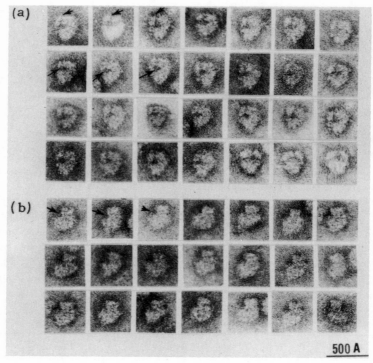

Fig. 4. Gallery of electron microscopic images from monomeric ribosomes
(13). (a) Front views; (b) side views.

The size of the ribosome is near the limit of electron microscopic resolution, and only recently has a clearer definition of its structure become available through the work of Sabatini and his group (13), who have presented a very careful analysis of liver ribosomes by electron microscopy. Dr. Sabatini has permitted me to discuss this work and to use some of his pictures, selected from a large number of electron micrographs. The first of the series (Fig. 4) presents a gallery of front and side views of liver ribosomes. In the side views, the smaller subunit appears to fill only about half the surface of the larger one. There is a ridge in the smaller which, together with one in the larger, forms a channel at a right angle to the long surface extension of the larger; it is not quite central but somewhat displaced sideways.

The mRNA is shown in the electron micrograph of Fig. 5 to extend between the units. The exact position has not been fixed. Two possibilities appear from Sabatini's evaluation of these data: (A) the mRNA may stretch between the two subunits along the longer diameter, or (B) it may thread through the channel.

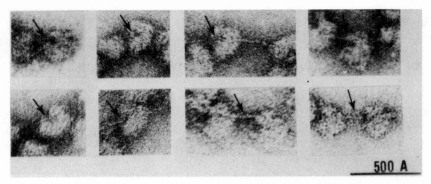

Fig. 5. Selected polysome images (13). The arrows indicate mRNA threading along between the subunits.

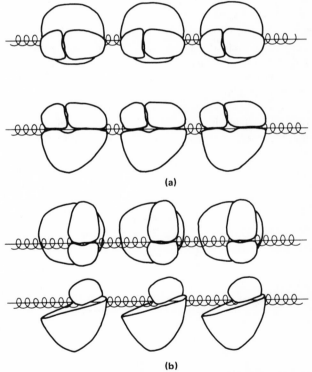

(a)

(b)

Fig. 6. Schematic representation of two possible relationships of the ribosomes with the messenger strand in polysomes (13). (a) The strand runs through the tunnel between the subunits; (b) it runs between the two subunits along the longer extension of the ribosome.

The two possibilities are shown schematically in Fig. 6, which also shows more clearly the interrelationship between the two subunits.

RECENT PROGRESS IN UNDERSTANDING TRANSLOCATION

To me, the most interesting part of the elongation phase is the translocation step, the energy derivation for which we attribute to the ribosome-linked GTPase catalyzed by the G factor. We visualize that the energy available from GTP breakdown should be used to move the ribosome along. We are now slowly beginning to see more clearly what might happen.

An earlier proposed possibility (14) that there was a similarity between muscle contraction and translocation has recently been taken up in some detail in a paper by Hill (15) which is too complex to discuss here. However, the finding that a specific ribosomal protein is essential in the ribosome-linked GTPase effect of the G factor is of special interest (16). It is the only acidic protein of the 50S (bacterial) subunit which is described as having an amino acid composition similar to that of contractile fiber proteins. In addition, recent observations indicate that a conformational change of the ribosome occurs parallel with the translocation step. A change in the sedimentation constant (17,18) has been reported, as well as an altered rate of hydrogen exchange with the medium by ribosomes in the translocation phase (18).

Recent observations have linked the GTP hydrolysis in the early phase of elongation when the ternary complex aminoacyl-tRNA-T_u-GTP binds to the ribosome, with the normally following G-GTP linked translocation. Using anti-

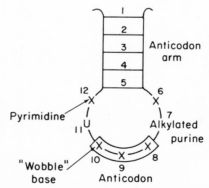

Fig. 7. Scheme of the anticodon arm of a tRNA (22). (1-5) Hydrogen bonds between two bases in the stem region; (6-12) the seven bases of the loop containing the anticodon triplet.

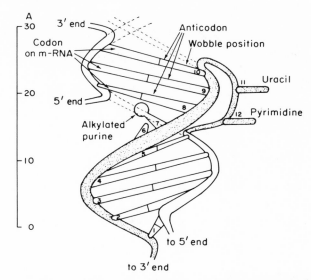

Fig. 8. *A double helical region composed of three codon and three anticodon bases, extending into the stem double helix (22).*

biotics of the siomycin-bryamycin-thiostrepton family, a number of workers reported simultaneously (19-21) that the ternary aminoacyl-T_u-GTP complex and G factor bind to an identical or overlapping site and that the antibiotic that inhibits protein synthesis also inhibits the GTP breakdown connected with both the binding of the ternary complex and the G factor-ribosome interaction. We might then conclude that when the ternary complex binds in the absence of G factor, breakdown of GTP may be due to uncoupling. However, when the presence of G factor allows the overall reaction to go to completion, GTP of the ternary complex may be used for producing translocation.

It was my intention to give some idea of the more complex parts of the overall scheme which, until relatively recently, were only very superficially understood. I would like to close by showing ways in which we can approach the understanding of the crucial reaction in the whole complex, namely, the interaction between the two tRNAs and the mRNA essential for production of a specific amino acid sequence.

Some time ago, Fuller and Hodgson (22) published a paper in *Nature* from which I have taken some figures that are attempts to map out the details of the triplet codon-anticodon interaction. Figure 7 is just for orientation and shows the lower part of the well-known tRNA cloverleaf, the anticodon arm with the relatively constant environment of the triplet. This anticodon chain is usually

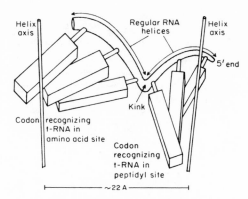

Fig. 9. Schematic diagram of two successive codon triplets in mRNA recognizing two tRNA anticodons (22).

schematized as circular. However, to fit it for bonding to the codon sequence in mRNA, it is assumed that the two triplets will form a short double helical stretch, as visualized in Fig. 8. To round out the discussion, Fig. 9 presents presumed positions of the two active triplet codons, both presumably interacting with their respective anticodons, as shown in Fig. 8. Of interest is the placing of a kink in mRNA between the two adjacent active triplets.

I have tried to present some glimpses of different stages where we are approaching a better specification in our still quite superficial scheme. We have to visualize that there are many unsolved problems in the interaction of the codon-anticodon. We do not understand the role of the ternary complex with the $GTP-T_u$ that binds the newly adding aminoacyl-tRNA to the ribosome—it may be involved in reinforcing the hydrogen bonding. In the placement of the two tRNAs on the ribosome, they should be centered around the transpeptidation enzyme, the location of which on the ribosome has not been very well defined. So far, it has not been possible to isolate the enzymatic function, which Monro's experiments (23) place indisputably in the large subunit of the ribosome.

It has been my intention to focus on those phases in which an extension of our knowledge seems to be developing, using for illustration examples of partial reactions where we are on the way to understanding more fully the dynamics of the process. I hope that eventually one may be able to compose a picture which will map out in all its details the biosynthesis of a protein. The feeling one might have on comprehending it completely I would like to compare to Mozart's description of his feeling on reviewing a finished piece of his music (24): "the whole, though it be long, stands almost complete and finished in my mind, so that I can survey it, like a fine picture, or a beautiful statue, at a glance. Nor do I hear in my imagination the parts *successively* but I hear them, as it were, all at once. What a delight this is, I cannot tell!"

ACKNOWLEDGMENTS

I should like to thank Dr. D. Sabatini for permitting me to show his electron micrographs and schemes, and Drs. W. Fuller and A. Hodgson for allowing me to reproduce their figures.

SUMMARY

This paper summarizes our present understanding of the machinery for sequential amino acid polymerization on ribosomes to yield the polypeptide chain of a protein through translation of the nucleotide sequence in the messenger ribonucleic acid. The three phases of the process, initiation, elongation, and release of the completed polymer, are outlined as being dependent on interaction between the ribosome, peptide- and amino acid-charged transfer ribonucleic acids, and cytoplasmic complements (supernatant factors). The repeating elongation cycles are concentrated on. They are catalyzed by enzyme-like functions: (a) T factor in aminoacyl-tRNA fixation, (b) a ribosomal protein complex in transpeptidation, and (c) peptidyl-tRNA translocation along the mRNA through G-factor-dependent GTP breakdown.

Although still relatively superficial, the understanding of these key reactions is now developing into more detailed comprehension. Through recent gains in the recognition of ribosomal structures by Sabatini and his group, the interaction between messenger RNA and ribosome has become better understood. Furthermore, advances in our knowledge of the manner in which energy from G-linked GTP breakdown may be used to move the ribosome are discussed, together with theories on mRNA codon-tRNA anticodon interaction.

RESUMEN

Este papel resume muestro presente conocimiento del mecanismo de la polimerización en secuencia de aminoácidos en los ribosomas, la cual resulta en una cadena polipeptídica mediante la traducción de la secuencia nucleótida en el ácido ribonucléico mensajero. Las tres fases del proceso, iniciación, elongación y liberación del polímero completado, son descritas como dependientes de la interacción entre el ribosoma, el péptide y los ácidos ribonucleicos de transferencia cargados, y los factores citoplasmáticos (factores en el supernadante). Hemos concentrado nuestra atención en los ciclos de elongación. Estos son catalizados por funciones similares a las enzimáticas: (a) el factor T en la fijación del aminoacil-tRNA, (b) el complejo proteico ribosomal en la transpeptidación, y (c) la translocación del peptidil-tRNA a lo largo del mRNA a través del factor G, dependiente de la disociación de GTP.

Aunque nuestra comprension de estas reacciones es todavía relativamente superficial, está desarrollándose un conocimiento más detallado. Como consecuencia de los resultados obtenidos recientemente por Sabatini y su grupo eon relación al reconocimiento de las estructuras ribosomales, la interacción entre el RNA mensajero y el ribosoma se comprende mejor. Más aún, los avances de nuestro conocimiento de la manera en que la energía del G ligado al GTP durante la disociación puede utilizarse para mover el ribosoma, son discutidos, conjuntamente con las teorías sobre las interacciones entre mRNA, codon-tRNA y el anticodon.

REFERENCES

1. Lucas-Lenard, J. and Lipmann, F., *Ann. Rev. Biochem., 40,* 409 (1971).
2. Lipmann, F., *Science, 164,* 1024 (1969).
3. Burgess, R. R., Travers, A.A., Dunn, J. J., and Bautz, E. K. F., *Nature, 221,* 43 (1969).
4. Roberts, J. W., *Nature, 224,* 1168 (1969).
5. Crick, F. H. C., *Sci. Am., 215,* 55 (1966).
6. Spirin, A., and Gavrilova, L. P., *The Ribosome,* Springer-Verlag, New York (1969), p. 121.
7. Iwasaki, K., Sabol, S., Wahba, A. J., and Ochoa, S., *Arch. Biochem. Biophys., 125,* 542 (1968).
8. Subramanian, A. R., Davis, B. D., and Beller, R. J., *Cold Spring Harbor Symp. Quant. Biol., 34,* 223 (1969).
9. Davis, B. D., *Nature, 231,* 153 (1971).
10. Guthrie, C., and Nomura, M., *Nature, 219,* 232 (1968).
11. Caskey, C. T., Tompkins, R., Scolnick, E., Caryk, T., and Nirenberg, M., *Science, 162,* 135 (1968); Scolnick, E., Tompkins, R., Caskey, T., and Nirenberg, M., *Proc. Natl. Acad. Sci. U.S.A., 61,* 768 (1968).
12. Wittmann, H. G., Stöffler, G., Hindennach, I., Kurland, C. G., Randall-Hazelbauer, L., Birge, E. A., Nomura, M., Kaltschmidt, E., Mizushima, S., Traut, R. R., and Bickle, T. A., *Mol. Gen. Genet., 111,* 327 (1971).
13. Nonomura, Y., Blöbel, G., and Sabatini, D., *J. Mol. Biol., 60,* 303 (1971).
14. Nishizuka, Y., and Lipmann, F., *Arch. Biochem. Biophys., 116,* 344 (1966).
15. Hill, T. L., *Proc. Natl. Acad. Sci. U.S.A., 64,* 267 (1969).
16. Kischa, K., Möller, W., and Stöffler, G., *Nature New Biol. 233, 62* (1971)
17. Schreier, M. H., and Noll, H., *Proc. Natl. Acad. Sci. U.S.A., 68,* 805 (1971).
18. Chuang, D.-M., and Simpson, M. V., *Proc. Natl. Acad. Sci. U.S.A., 68,* 1474 (1971).
19. Kinoshita, T., Liou, Y.-F., and Tanaka, N., *Biochem. Biophys. Res. Commun., 44,* 859 (1971).
20. Cundliffe, E., *Biochem. Biophys. Res. Commun., 44,* 912 (1971).
21. Modolell, J., Cabrer, B., Parmeggiani, A., and Vazquez, D., *Proc. Natl. Acad. Sci. U.S.A., 68,* 1796 (1971).
22. Fuller, W., and Hodgson, A., *Nature, 215,* 817 (1967).
23. Monro, R. E., Staehelin, T., Celma, M. L., and Vazquez, D., *Cold Spring Harbor Symp. Quant. Biol., 34,* 357 (1969).
24. Davenport, M., *Mozart,* Charles Scribner's Sons, New York (1956), p. 283.

2

Structure and Function
of Phage RNA:
A Summary of Current Knowledge

C. Weissmann, M. A. Billeter,
H. Weber, H. M. Goodman,
and J. Hindley

Institut für Molekularbiologie
Universität Zürich
Zürich, Switzerland
H. M. Goodman
Department of Biochemistry
University of California
San Francisco, California, U.S.A.
and
J. Hindley
Department of Biochemistry
University of Bristol
Bristol, England

The RNA-containing coliphages may be classified into three, possibly four, serological groups (1,2). The first of these is comprised of phages such as f2, R17, and MS2, which are quite similar among themselves and differ considerably from Qβ, a member of the third group. These four phages have been studied intensively in the last few years (3-6). Their RNAs consist of about 3500 nucleotides (7,8) and comprise three cistrons (10-12). The capsid consists of about 180 coat protein subunits (13) and at least one molecule of another virus-specific protein, the A or maturation protein (14-16). Qβ contains a further protein, designated A_1, which may arise by read-through from the coat cistron into the subsequent nucleotide sequence (17-19). The third viral cistron codes for the β subunit of the viral replicase (20,21). The cistron order is A-coat-replicase for both phage groups (23-25). The complete amino acid sequence of the coat proteins of several phages has been established (26-29); only the first few amino acids of the A proteins and the replicase subunits have been determined (18,30,31).

The nucleotide sequences of the phage RNAs are being studied in several laboratories (33-47). The strategy currently applied may be broken down into three phases: (1) reduction of the viral RNA into subsets of about 50-200 nucleotides in length, (2) determination of the nucleotide sequence of the subsets, and (3) alignment of the subsets in their natural order. Only the first of these steps will be discussed below (*cf.* ref. 48 for the latter steps).

REDUCTION OF THE VIRAL RNA TO SUBSETS

Two principal approaches have been used to obtain RNA segments susceptible to nucleotide sequence analysis. The degradative methods are based on the use of nucleases under conditions where only a limited number of the potentially cleavable phosphodiester bonds are split. Relative resistance to nucleolytic cleavage is inherent in the secondary and possibly tertiary structure of the RNA, since linkages between nucleotides located in double-helical regions are less susceptible to enzymatic attack than those present in single-stranded regions (46,49-51); it appears, however, that also the primary structure of the RNA confers relative resistance on some internucleotide bonds which in principle are susceptible to the nuclease in question (53). The isolation of pure RNA fractions from the mixture of degradation products is one of the main technical bottlenecks. Two main separation techniques have been developed for this purpose, namely,

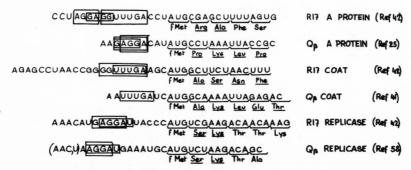

Fig. 1. The ribosome binding sites of RNA phage cistrons. The sequences of the underlined amino acids have been determined independently (*cf.* text for references); the others were deduced from the nucleotide sequence.

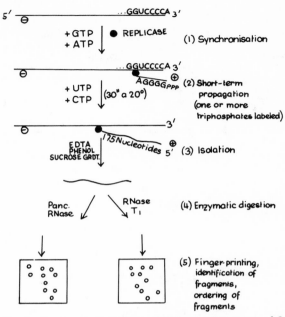

Fig. 2. *Synchronized synthesis of 5'-terminal segments of Qβ RNA* in vitro. (1) Synchronization of Qβ replicase. Qβ-minus strands, GTP, and ATP are incubated to give initiation and limited chain elongation up to the point where CTP is required for further synthesis. (2) UTP and CTP are added. (Any one or all of the substrates are α-^{32}P labeled.) Incubation is carried out under conditions where the elongation rate is about six nucleotides per second. Synthesis is stopped at any desired point by the addition of EDTA. (3) After deproteinization, the radioactive product is heat-denatured and purified by sucrose gradient centrifugation. (4) Aliquots are digested with pancreatic and T1 RNase, respectively. (5) the oligonucleotides are separated by two-dimensional electrophoresis and analyzed by Sanger's techniques.

polyacrylamide gel electrophoresis (50-52,54) and displacement chromatography (homochromatography) (55,56).

Specific protection of certain regions of viral RNA against nucleases can be attained by binding ribosomes to either intact or fragmented RNA. This procedure has allowed the isolation of the RNA segments corresponding to the ribosome binding sites of all cistrons of R17 (42) and of Qβ (25,41 58) (Fig. 1). A similar approach, in which Qβ replicase was bound to Qβ RNA prior to digestion with T1 RNase, has yielded a piece of RNA containing a binding site for the viral polymerase (59).

A synthetic approach to the preparation of viral RNA subsets has been reported by Billeter *et al.* (43). Qβ RNA is synthesized *in vitro* by Qβ replicase,

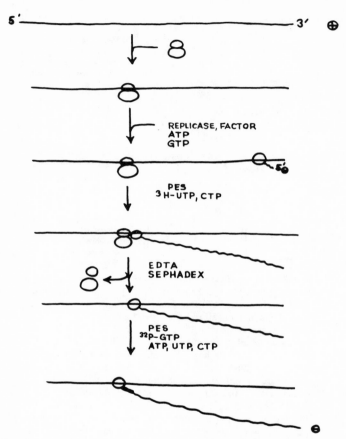

Fig. 3. Resynchronization of RNA synthesis at the beginning of the coat cistron. The Qβ RNA-ribosome complex is incubated with Qβ replicase factor, ATP, and GTP to give an early replicating complex. Polyethylene sulfonate is added to inactivate any free enzyme and thereby prevent initiation during the later phase of the experiment. Elongation is started by adding UTP and CTP (in some experiments ^{3}H-UTP was used to monitor the first phase of synthesis). After 5 min at 37° EDTA is added to remove the ribosome from the complex. EDTA and substrates are removed by Sephadex chromatography. The complex is then incubated with the four standard triphosphates, of which one or all are α-labeled with ^{32}P at high specific activity, for 15 sec at 20°, to allow synthesis of a labeled segment about 100 nucleotides in length.

using either a plus or a minus strand as template. Synthesis begins with the 5′ terminus and proceeds with an elongation rate of about six nucleotides per second at 20°. By synchronizing RNA synthesis and using a-^{32}P-labeled ribonucleoside triphosphates as substrates during defined periods of synthesis, it becomes possible in principle to synthesize either plus or minus strands, radioactively labeled in any desired segment (Fig. 2). In practice, however, synchrony diminishes as synthesis proceeds, so that the method has up to now been utilized only to examine the first few hundred nucleotides at the 5′ termini of both plus and minus strands. A new approach has been reported recently, allowing resynchronization of synthesis at an interior position of the RNA (60). A ribosome is bound to the coat cistron binding site [the only site ribosomes bind to in native Qβ RNA (41,58)]; and the RNA-ribosome complex is used as a template for Qβ replicase, with unlabeled ribonucleoside triphosphates as substrates. Elongation ceases when replicase reaches the ribosome. The ribosome is then removed from the RNA by treatment with EDTA, and the replicating complex is separated from substrates and EDTA by chromatography on Sephadex. On addition of radioactive substrates, synchronized synthesis ensues and a labeled minus strand segment is produced, which extends from the region complementary to the coat initiation site into the region complementary to the end of the A-protein cistron (Fig. 3). As first pointed out and illustrated by Bishop *et al.* (61), sequence determination on RNA labeled with a single, a-^{32}P-nucleotide allows exploitation of nearest-neighbor data, which offers many advantages, as discussed in detail by Billeter *et al.* (62).

PRIMARY STRUCTURE OF PHAGE RNAs: CURRENT STATUS

In the case of the RNA of phage group I (considering combined data obtained both from R17 by the Cambridge group and from MS2 by the Ghent group), three main segments have been elucidated. The first (Fig. 4) extends from the 5′ terminus into the beginning of the A cistron and contains 145 nucleotides (42,46,63,64); the second extends from the intercistronic region after the A cistron through the coat cistron (with a short stretch of 16 nucleotides still unknown) and into the beginning of the replicase cistron (about 420 nucleotides) (42,56,65,66), and the third is comprised of the last 104 nucleotides of the molecule (47,63). In total, about 680 nucleotides, or 20% of the genome, have thus been elucidated.

In the case of Qβ the two main segments known at present extend from the 5′ terminus to the 330th nucleotide (43), which is located well within the A cistron (see Fig. 5 for the first 175 nucleotides), and from the 160th to last nucleotide to the 3′ terminus (45). Moreover, a segment of 50 nucleotides corresponding to the intercistronic region between A and coat cistron and extending into the beginning of the coat cistron is known (59), as well as a segment of 27 nucleotides around the beginning of the replicase cistron. Thus the sequence of about 570 nucleotides (about 15% of Qβ RNA) has been established.

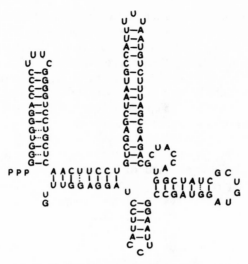

Fig. 4. Nucleotide sequence at the 5'-terminal
region of MS2 RNA (66).

SECONDARY STRUCTURE

Large parts of the sequences elucidated can be folded to give extensively hydrogen-bonded hairpins (43,46,52,56,57,63) using rules such as those advanced by Tinoco *et al.* (67). In the case of the MS2 coat cistron, about 70% of the nucleotides are believed to take part in such secondary interactions (66). The proposed structures are supported to some extent by the finding that, under conditions of partial digestion, nucleolytic splits are introduced predominantly (but not exclusively!) into single-stranded regions and into loops and bulges rather than into stem regions of the proposed hairpins.

ORGANIZATION OF THE GENOME

Since recombination does not occur among RNA phages, the order of their cistrons could not be elucidated by genetic techniques. This information was finally obtained by chemical techniques, in principle by searching for nucleotide sequences corresponding to the beginnings and ends of the phage proteins and locating the absolute or relative positions of these nucleotide sequences on the RNA strand (8,22,25). In all cases, the order of cistrons is A-coat-replicase. Extended noncoding nucleotide sequences are located at the beginning [62 nucleotides in Qβ (25), 129 in the MS2-R17 group (63)] and the end [at least 32 in Qβ (45) and not less than ten in the MS2-R17 group (47,63)] of the RNAs, as well as between the cistrons [for example, 36 nucleotides between coat and replicase cistron of R17 (65)].

DEDUCTIONS REGARDING THE GENETIC CODE

Since the sequences of amino acids of R17 coat protein and those of the nucleotides in the corresponding cistron are known, it is possible to deduce, at least in part, the genetic code independent of previous data. All assignments made in this fashion agree with the Nirenberg-Ochoa-Khorana code. In addition, it was found that for certain amino acids not all degenerate codons are used in the translation of the coat. For example, AUU and AUC are each used five times for

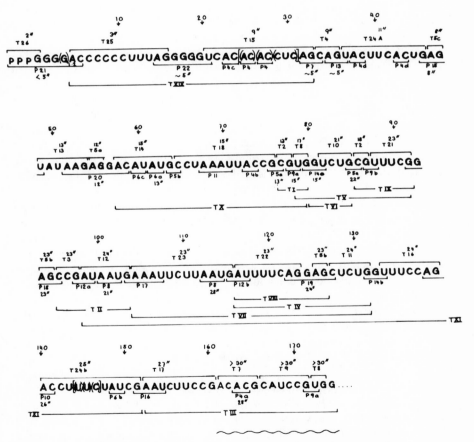

Fig. 5. Nucleotide sequence at the 5'-terminal region of Qβ RNA (43).

isoleucine, while AUA is not used at all; tyrosine is coded for four times by UAC and never by UAU (56,66).

RECOGNITION OF INITIATION SITES OF PROTEIN SYNTHESIS BY RIBOSOMES

The nucleotide sequences around the initiation sites of six different phage cistrons are now known (25,41,42,58). Initiation of phage cistrons always occurs at an AUG triplet, although GUG is also an efficient initiator codon *in vitro*. No extensive sequences are common to all initiation sites; however, certain short sequences precede the initiator AUG of some cistrons (for example, GGUUUGA occurs prior to both the A and the coat cistron of R17, and UUUGA before the Qβ coat cistron; UAAGAGGA precedes the A cistron of Qβ, UAGGAGG the A cistron of R17, GAGGA the replicase cistron of R17, and AGGA the replicase cistron of Qβ). If recognition of a determined nucleotide sequence rather than some three-dimensional structure is required for ribosome binding, it would seem that more than one such sequence is possible. Another remarkable aspect of ribosomal binding sites is that some are directly available [the coat cistron binding sites in both R17 (42) and Qβ (41)] while others are cryptic, i.e., not available on the mature, native RNA strand [for example, the A cistron binding site of Qβ, which only binds ribosomes detectably when present on an RNA fragment or on a nascent strand (25)]. It has been proposed that this unavailability of the binding site is due to the secondary and/or tertiary structure of the RNA (68,69), and in at least one case tentative structural evidence is forthcoming to support this view. Evidence has been presented that ribosomes do not initiate polypeptide synthesis at the replicase cistron of native viral RNA unless the coat cistron is being translated (69). Lodish and Robertson (69) proposed that an interaction between the replicase initiation site and a region of the coat cistron prevented ribosome attachment to the former. Translation of the coat cistron was thought to be instrumental in reversing this interaction, thereby allowing translation of the replicase cistron. Fiers and his colleagues (personal communication) have pointed out that a complementary relationship in fact exists between an RNA segment (nucleotides 72-96) of the coat cistron and the initiation site of the replicase cistron, lending strong support to the hypothesis described above.

INTERACTION OF Qβ REPLICASE WITH Qβ RNA

As first noted by Spiegelman and his colleagues, the viral replicases show a very high template specificity for the homologous, intact viral RNA (70), as well as for the complementary minus strand (71), to the exclusion of all other, unrelated viral RNAs and most other RNAs examined (70,71). It has been suggested that the nontranslatable regions at the termini of the viral RNAs are responsible for the recognitive interaction with the replicase (46,63), and some evidence has been offered that the integrity of the 3' terminus (up to the penultimate nucleotide) is required for template function (71). In order to explore the structural features required for template function, Spiegelman and his colleagues have taken advantage of the observation that, apart from the Qβ plus and minus strands, Qβ replicase also replicates (a) species of 6S RNA detected in Qβ-infected *Escherichia coli* (73) and (b) variants of Qβ RNA which were obtained by extensive *in vitro* replication of Qβ RNA, with repeated selection of the most rapidly replicated species (74,75). While the 6S RNA species appear to be unrelated to Qβ RNA inasmuch as they failed to hybridize to the latter (S. Spiegelman, personal communication), the variants are abbreviated Qβ RNA molecules, still sufficiently similar to Qβ RNA to hybridize with it. The determination of the 5'-terminal sequence of a Qβ variant (V-2, ref. 61) and of a 6S RNA (MV-I, ref. 76) has shown that there is only a restricted similarity between these termini and those of Qβ plus and minus strands, which does not extend beyond the first four or five nucleotides, the common feature being a cluster of three or four Gs followed by an A (Fig. 6). Since Qβ replicase initiates synthesis at the 3' end of its templates, it is likely that a cluster of Cs may be involved in the replicase-template interaction. However, this limited sequence cannot be the only requirement for initiation, since Qβ fragments (comprising the 3'-terminal region with an average chain length of several hundred nucleotides) do not elicit initiation of RNA synthesis (77).

It is interesting to note that despite the fact that MS2, R17, and f2 RNA also have clusters of C at their termini, they do not allow initiation by Qβ replicase, while on the other hand poly C directs the synthesis of poly G by the same enzyme (77-79).

It has been observed that Qβ replicase binds strongly and specifically to Qβ RNA (86). This binding entails protection of a segment of the RNA against nuclease digestion (59). Analysis of the protected RNA has revealed that it is derived from the intercistronic region between the A and the coat cistron and consequently comprises part of the ribosome binding site of the coat cistron

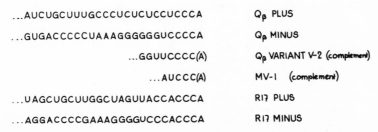

...AUCUGCUUUGCCCUCUCUCCUCCCA	Qβ PLUS
...GUGACCCCCUAAAGGGGGGUCCCCA	Qβ MINUS
...GGUUCCCC(A)	Qβ VARIANT V-2 (complement)
...AUCCC(A)	MV-I (complement)
...UAGCUGCUUGGCUAGUUACCACCCA	R17 PLUS
...AGGACCCCGAAAGGGGUCCCACCCA	R17 MINUS

Fig. 6. The 3' termini of several RNAs of biological interest. The nucleotide sequences were deduced from the 5'-terminal sequences of the complementary strands (43,45,61,66,76).

(59). This recognition therefore occurs at a position one-third strand length removed from the 5′ terminus. It will be shown below that this interaction allows a regulatory effect of Qβ replicase on the translation of the RNA; it is, however, not clear as yet whether it is required for RNA chain initiation.

Qβ REPLICASE AS REPRESSOR OF PROTEIN SYNTHESIS

After invading its host, the phage RNA serves first as messenger for phage-specific protein synthesis (80) and subsequently as template for its own replication (81,82). During the first process, the viral RNA is present as a polysome, with ribosomes traveling in the 5′ to 3′ direction (83-85). In replication, the viral

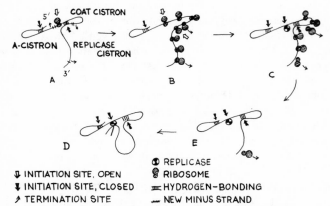

Fig. 7. Transition of Qβ RNA from polysome to replicating complex—repressor function of Qβ replicase (96). The order of cistrons in Qβ RNA is A protein-coat protein-replicase (22,24) with non-translatable segments preceding and following this region (43,45). (A) Ribosomes attach to Qβ RNA at the coat initiation site. The initiation site of the replicase cistron is unavailable because of the secondary structure of the RNA. (B) Translation of the coat cistron ensues, and the initiation site of the replicase cistron is exposed. The replicase cistron is translated. (C) When Qβ replicase becomes available, it attaches to the initiation site of the coat protein and blocks attachment of ribosomes in this position. The RNA can again refold, preventing initiation at the replicase cistron. (D) The RNA is cleared of ribosomes. (EO Qβ replicase can now attach to the 3′ terminus and initiate synthesis of the minus strand. The model supposes that the A-cistron initiation site of complete Qβ RNA is always unavailable to ribosomes because of the secondary structure of the mature RNA; it is believed to be translatable only on nascent RNA strands (88).

polymerase advances along the template in the 3′ to 5′ direction, i.e., on a collision course with translating ribosomes (86). Since replicase cannot dislodge ribosomes bound to Qβ RNA (87), a special mechanism must exist to free the parental RNA of ribosomes and render it competent as template for replication. It was found that Qβ replicase strongly and specifically inhibits binding of ribosomes to Qβ RNA while allowing translating ribosomes to terminate synthesis and detach (96). Since ribosome attachment at the A cistron of the mature RNA (69,88) does not occur to a significant extent, and since initiation at the replicase cistron is dependent on translation of the coat cistron (69), this process ultimately leads to a dismantling of the polysome (Fig. 7). As mentioned in a previous section, an RNA segment protected by Qβ replicase against RNase digestion has been isolated and shown to be derived from a region comprising the left half of the ribosome binding site (59). This finding provides a molecular basis for the repressor activity of Qβ replicase.

INTERACTION OF COAT PROTEIN WITH VIRAL RNA

It had been postulated (10,89), on the basis of the finding that amber mutants in the coat cistron overproduce replicase, that the phage coat protein functions as repressor of translation of the replicase cistron. This hypothesis has been strengthened by *in vitro* experiments showing that use of a complex of phage RNA and the homologous coat protein as messenger leads to a strongly decreased translation of the replicase cistron (90-95). So far, this finding has not been successfully exploited to isolate an RNA binding site for the coat protein.

EVOLUTIONARY ASPECTS OF VIRAL RNA STRUCTURE

Phage Qβ differs substantially in many regards from phages of group I, such as R17 and MS2. Although competition hybridization had not disclosed any relationship between the RNAs of the two phage groups (4), several significant homologies have since been found in their nucleotide sequences (40,45). Also, the coat proteins of the two groups show remarkable similarities (28), so that a common RNA phage ancestor has been considered (28,40,45).

Comparison of the nucleotide sequences of the coat cistrons of the closely related phages R17 and MS2 by Fiers *et al.* (66) has revealed that although the coat proteins differ by only one amino acid, there are at least nine nucleotide changes, i.e., one for about every 40 nucleotides. By contrast, the nontranslatable regions show no differences in their nucleotide sequence. The cistronic regions are thus subject to genetic drift, inasmuch as their phenotypic expression can be maintained unaltered by virtue of the degeneracy of the genetic code. As pointed out by Fiers *et al.* (66), base changes are also such that virtually no changes in the secondary structure are expected to occur. The as yet unknown function of the extracistronic regions is apparently stringently dependent on the primary structure of that RNA.

CONCLUDING REMARKS

Despite its apparent simplicity, the replication of RNA phages entails a number of sophisticated control mechanisms. Since the amount of genetic information encoded in the phage genome is limited to three cistrons, evolutionary pressure has imposed more than one function onto each of the phage components. The coat protein is not only a structural component of the particle but also serves to modulate translation of the viral genome; the replicase, endowed with a remarkable template specificity, not only distinguishes viral plus and minus strands from virtually all of the other RNAs present in the host cells but also fulfills the role of a translational repressor, a function essential in the early stages of viral replication. The viral RNA has evolved within the narrow constraints imposed by the multiple demands made on it (a) as a genome which is to be replicated, compactly folded, and encapsidated in a symmetrical particle and (b) as a messenger subjected to translational control and moreover required to retain its integrity in an aggressive environment. The hope of eventually understanding this plethora of functions at the molecular level sustains those engaged in the arduous task of elucidating the structure of the phage components.

SUMMARY

After invading its host, the RNA of RNA phages such as Qβ serves first as messenger for virus-specific protein synthesis and subsequently as template for its own replication. During the first process, the viral RNA is present as a polysome with ribosomes traveling in the 5′ to 3′ direction. In replication, the viral RNA polymerase (replicase) synthesizes a strand complementary to the parental RNA, with the enzyme advancing along the template in the 3′ to 5′ direction, i.e., on a collision course with translating ribosomes. Replicase cannot dislodge ribosomes bound to Qβ RNA; we have therefore searched for a mechanism which frees the RNA of ribosomes, allowing it to serve as template for replication. It was found that Qβ replicase binds strongly to Qβ RNA and thereby prevents attachment of ribosomes at the main ribosome binding site (at the beginning of the coat cistron). If replicase is added to a Qβ polysome, the ribosomes engaged in translation can terminate synthesis, but no new ribosomes attach: protein synthesis stops after a few minutes and the polysomes are dismantled. If Qβ replicase is bound to Qβ RNA, it protects a segment of Qβ RNA against digestion by T1 RNase. This segment was isolated and its nucleotide sequence determined. It was found that it comprised the right half of the main ribosome binding site. It has therefore been established that Qβ replicase acts as a repressor of Qβ RNA translation by attaching to and blocking the main ribosome binding site.

RESUMEN

Después de invadir a su huésped, el RNA de fagos a RNA tales como el Qβ sirve primero como mensajero para la síntesis de las proteínas específicas del virus, y posteriormente como patrón para su propia replicación. Durante el primer proceso el RNA del virus se presenta como un polisoma con ribosomas desplazándose en la dirección 5' a 3'. En la replicación la RNA polimerasa viral (replicasa) sintetiza una cadena complementaria al RNA paterno con la enzima que avanza a lo largo del patrón en la dirección 3' a 5' en un rumbo de colisión con los ribosomas que se encuentran traduciendo. La replicasa no puede dislocar los ribosomas unidos al RNA del Qβ; por ello hemos buscado un mecanismo que libere al RNA de los ribosomas perun mecanismo que libere al RNA de los ribosomas permitiéndole que sirva como patrón para su replicación. Se encontró que la replicasa de Qβ se une fuertemente al RNA del Qβ y así impide la unión de los ribosomas en el sitio principal de unión de ribosomas (al comienzo del cistrón de cubierta). Si se agrega la replicasa a un polisoma de Qβ los ribosomas que participan en la traducción pueden terminar la síntesis, pero no se unen nuevos ribosomas: la síntesis de proteínas se detiene después de unos pocos minutos y los polisomas se desagregan. Si la replicasa de Qβ se une al RNA de Qβ, protege un segmento del mismo contra la digestión por la RNasa T1. Este segmento se aisló y se determinó su secuencia de nucleótidos. Se encontró que comprende la mitad derecha del sitio principal de unión de los ribosomas. Se estableció por lo tanto que la replicasa de Qβ actúa como represor de la traducción del RNA de Qβ al unirse y bloquear el sitio principal de unión de los ribosomas.

REFERENCES

1. Watanabe, I., Miyaki, T., Sakurai, T., Shiba, T., and Ohno, T., *Proc. Japan Acad., 43,* 204 (1967).
2. Sakurai, T., Miyake, T., Shiba, T., and Watanabe, F., *Japan. J. Microbiol., 12,* 544 (1968).
3. Zinder, N. D., *Ann. Rev. Microbiol., 19,* 455 (1965).
4. Weissmann, C., and Ochoa, S., *Progr. Nucl. Acid Res. Mol. Biol., 6,* 353 (1967).
5. Lodish, H. F., *Proc. Biophys. Mol. Biol., 18,* 285 (1968).
6. Stavis, R. L., and August, J. T., *Ann. Rev. Biochem., 39,* 527 (1970).
7. Sinha, N. K., Fujimura, R. K., and Kaesberg, P., *J. Mol. Biol., 11,* 84 (1965).
8. Hindley, J., Staples, D. H., Billeter, M. A., and Weissmann, C., *Proc. Natl. Acad. Sci. U.S.A., 67,* 1180 (1970).
9. Boedtker, H., *Biochim. Biophys. Acta, 240,* 448 (1971).
10. Gussin, G. N., *J. Mol. Biol., 21,* 435 (1966).
11. Horiuchi, K., Lodish, H. F., and Zinder, N. D., *Virology, 28,* 438 (1966).
12. Horiuchi, K., and Matsuhashi, S., *Virology, 42,* 49 (1970).
13. Vasquez, C., Granboulan, N., and Franklin, R. M., *J. Bacteriol., 92,* 1779 (1966).
14. Nathans, D., Oeschger, M. P., Eggen, K., and Shimura, Y., *Proc. Natl. Acad. Sci. U.S.A., 56,* 1844 (1966).
15. Steitz, J. A., *J. Mol. Biol., 33,* 923 (1968).
16. Garwes, D., Sillero, A., and Ochoa, S., *Biochim. Biophys. Acta, 186,* 166 (1969).
17. Horiuchi, K., Webster, R. E., and Matsuhashi, S., *Virology, 45,* 429 (1971).
18. Weiner, A. M., and Weber, K., submitted to *Nature.*
19. Moore, C., Farron, F., Bohnert, D., and Weissmann, C., *Nature,* in press.
20. Kamen, R. I., *Nature, 228,* 527 (1970).
21. Kondo, M., Gallerani, R., and Weissmann, C., *Nature, 228,* 525 (1970).
22. Jeppesen, P. G. N., Argetsinger-Steitz, J., Gesteland, R. F., and Spahr, P.F., *Nature, 226,* 230 (1970).
23. Konings, R. N. H., Ward, R., Francke, B., and Hofschneider, P. H., *Nature, 226,* 604 (1970).

24. Hindley, J., Staples, D. H., Billeter, M. A., and Weissmann, C., *Proc. Natl. Acad. Sci. U.S.A., 67,* 1180 (1970).
25. Staples, D. H., Hindley, J., Billeter, M. A., and Weissmann, C., *Nature,* in press.
26. Weber, K., and Konigsberg, W., *J. Biol. Chem., 242,* 3563 (1967).
27. Wittmann-Liebold, B., *Z. Naturforsch., 21B,* 1249 (1966).
28. Konigsberg, W., Maita, T., Katze, J., and Weber, K., *Nature, 227,* 271 (1970).
29. Lin, J.-Y., Tsung, C. M., and Fraenkel-Conrat, H., *J. Mol. Biol., 24,* 1 (1967).
30. Lodish, H. F., *Nature, 220,* 345 (1968).
31. Lodish, H. F., *Biochem. Biophys. Res. Commun., 37,* 127 (1969).
32. Skogerson, L., Roufa, D., and Leder, P., *Proc. Natl. Acad. Sci. U.S.A., 68,* 276 (1971).
33. Weith, H. L., and Gilham, P. T., *J. Am. Chem. Soc., 89,* 5473 (1967).
34. De Wachter, R., and Fiers, W., *J. Mol. Biol., 30,* 507 (1967).
35. De Wachter, R., and Fiers, W., *Nature, 221,* 233 (1969).
36. Robinson, W. E., Frist, R. H., and Kaesberg, P., *Science, 166,* 1291 (1969).
37. Weith, H. L., and Gilham, P. T., *Science, 166,* 1004 (1969).
38. Glitz, D. G., *Biochemistry, 7,* 927 (1968).
39. Glitz, D. G., Bradley, A., and Fraenkel-Conrat, H., *Biochim. Biophys. Acta, 161,* 1 (1968).
40. Adams, J. M., Jeppesen, P. G. N., Sanger, F., and Barrell, B. G., *Cold Spring Harbor Symp. Quant. Biol., 34,* 611 (1969).
41. Hindley, J., and Staples, D. H., *Nature, 224,* 964 (1969).
42. Steitz, J. A., *Nature, 224,* 957 (1969).
43. Billeter, M. A., Dahlberg, J. E., Goodman, H. M., Hindley, J., and Weissmann, C., *Nature, 224,* 1083 (1969).
44. Gupta, S. L., Chen, J., Schaefer, L., Lengyel, P., and Weissman, S. M., *Biochem. Biophys. Res. Commun., 39,* 883 (1970).
45. Goodman, H. M., Billeter, M. A., Hindley, J., and Weissmann, C., *Proc. Natl. Acad. Sci. U.S.A., 67,* 921 (1970).
46. De Wachter, R., Merregaert, J., Vandenberghe, A., Contreras, R., and Fiers, W., *Europ. J. Biochem., 22,* 400 (1971).
47. Contreras, R., Vandenberghe, A., Min Jou, W., de Wachter, R., and Fiers, W., *FEBS Letters, 18,* 141 (1971).
48. Gilham, P. T., *Ann. Rev. Biochem., 39,* 227 (1970).
49. Penswick, J. R., and Holley, R. W., *Proc. Natl. Acad. Sci. U.S.A., 53,* 543 (1965).
50. Gould, H. J., *J. Mol. Biol., 29,* 307 (1967).
51. Min Jou, W., Hindley, J., and Fiers, W., *Arch. Internat. Physiol. Biochem., 76,* 194 (1968).
52. Adams, J. M., Jeppesen, P. G. N., Sanger, F., and Barrell, B. G., *Nature, 223,* 1009 (1969).
53. Pinder, J. C., and Gratzer, W. B., *Biochemistry, 9,* 4519 (1970).
54. De Wachter, R., and Fiers, W., in Grossman, L., and Moldave, K. (eds.), *Methods in Enzymology,* Vol. 21, Academic Press, New York (1971), p. 167.
55. Brownlee, G. G., and Sanger, F., *Europ. J. Biochem., 11,* 395 (1969).
56. Jeppesen, P. G. N., Nichols, J. L., Sanger, F., and Barrell, B. G., *Cold Spring Harbor Symp. Quant. Biol., 35,* 13 (1970).
57. Min Jou, W., Haegeman, G., and Fiers, W., *FEBS Letters, 13,* 105 (1971).
58. Staples, D. H., and Hindley, J., *Nature,* in press.
59. Weber, H., Billeter, M. A., Kahane, S., and Weissmann, C., *Experientia, 27,* 742 (1971).
60. Kolakofsky, D., Billeter, M. A., and Weissmann, C., V. Congreso Nacional de la Sociedad Española de Bioquìmica, Barcelona (1971), p. 359.
61. Bishop, D. H. L., Mills, D. R., and Spiegelman, S., *Biochemistry, 7,* 3744 (1968).

62. Billeter, M. A., Dahlberg, J. E., Goodman, H. M., Hindley, J., and Weissmann, C., *Cold Spring Harbor Symp. Quant. Biol., 34*, 635 (1969).
63. Cory, S., Spahr, P. F., and Adams, J. M., *Cold Spring Harbor Symp. Quant. Biol., 35*, 1 (1970).
64. Young, R. J., and Fraenkel-Conrat, H., *Biochim. Biophys. Acta, 228*, 446 (1971).
65. Nichols, J. L., *Nature, 225*, 147 (1970).
66. Fiers, W., Contreras, R., de Wachter, R., Haegeman, G., Merregaert, J., Min Jou, W., and Vandenberghe, A., *Biochimie, 53*, 495 (1971).
67. Tinoco, I., Jr., Uhlenbeck, O. C., and Levine, M. D., *Nature, 230*, 362 (1971).
68. Gussin, G. N., Capecchi, M. R., Adams, J. M., Argetsinger, J. E., Tooze, J., Weber, K., and Watson, J. D., *Cold Spring Harbor Symp. Quant. Biol., 31*, 257 (1966).
69. Lodish, H. F., and Robertson, H. D., *Cold Spring Harbor Symp. Quant. Biol., 34*, 655 (1969).
70. Haruna, I., and Spiegelman, S., *Proc. Natl. Acad. Sci. U.S.A., 54*, 579 (1965).
71. Feix, G., Pollet, R., and Weissmann, C., *Proc. Natl. Acad. Sci. U.S.A., 59*, 145 (1968).
72. Rensing, U., and August, J. T., *Nature, 224*, 853 (1969).
73. Banerjee, A. K., Rensing, U., and August, J. T., *J. Mol. Biol., 45*, 181 (1969).
74. Mills, D. R., Peterson, R. L., and Spiegelman, S., *Proc. Natl. Acad. Sci. U.S.A., 58*, 217 (1967).
75. Levisohn, R., and Spiegelman, S., *Proc. Natl. Acad. Sci. U.S.A., 60*, 866 (1968).
76. Kacian, D. L., Mills, D. R., and Spiegelman, S., *Biochim. Biophys. Acta, 238*, 212 (1971).
77. Haruna, I., and Spiegelman, S., *Proc. Natl. Acad. Sci. U.S.A., 54*, 1189 (1965).
78. Hori, K., Banerjee, A. K., Eoyang, L., and August J. T., *Proc. Natl. Acad. Sci. U.S.A., 57*, 1790 (1967).
79. Eikhom, T. S., and Spiegelman, S., *Proc. Natl. Acad. Sci. U.S.A., 57*, 1833 (1967).
80. Godson, G. N., and Sinsheimer, R. L., *J. Mol. Biol., 23*, 495 (1967).
81. Erikson, R. L., Fenwick, M. L., and Franklin, R. M., *J. Mol. Biol., 10*, 519 (1964).
82. Weissmann, C., Borst, P., Burdon, R. H., Billeter, M. A., and Ochoa, S., *Proc. Natl. Acad. Sci. U.S.A., 51*, 682 (1964).
83. Streisinger, G., Okada, Y., Emrich, J., Newton, J., Tsugita, A., Terzaghi, E., and Inouye, M., *Cold Spring Harbor Symp. Quant. Biol., 31*, 77 (1966).
84. Thach, R. E., Cecere, M. A., Sundararajan, T. A., and Doty, P., *Proc. Natl. Acad. Sci. U.S.A., 54*, 1167 (1965).
85. Salas, M., Smith, M. A., Stanley, W. M., Jr., Wahba, J., and Ochoa, S., *J. Biol. Chem., 240*, 3988 (1965).
86. August, J. T., Banerjee, A. K., Eoyang, L., Franze de Fernandez, M. T., Hori, K., Kuo, C. H., Rensing, U., and Shapiro, L., *Cold Spring Harbor Symp. Quant. Biol., 33*, 73 (1968).
87. Kolakofsky, D., and Weissmann, C., *Nature New Biol., 231*, 42 (1971).
88. Robertson, H. D., and Lodish, H. F., *Proc. Natl. Acad. Sci. U.S.A., 67*, 710 (1970).
89. Lodish, H. F., and Zinder, N. D., *J. Mol. Biol., 19*, 333 (1966).
90. Sugiyama, T., and Nakada, D., *Proc. Natl. Acad. Sci. U.S.A., 57*, 1744 (1967).
91. Ward, R., Shive, K., and Valentine, R. C., *Biochem. Biophys. Res. Commun., 29*, 8 (1967).
92. Sugiyama, T., and Nakada, D., *J. Mol. Biol., 31*, 431 (1968).
93. Robertson, H. D., Webster, R. E., and Zinder, N. D., *Nature, 218*, 533 (1968).
94. Eggen, K., and Nathans, D., *J. Mol. Biol., 39*, 293 (1969).
95. Ward, R., Strand, M., and Valentine, R. C., *Biochem. Biophys. Res. Commun., 30*, 310 (1968).
96. Kolakofsky, D., and Weissmann, C., *Biochim. Biophys. Acta, 246*, 596 (1971).

DISCUSSION

C. Vásquez (Buenos Aires, Argentina): Do you know something about how the A cistron is opened, since it is completely closed?

C. Weissmann (Zurich, Switzerland): If we take the isolated 5'-terminal region of Qβ RNA and present it to the ribosomes, then the ribosomes will attach at the A-cistron binding site. But if we take a long piece of RNA, then the ribosomes will not attach at that position. The idea is then, and this has been proposed by several people, in particular Lodish and Robertson, that the A cistron is only recognized when it is present as a short piece of RNA and cannot interact extensively with other regions of the RNA. Of course, the time when only a short piece is available is during synthesis. When you are making the plus strand on the minus strand, there is a time at which only the A cistron has been synthesized, and we think that that is when the A cistron is translated. This provides a nice regulation system, because only a small fraction of the RNA is in the nascent state at any one time. You do not need very much A protein, only about one molecule for every 180 coat protein molecules.

Speaker unidentified: Which of the subunits is involved in specific binding?

C. Weissmann: We know that a combination of α plus β, the two largest subunits, binds and gives the entire effect which we have described for repression. We do not know if α alone or β alone can do it. At present, it is difficult to get the two apart in a native state.

J. T. August (New York, U.S.A.): Have you done control experiments where you digested other RNA exposed to the enzyme? Do you get fragments with R17 RNA?

C. Weissmann: We have not yet attempted to protect R17 RNA with Qβ replicase; however, this will be done soon. We believe that our experiments with Qβ RNA are meaningful for the following reasons. Our digestion experiments are done under competition with a 24-fold excess of cold RNA so that we do not see any random fragments but only the specifically bound radioactive RNA. Moreover, we have recovered this protected piece of RNA and have bound it again to Qβ replicase, competing it against random fragments. Competition of ^{32}P binding site RNA by cold random fragments is very low, approximately in keeping with the expected frequency of this binding site in the random RNA fragments. We have also taken this same ^{32}P binding site which binds to replicase and shown that it binds specifically to ribosomes in an fMet-tRNA dependent reaction.

E. P. Geiduschek (La Jolla, U.S.A.): Is the A1 protein stable or is it broken down?

C. Weissmann: If you mean in the cell, I cannot say. We have tried very hard to dissociate this A1 protein *in vitro* using techniques such as oxidation or reduction, and urea and SDS, yet we cannot dissociate it into coat and something else. The disturbing thing about the A1 protein is that we can well envisage how it gets started, but we don't know how it is terminated at a rather precise position.

J. T. August: Is it suggested that this A2 protein is playing the role of a maturation protein?

C. Weissmann: The A2 protein has been characterized genetically as maturation protein by Horiuchi. Amber mutants in the A2 cistron give defective particles, as is the case with R17. The identification of the cistron can be made because the A2 protein has an amino terminal sequence which corresponds to the first cistron of the Qβ genome.

3

Host Proteins in the Replication of Bacteriophage RNA

J. T. August, Lillian Eoyang, M. T. Franze de Fernández, W. S. Hayward, C. H. Kuo, and P. M. Silverman

Department of Molecular Biology
Division of Biological Sciences
Albert Einstein College of Medicine
Bronx, New York, U.S.A.

In recent years, the bacteriophage Qβ RNA polymerase reaction has become a highly characterized system for studying the synthesis of genetic material. An outstanding feature of this reaction is the actual replication of infectious bacteriophage RNA, as first shown by Spiegelman *et al.* (1). All of the reaction components have now been isolated as discrete species:

(a) The *enzyme*, containing four proteins.
(b) A *host RNA binding factor*, composed of a single protein.
(c) A *basic protein factor*, of which there are many active species.
(d) *Qβ RNA*.
(e) *Qβ RNA complementary strand*.

Qβ RNA Polymerase

Only one fraction with RNA-dependent RNA polymerase activity has been detected in extracts of Qβ-infected cells. This enzyme has been extensively purified by Eoyang and August (2,3) and by Kamen (4).

The most highly purified active fractions contain four proteins, as shown by sodium dodecyl sulfate-polyacrylamide gel electrophoresis (4,5, unpublished observations of Eoyang and August). Three of these proteins are contributed by the *Escherichia coli* host and have molecular weights of approximately 70,000, 47,000, and 30,000. One, of approximately 62,000 molecular weight, is coded for by the phage genome. Although it has not been unambiguously proven that all four species are required for polymerase activity, it has been suggested that each is a component of the active polymerase since they demonstrate an associative interaction and are the minimum number present with active enzyme (4). However, the apparent molecular weight of the enzyme complex is 160,000, considerably less than the sum of the molecular weights of the individual proteins, and the relative concentrations of the four proteins in active enzyme are not constant. Moreover, multiple polymeric forms are produced by simple changes in ionic concentration. These findings suggest that the enzyme is made up of a complex of interacting factors or enzyme molecules rather than of subunits of a single active enzyme.

The role in host metabolism of the *E. coli* proteins associated with the enzyme has not been elucidated. It was reported that two of the proteins are active in stimulating the *in vitro* synthesis of ribosomal RNA catalyzed by the *E. coli* RNA polymerase (6), but at present this result is uncertain (K. Weber, personal communication).

Separation of the enzyme into "heavy" and "light" subunits or components has been reported by Eikhom *et al.* (7). The active proteins of these fractions have not been identified, but the heavy component appears to represent the enzyme and the light component the host cell factors described below.

The only catalytic activity of the purified enzyme is that of RNA-dependent RNA synthesis. The reaction mechanism seems to be common to that of other polymerase enzymes, i.e., the joining of the a phosphate of the nucleoside triphosphate substrate by phosphodiester linkage to the 3'-hydroxyl terminus of the nascent polynucleotide chain and the release of pyrophosphate. This conclusion is supported by evidence that chain growth, both *in vivo* and *in vitro*, is in the direction from the 5'-triphosphate to the 3'-hydroxyl terminus (8-12) and that pyrophosphate release in the reaction is stoichiometric to nucleotide incorporation (M. Strand and J. T. August, unpublished observations).

Another property of the Qβ enzyme is its specificity for template RNA. Only intact Qβ RNA (13), the strand complementary to Qβ RNA (14), RNA molecules described as variants of Qβ RNA (15), and a 6S RNA present in Qβ-infected *E. coli* (16) are known to undergo replication in the reaction catalyzed by the enzyme. Synthetic ribopolymers also act as template provided they contain cytidylate as one of the bases (17), but only the complementary strand is synthesized.

HOST FACTORS

Synthesis of Qβ RNA *in vitro* is also dependent on two protein factors that are present in both infected and uninfected *E. coli* (18,19). The function of these proteins is related to the template activity of Qβ RNA rather than to polymerization *per se,* as synthesis with other templates, most notably the Qβ complementary strand RNA, proceeds normally in the absence of either factor (8).

Factor I: An RNA-Binding Protein

Factor I, a heat-resistant protein, has been purified from uninfected *E. coli* to apparent homogeneity by Hayward (20) and Franze de Fernández *et al.* (21). When analyzed by sodium dodecyl sulfate-polyacrylamide gel electrophoresis, the purified protein migrates as a single band with an apparent molecular weight of 12,500. The molecular weight of the active factor is approximately 75,000, and it may therefore possess a hexameric subunit structure. The concentration of this factor required for the maximum rate of synthesis varies according to the amount of RNA added but is independent of enzyme concentration, suggesting that it acts directly on Qβ RNA rather than as an enzyme subunit. The stoichiometry of the reaction indicates that one molecule of factor is required per molecule of RNA. Binding of factor to several different types of phage RNA and *E. coli* RNA was demonstrated by zonal centrifugation. This binding appeared to be specific for single-stranded RNA since it did not occur with double-stranded reovirus RNA or with DNA (21).

Factor II: *E. coli* Basic Proteins and Histones

Factor II proteins in crude cell extracts of *E. coli* bind tightly to nucleic acid but are released upon extraction with guanidine hydrochloride and perchloric acid (22). Further purification is achieved by cation exchange chromatography, after which gel filtration on Sephadex yields five discrete protein fractions with molecular weights ranging from 5000 to greater than 30,000, each of which possesses factor activity. These proteins are highly basic and rich in arginine and lysine. The most active fraction contains at least eight different molecular species, as shown by polyacrylamide gel electrophoresis in the presence of urea. These proteins are not inactivated by urea and can be assayed after elution from the gel; all are active. This principal Sephadex fraction contains one third of the total initial factor activity and 1% of the total protein of the cell extract. Thus it seems that approximately 3% of the total proteins of *E. coli* serve as factor II in the Qβ polymerase reaction.

A few of these *E. coli* basic proteins act as phosphate acceptors *in vitro* in reactions catalyzed by animal cell protein kinases (23,24). The phosphate is incorporated into the acid-stable O-phosphoserine linkage characteristic of the protein kinase reaction. Analysis of the reaction product by polyacrylamide gel electrophoresis in sodium dodecyl sulfate suggests that there are at least two phosphorylated proteins; these have apparent molecular weights of approximately 15,000 and separate poorly because of their small sizes.

A remarkable finding is that of a functional similarity between the *E. coli* factor protein and histones. Various lysine-rich and arginine-rich calf thymus histones, and salmon sperm protamine sulfate, completely substitute for the bacterial factor II proteins required for replication of Qβ RNA (24). The maximum rate of nucleotide incorporation varies but in every case is achieved with approximately 1-3 μg protein per milliliter reaction mixture, as with factor II proteins. At greater concentrations, the rate of RNA synthesis is decreased. Zonal centrifugation of the RNA product synthesized in the presence of histones shows that the reaction yields intact, 32S molecules of phage RNA. Histones or protamine do not substitute for either factor I or polymerase.

The activity of the *E. coli* factor II proteins or of histones cannot be attributed to a nonspecific electrostatic interaction between Qβ RNA and any basic peptide. Several compounds were tested in the reaction, including basic proteins (lysozyme, cytochrome c, poly-L-lysine, and poly-L-arginine), bovine serum albumin, and polyamines (spermine, spermidine, and putrescine). None of these compounds showed any effect in amounts corresponding to the maximally effective concentrations of the *E. coli* basic proteins or calf thymus histones. At tenfold higher concentrations, a slight stimulation was observed with several of the compounds, particularly with spermine and lysozyme.

In order to determine the location in *E. coli* of the basic proteins active as factors II, we have lysed the cells and prepared fractions rich in DNA, RNA, and ribosomes (24). Factor II activity was measured after the fractions were extracted with guanidine hydrochloride and perchloric acid, since maximum activity was found in the acid-soluble fraction.

Bacteria treated with lysozyme and a nonionic detergent release most of the cellular ribosomes and RNA into a supernatant fraction and retain almost all of the DNA in a particulate fraction. Using this procedure, we have found that most of the basic proteins active as factor II were present in fractions rich in RNA and that almost all of the active proteins released into the supernatant fraction were present with the ribosomes isolated by high-speed centrifugation. After separating the DNA and RNA of the particulate fraction, about 15% of the basic proteins and factor activity was found associated with the DNA.

We have further fractionated the factor proteins associated with the ribosomal fraction. When the cells were ruptured by grinding with alumina and the crude extract was treated with DNase, most of the factor activity was present in the precipitate after high-speed centrifugation. Some active proteins became soluble when the ribosomes were washed with 1. 0 M NH$_4$Cl, but about 60% of the total activity was present in the final ribosomal fraction. The individual proteins of the washed ribosomes were then isolated by urea-polyacrylamide gel electrophoresis, and almost all were found to possess factor II activity. We conclude that many of the basic proteins of *E. coli* that are active in the replication of Qβ RNA *in vitro* are structural proteins of the ribosomes.

One of the active proteins released from the ribosomes by the washing procedure has been identified as the polypeptide chain initiation factor FII. This basic protein has factor II activity, whereas initiation factor FI does not.

Role of the Host Factors

These observations of the properties of the host factors suggest that the proteins act as regulators in the reaction controlling the utilization of template. This may also be related to the asymmetry of RNA synthesis in the reaction, the synthesis predominantly of Qβ RNA, not the complementary strand. At this time, the only known difference in the utilization of Qβ RNA or its complement as template is the requirement for factors with Qβ RNA but not with the complement (8).

The step in which the factors act is early in the polymerase reaction. They are absolutely required for pyrophosphate exchange, chain initiation, and polymerization when Qβ RNA is template (21; unpublished observations of C. H. Kuo). Thus it seems likely that they act prior to the initiation of synthesis. The apparent first step in the polymerase reaction is the binding of RNA by the enzyme. This binding, as described below, occurs at multiple sites on nontemplate as well as template RNA, is reversible, and does not require either of the two factors (8,25). It has recently been found, however, that if the enzyme-RNA complex is incubated with both of the factors and GTP, an irreversible complex is formed at a single site on template RNA (26). It is thus speculated that both factors are involved in the formation of a specific initiation complex of enzyme, RNA, factors, and GTP.

Our hypothesis is that the factors affect the secondary structure of Qβ RNA, serving to organize and maintain a structure required for template activity. Since only one molecule of factor I per molecule of RNA is required for synthesis, this RNA-binding protein appears to act on a limited region of the RNA, possibly the enzyme-binding site. In contrast, several molecules of the factor II proteins are required, and it can be speculated that these basic proteins act on much larger regions of RNA. The ability of such a wide diversity of basic proteins to function as factor II in the reaction makes it seem likely that the interaction of these proteins with Qβ RNA is not closely dependent on base sequence.

The role of HFI in the bacterial host is unknown. The protein can be distinguished from the other proteins known to be involved in RNA synthesis in *E. coli* by virtue of its molecular weight. These include the RNA polymerase and its σ subunit, the *lac* repressor, the ρ factor, and the host proteins associated with the Qβ polymerase. Nevertheless, the specific binding of HFI to single-stranded RNA and its role in regulating Qβ RNA replication suggest that this protein may be involved in RNA metabolism in *E. coli.* Factor II proteins in *E. coli* appear to be involved in many different functions, mainly those of ribosomal proteins. There is evidence of interaction with DNA and mRNA as well (24).

IN VITRO SYNTHESIS OF Qβ RNA

Recognition of Template RNA

The specific recognition of template RNA by the Qβ RNA polymerase is manifest in two of the properties of the enzyme. One is template specificity. As described above, the enzyme uses as template only a few natural RNA molecules specific to Qβ-infected cells or to the *in vitro* reaction, and polyribocytidylic acid or synthetic ribopolymer containing cytidylate. The second property is site specificity. The enzyme initiates synthesis exclusively at the 3'-hydroxyl terminal region of the natural RNA templates. This is shown by the observations that the products are predominantly intact molecules (1), that the direction of synthesis is from the 5' to the 3' terminus (8-12), and that the nucleotide sequence at the 5' end of the Qβ complementary strand is complementary in an antiparallel fashion to the 3'-terminal sequence of Qβ RNA (27).

The relationship between template and site specificities is as yet unknown. Two alternatives can be considered: One is that both are the result of a single reaction, which must then involve recognition by the enzyme of the 3'-terminal region of template RNA. The other is that these specificities are expressed in separate reactions involving different sites in template RNA.

There is considerable evidence that at least part of the enzyme recognition of template involves a specific sequence at the hydroxyl terminal region of the RNA. This is in contrast to the nonspecific initiation of synthesis at any hydroxyl terminus following recognition of some other RNA sequence. For one thing, it was found by Rensing and August (28) that the penultimate nucleotide, the cytidylate of the $CCCA_{OH}$ terminus, is required for template activity, as it is for infectivity (29). Other evidence has come from the work of Fiers *et al.* (12), Dahlberg (30), and Adams and Cory (31), who have shown that there is extensive complementarity between the sequences at the 5' and 3' termini of MS2 and R17 RNA:

$$MS2: pppGGGU \quad \ldots \quad ACCCA_{OH}$$
$$R17: pppGGGUGG \ldots \quad CCACCCA_{OH}$$

It thus is almost certain that the 3' termini of the parent and minus strands corresponding to the complementary regions have identical sequences, thus providing a possible specific recognition sequence common to the two RNA templates.

There are other observations that require further explanation, however. One is the finding by Haruna and Spiegelman (32) that fragments of Qβ RNA do not serve as template, suggesting that recognition of the template itself or of the initiation site involves more than just the primary structure of a limited region of the RNA. This could possibly be included in the terminal sequence model for template recognition if base pairing of the terminal complementary regions is required for template activity, as suggested by Fiers et al. (12). But it may be that other regions are involved as well. Another problem is that the only complementary terminal sequences found in the natural Qβ RNA templates is pppGGG . . . $CCCA_{OH}$ (12,27,28,30-37). This $CCCA_{OH}$ region is not unique to Qβ RNA but is common to all phage RNA. Thus it would appear that specific recognition of Qβ template by the enzyme must depend on some other feature of primary, secondary, or tertiary structure. In the case of Qβ RNA, the last is implicated, because of the requirement for the host cell factors in an early step possibly related to the recognition process (21,26). One additional complication is that the enzyme also recognizes synthetic polymers containing as little as approximately 10% cytidylate (17). It is remarkable that a recognition sequence is available with these copolymers but not with natural, nontemplate RNA.

Binding of Template RNA

The role of enzyme binding of RNA in the mechanism of template recognition has been extensively studied (8,25,38). Enzyme and RNA form a stable complex in the absence of any of the other components required for synthesis, i.e., the ribonucleoside triphosphates, Mg^{2+}, or host factors. The reaction is reversible and is inhibited by salt. Under standard ionic conditions (I equal to 0.26 M) in a 4.5% dextran-5.0% polyethylene glycol phase mixture, the K_a for binding to Qβ RNA was estimated to be $1.3 \times 10^9 M^{-1}$ at $0°$, corresponding to a standard free energy change of -11.5 kcal/mole (25). The enzyme shows a preference for binding to Qβ RNA, but it appears unlikely that either the template specificity or site specificity can be totally attributed to the formation of this reversible complex, since the enzyme binds with high affinity to multiple sites on any RNA, approximately 32, 26, and 12 sites for Qβ RNA, f2 RNA, and 16S rRNA, respectively (25).

The specificity of the enzyme for a single template site must then depend on some other interaction. One possibility is that there is a unique Qβ RNA site for which the enzyme has an extremely high affinity but that binding to this site is obscured by the multiple, nonspecific interactions. Another possible mechanism is that the enzyme recognition of a single site occurs after the initial binding reaction. It has recently been observed that once RNA synthesis begins the enzyme is irreversibly bound to template RNA and that the reaction yielding this nondissociable complex can easily be distinguished from the initial binding reaction (26). This irreversible complex is formed when enzyme and RNA are incubated in the presence of GTP and host factors. The reaction is highly specific, being detected only with template RNA, and involves only a single RNA site. Therefore, two steps in the binding of Qβ RNA by the polymerase can be distinguished. One is the formation of a complex between enzyme and RNA, a reversible reaction which occurs with any RNA. The second requires the presence of GTP and host factors and is irreversible and specific for a single site on template RNA.

Paradox of the Terminal Adenosine

Another of the remarkable features of the reaction is that replication of Qβ RNA is not the simple end-to-end copying of the RNA template. If synthesis of RNA were to begin precisely at the 3′-adenosine terminus of the template, a complementary relationship between the 3′ terminus of the viral strand and the 5′ terminus of the complementary strand would be expected. In fact, the 5′ terminus of the Qβ complementary strand is pppG, not pppU, and the initiation of synthesis is directed by the penultimate cytidylate (8-10,27). What then is the role of the 3′-terminal adenosine? This question remains unanswered. Kamen (29) found that infectivity of R17 RNA was not lost when the terminal adenosine was removed, indicating either that it was not required or that it was replaced in the bacterium. Furthermore, the primary structure of the terminal adenosine or even the actual presence of this base is not critical for template activity, since Rensing and August (28) and Fiers et al. (12) found that neither oxidation, oxidation and reduction, nor even removal of the adenosine terminus destroyed template activity.

How then does Qβ RNA come to contain adenosine, since its incorporation cannot be directed by the appropriate terminal complementary base of the template strand? The synthesis of the terminal adenosine appears to be a general feature of the Qβ polymerase reaction with natural RNA templates. Rensing and August (28) found that both Qβ RNA and Qβ 6S RNA were terminated predominantly with adenosine even when synthesized in vitro with a highly purified reaction system, and the same was found by Weber and Weissmann (35) with the Qβ complementary strand. This was true even when adenosine was removed from the Qβ RNA template. Because of these findings with the in vitro system, it is unnecessary to invoke anything other than the activity present in the purified polymerase system as an explanation for the terminal adenosine. Moreover, the two host factors are not implicated, since the Qβ 6S RNA is replicated without these factors and contains the $pppG \ldots A_{OH}$ terminus

(28,37). It may be concluded that synthesis of the terminal adenosine is catalyzed by the Qβ polymerase itself. There are several ways by which this may be explained (28). For example: (a) The enzyme could utilize RNA as a primer, catalyzing addition to the hydroxyl terminus in a reaction divorced from synthesis; this has not been detected, however (35). (b) It might be ascribed to the secondary or tertiary structure of the RNA whereby the enzyme transcribes an internal uridylate as a result of intra- or intermolecular hydrogen bonding. An attractive feature of this hypothesis is that it adheres to the basic transcriptional function of the enzyme and may not require additional enzyme-active sites. Moreover, a more extensive heterogeneity that is found in the Qβ 6S RNA which is predominantly, but not solely, double-stranded may be explained in the same way. (3) A third alternative, which is attractive because the terminal adenosine is found in all RNA products (except those from synthetic polymer templates), is that synthesis of the adenosine is a feature of chain termination. This could be in accord with the fact that termination is a unique event, since fragments of RNA, are rarely, if ever, synthesized. This would implicate a special mechanism, perhaps one analogous to the specific initiation of synthesis and involving an enzyme-active site that recognizes a unique termination signal.

The Replicative Complex

There is as yet no unequivocal model for the structure of the replicative enzyme-RNA complex that gives rise to Qβ RNA. For example, the secondary structure of the molecules, the number of nascent strands per template, and the mechanism of displacement of Qβ RNA and the complementary strand are unknown. Double-stranded and partially double-stranded forms of RNA can be isolated from the reaction mixture, but it is not clear whether any of these is the actual replicative structure, or whether they represent intermediates in the reaction or artifacts of the isolation procedures. When the untreated mixture containing progeny RNA is fractionated by zone centrifugation, several different components are found (39,40). One is a 40S to 50S complex which recently was shown by Hori (40) to contain most of the active enzyme, template, progeny RNA, and probably the host cell factors as well. This 45S structure appears to be the actively replicating complex. RNA sedimenting at 22S and 15S did not appear to play any role in replication; these molecules developed late in the reaction, were not associated with enzyme, and could be derived from the 45S form by deproteinization. By their sedimentation properties and ribonuclease resistance, the 22S and 15S forms are similar to molecules termed "replicative intermediates" or "replicative forms," but they may instead be molecules derived from the actual replicating complex of unknown structure by denaturation or by loss of enzyme and related factors.

Weissmann *et al.* (41) have proposed that the replicative template is not a double-stranded structure but rather is the free complementary strand base-paired with nascent Qβ RNA over a relatively small region. This model is supported by the observations that very little RNase-resistant RNA is found in the reaction mixture unless it is first treated with phenol and that the free complementary strand serves as template for the enzyme whereas the double-stranded or partially double-stranded RNA molecules do not. This would imply that some reaction mechanism other than the usual conservative or semiconservative displacement of product is operating in the Qβ reaction to separate the nascent strand from the template. The most likely candidate for this role is factor II. These basic proteins could act by denaturing base-paired regions as may be necessary both for initiation of synthesis and for replication. These details of the replication mechanism remain to be elucidated.

ACKNOWLEDGMENTS

This work was supported in part by grants from the National Institute of General Medical Sciences, National Institutes of Health (GM 11301 and GM 11936). This is Communication No. 267 from the Joan and Lester Avnet Institute of Molecular Biology.

SUMMARY

In recent years, the bacteriophage Qβ RNA polymerase reaction has become a highly characterized system for studying the synthesis of genetic material. An outstanding feature of this reaction is the actual replication of infectious bacteriophage RNA. All of the reaction components have now been isolated as discrete species: the enzyme containing four proteins, a host RNA binding factor composed of a single protein, a basic protein factor of which there are many active species, Qβ RNA, and Qβ RNA complementary strand. The properties of these components and of the reaction are described.

RESUMEN

En años recientes la reacción de la RNA polimerasa del bacteriófago Qβ ha llegado a ser un sistema altamente caracterizado para el estudio de la síntesis de material genético. Una característica sobresaliente de esta reacción es que se produce una verdadera replicación del RNA del bacteriófago infectivo. Todos los componentes de la reacción han sido aislados como especies separadas: la enzima que contiene cuatro proteínas, un factor de unión del RNA, proveniente del huésped, constituido por una única proteína, un factor proteico básico del que existen muchas especies activas, RNA de Qβ, y la cadena complementaria del RNA de Qβ. Se describen las propiedades de estos componentes y de la reacción.

REFERENCES

1. Spiegelman, S., Haruna, I., Holland, I., Beaudreau, G., and Mills, D., *Proc. Natl. Acad. Sci. U.S.A.*, *54*, 949 (1965).

2. Eoyang, L. and August, J. T., in Colowick, S. P., and Kaplan, N. O., *Methods in Enzymology*, Vol. XIIB, Academic Press, New York (1968), p. 530.
3. Eoyang, L. and August, J. T., in Cantoni, G., and Davies, D., *Procedures in Nucleic Acid Research*, Harper and Row, New York (1971), p. 829.
4. Kamen, R., *Nature, 228*, 527 (1970).
5. Kondo, M., Gallerani, R., and Weissmann, C., *Nature, 228*, 525 (1970).
6. Travers, A. A., Kamen, R. I., and Schleif, R. F., *Nature, 228*, 748 (1970).
7. Eikhom, T. S., Stockley, D. J., and Spiegelman, S., *Proc. Natl. Acad. Sci. U.S.A., 59*, 506 (1968).
8. August, J. T., Banerjee, A. K., Eoyang, L., Franze de Fernández, M. T., Hori, K., Kuo, C. H., Rensing, U., and Shapiro, L., *Cold Spring Harbor Symp. Quant. Biol., 33*, 73 (1968).
9. Banerjee, A. K., Kuo, C. H., and August, J. T., *J. Mol. Biol., 40*, 445 (1969).
10. Spiegelman, S., Pace, N. R., Mills, D. R., Levisohn, R., Eikhom, T. S., Taylor, M. M., Peterson, R. L., and Bishop, D. H. L., *Cold Spring Harbor Symp. Quant. Biol., 33*, 101 (1968).
11. Robertson, H. D. and Zinder, N. D. *Nature, 220*, 69 (1968).
12. Fiers, W., Van Montagu, M., De Wachter, R., Haegeman, G., Min Jou, W., Messens, E., Remaut, E., Vandenberghe, A., and Van Styvendaele, B., *Cold Spring Harbor Symp. Quant. Biol., 34*, 697 (1969).
13. Haruna, I., and Spiegelman, S., *Proc. Natl. Acad. Sci. U.S.A., 54*, 579 (1965).
14. Feix, G., Pollet, R., and Weissman, C., *Proc. Natl. Acad. Sci. U.S.A., 59*, 145 (1968).
15. Mills, D., Peterson, R. L., and Spiegelman, S., *Proc. Natl. Acad. Sci. U.S.A., 58*, 217 (1967).
16. Banerjee, A. K., Rensing, U., and August, J. T., *J. Mol. Biol., 45*, 181 (1969).
17. Hori, K., Eoyang, L., Banerjee, A. K., and August, J. T., *Proc. Natl. Acad. Sci. U.S.A., 57*, 1790 (1967).
18. Franze de Fernández, M. T., Eoyang, L., and August, J. T., *Nature, 219*, 588 (1968).
19. Shapiro, L., Franze de Fernández, M. T., and August, J. T., *Nature, 220*, 478 (1968).
20. Hayward, W. S., and Franze de Fernández, M. T., in Cantoni, G., and Davies, D., *Procedures in Nucleic Acid Research*, Harper and Row, New York (1971), p. 840.
21. Franze de Fernández, M. T., Hayward, W. S., and August, J. T., *J. Biol. Chem.*, in press.
22. Kuo, C. H. in Cantoni, G., and Davies, D., *Procedures in Nucleic Acid Research*, Harper and Row, New York (1971), p. 846.
23. Kuo, C. H., and August, J. T., *Fed. Proc. 30*, 1316 Abst. (1971).
24. Kuo, C. H., and August, J. T., *Nature New Biol. 237*, 105 (1972).
25. Silverman, P. M., *Fed. Proc., 30*, 1316 (1971).
26. Silverman, P. M. and August, J. T., *Fed. Proc. 29*, 340 Abst. (1970).
27. Goodman, H. M., Billeter, M. A., Hindley, J., and Weissmann, C., *Proc. Natl. Acad. Sci. U.S.A., 67*, 921 (1970).
28. Rensing, U., and August, J. T., *Nature, 224*, 853 (1969).
29. Kamen, R., *Nature, 221*, 321 (1969).
30. Dahlberg, J. E., *Nature, 220*, 548 (1968).
31. Adams, J. M., and Cory, S., *Nature, 227*, 570 (1970).
32. Haruna, I. and Spiegelman, S., *Proc. Natl. Acad. Sci. U.S.A., 54*, 1189 (1965).
33. De Wachter, R. and Fiers, W., *Nature, 221*, 233 (1969).
34. Weith, H. L., and Gilham, P. T., *Science, 166*, 1004 (1969).
35. Weber, H., and Weissmann, C., *J. Mol. Biol., 51*, 215 (1970).
36. Bishop, D. H. L., Mills, D. R., and Spiegelman, S., *Biochemistry, 70*, 3744 (1968).
37. Kacian, D. L., Mills, D. R., and Spiegelman, S., *Biochim. Biophys. Acta, 238*, 212 (1971).

38. Okada, Y., Ohno, T., and Haruna, I., *Virology, 43,* 69 (1971).
39. Feix, G., Slor, H., and Weissmann, C., *Proc. Natl. Acad. Sci. U.S.A., 57,* 1401 (1967).
40. Hori, K., *Biochim. Biophys. Acta, 217,* 394 (1970).
41. Weissmann, C., Feix, G., and Slor, H., *Cold Spring Harbor Symp. Quant. Biol., 33,* 83 (1968).

DISCUSSION

C. Weissmann (Zurich, Switzerland): Where did those proteins come from in the last data you showed? There were two bands on a gel and then the phosphorylating activity. What was the origin of that protein?

J. T. August (New York, U.S.A.): The slide showed the urea-polyacrylamide electrophoresis pattern of the major factor component and those proteins which were labeled with phosphate.

C. Weissmann: Those are factor II proteins?

J. T. August: Yes, these are factor II proteins which were then used as substrates for phosphorylation *in vitro* with an animal cell protein kinase. The molecular weights of the proteins which are phosphorylated are approximately 15,000, and because of their low molecular weight they separate poorly. Two proteins can be distinguished, although there may be more than two. Most likely, at least one of them is a ribosomal protein.

R. Soeiro (New York, U.S.A.): Can you get these factor II proteins to exchange with the ribosomes and Qβ RNA during the course of the reaction?

J. T. August: Are you asking about what is going on in the cell? We are now studying the effect of ribosomes in the reaction in relation to the role of factor II and to enzyme activity. I don't wish to elaborate on these findings now because Dr. Weissmann is going to describe his results in a moment.

E. Bustamente (Lima, Peru): Do these basic proteins ever become phosphorylated, as do the histones of eukaryotic organisms?

J. T. August: I believe you're asking whether they are phosphorylated *in vivo*. I don't know anyone who has detected a protein phosphorylating activity from *E. coli.* Dr. Phil Silverman at Albert Einstein College in New York looked for ^{32}P-labeled proteins in *E. coli* but didn't find any. We have looked for a protein kinase in *E. coli* and, with others, have failed to find such an activity. At this time, we can't attribute any biological role to the phosphorylation of the proteins that we show here.

E. P. Geiduschek (La Jolla, U.S.A.): Did you find any nonribosomal proteins as factor?

J. T. August: We showed that after the cells were lysed with detergent and EDTA, factor activity was present in the precipitate along with all of the cell DNA and about 30% of the RNA. We then separated the DNA from the RNA and found basic proteins with factor activity associated with the DNA. In all of these fractions, the relative concentration of factor to nucleic acid, whether DNA or RNA, was approximately the same. However, I can't say whether these basic proteins, active as factor and associated with DNA, are ribosomal or nonribosomal, since there is no way to rule out the possibility that there was an exchange of proteins from ribosomal-associated elements to DNA during the course of extraction. There is an apparent association of the active basic proteins with DNA in *E. coli,* but whether this results from the isolation procedures or is a biologically significant relationship remains to be elucidated.

G. Feix (Freiburg, Germany): Is it possible to differentiate between the activity of both factors? Do you see anything in the first step of the reaction if you omit one of the factors?

J. T. August: These studies have been carried out by Dr. Phil Silverman, and he has thus far not found steps in the reaction that can be related specifically to factor I or to factor II. The basic observation is that in the presence of both factors he can measure the specific association of enzyme to RNA, the conversion of a reversibly bound enzyme to one that is tightly bound to a unique site and which proceeds to the initiation of synthesis. If you leave out one of the factors, you do not get this reaction. At this time, we don't have any additional assays between those two steps in the reaction. We have looked for changes in RNA conformation and for other reactions in association with one or the other of these proteins but have not identified the primary role of the proteins. We believe it is very likely that both of these proteins act on the RNA. The stoichiometry of the reaction shows that both of these structures act on RNA, in one case to a specific site with factor I and in the case of factor II to many sites on the RNA.

P. Chambon (Strasbourg, France): When you speak about stoichiometry, is this in respect to the enzyme concentration or RNA concentration?

J. T. August: The requirement of the reaction for factor I and factor II is stoichiometric with the concentration of the RNA and not with enzyme concentration.

4

On the Regulation of RNA Synthesis in *Escherichia coli*

Andrew Travers

Laboratory of Molecular Biology
Medical Research Council
Cambridge, England

The accumulation of the stable RNA species, ribosomal RNA (rRNA) and transfer RNA (tRNA), in bacteria is regulated in accordance with the physiological state of the cell. (This subject is extensively reviewed in refs. 1-4.) Thus at high growth rates ribosomal RNA is accumulated rapidly, the synthesis of ribosomal RNA accounting for up to 40% of the instantaneous rate of RNA synthesis (5,6), although the cistrons coding for these RNA species comprise less than 0.5% of the bacterial genome (7,8). However, at low growth rates, when, for example, the carbon source is restricted, the accumulation of rRNA may proceed at less than 20% of the rate approached during maximal exponential growth. This type of regulation occurring during balanced growth of the bacterium may be regarded as a "fine tuning" (9).

A second mode of regulation of rRNA accumulation, "stringent" control, is defined genetically by the *rel* or RC locus (10). When *rel*+ strains of *Escherichia coli* are functionally deprived of amino acid, either by starvation of an amino acid auxotroph (11-14) or by restriction of amino acylation of a tRNA species even in the presence of the required amino acid (15), the rate of rRNA accumulation is reduced at least tenfold (6). Mutants of the *rel* gene (rel⁻) exist which are unable to restrict rRNA accumulation during amino acid starvation and are said to possess "relaxed" control. It is probable that the *rel*⁻ mutation permits constitutive synthesis of rRNA during amino acid starvation. In diploids, *rel*+ is dominant to the *rel*⁻ allele (16), consistent with the existence of a functional inhibitor of rRNA accumulation. Although *rel*⁻strains cannot control the rate of accumulation under conditions of amino acid starvation, it should be emphasized that most *rel*⁻strains regulate rRNA accumulation normally during a carbon source transition (17). The existence of other mutants having a relaxed phenotype but mapping at different loci has been reported (18). The implications of these and other mutants will be discussed below.

To what extent are other species of RNA regulated in a manner similar to rRNA? The accumulation of tRNA is restricted to an extent comparable to that of rRNA during the stringent response (7,19-21). Thus it is probable that rRNA and tRNA are regulated coordinately, at least by the system responsible for effecting stringent control. Nevertheless, there is some evidence that at low growth rates the accumulation of rRNA and tRNA may not be coordinately regulated (22). With regard to mRNA synthesis, although there are some indications that certain mRNA species may be subject to stringent control (9) and that certain other mRNA species are not (20), the data at present available are too scanty to resolve the question of the extent to which different mRNA species are subject to degrees of stringent control (23).

A very early and apparently invariant manifestation of *rel*⁺ gene function during amino acid starvation is the accumulation of an unusual nucleotide, MS1 (24,25), for which the structure guanosine 5′-diphosphate 2′- (or 3′-) diphosphate has been proposed (26). The accumulation of MS1 after amino acid starvation is very rapid in cells bearing *rel*⁺ but not *rel*⁻ alleles, the *in vivo* concentration of the nucleotide attaining and usually exceeding the levels of GTP within 2 min (9,25). Conversely, on amino acid resupplementation, MS1 rapidly disappears (26). In the case of carbon source deprivations and growth rate transitions, *rel*⁺ as well as *rel*⁻strains restrict rRNA accumulation and both cell types also accumulate MS1 (27). Furthermore, even the basal level of MS1 found in *rel*⁺ and *rel*⁻strains during balanced growth can be correlated with the RNA content and growth rate of the cells (27). Such correlations would be obtained if MS1 accumulation were either a cause or a consequence of restricted rRNA synthesis. In addition to MS1, a second guanine nucleotide, MS2, tentatively identified as a guanosine pentaphosphate (26), accumulates in *rel*⁺ cells during the stringent response (24,25). However, bacterial strains exist which, although accumulating MS1, fail to accumulate MS2 on amino acid starvation (25). Such strains have stringent control of rRNA accumulation.

The accumulation of specific RNA species could be regulated at the level either of synthesis or of degradation (or both). In the case of the most drastic reduction in the accumulation of the stable RNA species, i.e., during the stringent response, Lazzarini and Dahlberg (19) have argued that this effect is most probably a consequence of the restriction of synthesis. The basis of their argument is that the rate of accumulation of RNA which they observe is that which would be predicted from the measured instantaneous rate of synthesis and, further, that under these conditions of growth, no turnover of newly synthesized rRNA could be detected. Nevertheless, *in vivo* degradation of rRNA and tRNA has been observed under certain conditions (28-30), and it is possible to interpret Lazzarini and Dahlberg's data in terms of a model postulating control by degradation.

Control of RNA synthesis can be exerted principally during initiation or elongation of RNA molecules. Winslow and Lazzarini (31) have concluded that the rate of RNA chain elongation is lowered, on the average, by three- to fourfold (and perhaps up to ninefold) during the stringent response. However, the data of Primakoff and Berg (20), showing that the total rate of $\phi80$ mRNA synthesis is unaffected by the stringent response, argue that if this reduction in the rate of elongation is general it is exactly compensated for by an increase in the rate of initiation of $\phi80$ mRNA. An alternative explanation is that the rates of elongation of different RNA species are affected to varying extents by the stringent response. The most compelling argument that the principal effect of the stringent response on RNA synthesis is at the level of chain initiation is provided by Stamato and Pettijohn (32), who showed that the synthesis of 16S RNA resumes within 40 sec after the restoration of a required amino acid to a starved culture of *rel*[+] cells. The synthesis of 23S RNA then succeeds that of 16S RNA. Since the 16S sequence is proximal to the rRNA promoter (33-35), it is probable that the resumption of rRNA synthesis results from an increased rate of initiation. The only model invoking degradation as the principal mode of control that is compatible with the observed results would have to postulate that the degrading nuclease followed immediately behind the transcribing polymerase. Further, such a nuclease, once activated to degrade a particular rRNA molecule, could not subsequently be deactivated until the whole molecule had been degraded.

What is the molecular mechanism for the control of the synthesis of the stable RNA species? Dennis (36) has presented evidence that the control of rRNA synthesis is not dependent on gene dosage, and he suggests that cytoplasmic elements may therefore be involved in its regulation. This conclusion is, however, dependent on the genes for rRNA being clustered, a point on which the experimental evidence is conflicting (37,38).

One possibility which cannot be excluded is that the observed pattern of control is a consequence of the independent actions of several regulatory mechanisms directly affecting the activity of the rRNA promoters. More attractive is the hypothesis that the initiation of rRNA synthesis is primarily controlled by a simple regulatory protein. If it is assumed that control of RNA synthesis during the stringent response and during carbon source transitions is mediated by the same regulatory system, this system would have as its primary target the control of stable RNA synthesis. Now although the synthesis of the stable RNA species is preferentially curtailed during the stringent response, the synthesis of certain mRNA species may also be reduced, although to a lesser degree. Accordingly, it is conceivable that the regulatory system for stable RNA species might also control the synthesis of certain mRNA species. In this case, the regulatory system would lack the specificity which characterizes such transcriptional regulatory proteins as the *lac* repressor (39) and the CAP protein (40). Such a lack of specificity might well be an inherent property of the RNA polymerase itself or of a transcription factor interacting directly with the polymerase.

The known components of the transcriptional machinery of *E. coli* comprise the core RNA polymerase, which synthesizes the internucleotide bonds of the RNA molecule (41,42): the σ factor, an initiation factor (42) required for accurate initiation on phage DNA templates (43-45); the ψ factor, an initiation factor which increases initiation efficiency with bacterial DNA templates (46,47); and the ρ factor, which acts as a termination factor (48). We must ask whether it is possible to explain the control of transcription of stable RNA species in terms of these components.

Originally, it was reported that the RNA polymerase containing σ factor was by itself unable to synthesize detectable quantities of rRNA with *E. coli* DNA as template (46-49). However, it has recently been shown (ref. 50 and Haseltine, personal communication) that RNA polymerase can, under certain conditions, transcribe *E. coli* DNA so that rRNA comprises about 10% of the total transcript. In addition, Zubay *et al.* (51) have shown that tRNA^{Tyr} can be transcribed *in vitro*. The resolution of this apparent conflict springs from a recent observation that the amount of rRNA synthesized *in vitro* is dependent, in part, on the state of a reactive sulfydryl group in the RNA polymerase itself (Travers, unpublished observations). In this context, it is interesting to note that those workers who initially failed to observe rRNA synthesis *in vitro* used 2-mercaptoethanol as their thiol reagent, employing concentrations of 2 mM (49) or 6 mM (46). In contrast, those workers who observed either rRNA or tRNA synthesis *in vitro* used dithiothreitol as their thiol reagent (50-52). The implication is that RNA polymerase can exist in two forms, one which can synthesize rRNA efficiently and one which cannot.

Clearly, one method of controlling the synthesis of rRNA would be to control the transition between the two forms of RNA polymerase. To effect a change in the operative thiol concentration *in vivo* might adversely affect the activity of other essential enzymes. Another plausible mechanism by which the change might be effected is for the RNA polymerase to interact with an effector molecule. Such an effector could be either a low molecular weight compound or a protein factor. A candidate for such a protein factor is the ψ factor.

The ψ factor was originally characterized as an activity in crude extracts that preferentially stimulated total RNA synthesis on an *E. coli* DNA template, having little effect on the synthesis of RNA from phage DNA templates (46). Interestingly, ψ activity is also exhibited by a host-specified component of the

Qβ replicase (47). The ψ factor prepared from Qβ replicase contains two polypeptide chains of molecular weights 45,000 and 35,000 (52). However, it is not known whether both or only one of these chains is required for ψ activity. Nor has it been rigorously proven that the ψ activity isolated from uninfected cells and that isolated from Qβ replicase are physically identical.

In addition to stimulating total RNA synthesis, the ψ factor also altered the spectrum of RNA species transcribed (46). In its absence, little or no rRNA synthesis was observed, whereas in its presence about 20-30% of the labeled *in vitro* RNA product hybridizing to *E. coli* DNA was competable by unlabeled rRNA (46). This amount of competition suggests that rRNA comprised about 10-15% of the total transcript. Since the rRNA cistrons comprise less than 0.5% of the bacterial genome, this indicates that rRNA is being preferentially tran-scribed *in vitro*. This result suggests that under the appropriate conditions ψ factor can effect a conformational change in the RNA polymerase, enabling it to transcribe rRNA. It is perhaps significant that under the same conditions wherein ψ preferentially increases the proportion of rRNA synthesized, the factor also decreases the apparent initiation K_m of the polymerase for GTP by about fivefold while having little effect on the apparent K_m value of the other three nucleoside triphosphates (Travers, unpublished observations). Clearly, if one function of ψ factor is to convert RNA polymerase from a form in which it cannot synthesize rRNA efficiently to a form in which it can, then it follows that in the condition of RNA polymerase being already in the form that can synthesize rRNA, ψ factor would have no preferential effect on rRNA synthesis. This has in fact been observed to be the case (Haseltine, personal communication; Travers and Pedersen, manuscript in preparation).

The rapidity of the response of rRNA synthesis *in vivo* to amino acid starvation or to its relief suggests that the control may be effected by a low molecular weight compound interacting directly with a component of the transcription. A candidate for such an effector is MS1. This compound has been shown to interact both with RNA polymerase (53) and with ψ factor (47). Cashel (53) has shown that MS1 inhibits RNA synthesis by RNA polymerase alone *in vitro*, with a variety of DNA templates, by inhibiting both chain elongation and chain initiation. Interestingly, MS1 affects initiation by selective-ly inhibiting a fraction of the RNA chains that contain a 5′-terminal pppG residue. The effect of MS1 on chain elongation could account, in part, for the observed decrease in the rate of chain elongation during the stringent response. However, the significance of the effect of interaction of MS1 with RNA polymerase on chain initiation is less clear.

The effect of MS1 on ψ factor is also complex. Under conditions where ψ preferentially turns on rRNA synthesis, MS1 inhibits ψ activity at the level of initiation of RNA synthesis. It should be emphasized that the inhibition of the ψ stimulation of rRNA synthesis by MS1 is the only evidence against the proposition that ψ is in some way altering the *in vitro* environment in a nonspecific manner and so allowing the RNA polymerase to alter its conformation. When the *in vitro* conditions are such that RNA polymerase synthesizes rRNA efficiently in the absence of ψ, MS1 has no preferential effect on the synthesis of rRNA (Haseltine, personal communication; Travers and Pedersen, manuscript in preparation) or of tRNA (51).

We can now formulate a model for the control of the synthesis of stable RNA species in *E. coli*. This model has three major postulates:

(a) RNA polymerase can exist in two forms, one which can initiate synthesis of stable RNA species efficiently and one which cannot. These forms are termed $(E\sigma)_G$ and $(E\sigma)_A$, respectively. The change in specificity is a consequence of a conformational change in the enzyme.

(b) The function of ψ factor is principally to convert $(E\sigma)_A$ to $(E\sigma)_G$. In addition, ψ may increase the initiation efficiency of RNA polymerase.

(c) MS1 acts as an inhibitor of the ψ-mediated conversion of $(E\sigma)_A$ to $(E\sigma)_G$.

A minor postulate, which is not a necessary consequence of the model, is that the $(E\sigma)_G$ form will initiate RNA chains with pppG more efficiently than will the $(E\sigma)_A$ form.

This model predicts that three classes of relaxed mutations might exist:

Class 1. A mutant defective in MS1 accumulation. This includes the *rel⁻* mutants, which are *recessive* to normal *rel⁺*.

Class 2. A mutant ψ factor in MS1 binding. Such a mutant should be *dominant* to *rel⁺*. However, in addition to binding MS1, ψ also binds guanine nucleotides such as GTP (Blumental, personal communication). Since it is conceivable that GTP might act as a positive effector in this system and that a mutation affecting MS1 binding might also affect GTP binding, such a mutation might be lethal.

Class 3. A mutant RNA polymerase stabilized in the $(E\sigma)_G$ form, i.e., ψ is not required for the conversion. Such a mutant should synthesize rRNA constitutively and should be dominant to *rel⁺*.

In addition, the model predicts that there should exist polymerase mutants that preferentially shut off RNA synthesis under restrictive conditions.

In conclusion, the observed *in vitro* effects of RNA polymerase, ψ factor, and MS1 on the *in vitro* transcription of stable RNA species can explain in large part the control of stable RNA synthesis observed *in vivo*. Such a correspondence does not, however, constitute rigorous proof that ψ and RNA polymerase act as regulatory proteins or that MS1 acts as a regulatory low molecular weight effector in this control. A final elucidation of this problem clearly requires the isolation of suitable mutants.

SUMMARY

A model is proposed for the regulation of the synthesis of stable RNA species in *E. coli*. This model has three principal postulates: (a) that RNA polymerase can exist in two forms, one $(E\sigma)_G$, which can initiate the synthesis of stable RNA species, efficiently, and one, $(E\sigma)_A$, which cannot; (b) that one function of the ψ factor is to effect the transition from $(E\sigma)_A$ to $(E\sigma)_G$; (c) that the ψ-mediated transition of the RNA polymerase is inhibited by the guanine nucleotide, MS1.

RESUMEN

Se presenta un modelo para la regulación de la síntesis de especies de RNA estables en' E. coli. Este modelo contiene tres postulados principales: (a) La RNA polimerasa puede existir en dos formas, una $(E\sigma)_G$, la cual inicia la síntesis de las especies estables de RNA eficientemente, y la otra $(E\sigma)_A$, la cual no puede iniciar la síntesis. (b) La unica función del factor psi es afectar la trasición de $(E\sigma)_A$ a $(E\sigma)_G$. (c) La transición por ψ de la RNA polimerasa es inhibida por el nucleótido de guanina, MS1.

REFERENCES

1. Neidhardt, F. C., *Progr. Nucleic Acid Res., 3,* 145 (1964).
2. Maaløe, O., and Kjeldgaard, N. O., *Control of Macromolecular Synthesis,* W. A. Benjamin, New York, (1966).
3. Edlin, G., and Broda, P., *Bacteriol. Rev., 32,* 206 (1968).
4. Ryan, A., and Borek, E., *Progr. Nucleic Acid Res., 2,* 212 (1971).
5. Salser, W., Janin, J., and Levinthal, C., *J. Mol. Biol., 31,* 237 (1968).
6. Lazzarini, R. A., and Winslow, R. M., *Cold Spring Harbor Symp. Quant. Biol., 35,* 383 (1970).
7. Yankofsky, S. A., and Spiegelman, S., *Proc. Natl. Acad. Sci. U.S.A., 48,* 1466 (1962).
8. Kennell, D., *J. Mol. Biol., 34,* 85 (1968).
9. Gallant, J., Erlich, H., Hall, B., and Laffler, T., *Cold Spring Harbor Symp. Quant. Biol., 35,* 397 (1970).
10. Stent, G. S., and Brenner, S., *Proc. Natl. Acad. Sci. U.S.A., 47,* 2005 (1961).
11. Sands, M. K., and Roberts, R. B., *J. Bacteriol., 63,* 505 (1952).
12. Gale, E. F., and Folkes, J. P., *Biochem. J., 53,* 493 (1953).
13. Gros, F., and Gros, F., *Exptl. Cell Res., 14,* 104 (1958).
14. Pardee, A. B., and Prestidge, L. S., *J. Bacteriol., 71,* 677 (1956).
15. Neidhardt, F. C., *Bacteriol. Rev., 30,* 701 (1966).
16. Fiil, N., *J. Mol. Biol., 45,* 195 (1969).
17. Neidhardt, F. C., *Biochim. Biophys. Acta, 68,* 380 (1963).
18. Lavalle, R., *Bull. Soc. Chim. Biol., 47,* 1567 (1965).
19. Lazzarini, R. A., and Dahlberg, A. E., *J. Biol. Chem., 246,* 420 (1971).
20. Primakoff, P., and Berg, P., *Cold Spring Harbor Symp. Quant. Biol., 35,* 391 (1970).
21. Neidhardt, F. C., and Eidlie, L., *Biochim. Biophys. Acta, 68,* 380 (1963).
22. Kurland, C. G., and Maaløe, O., *J. Mol. Biol., 4,* 193 (1962).
23. Travers, A., in Sussman, M. (ed.), *Molecular Genetics and Developmental Biology,* Prentice-Hall, New York, in press.
24. Cashel, M., and Gallant, J., *Nature, 221,* 838 (1969).
25. Cashel, M., *J. Biol. Chem., 244,* 3133 (1969).
26. Cashel, M., and Kalbacher, B., *J. Biol. Chem., 245,* 2309 (1970).

27. Lazzarini, R. A., Cashel, M., and Gallant, J., *J. Biol. Chem., 246,* 4381 (1971).
28. Dubin, D. T., and Elkort, A. T., *Biochim. Biophys. Acta, 103,* 355 (1965).
29. Lazzarini, R. A., and Santangelo, E., *J. Bacteriol., 95,* 1212 (1968).
30. Lazzarini, R. A., and Peterkofsky, A., *Proc. Natl. Acad. Sci. U.S.A., 53,* 549 (1965).
31. Winslow, R. M., and Lazzarini, R. A., *J. Biol. Chem., 244,* 3387 (1970).
32. Stamato, T. D., and Pettijohn, D. E., *Nature New Biol. 234,* 99 (1971).
33. Pato, M., and von Meyenburg, K., *Cold Spring Harbor Symp. Quant. Biol., 35,* 494 (1970).
34. Doolittle, W. F., and Pace, N. R., *Proc. Natl. Acad. Sci. U.S.A., 68,* 1786 (1971).
35. Kossman, C. R., Stomato, T. D., and Pettijohn, D. E., *Nature New Biol. 234,* 102 (1971).
36. Dennis, P., *Nature New Biol., 232,* 43 (1971).
37. Yu, M. T., Vermeulen, C. W., and Atwood, K. C., *Proc. Natl. Acad. Sci. U.S.A., 67,* 26 (1970).
38. Gorelic, L., *Mol. Gen. Genet., 106,* 323 (1970).
39. Gilbert, W., and Müller-Hill, B., *Proc. Natl. Acad. Sci. U.S.A., 57,* 2415 (1967).
40. de Crombrugghe, B., Chem, B., Goltesman, M., Pastan, I., Varmus, H. E., Emmer, M., and Perlman, R. L., *Nature New Biol. 230,* 37 (1971).
41. Burgess, R. R., Travers, A. A., Dunn, J. J., and Bautz, E. K. F., *Nature, 221,* 43 (1969).
42. Travers, A. A., and Burgess, R. R., *Nature, 222,* 537 (1969).
43. Bautz, E. K. F., Bautz, F. A., and Dunn, J. J., *Nature, 223,* 1022 (1969).
44. Goff, C. G., and Minkley, E. G., in Silvestri, L. (ed.), *Lepetit Colloquium on RNA Polymerase and Transcription,* North-Holland, Amsterdam (1970), p. 124.
45. Sugiura, M. T., Okamoto, T., and Takanami, M., *Nature, 225,* 598 (1970).
46. Travers, A. A., Kamen, R. I., and Schleif, R. F., *Nature, 228,* 748 (1970).
47. Travers, A. A., Kamen, R. I., and Cashel, M., *Cold Spring Harbor Symp. Quant. Biol., 35,* 415 (1970).
48. Roberts, J. W., *Nature, 224,* 1168 (1969).
49. Pettijohn, D. E., Clarkson, K., Kossman, C. R., and Stonington, C. R., *J. Mol. Biol., 52,* 281 (1970).
50. Hussey, C., Pero, J., Shorenstein, R. G., and Losick, R., *Proc. Natl. Acad. Sci. U.S.A., 69,* 407 (1972).
51. Zubay, G., Cheong, L., and Gefter, M. L., *Proc. Natl. Acad. Sci. U.S.A., 68,* 2195 (1971).
52. Kamen, R. I., *Nature, 228,* 527 (1970).
53. Cashel, M., *Cold Spring Harbor Symp. Quant. Biol., 35,* 407 (1970).

DISCUSSION

J. T. August (New York, U.S.A.): To what extent have you purified the ψ factor from uninfected cells?

A. A. Travers (Cambridge, England): In our most highly purified ψ preparations from uninfected *E. coli*, we observe that on a polyacrylamide gel there are two bands which have the same mobility as subunits 3 and 4 and which comprise about 25-40% of the total protein. So we do not have ψ pure as yet.

G. D. Novelli (Oak Ridge, U.S.A.): You started your discussion by saying that you were going to discuss the control of stable RNA species, ribosomal and transfer RNA, but you've talked exclusively about ribosomal RNA. I'd like to ask what is the status of the ψ factor with respect to transcription of the tRNA genes.

A. A. Travers: We have some preliminary results. Under conditions where we see the ψ stimulation of ribosomal RNA synthesis, we have tested the effect of ψ on the *in vitro* transcription of $\phi80_{psu^+}$ DNA. This DNA contains in it the gene for tyrosine suppressor tRNA. We find that without the ψ factor we see little or no tRNA synthesis. With the ψ factor there is a stimulation of synthesis of this tRNA, which is reversed by guanosine tetraphosphate. These data are based on hybridization to the separated strands of $\phi80_{psu^+}$ DNA. I believe that Ikeda at Harvard has found that, using high thiol concentration, tRNA is synthesized without ψ factor. So the situation for tRNA may well be very much the same as for ribosomal RNA.

F. Lipmann (New York, U.S.A.): Do you think that guanosine tetraphosphate competes with GTP?

A. A. Travers: Since I have done no experiments to test whether it competes with GTP or not, I can't say. The ψ factor decreases the apparent K_m for GTP for the polymerase, and the effect of ψ is reversed by guanosine tetraphosphate. I don't know whether GTP actually works on ψ factor itself.

F. Lipmann: Where do you get your guanosine tetraphosphate?

A. A. Travers: I get it from Mike Cashel and from Harvard.

F. Lipmann: You seem to assume that one of the diphosphate chains is on the 2' or 3' position, the other on 5'. How much has been done to confirm this?

A. A. Travers: It's not clear whether it is on the 3' or 2' position. I think guanosine tetraphosphate has been chemically synthesized in Europe, but it is not known whether the synthetic material is biologically active.

R. M. Bock (Madison, U.S.A.): I think that Dr. Lipmann's comments are particularly important because what is referred to in all the data presented as ppGpp has not reached the state where I feel that that label is justified. It should now only be called "magic spot 1." The necessary evidence to identify it as ppGpp is still lacking. In fact, there are some severe discrepancies between the chemical stability in alkali and the proposed structure.

I. D. Algranati (Buenos Aires, Argentina): Do you know the intracellular level of ppGpp in stringent bacteria?

A. A. Travers: In starved stringent bacteria, I believe Gallant has shown that the level is of the order of 0.5-2 mM.

E. P. Geiduschek: (La Jolla, U.S.A.): If you take the ATP concentration very much below the K_m for initiation and GTP concentration up to 1 mM, can you force a ribosomal RNA synthesis in the absence of DTT and in the absence of ψ?

A. A. Travers: I don't know, we have yet to do the experiment.

J. T. August: Do you know how your studies relate to the observations of Pettijohn? As I understand it, in the work that Pettijohn has carried out he isolates a complex of RNA polymerase and *E. coli* DNA that is actually making a high proportion of ribosomal RNA. When he dissociates this complex into free DNA and free enzyme, he no longer observes that high rate of ribosomal RNA synthesis. Can you correlate these results with your findings?

A. A. Travers: First, I don't know the conditions under which Pettijohn carries out his experiments. I believe that the conversion between the A and the G forms is very fast and reversible. If his conditions for synthesis were such as to favor the A form when he freed the enzyme, then he would see little or no further initiation of rRNA synthesis. When the enzyme is actually transcribing, it doesn't matter which if any of these forms it is in, if indeed it's at all meaningful.

P. Lengyel (New Haven, U.S.A.): I would like to make a comment on ppGpp. We wanted to test *in vivo* experiments the possible involvement of ppGpp in the regulation of methionine tRNA synthesis. We did this on the basis of the finding that inhibition of stable RNA synthesis in stringent strains can be caused not only by the deprivation of the required amino acid but also by an inhibitor of peptide chain initiation, trimethoprim. Also, it was found recently that trimethoprim, which selectively blocks methionine tRNA accumulation in stringent strains but not in relaxed strains, has no effect on the ppGpp levels. That means it does not cause an increase in ppGpp levels and furthermore means it doesn't interfere with the increase in ppGpp levels which is accomplished by deprivation from a required amino acid. In view of this, we wonder whether ppGpp is indeed involved or not.

R. P. Perry (Philadelphia, U.S.A.): Is there any evidence that there might be different kinds of control which would result in different amounts of loading of a ribosomal gene with polymerase molecules? For example, in cells with different growth rates, you might expect an initiation type of control which might respond to changes slowly. In a situation where we want a quick response, it is probably not a good idea to regulate at the level of initiation, since one would have to load the whole cistron with RNA polymerases again. Do you have any comments relative to the existence of different kinds of regulation which might be related to the extent of loading of the ribosomal RNA genes with polymerase molecules?

A. A. Travers: Cashel has suggested that guanosine tetraphosphate may affect the rate of chain elongation as well as initiation. In addition, the scheme which we have here can accommodate other methods of regulation. One mode of regulation may be by guanosine tetraphosphate, but it is also possible that a factor exists which could, for example, convert the enzyme from G form to A form. There could be additional controls in the cell, but they can't be elucidated by studying the test tube reaction.

F. Lipmann: Why do you call the Eσ complex a holoenzyme? Does σ also have an influence on elongation; Is the ρ enzyme complex also a holoenzyme?

A. A. Travers: The σ factor has no direct effect on chain elongation, although it may allow polymerase to initiate more accurately, and once the polymerase has initiated more accurately, it may make longer chains. The interaction of ρ with RNA polymerase is not clear; some workers claim that ρ binds to RNA polymerase.

C. Weissmann (Zurich, Switzerland): Do you have any indications whether the effect of ψ is catalytic or stoichiometric, which could be tested by incubating with only three triphosphates prior to letting elongation proceed? In the experiment designed to localize the time at which ψ exerts its effect, did you show that it was actually ribosomal RNA which was being stimulated, or was that just *net* synthesis?

A. A. Travers: I have little information on whether ψ is catalytic or stoichiometric. Using the ψ from Qβ replicase, there are a couple of experiments which say that the maximum stimulation of RNA synthesis is attained at ψ levels where the amount of ψ is about one tenth of the molar amount of polymerase. In this system, only about 40 or 50% of the polymerase molecules were active. Therefore, it looks as though ψ can act catalytically, but it's not entirely clear. The answer to your second question is, it was *net* synthesis I was looking at.

5

Interconvertible Forms of Bacterial RNA Polymerase

Pedro Ezcurra, Eduardo M. De Robertis, Norberto Judewicz, and Héctor Torres

Instituto de Investigaciones Bioquímicas "Fundación Campomar"
and
Facultad de Ciencias Exactas y Naturales
Buenos Aires, Argentina

Transcription of phage and bacterial genes seems to be regulated by two types of control mechanisms. One of them stimulates the ability of the RNA polymerase to transcribe specific DNA sequences. This is a positive mechanism of control that requires the presence of different factors such as σ, CAP or ψ (1-3). The other is a negative control exerted by the repressor proteins (4,5).

In addition, some evidence indicates that bacterial RNA polymerase is modified during phage infection. This modification leads to a change in the specificity and catalytic activity of the enzyme (6,6,).

This work reports the existence of two interconvertible forms of bacterial RNA polymerase. In addition, evidence is presented on the properties of the adenylylating system found in bacterial extracts.

INTERCONVERSIONS

The existence of interconvertible forms of RNA polymerase was explored in three systems. These experiments were done in collaboration with Drs. Ezcurra, Chelala, and Hirschbein.

Escherichia coli **A19**

RNA polymerase was purified from *Escherichia coli A19* as previously described (8). Incubation of an RNA polymerase preparation in the presence of ATP-Mg^{2+} led to a time-dependent inactivation of the enzyme (Fig. 1). This effect is reversible, since the activity was restored to a large extent by addition of a fraction found in the same extracts. This reactivation was also time dependent, and the effect could be due to the removal of ATP, since this fraction contains both an active adenylate kinase and a $5'$-nucleotidase. On the other hand, the maximum rate of inactivation was observed at equimolar concentration of ATP and Mg^{2+}. When Mg^{2+} was added at concentrations above those of ATP, the rate of inactivation diminished. This evidence might indicate that RNA polymerase exists in two interconvertible forms, according to the following scheme:

$$\text{Polymerase (active)} \underset{Mg^{2+}}{\overset{ATP-Mg^{2+}}{\rightleftharpoons}} \text{Polymerase (inactive)}$$

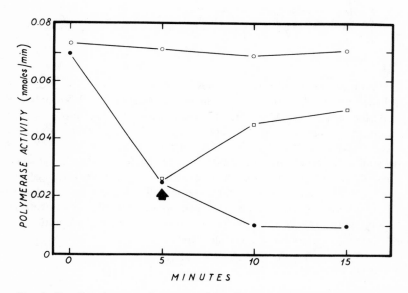

Fig. 1. E coli *polymerase interconversions.* The enzyme was incubated in the presence (●) or absence (○) of 4.1 mM ATP-Mg^{2+}. At the time indicated by the arrow, some reaction mixtures (□) received an enzyme fraction containing adenylate kinase and $5'$-nucleotidase activity. Other conditions were as previously described(8).

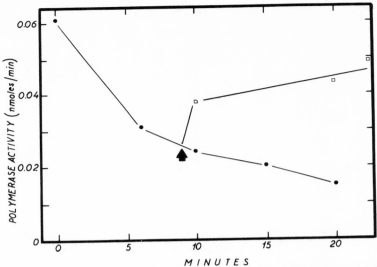

Fig. 2. B. subtilis *RNA polymerase interconversions.* Fraction ASI (9) containing 250 μg protein was incubated at 37° in the presence of 5 mM ATP-Mg^{2+} (●). At the indicated times, aliquots were removed, diluted in a cold solution containing 50 mM Tris-HCl buffer (pH 7.8), 1 mM EDTA, 5 mM NaF, 5 mM and bovine serum albumin (0.5 mg/ml) and assayed for polymerase activity. Conditions for this assay were as previously indicated (9) except for the presence of 5 mM MnCl$_2$ instead of MgCl$_2$ and 0.05 mM ATP, GTP, CTP, and 0.1 mM ^{14}C-UTP (2.5 μc/μmole) instead of 0.2 mM nucleoside triphosphates. At the time indicated by the arrow, some incubations (□) carried out in the presence of ATP-Mg^{2+} received MgCl$_2$ to a final concentration of 40 mM.

It is important to emphasize that these changes in the enzyme activity were observed only if the assay was performed in the presence of limiting amounts of Mn^{2+}. That is, in the conditions of the assay mixture, only one half of the nucleoside triphosphates could be complexed with Mn^{2+}. When the concentration of this cation was above that of the corresponding nucleoside triphosphate concentration, the effect of ATP-Mg^{2+} in the preincubation reaction was not observed. This suggests that in this condition the enzyme rapidly returns to the active form.

Bacillus subtilis Extracts

Experiments with *Bacillus subtilis* extracts were performed in collaboration with Drs. Salas, Avila, and Viñuela in the Instituto Marañon (Madrid). RNA polymerase from *B. subtilis* was prepared as described elsewhere (9). As shown in Fig. 2, there was a decrease in the RNA polymerase activity by incubation

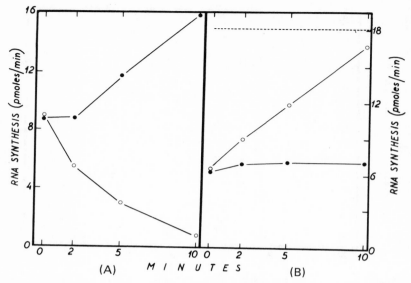

Fig. 3. Activation and inactivation of RNA synthesis in toluene-treated E. coli. Cells from an exponential culture of *E. coli* A19 were collected and resuspended in 50 mM Tris-HCl buffer, pH 7.5, to give an optical density (550 mμ) of about 7. Then 1% toluene (v:v) was added, and the suspension was mixed and left for 15 min in the cold. After that, the suspension was centrifuged for 15 min at 10,000 × g, and the cellular precipitate was resuspended in Tris-toluene to give an optical density of about 14. (A) Aliquots of the cell suspension (0.1 ml) were incubated at 37° for the indicated times in the presence (○) or absence (●) of 1 mM ATP-Mg^{2+}. The total volume was 0.11 ml. The reactions were stopped by dilution with 0.4 ml of a cold solution containing 50 mM Tris-HCl buffer (pH 7.5), 11.5 mM EDTA, 15 mM KF, 0.2 mM dithiothreitol, and 1% toluene (v:v). RNA synthesis was assayed on 0.02 ml aliquots of these diluted samples in a mixture containing 0.2 mM each of ATP, CTP, GTP, and ^{3}H-UTP (30 μc/μmole), 50 mM Tris-HCl buffer (pH 7.5), 150 mM KCl, 5 mM MnCl$_2$, and 0.2 mM dithiothreitol. The total volume was 0.1 ml. Incubations were carried out for 10 min at 37°. The reactions were stopped by the addition of 1 ml cold trichloroacetic acid, and the precipitates were collected on nitrocellulose filters and counted as described previously (8). (B) A toluene-treated cell suspension was incubated for 10 min at 37° in the presence of ATP-Mg^{2+} as described above, except that the amount of cells and reagents was increased tenfold. The reaction was stopped by the addition of 1 ml Tris-EDTA-KF-DTT-toluene cold buffer solution, and the suspension was centrifuged at 10,000 × g for 15 min. Then the cellular precipitate was resuspended in 1 ml of cold 50 mM Tris-HCl buffer, pH 7.5, containing 0.2 mM dithiothreitol and centrifuged again. After resuspension in 0.5 ml of the same cold buffer, aliquots of this suspension (0.02 ml) were further incubated at 37° for the indicated periods with 50 mM Tris-HCl buffer (pH 7.5) and 0.2 mM dithiothreitol in the presence (○) or absence (●) of 20 mM MgCl$_2$. The total volume was 0.1 ml. Reactions were stopped by the addition of 0.2 ml of cold Tris-EDTA-KF-DTT buffer solution and centrifuged for 15 min at 10,000 × g. Synthesis of RNA was determined on the cellular precipitates as described above.

with ATP-Mg^{2+}. As in the case of *E. coli* enzyme, the activity was restored to a large extent, in this case by addition of Mg^{2+}.

E. coli Cells Treated with Toluene

Recent evidence indicated that the treatment of bacterial cells with toluene renders preparations no longer viable, but permeable to a variety of compounds including ribonucleoside and deoxyribonucleoside triphosphates. These preparations were found to be able to catalyze the synthesis of RNA and DNA (10,11). The following experiments were carried out in collaboration with Dr. Cantarella. As can be seen in Fig. 3, treatment of toluenized cells with ATP-Mg^{2+} led to inactivation of the capacity of these cells to carry out further synthesis of RNA, using nucleoside triphosphates as precursors. This capacity increased when the toluene-treated cells were preincubated in the absence of ATP-Mg^{2+}. Reincubation of the ATP-Mg^{2+} inactivated cells in the presence of Mg^{2+} partially restored the ability of the cells to synthesize RNA.

ADENYLYLATION BY EXTRACTS FROM *E. Coli*

These experiments were carried out in collaboration with Drs. Ezcurra, De Robertis, Leoni, and Judewicz. When enzyme extracts from *E. coli* or *B. subtilis* were incubated with α-^{32}P-ATP-labeled ATP in the presence of limiting amounts of Mg^{2+}, radioactivity was incorporated into a trichloroacetic acid insoluble product. This product was resistant to RNase, but a great proportion of it remained in the aqueous phase after phenol extraction. This suggests that this radioactive product is a complex mixture of adenylylated protein and a nucleic acid, perhaps polyadenylate.

Some insights into the properties of the system responsible for the adenylylation reaction(s) were obtained from DEAE-cellulose column chromatograhy of unlabeled extracts. Usually, when an extended linear gradient of KCl was used, the elution pattern gave two peaks with RNA polymerase activity (Fig. 4). The ability of each fraction from this column to catalyze the adenylylating reaction was studied. As can be seen, the adenylylating capacity was observed at the level of peak II. However, addition of a portion of the unabsorbed fraction to the assay mixture gave a pattern of activity similar to that of the polymerase activity.

Figure 5 shows a titration curve for adenylylating activity keeping the peak I fraction constant and varying the amount of the unabsorbed ("percolate") fraction, and *vice versa*. In the same figure it can be observed that, whereas the peak I fraction is labile to heat treatment (100°, 5 min), the unabsorbed fraction is stable to this condition.

Some work was carried out in order to characterize the structure of the

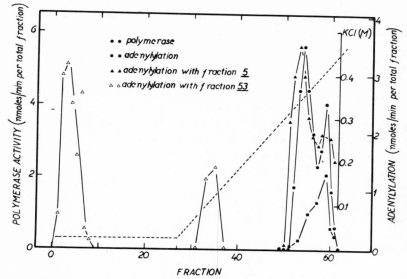

Fig. 4. DEAE-cellulose column chromatography of an E. coli *extract.* The enzyme extract purified to step SI (8) containing 186 mg of protein was diluted in 380 ml of a cold buffer solution containing 10 mM Tris-HCl (pH 8.4), 25 mM KCl, 5 mM mercaptoethanol, 1 mM EDTA, and 15% glycerol (TKMEG). The diluted protein was loaded on a DEAE-cellulose column (12 by 2.9 cm) equilibrated with the TKMEG buffer solution. The column was eluted with a linear KCl gradient (500 ml) from 0.025 to 0.50 M, in the same buffer. RNA polymerase activity (●) was assayed on 0.02 ml aliquots of each fraction. Adenylylating activity (△, □, ▲) was assayed with 0.02 ml aliquots of each fraction. The assay mixture contained 0.0154 mM α-^{32}P-labeled ATP (specific activity 3 μc/nmole), 0.065 mM MgCl$_2$, and enzyme fractions (0.02 or 0.04 ml). The total volume was 0.065 ml. Incubations were carried out for 10 min at 37°. The reaction was stopped by the addition of cold 5% trichloroacetic acid. The precipitates were collected on nitrocellulose filters and counted for radioactivity as previously described (8) ■, 0.02 ml of each fraction plus 0.02 ml TKMEG buffer; ▲, 0.02 ml of each fraction plus 0.02 ml of fraction 5; △, 0.02 ml of each fraction plus 0.02 ml of fraction 53.

active components on this last column chromatography. This characterization was performed by electrophoresis in polyacrylamide gels in the presence of sodium dodecyl sulfate. The result is shown in Fig. 6. Peak I fractions gave a polypeptide composition similar to peak II, but this latter fraction showed two additional bands, with mobilities μ and ω. Since peak II fraction but not peak I fraction was able to adenylylate itself, it seemed of interest to explore the composition of the unabsorbed thermostable fraction. This is shown in Fig. 7. Gel electrophoresis of the thermostable fraction showed only two bands, one of them with the mobility of ω. The latter fraction showed some unexpected

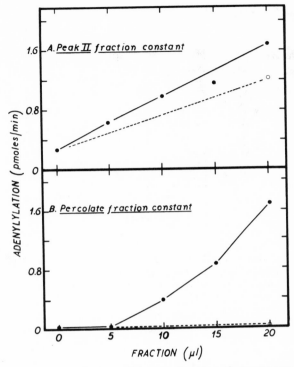

Fig. 5. Adenylylating activity as a function of enzyme concentration. The assay for adenylylating activity was carried out as described in Fig. 5 in the presence of a constant amount (0.02 ml) of fraction 61 (A) or fraction 2 (B), varying that of the other. The open circle indicates the activity of each fraction after treatment for 5 min at 100°.

similarities to the factor required for the activity of polymerase studied by Franze de Fernández *et al.* (13) in the laboratory of Dr. J. T. August. This factor is thermostable, was purified from uninfected cells, and migrates as a single band with a molecular weight of 12,000 when subjected to polyacrylamide gel electrophoresis in the presence of sodium dodecyl sulfate.

SUMMARY

E. coli and *B. subtilis* RNA polymerase exists in two different forms, one less active than the other under standard assay conditions. Conversion of the active to the inactive form requires Mg^{2+}. Covalently bound adenylic residue(s) are contained in the inactive form. Using α-^{32}P-ATP or ^{14}C-ATP as substrate for the polymerase inactivation, the radioactivity

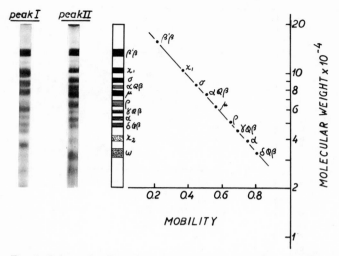

*Fig. 6. Polyacrylamide gel electrophoresis of fractions 53 (peak I)
and 59 (peak II) from the DEAE column chromatography.* The
electrophoreses were carried out using 5.2% gels in the presence of
sodium dodecyl sulfate (12).

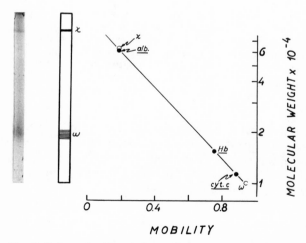

*Fig. 7. Polyacrylamide gel electrophoresis of the unabsorbed
fraction treated for 5 min at 100°.* Electrophoresis was
carried out using a 10.4% gel according to the conditions
described in Fig. 6.

is incorporated into a polypeptide of low molecular weight. When subjected to polyacrylamide gel electrophoresis in the presence of sodium dodecyl sulfate, this polypeptide has a mobility nearly equivalent to that of cytochrome c.

Some evidence indicates that the enzyme(s) responsible for this radioactivity incorporation is tightly bound to the polymerase, whereas the enzyme(s) catalyzing the reverse reaction is loosely associated with polymerase.

Preparations from toluenized cells, catalyzing rifampicin-sensitive RNA synthesis in the presence of the four ribonucleoside triphosphates, are much less active when they are preincubated with ATP-Mg^{2+}.

RESUMEN

La RNA polimerasa de *E. coli* y *B. subtilis* existe en dos formas diferentes, una menos activa que la otra en las condiciones normales de ensayo. La conversión de la forma activa en la inactiva requiere ATP-Mg^{2+}. La transformación inversa requiere sólo Mg^{2+}. La enzima inactiva tiene residuos adenílicos unidos covalentemente. Usando ATP-α-^{32}P ó ATP-^{14}C como sustrato para la inactivación de la polimerasa, la incorporación de la radioactividad tiene lugar en un polipéptido de bajo peso molecular. En electroforesis en gel de poliacrilamida con dodecil sulfato de sodio, la movilidad de este polipéptido es aproximadamente equivalente a la del citocromo c.

Algunas evidencias indican que la(s) enzima(s) responsable de la incorporación de la radioactividad está fuertemente unida a la polimerasa, mientras que la enzima que cataliza la reacción inversa está asociada débilmente con ella.

Las preparaciones de células toluenizadas que catalizan la síntesis de RNA rifampicina-sensible en presencia de los cuatro ribonucleósidos trifosfato, son mucho menos activas cuando se preincuban con ATP-Mg^{2+}.

REFERENCES

1. Burgess, R. R., Travers, A. A., Dunn, J. J., and Bautz, E. K. F., *Nature, 221,* 43 (1969).
2. Emmer, M., Crombrugghe, B., Pastan, I., and Perlman, R., *Proc. Natl. Acad. Sci., U.S.A., 66,* 480 (1970).
3. Travers, A. A., *Nature, 223,* 1107 (1969).
4. Gilbert, W., and Müller-Hill, B., *Proc. Natl. Acad. Sci. U.S.A., 56,* 1891 (1966).
5. Ptashne, M., *Proc. Natl. Acad. Sci. U.S.A., 57,* 306 (1967).
6. Seifert, W., Qasba, P., Walter, G., Palm, P., Schachner, M., and Zilling, W., *Europ. J. Biochem., 9,* 319 (1969).
7. Goff, C. G., and Weber, K., *Cold Spring Harbor Symp. Quant. Biol., 35,* 101 (1970).
8. Chelala, C. A., Hirschbein, L., and Torres, H. N., *Proc. Natl. Acad. Sci. U.S.A., 68,* 152 (1971).
9. Avila, J., Hermoso, J. M., Viñuela, E., and Salas, M., *Europ. J. Biochem. 21,* 526 (1971).
10. Moses, R. E., and Richardson, C. C., *Proc. Natl. Acad. Sci. U.S.A., 67,* 179 (1970).
11. Peterson, R. L., Radcliffe, C. W., and Pace, N. R., *J. Bacteriol., 107,* 585 (1971).
12. Schapiro, A., Viñuela, E., and Maizel, J. V., *Biochem. Biophys. Res. Commun., 28,* 815 (1967).
13. Franze de Fernández, M. T., Hayward, W. S., Shapiro, L., and August, J. T., *J. Biol. Chem., 247,* 824 (1972).

DISCUSSION

H. N. Torres (Buenos Aires, Argentina): Our hypothesis predicts that we have two inter-convertible forms of RNA polymerase, the active form and the inactive form. Equilibrium between the two forms is displaced to the inactive form in the presence of ATP-Mg^{2+} and is displaced to the active form by the action of a divalent cation. Perhaps the effector for the inactivation reaction is ppGpp, and some results indicate that the reactivation reaction requires inorganic phosphate. Our enzyme preparations catalyze the synthesis of RNA in the presence of nucleoside triphosphates, but when UTP, CTP, and CTP are omitted in the incubation mixture, in some conditions these preparations catalyze the synthesis of polya-denylic acid. This latter reaction requires a protein factor with a mobility in polyacrylamide gels equivalent to that of ω. Perhaps ω is involved in the inactivation reaction, and perhaps this ω factor is required for the activity of Qβ polymerase and other similar enzyme activities.

C. Weissmann (Zurich, Switzerland): I did not understand the last slide. What were the two peaks which you were analyzing on gel? I did not understand where they came from.

H. N. Torres: "When an *E. coli* extract is chromatographed in a DEAE-cellulose column and the enzyme is eluted with an extended linear gradient, two peaks of polymerase are obtained: peaks 1 and 2. In polyacrylamide gel electrophoresis, the pattern is almost the same for peak 1 and peak 2, but there are two differences: in peak 2, there are ω and μ; ω is one of the factors responsible for polyadenylate synthesis and μ may be the factor responsible for the deadenylylating reaction.

C. Weissmann: How were the Qβ subunits identified?

H. N. Torres: Qβ subunits were identified by their mobilities in polyacrylamide gels.

C. Weissmann: And what is the material you put on the DEAE column? Is that a relatively crude extract?

H. N. Torres: A very crude extract. It was purified by phase distribution between poly-ethylene glycol and dextran and then directly precipitated with ammonium sulfate and purified by column chromatography.

A. A. Travers (Cambridge, England): I'd like to ask whether you tested the activity of the active and the inactive forms on a variety of DNA templates or only one one.

H. N. Torres: Usually, we use thymus DNA in order to detect polymerase activity, but our assay was performed with the following steps: the first step is the incubation with ATP-Mg^{2+}, the second step is dilution, and the third step is the assay in these conditions—using Mn^{2+} as divalent cation. It is important to emphasize that in order to detect the conversion to the inactive form in the preincubation, Mn^{2+} in the assay must be in limiting amount compared with the concentration of nucleoside triphosphate. The relation between the concentration of nucleoside triphosphate is about 1 for nucleoside triphosphate and 0.5 for Mn^{2+}. When Mn^{2+} is increased over the concentration of nucleoside triphosphate, there is an effect: all the inactive enzyme is converted to the active enzyme. The effect was observed with thymus DNA, with *E. coli* DNA, with *B. subtilis* DNA, with ϕ29 DNA, and with DNA from T4 phage. With all these templates, inactivation was observed.

6

Visualization of Genetic Transcription

Barbara A. Hamkalo and O. L. Miller, Jr.

Biology Division
Oak Ridge National Laboratory
Oak Ridge, Tennessee, U.S.A.

Transcription of structural genes by RNA polymerase to produce messenger RNAs (mRNAs) and the translation of such messengers by polyribosomes to produce proteins are intimately coupled processes in bacterial cells (1). In fact, it is possible to reconstruct coupled transcription and translation systems *in vitro* from separated bacterial components (2,3). Using techniques developed by Miller and Beatty (4) to prepare the nuclear contents of amphibian oocytes for electron microscopy, we can now directly visualize genetically active bacterial chromosomes. In these studies, we have identified both structural genes and ribosomal RNA (rRNA) genes (5,6).

TECHNIQUE

Bacterial cultures in log phase are rendered osmotically sensitive by a brief treatment with T4 lysozyme in the presence of sucrose at $4°$. The protoplasts are then osmotically shocked by rapid dilution into distilled water, and a sample of burst cells is deposited onto a carbon-coated electron microscope grid by low-speed centrifugation. Preparations are stained with phosphotungstic acid (PTA) under conditions that stain net positive groups of proteins (7). Therefore, all the structures observed have protein associated with them.

STRUCTURAL GENES

At low magnification, the extruded contents of a shocked bacterial cell

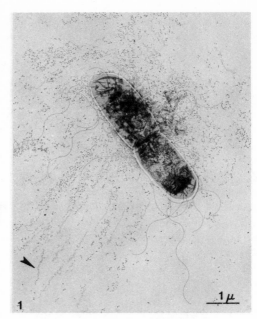

*Fig. 1. Low magnification of the extruded con-
tents of an osmotically shocked* Salmonella ty-
phimurium *cell from a log phase, broth-grown culture.* The arrow designates one of the 19 rRNA loci
in the field.

appear as a network of deoxyribonuclease-digestible fibers with attached ribo-
nuclease-sensitive polyribosomes (Fig. 1). The fibers are stained with PTA and
measure approximately 40 Å in diameter, twice the diameter of duplex DNA.
Thus the bacterial chromosome appears to be uniformly coated with protein.
The protein may become associated with the DNA during isolation, or the DNA
may in fact exist as a deoxyribonucleoprotein complex in the cell, as suggested
by the experiments of Zubay and Watson (8). In Chapter 3 of this volume,
August *et al.* (9) describes the isolation of several classes of histone-like proteins
that could associate with the bacterial chromosome.

Figures 2 and 3 show relatively long regions of the genome exhibiting
short-to-long polyribosome gradients. Since the length of genetically active DNA
in both figures is sufficient to code for several proteins,* we conclude that these
active segments are operons exhibiting intimately coupled transcription and
translation. The absence of free polyribosomes on grids or in the supernatant

---

* Lactose operon (three genes), approximately 1.4 μ; tryptophan operon (five genes),
approximately 2.3 μ.

fraction after centrifugation and the presence of short polyribosomes distal to the longest polyribosome of a gradient (Fig. 3) strongly suggest that mRNAs are degraded while attached to the DNA. There is biochemical evidence (10-12) substantiating the degradation of bacterial messengers from the $5'$-PO_4 to the $3'$-OH end, as would be required in this case.

Polyribosomes on active loci typically are unequally spaced, possibly because the initiation of transcription is aperiodic. If initiation were periodic, however, polyribosomes could become irregularly spaced during transcription, provided that individual polymerases transcribe at different rates.

A comparison of the number of ribosomes within a polyribosome with its relative distance from the initiation site of the locus permits an estimate of the average length of mRNA associated with a ribosome. This estimate takes into consideration the fact that, when transcribed, 1 μ of duplex DNA in the B conformation gives rise to a single-stranded RNA molecule which, if fully extended, would measure 2 μ. Based on several measurements, approximately 1000-1500 Å (150-200 nucleotides) of messenger is associated with each ribosome. Since the diameter of a ribosome would protect only about one twentieth of this amount of extended mRNA, the messenger must be rather extensively coiled in the normal polyribosome configuration. In fact, we have measured lengths of mRNA up to 2000 Å between adjacent ribosomes within polyribosomes that have been stretched during preparation.

In unstretched polyribosomes, the first ribosome attached to the mRNA

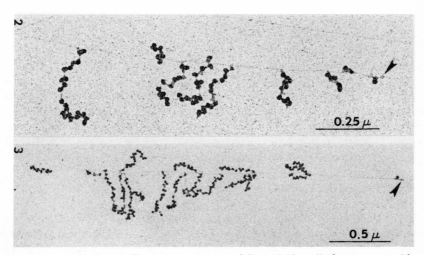

Figs. 2 and 3. Genetically active segments of Escherichia coli *chromosome with attached polyribosomes.* The arrows indicate RNA polymerase molecules on or very near the initiation sites for transcription.

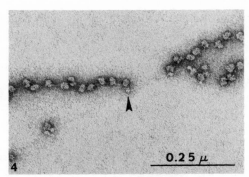

Fig. 4. Negatively stained (uranyl acetate) portion of E. coli genome showing polyribosomes
attached to chromosome by RNA polymerase
molecules (arrow).

typically is closely apposed to the bacterial chromosome. However, when polyribosomes are slightly stretched during preparation, a granule about 80 Å in
diameter can be seen at each site of polyribosome attachment to the genome
(Figs. 2 and 3). These granules undoubtedly are RNA polymerases that were
actively transcribing at the time of isolation. Figure 4 shows, at higher magnification, a portion of a negatively stained preparation. The RNA polymerases can
be seen as lightly stained granules smaller than individual ribosomes. In some
cases, the individual 30S and 50S subunits of a single ribosome can be resolved.
The mRNA strand is seen associated primarily with the 30S subunits, in
agreement with biochemical data (13).

Granules about the same size as active RNA polymerases also are bound to
genetically "silent" regions of the genome, as defined by the absence of polyribosomes. This suggests that RNA polymerases are associated with inactive
portions of the genome, awaiting the proper initiation signals. Although only
qualitative estimates can be made from micrographs of burst cells, it appears that
a relatively small percentage of the bacterial chromosome is active at any one
instant. This observation is in agreement with a similar conclusion by Kennel
(14), based on DNA-RNA hybridization with *Escherichia coli* nucleic acids.

RIBOSOMAL RNA GENES

Hybridization data indicate that bacterial rRNA genes reside in DNA segments containing three contiguous cistrons: 16S-23S-5S (15). There are about
six such segments per *E. coli* chromosome (16), and it has been calculated
(17,18) that under optimal growth conditions 80-90 RNA polymerases must
simultaneously transcribe each region in order to meet cellular requirements for

ribosomes. The molecular weights of the three rRNA molecules are 16S, 0.55×10^6; 23S, 1.1×10^6; and 5S, 0.04×10^6 daltons (19,20). Since 1 μ of duplex DNA codes for a 1×10^6 dalton single-stranded polyribonucleotide, the length of B-conformation DNA required to accomodate the three cistrons is approximately 1.7 μ. These considerations can be used to predict the structure of active rRNA genes—i.e., chromosomal segments approximately 1.7 μ long, which under optimal growth conditions are transcribed simultaneously by a large number of closely spaced RNA polymerases and which can be distinguished from structural genes by attached ribonucleoprotein (RNP) fibrils rather than polyribosomes.

The extruded contents of the burst cell shown in Fig. 1 exhibit a number of such regions. Positive identification of these regions as rRNA genes rests on the use of a temperature-sensitive mutant of *E. coli* isolated and characterized by A. G. Atherly (unpublished data). At the permissive temperature, the mutant synthesizes normal amounts of rRNA; however, after a shift to the nonpermissive temperature, no rRNA synthesis can be detected biochemically. The rRNA loci in preparations of mutant cultures grown at $30°$ are normal in appearance, but at $42°$ no rRNA segments are visible, although structural gene activity appears to be normal.

Figure 5A shows a single rRNA segment. The length of such regions is about

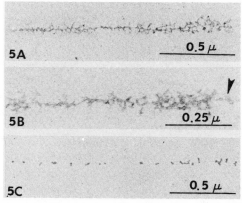

Fig. 5. rRNA loci. (A) An rRNA locus showing activity of 16S (short fibril gradient) and 23S (longer gradient) in log phase, broth-grown *E. coli.* (B) An rRNA locus showing RNA polymerases (arrow) distal to the 23S cistron in *E. coli.* Linkage data indicate that this site may be the location of the 5S rRNA cistron. (C) Activity of an rRNA locus from *E. coli* grown under suboptimal conditions (synthetic medium with glycerol and 0.05% Casamino acids).

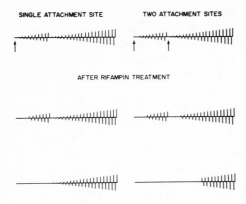

Fig. 6. Schematic representation of rifampin readouts of rRNA cistrons based on one and on two RNA polymerase binding sites per 16S-23S doublet.

1.3 μ, shorter than the DNA length expected from the combined molecular weights of the products. A large number of RNA polymerases transcribing adjacent to one another might foreshorten the DNA relative to its B-conformation length, because of extensive local denaturation at each polymerase site.

Each rRNA segment is composed of 60-70 RNP fibrils, which form two contiguous short-to-long fibril gradients. The first gradient is half as long as the second, in agreement with expectations based on the molecular weight differences between the 16S and 23S rRNAs. A few polymerases are sometimes seen (Fig. 5B) beyond the 23S gradient; biochemical data suggest that these regions could be active 5S rRNA cistrons (15).

When cellular growth rate is reduced, the rRNA segments become increasingly difficult to visualize, because the number of RNP fibrils decreases (Fig 5C). If one assumes that all polymerases travel at approximately the same speed, the initiation of transcription of these genes must be aperiodic, since the fibrils on these loci are unevenly spaced.

The fact that the rRNA segments are composed of two fibril gradients (Fig. 5A) suggests the occurrence of two RNA polymerase initiation sites per region but does not exclude the existence of only one initiation site. Rifampin, a drug that inhibits initiation but not elongation by RNA polymerase (21), can be used to distinguish between these two alternatives. Figure 6 schematically depicts the configuration of rRNA genes after addition of the drug, based on one and on two polymerase binding sites. With appropriate sampling times, it can be seen that the 16S fibril gradient disappears first, and only then does the 23S gradient begin to disappear. In Figure 7, a complete 23S cistron is evident, although the entire 16S cistron has been cleared of fibrils. Thus there is a single initiation site for the transcription of the linked rRNA cistrons. These observations agree with data based on the relative amounts of labeled uridine in the two rRNA molecules after addition of rifamycin (22) and the appearance of label first in the 16S

Fig. 7. An E. coli rRNA locus 40 sec after
rifampin (200 μg/ml) treatment. The 16S cistron
is essentially cleared, whereas the 23S cistron
shows a normal complement of fibrils.

rRNA when amino acid starved cells synthesizing no rRNA (under stringent
RNA synthesis control) are supplied with the required amino acid (23).

The relative physical location of bacterial rRNA segments on the chromosome is unclear. Data of Yu *et al.* (24) suggest that all regions are virtually
contiguous, while Birnbaum and Kaplan (25) localize only half of the genes in a
region about 30 μ long, and Spadari and Ritossa (26) conclude that there is some
nonribosomal DNA between bacterial rRNA segments. Figure 8 illustrates a

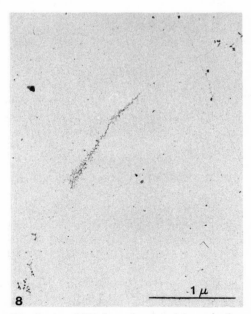

Fig. 8. An rRNA locus bracketed by polyribosomes attached to active structural genes in E.
coli.

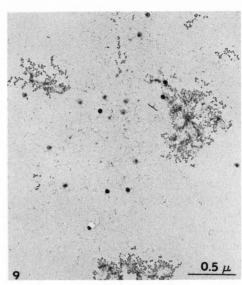

Fig. 9. Extruded contents from an E. coli *cell infected with bacteriophage T7,* with rifampin (200 μg/ml) added 2 min after infection to inhibit bacterial RNA polymerase. The preparation was made 8 min after infection at 37°, lysis occurs at 12 min.

single rRNA region bracketed by structural gene activity. Similar regions over 10 μ long have been seen, an observation which excludes the possibility that bacterial rRNA genes are closely adjacent, as are rRNA genes of most eukaryotic cells.

BACTERIOPHAGE TRANSCRIPTION AND TRANSLATION

Biochemical studies of the genetic activity of *E. coli* cells infected with bacteriophage T7 suggest that it should be relatively simple to identify active viral genomes. First, host transcription ceases after infection, due to a viral function (27); second, the phage-induced RNA polymerase, unlike the host enzyme, is totally insensitive to inhibition by rifamycin and its derivatives, such as rifampin (28). Therefore, any transcription occurring early in the infection cycle in the presence of the drug, and all transcription later in the cycle, must be directed by the viral enzyme.

Preliminary observations indicate that our isolation procedures do permit visualization of phage genetic activity and maturation. Figure 9 shows the extruded contents of a cell late in the infection cycle. Large quantities of genetically silent DNA, with phage-sized particles in the midst of this DNA, are visible. The densely stained particles are mature phage, and the paler particles most probably are phage heads being filled with DNA. Unlike the extruded contents of uninfected cells, nearly all polyribosomes in these preparations appear to be associated with membrane fragments. Although no direct attachment between membrane and polyribosomes has been seen, there are several possible explanations for such a configuration: (1) the polyribosomes of infected cells associate with the membrane artifactually, during isolation; (2) the phage DNA, a molecule only 12 μ long, is attached to the bacterial membrane, and consequently structures associated with the viral DNA are found in close proximity to the membrane; or (3) T7 mRNAs are translated on membrane-associated polyribosomes. No evidence that favors any of these possibilities is available at present. However, this unique prokaryotic polyribosome configuration may be relevant to the long half-life (approximately 20 min) of T7 mRNAs (29), at the same time that at least some host messengers decay with their normal half-lives (approximately 3 min) (30).

CHLOROPLAST GENETIC ACTIVITY

Based on the differences in drug sensitivities between the RNA- and protein-synthesizing systems of chloroplasts and the corresponding nuclear and cytoplasmic systems (31,32), as well as the size of chloroplast rRNAs and ribosomes (33), it has been suggested that genetic activity in these organelles is prokaryotic in nature—i.e., transcription and translation are closely coupled. Opposing evidence, however, is also available (34). Figure 10 shows the contents extruded from a *Euglena gracilis* chloroplast by osmotic shock. The extruded fibers are portions of the chloroplast genome, and structures closely resembling polyribosomes appear to be attached to the genome. Although preliminary in

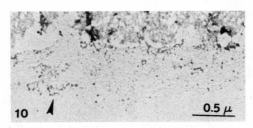

Fig. 10. Portion of an osmotically shocked chloroplast, showing extruded genome with associated structures resembling polyribosomes (arrow) in Euglena gracilis.

nature, these observations are direct visual support for the suggestion that transcription and translation are coupled in this system.

CONCLUSIONS

Development of rapid and simple preparative techniques has made it possible to visualize directly the structure of active genes in both eukaryotic and prokaryotic chromosomes (5). The vast amount of indirect data that have been accumulated in biochemical and genetic studies of prokaryotic chromosomes provides a background of information that can be complemented by observations of the structure of active loci, in order to analyze problems of the coordination and control of transcription and translation under different growth conditions or in strains which harbor mutations altering the coupling between these processes (e.g., polar mutants). With this multidisciplinary approach, the mechanism of action of drugs affecting transcription and translation can also be elucidated.

Finally, refinement of our preparative methods should allow visualization of the mechanism of integration of viral DNA into the bacterial genome. Such a study in the simple microbial system may provide guidelines that will be helpful in the visualization of the structural aspects of the integration of viral nucleic acid into human chromosomes.

ACKNOWLEDGMENTS

This research was sponsored by the U.S. Atomic Energy Commission under contract with the Union Carbide Corporation.

SUMMARY

Electron microscopic observations of the extruded contents of osmotically shocked bacterial cultures permit the direct study of microbial genetic activity. The bacterial chromosome, approximately 40 Å in diameter, is stained by a protein-specific stain, suggesting that the genome is a deoxyribonucleoprotein complex. Transcription-translation complexes at sites of structural gene activity are seen as irregularly spaced chains of polyribosomes attached to the bacterial genome by RNA polymerase molecules. Putative RNA polymerases, granules approximately 80 Å in diameter, appear to be bound also to genetically "silent" regions of the genome.

Bacterial ribosomal RNA genes are identified as segments of the chromosome about 1.3 μ in length, with ribonucleoprotein fibrils rather than polyribosomes attached. Under rapid growth conditions, these ribonucleoprotein fibrils are closely spaced and number 60-80 per region. Although the ribonucleoprotein fibrils form two contiguous gradients, corresponding to the 16S and 23S ribosomal RNA cistrons, respectively, there is a single initiation site for the transcription of these two linked cistrons. There are several 16S-23S doublets per bacterial chromosome; however, unlike eukaryotic ribosomal RNA genes, these regions are separated by chromosomal segments that contain structural genes.

RESUMEN

Las observaciones de microscopía electrónica del contenido extraído de cultivos de bacterias tratadas con choque smótico, permiten el estudio directo de la actividad génica microbiana. El cromosoma bacteriano tiene un diámetro de aproximadamente 40 Å y es teñido por un reactivo específico para proteínas, lo que sugiere que el genoma es un complejo de desoxiribonucleoproteína. Los complejos de transcripción-traducción en los sitios de actividad de genes estructurales se ven como cadenas de poliribosomas espaciados en forma irregular, unidos al genoma por moléculas de RNA polimerasa. RNA polimerasas putativas, gránulos de aproximadamente 80 Å de diámetro, aparecen unidos también a regiones del genoma genéticamente "silenciosas."

Los genes del RNA ribosómico bacteriano se identifican como segmentos de una longitud aproximada de 1.3 μ, a los que están unidas fibrillas de ribonucleoproteína en vez de poliribosomas. En condiciones de crecimiento rápido, estas fibrillas de ribonucleoproteína están distribuidas muy cerca las unas de las otras, de 60 a 80 por región. Aún cuando las fibrillas de ribonucleoproteína forman dos gradientes contiguos, que respectivamente corresponden a los cistrones 16S y 23S del RNA ribosójico, existe un solo sitio para la iniciación de la transcripción de estos dos cistrones eslabonados. Hay varios dobletes de 16S y 23S por cromosoma bacteriano, pero diferente de los genes del RNA ribosomal eucariótico; estas regiones están separadas por segmentos de cromosoma que contienen genes estructurales.

REFERENCES

1. Stent, G. S., *Science, 144,* 816 (1964).
2. Byrne, R., Levin, G., Bladen, H. A., and Nirenberg, M. W., *Proc. Natl. Acad. Sci. U.S.A., 52,* 140 (1964).
3. Zubay, G., and Chambers, D. A., *Cold Spring Harbor Symp. Quant. Biol., 34,* 753 (1969).
4. Miller, O. L., Jr., and Beatty, B. R., *Science, 164,* 955 (1969).
5. Miller, O. L., Jr., Hamkalo, B. A., and Thomas, C. A., Jr., *Science, 169,* 392 (1970).
6. Miller, O. L., Jr., Beatty, B. R., Hamkalo, B. A., and Thomas, C. A., Jr., *Cold Spring Harbor Symp. Quant. Biol., 35,* 505 (1970).
7. Silverman, L., and Glick, D., *J. Cell. Biol., 40,* 761 (1969).
8. Zubay, G., and Watson, M. R., *J. Biophys. Biochem. Cytol., 5,* 51 (1959).
9. August, J. T., Eoyang, L., Franze de Fernández, M. T., Hayward, W. S., Kuo, C. H., and Silverman, P. M., this symposium.
10. Kuwano, M., Kwan, C. N., Apirion, D., and Schlessinger, D., *Lepetit Colloq. Biol. Med., 1,* 222 (1969).
11. Morikawa, N., and Imamoto, F., *Nature, 223,* 37 (1969).
12. Morse, D., Mosteller, R., Baker, R., and Yanofsky, C., *Nature, 223,* 40 (1969).
13. Moore, P., *J. Mol. Biol., 22,* 145 (1966).
14. Kennel, D., *J. Mol. Biol., 34,* 85 (1968).
15. Doolittle, W. F., and Pace, N. R., *Proc. Natl. Acad. Sci. U.S.A., 68,* 1786 (1971).
16. Purdom, I., Bishop, J. O., and Birnstiel, M. L., *Nature, 227,* 239 (1970).
17. Bremer, H., and Yuan, D., *J. Mol. Biol., 38,* 163 (1968).
18. Manor, H., Goodman, D., and Stent, G. S., *J. Mol. Biol., 39,* (1969).
19. Kurland, C. G., *J. Mol. Biol., 2,* 83 (1960).
20. Smith, I., Dubnau, D., Morell, P., and Marmur, J., *J. Mol. Biol., 33,* 123 (1968).
21. Lill, H., Lill, U., Sippel, A., and Hartmann, G., *Lepetit Colloq. Biol. Med., 1,* 55 (1969).

22. Pato, M., and von Meyenburg, K., *Cold Spring Harbor Symp. Quant. Biol., 35,* 497 (1970).
23. Kossman, C. R., Stamato, T. D., and Pettijohn, D. E., *Nature New Biol., 234,* 102 (1971).
24. Yu, M. T., Vermeulen, C. W., and Atwood, K. C., *Proc. Natl. Acad. Sci. U.S.A., 67,* 26 (1970).
25. Birnbaum, L. S., and Kaplan, S., *Proc. Natl. Acad. Sci. U.S.A., 68,* 925 (1971).
26. Spadari, S., and Ritossa, F., in *Proceedings of the 7th FEBS Symposium, 23,* 337 (1972).
27. Summers, W. C., and Siegel, R. B., *Cold Spring Harbor Symp. Quant. Biol., 35,* 253 (1970).
28. Chamberlin, M., McGrath, J. M., and Waskell, L., *Nature, 228,* 227 (1970).
29. Summers, W. C., *J. Mol. Biol., 51,* 671 (1970).
30. Marrs, B. L., and Yanofsky, C., *Nature New Biol., 234,* 168 (1971).
31. Hawley, E. S., and Greenawalt, J. W., *J. Biol. Chem., 245,* 3573 (1970).
32. Ellis, R. J., and Hartley, M. R., *Nature New Biol., 233,* 193 (1971).
33. Ashwell, M., and Work, T. S., *Ann. Rev. Biochem., 39,* 251 (1970).
34. Summers, D. F., Maizel, J. V., and Darnell, J. E., *Proc. Natl. Acad. Sci. U.S.A., 54,* 505 (1965).

DISCUSSION

F. L. Sacerdote (Mendoza, Argentina): I would like to ask Dr. Hamkalo how she prepared her grids. Did you coat them with something?

B. A. Hamkalo (Oak Ridge, U.S.A.): Yes, the grids (300 or 400 mesh) have a coating of either carbon alone or plastic (parlodion or formvar) and carbon; carbon alone gives the best preparations, because it's the thinnest film and contrast is maximal.

C. Vasquez (Buenos Aires, Argentina): Was the material fixed?

B. A. Hamkalo: Yes, material is centrifuged onto the grid through a formalin solution; therefore, fixation occurs at this step.

7

Structural and Functional Studies on Mammalian Nuclear DNA-Dependent RNA Polymerases

P. Chambon, M. Meilhac, S. Walter, C. Kedinger, J. L. Mandel, and F. Gissinger

Institut de Chimie Biologique
and
Centre de Neurochimie du CNRS
Faculté de Médecine
Strasbourg, France

Although DNA-dependent RNA polymerase was first identified in rat liver nuclei (1), this enzyme has only recently been solubilized and purified from eukaryotic cells, due to difficulties in separating the enzyme from nuclear chromatin, the relatively small amounts of enzyme in animal cells, and its marked instability when separated from chromatin. One of the most interesting findings was the existence of multiple nuclear DNA-dependent RNA polymerases [for references, see (2)], which suggested that gene expression in animal cells could be regulated, at least in part, by distinct RNA polymerases with different template specificities. Three lines of evidence supported the existence of multiple RNA polymerases. Several peaks of enzyme activity were obtained by chromatography on substituted cellulose columns (3,4,7), and these activities appeared to have distinctive intranuclear localizations (4-6). Furthermore, two classes of enzyme were distinguished, according to the inhibitory effect of a-amanitin (7,15), a toxin of the toadstool *Amanita phalloïdes*. More recently, complete purification

Table I. Proposed Terminology for the Various Animal RNA Polymerases

Class of enzyme	Proposed terminology	Large subunits	Localization	Other terminology
A (insensitive to amanitin)	Enzyme AI	A1, A2	Nucleolar (3-6)	Enzyme Ia (3,4)
	Enzyme AII	?	Nucleolar	Enzyme Ib (3,4)
	Enzyme AIII	?	Nucleoplasmic (6)	Enzyme III (3)
B (sensitive to amanitin)	Enzyme BI	B1, B3	Nucleoplasmic (5,6)	Enzyme II (3)
	Enzyme BII	B2, B3	Nucleoplasmic	Enzyme II (3)

and structural analysis of some of the RNA polymerase activities have firmly established the multiplicity of RNA polymerases in animal tissues (8,9). This led us to propose a terminology for animal DNA-dependent RNA polymerase based both on the inhibitory effect of amanitin and the subunit structure of the enzyme (8) (Table I).

In this paper, we first report our recent studies on the subunit structure of the three DNA-dependent RNA polymerases that we have purified from calf thymus and then discuss some of our results which suggest that these enzymes have different template specificities.

STRUCTURE OF RNA POLYMERASES AI, BI, AND BII FROM CALF THYMUS

Enzymes AI, BI, and BII from calf thymus were purified by modifications of methods outlined previously (8,10) which will be reported in detail elsewhere. The specific activities of the purified enzymes were 200-400 units per milligram of protein when assayed under optimum conditions (8,10). One unit corresponds to the incorporation of 1 nmole of ^{32}P-GMP in 10 min at 37°. Figure 1 shows that each enzyme moves essentially as a single band when electrophoresed on polyacrylamide gels under nondenaturing conditions, enzyme BII being still lightly contaminated by traces of enzyme BI. Since the molecular weight of the three enzymes is in the range of 500,000, their different behaviors during electrophoresis are mainly related to charge differences. The subunit composition of enzymes AI, BI, and BII was investigated by polyacrylamide gel electrophoresis in the presence of sodium dodecyl sulfate (SDS) (8). Mixed gels, 5 and 10% in the upper and the lower part, respectively, were used in order to resolve both the high and the low molecular weight subunits. Figure 2 shows that enzyme AI contains two high molecular weight (A1 and A2) and several low molecular weight subunits. (A3, A4, A5, and A6). Enzyme BI contains two high molecular weight (B1 and B3) and at least three low molecular weight subunits (B4, B5, and B6). Enzyme BII possesses two high molecular weight (B2 and B3) and also at least three low molecular weight subunits (B4, B5, and B6). The molecular weights of these subunits were estimated by electrophoresis in the presence of SDS in 4% polyacrylamide gels (high molecular weight components) or 10% gels (low molecular weight components) (11,12). Table II summarizes our results, giving the probable stoichiometries of the various subunits. These values were obtained by densitometry of the various bands after staining of the mixed SDS gels. Similar values were obtained using either Coomassie Blue or Amido Black, indicating that the proposed stoichiometries do not reflect a preferential binding of the dye to some of the subunits. We also verified that under our conditions the areas of the peaks were proportional to protein concentration. The values for the stoichiometry of the small subunits should nevertheless be considered as tentative, when compared to the stoichiometry of the large subunits, since the standard error is very large when measuring by densitometry the stoichiometry of polypeptide chains whose molecular weights differ by an order of magnitude.

Our results demonstrate very clearly that enzyme AI is quite different from enzymes BI and BII. They firmly establish, on structural grounds, the multiplicity of nuclear RNA polymerases. It is interesting that subunits A5 and A6 appear

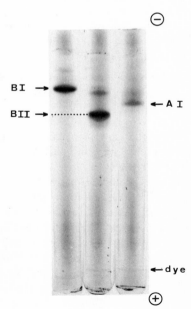

Fig. 1. Polyacrylamide gel electrophoresis under nondenaturing conditions of purified calf thymus RNA polymerases AI, BI, and BII. About 0.8 unit of each enzyme was run and stained with Coomassie Blue as previously described (8). Enzyme AI has a marked tendency to aggregate during electrophoresis under these conditions.

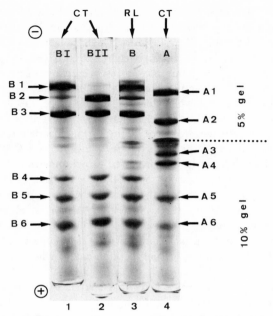

Fig. 2. Subunit pattern of calf thymus RNA polymerase AI (gel 4), BI (gel 1), and BII (gel 2) and of a mixture of purified rat liver B enzymes (gel 3). About 2.5 units of each enzyme was denatured, and SDS-polyacrylamide gel electrophoresis was carried out as previously described (8) using mixed gels (5 and 10% in the upper and the lower parts of gel, respectively). Gels were stained with Coomassie Blue for 24 hr and destained by repeated washing at 37°.

to have the same molecular weight as subunits B5 and B6, respectively. Whether these subunits are in fact identical remains to be seen, since charge differences are not revealed by polyacrylamide gel electrophoresis in the presence of SDS. Enzymes BI and BII seem closely related, since they have the same affinity for α-amanitin (8) and four of their subunits (B3, B4, B5, and B6) are similar, at least with respect to molecular weight. Possible charge differences are currently under investigation. It is not known whether subunits B1 and B2 are completely different or if B2 is derived from B1 by specific proteolytic cleavage, which may occur either *in vivo* or *in vitro* during the first steps of the purification (Rutter, personal communication). Further studies are presently under way in our laboratory to ascertain whether enzymes BI and BII are both present *in vivo* or if enzyme BII is an *in vitro* artifact.

Table II. Molecular Weight (Mol wt) and Stoichiometry (S) of the Various Subunits of Calf Thymus RNA Polymerases AI, BI, and BII[a]

	Enzyme AI			Enzyme BI			Enzyme BII		
Subunit	Mol wt ± 5%	S	Subunit	Mol wt ± 5%	S	Subunit	Mol wt ± 5%	S
A1	197,000	1	B1	214,000	1	B2	180,000	1
A2	126,000	1	B3	140,000	1	B3	140,000	1
A3	51,000	1	B4	34,000	1-2	B4	34,000	1-2
A4	44,000	1	B5	25,000	2	B5	25,000	2
A5	25,000	2	B6	16,500	3-4	B6	16,500	3-4
A6	16,500	2						

a The molecular weights were determined by electrophoresis in SDS-polyacrylamide gel as described in the text and in refs. 11 and 12. The marker proteins were rabbit myosin (mol wt 220,000), human γ-globulin (mol wt 160,000) (run without reduction by 2-mercaptoethanol), E. coli β-galactosidase (mol wt 130,000), phosphorylase a (mol wt 94,000), ovalbumin dimer (mol wt 90,000), ovalbumin monomer (mol wt 45,000), bovine pepsin (mol wt 35,000), bovine chymotrypsinogen A (mol wt 25,700), sperm whale myoglobin (mol wt 17,200), horse heart cytochrome c (mol wt 12,400), and chymotrypsin C chain (mol wt 10,150). Under our conditions, using these markers, we found the molecular weights of the β', β, σ, and α subunits of E. coli RNA polymerase to be 163,000, 153,000, 94,000, and 39,000. These values are close to those determined by Burgess (22).

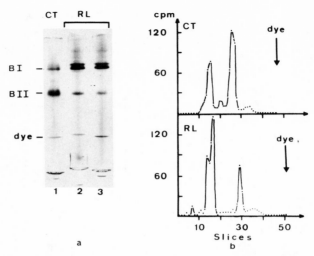

Fig. 3. Electrophoreses. (a) Comparison by nondenaturing polyacrylamide gel electrophoresis of the components of purified rat
liver RNA polymerase B activity (RL) (gels 2 and 3) and RNA
polymerases BI and BII of calf thymus (CT) (gel 1). [Repro-
duced from *FEBS Letters, 15,* 175 (1971).] (b) In parallel
electrophoresis, RL and CT enzyme B activities were run after
incubation in the presence of [14] C-methyl γ-amanitin. The gels
were sliced immediately after the electrophoresis, and the slices
(1 mm width) were counted in a scintillation counter. [Repro-
duced from *FEBS Letters, 15,* 175 (1971).]

COMPARISON OF B ENZYMES FROM CALF THYMUS AND RAT LIVER

Tissue specificity of at least some of the DNA-dependent RNA polymerases
could be one of the mechanisms involved in differentiation. For instance, one
enzyme could be specific for a given tissue in order to transcribe the genes which
are specifically expressed in that tissue. For technical convenience we decided,
as a first attempt, to explore this possibility by comparing components of RNA
polymerase B activity from calf thymus and rat liver (9). Nondenaturing polyacrylamide gel electrophoresis of purified rat liver B activity (Fig. 3a) revealed
that two components similar to calf thymus BI and BII enzymes were also
present in rat liver. This similarity was confirmed by subunit analysis of a
mixture of purified rat liver B enzymes, where polypeptide chains corresponding
to calf thymus subunits B1, B2, B3, B4, B5, and B6 (Fig. 2, gel 3) were
observed. The identity of the two rat liver components with calf thymus
enzymes BI and BII was also confirmed by the migration of labeled amanitin

with the two bands (Fig. 3b). It is interesting that the ratio of enzyme BI to enzyme BII is much higher in rat liver than in calf thymus. A similar ratio was also reported by Chesterton and Butterworth (13) for the liver B activities. Whether this difference is a characteristic of the tissues (or of the animals) or is due to artifacts occurring during the purification remains to be seen. The presence of a third band which follows enzyme BI during electrophoresis of purified rat liver B activity (Fig. 3a) is noteworthy, since labeled amanitin was also associated with this band (Fig. 3b). This suggests that rat liver could contain a B-type enzyme not found in calf thymus.

EVIDENCE THAT CALF THYMUS RNA POLYMERASE RECOGNIZES SPECIFIC INITIATION SITES

Neither enzyme AI nor B enzymes were able to initiate RNA synthesis on T4 and λ phage DNAs (10,14). These results suggested either that an initiation factor analogous to the bacterial σ factor was lost during the purification of enzymes A and B or that the lack of recognition of the initiation signals present in phage DNAs is an intrinsic property of the animal enzymes, which thus could have an active role in the control of transcription by recognizing only specific initiation signals. The most direct way to support this latter hypothesis would be to demonstrate that the various enzymes transcribe specifically different parts of the chromosomal DNA. Such experiments cannot be carried out at present for several reasons. Most purified animal DNAs contain a substantial number of nicks where RNA synthesis could be initiated unspecifically (10,16). For most RNAs, comparison of the *in vitro* products with the *in vivo* RNAs is not possible, since, in most cases, pure RNA species cannot be isolated. Moreover, DNA-RNA hybridization methods are inadequate to detect unique species of RNA due to the high complexity of the animal genome. In the only case where the *in vivo* product is easily available, i.e., ribosomal RNA, the corresponding genes cannot be readily isolated from chromosomal DNA. Where they have been isolated, their transcription did not exhibit any specificity with respect to the origin of the enzyme (17).

The discovery that some semisynthetic derivatives of rifamycin are inhibitors of the initiation but not of the elongation of RNA synthesis catalyzed by animal RNA polymerases (18) enabled us to show that the animal enzymes could play an active role in the control of the transcription by recognizing specific initiation sites on the chromosomal DNA. Previous studies on *Escherichia coli* RNA polymerase have shown that preincubation of enzyme and phage DNAs resulted in rifampicin resistance of RNA synthesis when the antibiotic was added together with the nucleoside triphosphates after the preincubation period (19,20). The appearance of this rifampicin resistance required the σ factor and was time and temperature dependent, suggesting that a local melting of the double helix was required for rifampicin-resistant RNA synthesis (19,20). Moreover, Bautz and Bautz (20) showed that only a very limited number of sites on phage DNAs can confer rifampicin resistance. This observation suggested that these sites could correspond to the true promoter sites (20).

Results presented in Table III show that, at least in the case of the B enzymes, preincubation of enzyme and calf thymus DNA for 10 min at 37° makes RNA synthesis almost completely resistant to the semisynthetic derivative of rifamycin AF/013. The amount of RNA synthesis was indeed similar whether AF/013 was added together with the nucleoside triphosphates or 15 sec after the

Table III. Resistance of RNA Synthesis to AF/013 After Preincubation of Enzyme and DNA at 37° or 0° [a]

Conditions of preincubation and incubation	Incorporation of ^{32}P-GMP, 10 min at 37° (pmoles)				
	Enzyme AI AF/013	Enzyme BI AF/013	Enzyme BII AF/013	E. coli holoenzyme	
				AF/013	Rif
Enzyme + DNA 10 min 37°, then NTP + DMF	31.5	42.2	31.9	320	320
Enzyme + DNA 10 min 37°, then NTP, AF/013 or Rif 15 sec after NTP	4.5	18.6	15.6	190	203
Enzyme + DNA 10 min 37°, then NTP + AF/013 or Rif	4.0	15.9	11.8	145	144
Enzyme + DNA 10 min 0°, then NTP + AF/013 or Rif	5.0	2.3	2.1	14.0	10.2
Enzyme + DNA + AF/013 or Rif 10 min 37°, then NTP	0	0	0	0	0

[a] Preincubation (0.18 ml) and incubation (0.25 ml) mixtures contained 80 mM Tris-HCl (pH 7.9), 3 mM Mn^{2+}, 50 mM ammonium sulfate, bovine serum albumin (200 μg/ml), 0.1 mM dithiothreitol, 4 mM thioglycerol, and 12% glycerol (final concentrations). In addition, the preincubation medium contained 0.625 μg calf thymus (CT) DNA and 0.5 μg purified enzyme in the case of enzymes BI and BII, 5 μg CT DNA and 0.5 μg purified enzyme in the case of enzyme AI, and 1.25 μg CT DNA and 1.5 μg purified enzyme (21) in the case of E. coli holoenzyme. After the preincubation period, nucleoside triphosphates (NTP) were added at a concentration of 1 mM (one NTP was labeled with ^{32}P). Where indicated, AF/013 (50 μg) or rifamicin (Rif, 10 μg) was added together with or 15 sec after the NTP. The assay tubes were incubated at 37° for 10 min, and RNA synthesis was stopped by addition of cold TCA. Since AF/013 and Rif were solubilized in 10 μl of dimethylformamide (DMF), 10 μl DMF was added to control incubations. AF/013 is 3-formyl rifamycin SV:O-n-octyloxime.

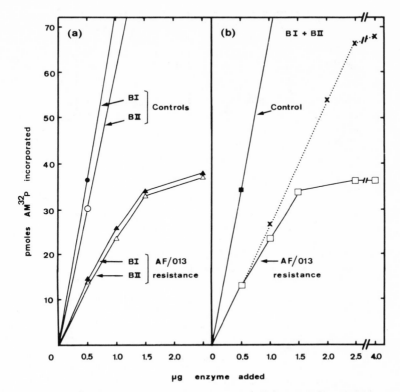

Fig. 4. AF/013-resistant RNA synthesis catalyzed by calf thymus (CT) B enzymes on CT DNA. AF/013-resistant RNA synthesis was determined as described in the footnote to Table III after preincubation of various amounts of enzyme for 10 min at 37° in the presence of 0.625 μg CT DNA. (a) •, Enzyme BI, control; ▲, enzyme BI, AF/013-resistant RNA synthesis; ○, enzyme BII, control; △, enzyme BII, AF/013-resistant RNA synthesis. (b) ■, Mixture of enzymes BI and BII (1:1), control; □, mixture of enzymes BI and BII (1:1), AF/013-resistant RNA synthesis; X, mixture of enzymes BI and BII (1:1), AF/013-resistant RNA synthesis in the presence of 1.25 μg of CT DNA.

onset of RNA synthesis. Table III shows also that similar resistances to AF/013 or rifampicin were obtained by preincubating DNA and *E. coli* holoenzyme for 10 min at 37°. In the case of enzyme AI, some resistance was also observed, but the same values were obtained whether the preincubation temperature was 37° or 0°, suggesting that the initiation process on calf thymus DNA could be different for the AI and the B enzymes. In the case of the B enzymes, it is most likely that the initiation takes place on double-stranded DNA when the strands

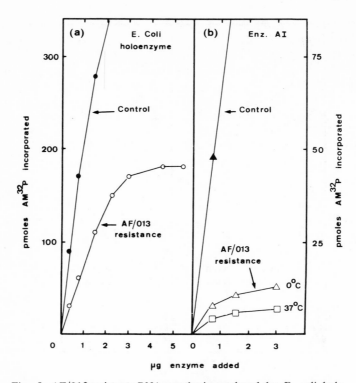

Fig. 5. AF/013-resistant RNA synthesis catalyzed by E. coli holo-enzyme and calf thymus (CT) enzyme AI on CT DNA. AF/013-resistant RNA synthesis was determined as described in the foot-note to Table III after preincubation of various amounts of enzyme for 10 min at 37° or 0° in the presence of 1.25 μg CT DNA for *E. coli* holoenzyme and 5 μg CT DNA for CT enzyme AI. (a) ●, *E. coli* holoenzyme, control; ○, *E. coli* holoenzyme, AF/013-resistant RNA synthesis after 10 min preincubation at 37°. (b) ▲ Enzyme AI, control; △, enzyme AI, AF/013-resistant RNA synthesis after 10 min preincuba-tion at 0°; □, enzyme AI, AF/013-resistant RNA synthesis after 10 min preincubation at 37°.

have been opened over a short local region, since the appearance of resistance to AF/013 is temperature (Table III) and time dependent (18).

Can any site on the DNA confer resistance on the polymerase molecules bound? Figure 4a shows that only a limited number of DNA sites could protect RNA synthesis catalyzed by B enzymes against the inhibitory effect of AF/013: the resistant RNA synthesis increased linearly with the ratios of enzyme to DNA until a plateau level was reached. Figure 4b indicates that the sites of calf thymus DNA which conferred resistance on enzyme BI were the same as those conferring resistance on enzyme BII, for no increase in the plateau level was observed when saturating amounts of enzyme BI and BII were incubated together. Similar results were obtained when the concentration of DNA was doubled, but as expected the plateau level of resistant RNA synthesis was doubled (Fig. 4b). Figure 5a shows that RNA synthesis catalyzed by *E. coli* holoenzyme can also be protected against the inhibitory effect of AF/013 by preincubation of the enzyme and calf thymus DNA for 10 min at 37°. In this case, a plateau level was also observed when the enzyme concentration was increased, suggesting that only a limited number of calf thymus DNA sites could confer resistance on *E. coli* holoenzyme. On the contrary, no clear plateau level was observed with enzyme AI (Fig. 5b).

Table IV. Calf Thymus DNA Sites Conferring AF/013 Resistance on Calf Thymus B Enzymes are Specific[a]

Conditions of preincubation and incubation	Incorporation of ^{32}P-GMP, 10 min at 37° (pmoles)		
	No α-amanitin	α-Amanitin (10 μg)	α-Amanitin-sensitive RNA synthesis
B enzymes + DNA 5 min 37°, then NTP + AF/013	56.5	0	56.5
E. coli enzyme + DNA 5 min 37°, then NTP + AF/013	236.0	236.0	0
B enzymes + DNA 5 min 37°, then *E. coli* enzyme 5 min 37°, then NTP + AF/013	291.0	232.0	59.0
E. coli enzyme 5 min 37°, then B enzymes 5 min 37°, then NTP + AF/013	278.0	223.0	55.0
E. coli enzyme + B enzymes 5 min 37°, then NTP + AF/013	289.0	231.0	58.0

[a] Preincubation and incubation mixtures were as described in the footnote legend to Table III, except that 1.25 μg calf thymus DNA was added per incubation medium. Saturating amounts of a mixture of purified B enzymes (2.5 μg) and of purified *E. coli* RNA polymerase (21) were added as described in the table. Where indicated, 10 μg α-amanitin was added together with the NTP and AF/013 in order to estimate RNA synthesis catalyzed by the B enzymes, which are specifically inhibited by α-amanitin (7,8).

These observations offer a unique opportunity to determine whether B enzymes and *E. coli* holoenzyme initiate at the same sites on double-stranded calf thymus DNA. Results presented in Table IV demonstrate that most of, if not all, the sites which conferred resistance on calf thymus RNA polymerase B activities were different from those which conferred resistance on *E. coli* RNA polymerase holoenzyme. It is clear that profound changes in the nature of the initiation sites have occurred during evolution, since the initiation sites recognized by *E. coli* holoenzyme on calf thymus DNA are completely different from those recognized by the homologous enzyme. A similar conclusion was also recently reached by Butterworth *et al.* (23), who suggested that *E. coli* holoenzyme and rat liver B enzymes do not initiate at the same sites on rat liver chromatin. There is therefore very little hope of synthesizing specific RNAs by transcribing animal DNAs or chromatin with a bacterial RNA polymerase. Similar experiments (Table V) conducted with the two types of calf thymus RNA polymerase activities show that enzyme AI does not bind or binds very

Table V. Calf Thymus Enzymes AI and B Do Not Initiate at the Same Sites on Calf Thymus DNA[a]

Conditions of preincubation and incubation	Incorporation of ^{32}P-AMP, 10 min at 37° (pmoles)	
	No α-Amanitin	α-Amanitin (10 μg)
B enzymes + DNA 5 min 37°, then NTP + AF/013	36.0	0
Enzyme AI (2 μg) + DNA 5 min 37°, then NTP	160.0	160.0
Enzyme AI (2 μg) + DNA 5 min 37°, then NTP + AF/013	1.5	1.7
Enzyme AI (2 μg) + DNA 5 min 37°, then B enzymes 5 min 37°, then NTP + AF/013	39.5	1.5
Enzyme AI (4 μg) + DNA 5 min 37°, then B enzymes 5 min 37°, then NTP + AF/013	38.5	1.4

[a] Preincubation and incubation mixtures were as described in footnote to Table III, except that 1.25 μg calf thymus DNA was added per incubation medium. Enzyme AI and a mixture of purified B enzymes (2.5 μg) were added as described in the table.

loosely to the sites of double-stranded calf thymus DNA which confer resistance on B enzymes. Results which will be presented elsewhere (18) suggest that in fact the RNA synthesis catalyzed by enzyme AI on calf thymus DNA is mainly initiated at nicks. This could mean either that enzyme AI lacks an initiation factor required for initiation on double-stranded calf thymus DNA or that the sites at which A enzymes can initiate specifically are very rare, which could be the case if enzyme AI is involved specifically in the transcription of the ribosomal cistrons, as suggested by its intranucleolar localization. In any case, our results suggest very strongly that, like the bacterial enzyme, animal nuclear DNA-dependent RNA polymerases can play an active role in the selection of the transcribed region of the chromosomal DNA.

ACKNOWLEDGMENTS

We are greatly indebted to Drs. Silvestri and Lancini (Lepetit, Milan) for a gift of derivatives of rifamycin and to Drs. Wieland and Faulstich (Heidelberg) for a gift of labeled amanitin. The technical assistance of Mrs. M. Acker, Mrs. C. Hauss, and Mr. G. Dretzen is gratefully acknowledged. M. Meilhac and F. Gissinger are Attachés de Recherche CNRS; S. Walter's permanent address is Institute of Biochemistry and Physiology, University of Lodz, Poland. This investigation was supported by grants from the Délégation Générale à Recherche Scientifique et Technique, the Commissariat à l'Energie Atomique, the Ligue Nationale Francaise contre le Cancer, the Fondation pour la Recherche Médicale Francaise, and the Institut National pour la Santé et la Recherche Médicale.

SUMMARY

Three DNA-dependent RNA polymerases AI, BI, and BII were purified from calf thymus. These enzymes were characterized by their sensitivity to amanitin, their subunit pattern, and their template specificities. Enzyme AI is resistant to amanitin, while B enzymes are inhibited by this poison. Each of these enzymes contains two subunits of high molecular weight: A1 (mol wt 197,000) and A2 (mol wt 126,000) for enzyme AI, B1 (mol wt 214,000) and B3 (mol wt 140,000) for enzyme BI, and B2 (mol wt 180,000) and B3 for enzyme BII. In addition, each enzyme contains several subunits of lower molecular weight. Purification of B enzymes from rat liver showed the presence of two enzymes similar to calf thymus RNA polymerases BI and BII and suggested the existence of an additional B enzyme in rat liver.

Studies with derivatives of rifamycin indicated that calf thymus B enzymes were able to recognize specific initiation sites on calf thymus DNA, which were different from those recognized by enzyme AI or *E. coli* RNA polymerase. These results favor the hypothesis that the multiplicity of animal RNA polymerases could play an active role in the control of transcription.

RESUMEN

Se purificaron tres RNA polimerasas-DNA dependientes, AI, BI, y BII, del timo de ternero. Estas enzimas se caracterizaron según su sensibilidad a la amanitina, su patrón de subunidades, y sus especificidades con respecto a los patrones. La enzima AI es resistente a la amanitina, mientras que las enzimas B son inhibidas por esta droga. Cada una de estas enzimas contiene dos subunidades de peso molecular alto: A1 (P. M. 197,000) y A2 (P.M. 126,000) para la enzima AI, B1 (P. M. 214,000) y B3 (P. M. 140,000) para la enzima BI, B2 (P. M. 180,000) y B3 para la enzima BII. Además cada enzima contiene varias subunidades de peso molecular más bajo. La purificación de las enzimas B del hígado de ternero demostró la presencia de dos enzimas similares a las RNA polimerasas del timo de ternero, BI y BII, y sugirió la existencia de una enzima B adicional en el hígado de rata.

Estudios con derivados de rifamacina indicaron que las enzimas B del timo de ternero son capaces de reconocer sitios específicos en el DNA del timo de ternero, los cuales son diferentes a los reconocidos por la enzima AI o la RNA polimerasa de *E. coli*. Estos resultados apoyan la hipótesis de que la multiplicidad de RNA polimerasas animales podría jugar un papel activo en el control positivo de la transcripción.

REFERENCES

1. Weiss, S. B., and Gladstone, L., *J. Am. Chem. Soc., 81,* 4118 (1959).
2. *Cold Spring Harbor Symp. Quant. Biol., 35,* (1970).
3. Roeder, R. G., and Rutter, W. J., *Nature, 224,* 234 (1969).
4. Chesterton, C. J., and Butterworth, P. H. W., *FEBS Letters, 12,* 301 (1971).
5. Jacob, S. T., Sajdel, E. M., and Munro, H. N., *Biochem. Biophys. Res. Commun., 38,* 765 (1970).
6. Roeder, R. G., and Rutter, W. J., *Proc. Natl. Acad. Sci. U.S.A., 65,* 675 (1970).
7. Kedinger, C., Gniazdowski, M., Mandel, J. L., Gissinger, F., and Chambon, P., *Biochem. Biophys. Res. Commun., 38,* 165 (1970).
8. Kedinger, C., Nuret, P., and Chambon, P., *FEBS Letters, 15,* 169 (1971).
9. Mandel, J. L., and Chambon, P., *FEBS Letters, 15,* 175 (1971).
10. Chambon, P., Gissinger, F., Mandel, J. L., Kedinger, C., Gniazdowski, M., and Meilhac, M., *Cold Spring Harbor Symp. Quant. Biol., 35,* 693 (1970).
11. Weber, K., and Osborn, M., *J. Biol. Chem., 244,* 4406 (1969).
12. Dunker, A. K., and Rueckert, R. R., *J. Biol. Chem., 244,* 5074 (1969).
13. Chesterton, C. J., and Butterworth, P. H. W., *FEBS Letters, 15,* 181 (1971).
14. Gniazdowski, M., Mandel, J. L., Gissinger, F., Kedinger, C., and Chambon, P., *Biochem. Biophys. Res. Commun., 38,* 1033 (1970).
15. Meilhac, M., Kedinger, C., Chambon, P., Govidan, V., Faulstich, H., and Wieland, T., *FEBS Letters, 9,* 258 (1970).
16. Vogt, V., *Nature, 223,* 854 (1969).
17. Roeder, R. G., Roeder, R. H., and Brown, D. D., *Cold Spring Harbor Symp. Quant. Biol., 35,* 727 (1970).
18. Meilhac, M., Tysper, S., and Chambon, P., *Eur. J. Biochem., 28,* 291 (1972).
19. Sippel, E. A., and Hartman, G. R., *Europ. J. Biochem., 16,* 152 (1970).
20. Bautz, E. K. F., and Bautz, F. A., *Nature, 226,* 1219 (1970).
21. Chamberlin, M., and Berg, P., *Proc. Natl. Acad. Sci. U.S.A., 48,* 81 (1962).
22. Burgess, R. R., *J. Biol. Chem., 244,* 6168 (1969).
23. Butterworth, P. H. W., Cox, R. F., and Chesterton, C. J., *Europ. J. Biochem., 23,* 229 (1971).

DISCUSSION

E. G. Bade (Cold Spring Harbor, U.S.A.): Have you been able to identify a specific transcription product of any of your enzymes transcribing calf thymus DNA?

P. Chambon (Strasbourg, France): We determined the base composition of the synthesized RNAs and found that the RNA synthesized by enzyme AI had a base composition complementary to that of calf thymus DNA, as is the case with the RNA synthesized by *E. coli* holoenzyme, while the RNA synthesized by the B enzymes presented a characteristic base composition close to that of the so-called nuclear heterogeneous RNA (10). This observation is exactly what one would expect if enzyme AI is initiating at random on nicks or ends and B enzymes at specific sites, as suggested by the experiments carried out with the rifamycin derivatives.

R. P. Perry (Philadephia, U.S.A.): Have you tried any experiments with DNA which has protein associated?

P. Chambon: Yes, we tried calf thymus chromatin, but it was a very bad template. The amount of RNA which was synthesized was very low with both enzymes AI and B. This result disagrees with the recent finding of Butterworth *et al.* (23) that rat liver chromatin was an efficient template for B enzymes but not for enzyme AI. As you know, chromatin is a very poorly defined material, and a difference in the extent of the shearing could explain this discrepancy. In any case, the results of Butterworth *et al.* could be explained, in the light of our results, by assuming that there were no accessible nicks in the DNA of their chromatin preparation and therefore enzyme AI was unable to initiate efficiently.

E. P. Geiduschek (La Jolla, U.S.A.): Did you determine the number of sites on calf thymus DNA which could confer resistance on B enzymes against AF/013?

P. Chambon: Yes, we measured the number of RNA chains initiated with a saturating amount of enzyme. This number was obtained by the determination of the incorporated γ-^{32}P-labeled nucleoside triphosphates. There were about 50,000 of such sites per haploid genome.

E. P. Geiduschek: Was the number of sites dependent on the size of the DNA template?

P. Chambon: I don't know; we used a calf thymus DNA with an average molecular weight of 12×10^6 daltons.

E. P. Geiduschek: Isn't it possible that most of these sites could correspond to the ends of the molecules?

P. Chambon: This possibility is unlikely, since the amount of resistant RNA synthesis measured after preincubation at $0°$ was very low. In fact, we observed that when sonicated calf thymus DNA was a template, initiation at ends was correlated with a very large increase of resistant RNA synthesis induced by preincubation at $0°$ [up to 50% of the resistance observed after preincubation at $37°$ (18)]. Furthermore, no increase in the amount of resistant RNA synthesis occurred after preincubation at $37°$ when an equivalent amount of sonicated calf thymus DNA was used instead of "native" DNA. I would like to emphasize that the number 50,000 should be taken only as an estimate. It could be higher if some sites were occupied by inactive enzyme molecules which were able to bind but not to synthesize. The number could be lower if several polymerase molecules were lined up close to the initiation site and could initiate in rapid sequence when AF/013 and the nucleoside triphosphates were added to the incubation medium.

8

Regulation of Nucleolar DNA-Dependent RNA Polymerase by Amino Acids in Ehrlich Ascites Tumor Cells

M. T. Franze de Fernández, and A. O. Pogo

Departamento de Química Biológica
Facultad de Farmacia y Bioquímica
Universidad de Buenos Aires
Buenos Aires, Argentina
and
A. O. Pogo
Laboratory of Cell Biology
New York Blood Center
New York, New York, U.S.A.

The factors controlling the synthesis of ribosomal RNA (rRNA) in eukaryotic systems are not well understood. Absences of amino acids in the incubation medium have been reported to cause a marked reduction in the rate of appearance of newly formed ^{3}H-uridine-labeled ribosomal subunits in the cytoplasm of Landschütz cells (1). Studies in HeLa cells indicated that both synthesis and maturation of 45S rRNA are depressed in the absence of protein synthesis (2,3) and also when the cells are cultured in media deprived of an essential amino acid (4-6). Nevertheless, Smulson (7) failed to find any difference in the RNA polymerase activity of isolated nuclei of HeLa cells cultured in the presence or absence of amino acids in the incubation medium. However, Smulson did not indicate which RNA polymerase activity was measured in his experiments.

Taking advantage of the fact that it is now possible to select conditions for

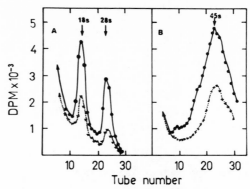

Fig. 1. Incorporation of ^{3}H-uridine into RNA in Ehrlich ascites cells. Preparation of the incubation media, cell fractionation, RNA extractions, and sucrose gradient analyses were as described elsewhere (18). (A) Cells were taken from the abdominal cavity of mice and incubated for 1 hr in Eagle's medium with or without amino acids. At this time, 5 μc/ml of ^{3}H-uridine (specific activity 27 c/mM) was added and incubation continued for 90 min. RNA was extracted from the cytoplasmic fraction, and aliquots corresponding to 1×10^6 cells were layered on a sucrose gradient and centrifuged at 32,000 rpm for 16½ hr in the Spinco SW40 rotor. (B) Cells were incubated as in (A) but were pulse labeled with ^{3}H-uridine for 25 min. Fractions of total cellular RNA corresponding to 1×10^7 cells were layered on a sucrose gradient and centrifuged at 23,000 rpm for 16 hr in the Spinco SW40 rotor. •, RNA from cells incubated in Eagle's medium; x, RNA from cells incubated in Eagle's medium without amino acids.

assaying different RNA polymerases in isolated, intact nuclei (8,9), we have explored the possibility that the amount of amino acids in the incubation medium may be one of the regulatory factors controlling nucleolar RNA polymerase activity (polymerase I or polymerase A; see refs. 10 and 11).

RESULTS

We first studied RNA synthesis in Ehrlich ascites cells incubated in media with or without amino acids. Figure 1A illustrates the incorporation of ^{3}H-uridine into the 18S and 28S rRNA species after 90 min of labeling. There was a higher incorporation of label into RNA of cells incubated in a medium with added amino acids. Furthermore, the ratio of the rates of incorporation of ^{3}H-uridine into the two RNA species was not affected by the presence of amino acids in the incubation media. This observation was similar to that reported for Landschütz cells (1) and indicated that lack of amino acids did not change the processing of the 45S rRNA precursor. Figure 1B illustrates the incorporation of ^{3}H-uridine into 45S rRNA after 25 min of labeling. A higher accumulation of labeled 45S rRNA occurred in cells incubated in a medium enriched with amino acids than in a medium without amino acids.

Table I lists the amounts of radioactivity incorporated into RNA species other than rRNA. This experiment was done by adding actinomycin D (0.04 μg/ml) to the incubation medium in order to suppress rRNA synthesis (12). It was found that cells incubated with or without amino acids had similar amounts of ^{3}H-uridine incorporated into RNA species other than 45S rRNA. Also, there was no difference in ^{3}H-uridine-labeled RNA at various times of cell incubation in the different media. The action of the amino acids on the accumulation of the 45S rRNA precursor was rather selective, because at least the amount of heterogeneous nuclear RNA synthesized in a 10 min pulse was not affected.

Table I. Incorporation of ^{3}H-Uridine into
RNA in Cells Incubated with Low
Amounts of Actinomycin D[a]

Time (hr)	Conditions of incubation	
	Eagle's medium	Eagle's medium minus amino acids
1	9,340	9,420
1½	11,000	10,560
2½	8,320	8,650

[a] All data are counts per minute incorporated in a 10 min pulse. The cells were incubated in the presence of 0.04 μg/ml of actinomycin D as described (18). At the times indicated, triplicate samples containing 1.2×10^6 cells were pulsed for 10 min with 5 μc/ml of ^{3}H-uridine. The cells were harvested, washed twice with cold saline, and precipitated with 7 ml of 10% trichloroacetic acid containing 0.2 μmole of cold uridine. The precipitate was collected by filtration and washed four times with 7 ml of 10% trichloroacetic acid. The Millipore filters were placed in vials, and the precipitate was dissolved in 0.4 ml of concentrated formic acid and counted as described (14).

Table II. Properties of the DNA-Dependent RNA Polymerase Reaction
in Isolated Nuclei of Ehrlich Ascites Tumor Cells[a]

	RNA polymerase assay		
Cell culture medium	Antibiotics[b]	Activity (%)	Ratio $\frac{UMP}{GMP}$
Eagle's	–	100	0.39
Eagle's	100μg actinomycin D	2	–
Eagle's	20μg α-amanitin	90	–
Eagle's	30μg α-amanitin	90	–
Eagle's without amino acids	–	50	0.57
Eagle's without amino acids	30μg α-amanitin	4	–

[a] Cells were incubated for 50 min and nuclei isolated as described elsewhere (18). RNA polymerase was measured by the incorporation of ^{3}H-GMP or ^{3}H-UMP into RNA. Aliquots of the crude nuclear fraction containing 80-90 μg DNA were added to the assay mixture (final volume 0.25 ml) containing 0.02 M Tris-HCl buffer, pH 8.0 (at 23°), 0.06 M NaCl, 4 mM MgCl$_2$, 1 mM dithiothreitol, 4 mM phosphoenolpyruvate, 1 μg pyruvate kinase, and 0.2 μmole each of ATP, CTP, UTP, and ^{3}H-GTP (specific activity 100 μc/μmole). Unless otherwise indicated, incubation was for 15 min at 37°. The reaction was stopped by adding 7 ml of 10% cold trichloroacetic acid containing 0.04 M sodium pyrophosphate. The precipitate was collected by centrifugation and was washed three times with 7 ml of the cold trichloroacetic acid-pyrophosphate solution. The final precipitate was dissolved in 0.4 ml of concentrated formic acid, and the radioactivity was counted as described elsewhere (14). All of the assays were done in triplicate.
[b] Total added in a final volume of 0.25 ml.

The low incorporation of ^{3}H-uridine into the 45S rRNA in cells incubated with no amino acids could be caused by an increase in RNA degradation or by a decrease in RNA synthesis. We investigated this last possibility by examining the activity of the DNA-dependent RNA polymerase in nuclei obtained from cells incubated in media with or without amino acids.

As carried out under the conditions described in Table II, the RNA polymerase activity was inhibited by actinomycin D, which showed its DNA dependence. The reaction was dependent on the presence of all four ribonucleoside triphosphates. The uptake of nucleotides into RNA proceeded optimally at pH 7.9 and was Mg^{2+} dependent. At a low salt concentration and 4 mM Mg^{2+}, the reaction was slightly inhibited by α-amanitin. This drug inhibits only RNA polymerase II (9). The small inhibition was observed in nuclei obtained from cells incubated with or without amino acids in the medium (Table II). The ratio of incorporation of UMP and GMP into the newly synthesized RNA was what would be expected for rRNA synthesis, assuming that in 45S RNA there is approximately

66% guanylic and cytidylic acids compared to 34% adenylic and uridylic acids. These results were consistent with previous observations (13,14) that incubation of isolated nuclei with a low salt concentration and Mg^{2+} mainly assayed the RNA polymerase which synthesized rRNA (nucleolar RNA polymerase). The activity of the enzyme was consistently higher in nuclei obtained from cells incubated in a medium enriched with amino acids than in a medium with low amino acid content. Furthermore, nucleolar RNA polymerase activity was proportional to the amino acid content in the incubation medium (Fig. 2).

In the experiment described in Fig. 3, it was shown that the kinetics of GMP incorporation had a similar time course in nuclei isolated from cells incubated in media with or without amino acids. However, the rate of GMP incorporation and final plateau level were less in nuclei isolated from cells incubated with low amounts of amino acids. The reaction stopped very soon in both cases, which suggests that elongation and termination of ribonucleotide chains were the only RNA polymerase activities of the isolated nuclei (15).

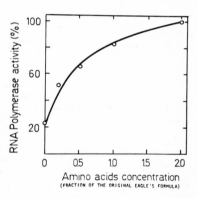

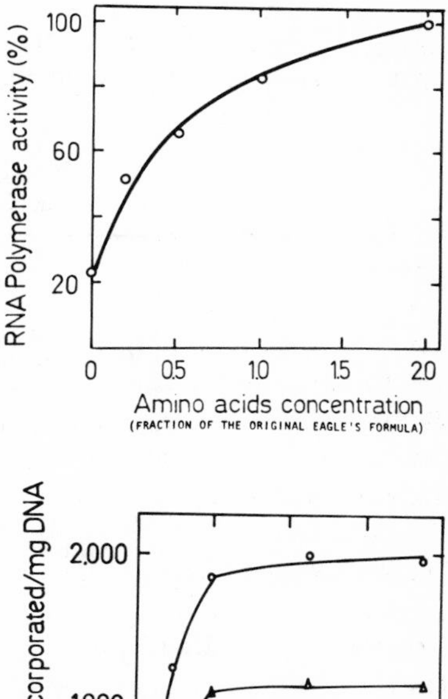

Fig. 2. Plot of nucleolar RNA polymerase activity against amino acid concentration in the medium. Cells were incubated for 50 min in the different media. At that time, the nuclei were isolated and the RNA polymerase activity was measured as described in Table II.

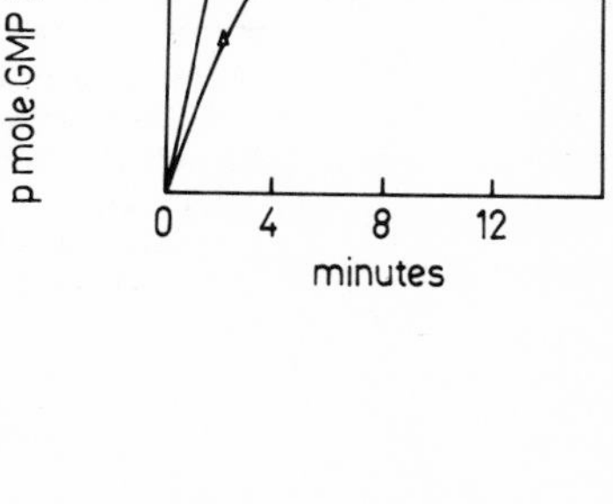

Fig. 3. Kinetics of the RNA polymerase reaction in isolated nuclei from Ehrlich ascites cells. The cells were incubated in Eagle's medium with or without amino acids for 40 min. At that time, the nuclei were isolated and the RNA polymerase activity was measured as described in Table II. ○, Nuclei from cells incubated in Eagle's medium; △, nuclei from cells incubated in Eagle's medium, without amino acids.

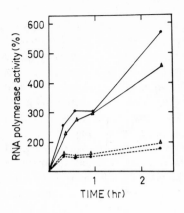

Fig. 4. Kinetics of RNA polymerase activation by amino acids. RNA polymerase activity of nuclei isolated from Ehrlich ascites cells incubated for different times in Eagle's medium with (——————) or without (——————) amino acids. At the times indicated, the nuclei were isolated and the RNA polymerase activity was measured as described in Table II. The results are expressed in percent of RNA polymerase activity; 100% is the RNA polymerase activity in the nonincubated cells. ● and △ are two separate experiments.

The time course of the augmentation of nucleolar RNA polymerase activity of isolated nuclei is shown in Fig. 4. Soon after the cells were exposed to a medium high in amino acids, a rapid increase in activity of the enzyme occurred. After approximately 20 min of incubation, this activity leveled off, but a second burst of enzymatic activity was detected after 60 min of incubation. A similar pattern of increased enzymatic activity was seen in cells incubated with no

Table III. Effect of Nucleosides on RNA Polymerase Activity[a]

Cells culture medium	RNA polymerase assay (pmoles GTP incorporated/mg DNA)
Eagle's + 0.1 mM uridine and 0.1 mM inosine	1030
Eagle's without amino acids + 0.1 mM uridine and 0.1 mM inosine	380
Eagle's	1150
Eagle's without amino acids	310

[a] Cells were incubated either in Eagle's medium with or without amino acids or in media supplemented with 0.1 mM uridine and 0.1 mM inosine with or without amino acids. Incubation was for 50 min. Nuclei were prepared and RNA polymerase was assayed as described in Table II.

amino acids in the medium. However, the amount of GMP incorporated into RNA was consistently higher in cells incubated in a medium with amino acids than in a medium with no amino acids. The nonlinear nature of the elevation in enzymatic activity occurring during incubation with amino acids indicates the complexity of this phenomenon and suggests that more than one metabolic process may be involved.

The activation of the nucleolar RNA polymerase by amino acids could be mediated by an increased synthesis of the purine and pyrimidine precursors normally derived from amino acids. This possibility was tested in the experiment described in Table III. Cells were incubated with or without amino acids in media containing uridine and inosine. These nucleosides are used preferentially for the synthesis of nucleic acids and inhibit the *de novo* formation of purines and pyrimidines (16). The results indicated that the effect of amino acids on the nucleolar RNA polymerase activity persists in the presence of exogenous uridine and inosine and cannot be ascribed to an increased synthesis of nucleoside precursors.

The data presented here clearly indicate that the nucleolar RNA polymerase activity is highly sensitive to the amino acid content of the incubation medium of the cells. One of the questions that emerges is whether amino acids activate the nucleolar RNA polymerase by their effect on protein synthesis. For example, they may act by increasing the synthesis of the RNA polymerase or some of its subunits or factors that may be in diminishing amounts within the cell. This possibility, however, seems unlikely due to the fact that partial inhibition of protein synthesis did not prevent the activation of the nucleolar RNA polymerase by amino acids (M. T. Franze de Fernández, unpublished results). The similarity between this amino acid control of nucleolar RNA polymerase and the stringent control of rRNA synthesis in bacterial cells (17) makes it attractive to assume that a similar phenomenon underlies both processes.

ACKNOWLEDGMENTS

This work was supported by grant No. HE-09011 from the National Institutes of Health, Heart and Lung Institute and Division of Research Resource, and by grant No. 4796/71 from the Consejo Nacional de Investigaciones Científicas y Técnicas de la República Argentina. Dr. Franze de Fernández is a member of the Investigator Career, Consejo Nacional de Investigaciones Científicas y Técnicas de la República Argentina.

SUMMARY

Lack of amino acids in the incubation medium of Ehrlich ascites cells caused a marked reduction in the apperance of 28S and 18S rRNA in the cytoplasm. The incorporation of

[3]H-uridine into the 45S rRNA precursor was also diminished, but the incorporation of label into RNA other than ribosomal was not altered. Nucleolar RNA polymerase activity rapidly increased when the cells were exposed to a medium rich in amino acids. The activity of the enzyme was proportional to the amino acid content of the incubation medium. The effect of amino acids on the RNA polymerase activity cannot be ascribed to an increased synthesis of nucleoside precursors.

RESUMEN

La falta de aminoácidos en el medio de incubación de las células de tumor ascítico de Ehrlich producen una reduccción marcada en la aparición del 28S y 18S RNA ribosomal (rRNA) en el citoplasma. La incorporación de uridina-^{3}H en el 45S rRNA precursor también está disminuída, pero la incorporación del radioactivo en otras especies de RNA no se encuentra alterada. La actividad de la RNA polimerasa nucleolar aumenta rápidamente cuando se exponen las células a un medio rico en aminoácidos. La actividad del enzima es proporcional al contenido de aminoácidos en el medio de incubación. El efecto de los aminoácidos en la actividad de la RNA polimerasa no se debe a una sintesis aumentada de los nucleósidos precursores.

REFERENCES

1. Shields, R., and Korner, A., *Biochim. Biophys. Acta, 204,* 521 (1970).
2. Soeiro, R., Vaughan, H., and Darnell, J. E., *J. Cell Biol., 36,* 91 (1968).
3. Willems, M., Penman, M., and Penman, S., *J. Cell Biol., 41,* 177 (1969).
4. Vaughan, M. H., Soeiro, R., Warner, J. R., and Darnell, J. E., *Proc. Natl. Acad. Sci. U.S.A., 58,* 1527 (1967).
5. Maden, B. E. H., Vaughan, M. H., Warner, J. R., and Darnell, J. E., *J. Mol. Biol. 45,* 265 (1969).
6. Maden, B. E. H., *Biochem. J., 123,* 36P (1971).
7. Smulson, M. E., *Biochim. Biophys. Acta, 199,* 537 (1970).
8. Widnell, C. C., and Tata, J. R., *Biochim. Biophys. Acta, 123,* 478 (1966).
9. Lindell, T., Weinberg, F., Morris, P. W., Roeder, R. G., and Rutter, W. J., *Science, 170,* 447 (1970).
10. Roeder, R. G., and Rutter, W. J., *Proc. Natl. Acad. Sci. U.S A., 65,* 675 (1970).
11. Kedinger, C., Nuret, P., and Chambon, P., *FEBS Letters, 15,* 169 (1971).
12. Roberts, W. K., and Newman, J. F. E., *J. Mol. Biol., 20,* 63 (1966).
13. Pogo, A. O., Littau, V. C., Allfrey, V. G., and Mirsky, A. E., *Proc. Natl. Acad. Sci. U.S.A., 57,* 743 (1967).
14. Pogo, A. O., *Biochim. Biophys. Acta, 182,* 57 (1969).
15. Maul, G. G., and Hamilton, T. M., *Proc. Natl. Acad. Sci. U.S.A., 57,* 1371 (1967).
16. Salzman, N. P., and Sebring, E. D., *Arch. Biochem. Biophys., 84,* 143 (1959).
17. Eden, G., and Broda, P., *Bacteriol. Rev., 32,* 206 (1968).
18. Franze-Fernández, M. T., and Pogo, A. O., *Proc. Natl. Acad. Sci. U.S.A., 68,* 3040 (1971).

DISCUSSION

Unidentified speaker: Did you try incomplete amino acid mixtures or isolated amino acids?

M. T. Franze de Fernández (Buenos Aires, Argentina): Yes, I found full activation of the enzyme with all the amino acids. Any amino acids removed from the incubation medium, even if they are not metabolically related, have the same effect of lowering the activity of the enzyme.

R. P. Perry (Philadelphia, U.S.A.): Have you explored the possibility that in the amino acid starved cells you get some sort of a polymerase inhibitor rather than activation? Have you done a reconstruction experiment?

M. T. Franze de Fernández: No, I have not.

G. D. Novelli (Oak Ridge, U.S.A.): In the experiment in which you exposed the cells to cycloheximide or different amino acid concentrations, did RNA synthesis continue or were you just talking about the activity of the RNA polymerase?

M. T. Franze de Fernández: I was just talking about the activity of the RNA polymerase. I have to test RNA synthesis.

J. E. Allende (Santiago, Chile): Have you explored the possibility that aminoacyl-tRNA may have something to do with the phenomenon?

M. T. Franze de Fernández: This subject is very interesting, but I have not explored it.

P. Chambon (Strasbourg, France): Did you try to extract the enzyme to see if the actual amount of enzyme is increased?

M. T. Franze de Fernández: No, I did not.

P. Chambon: What are your proofs that all the RNA which is synthesized in the nucleus is ribosomal RNA?

M. T. Franze de Fernández: I do not know if the synthesis is of ribosomal RNA. Because of the inhibition by a-amanitin, which inhibits only 10% of the activity of the enzyme assayed at low salt and 4 mM Mg^{2+}, I think that the activity corresponds to the so-called polymerase I or polymerase A. That is the only evidence I have.

P. Chambon: Yes, because there is no real evidence that polymerase I or A is the one that synthesizes ribosomal RNA.

C. Weissmann (Zurich, Switzerland): When you use isolated nuclei for incorporation, is it clear that you can overcome the complication which might arise if there are larger or smaller amounts of cold substrates in nucleus?

M. T. Franze de Fernández: This problem is overcome by the assay system. I use excess substrate in these assays, and the reaction is dependent on all four ribonucleosides.

9

Rhynchosciara angelae Salivary Gland DNA: Kinetic Complexity and Transcription of Repetitive Sequences

J. Bálsamo, J. M. Hierro, M. L. Birnstiel, and F. J. S. Lara*

Departamento de Bioquímica
Instituto de Química
Universidade de São Paulo
Caixa Postal 20780
São Paulo, Brasil
and
M. L. Birnstiel
Institut für Molekularbiologie
Universität Zürich
Zürich, Switzerland

Flies of the genus *Rhynchosciara*, in common with other Diptera, have polytene chromosomes of large size and clearly defined morphology in cells of many tissues. Because the larvae originating from a clutch of eggs develop synchronously, it is possible to obtain material in large enough quantities for biochemical experimentation, even from specialized tissues such as the salivary glands. This makes it possible to correlate biochemical and morphological events taking place in defined tissues. In this organism, we also have the "DNA puffs," which develop in the salivary gland chromosomes. It is this aspect of *Rhynchosciara* that makes it an especially interesting system for the study of gene action in higher organisms.

Breuer and Pavan (1) and Ficq and Pavan (2) indicated that DNA synthesis in puffs occurs at a faster rate than in other chromosomal regions. These

* Address correspondence and reprint requests to Dr. Lara.

observations were confirmed by the cytospectrophotometric measurements of Rudkin and Corlette (3). Similar observations are also available for related flies (4). Clearly, we have here a case of gene amplification in somatic cells, which might be a mechanism of importance in achieving the differentiated state. Indeed, such a mechanism might normally exist in other animals but goes undetected.

Previous studies with *Rhynchosciara* (5) confirmed the work of cytologists, providing biochemical evidence for the existence of gene amplification in the salivary gland at the time of appearence of the giant chromosomal puffs. These studies were also of importance in establishing a correlation of the amplification phenomenon with reiterated DNA and nuclear RNA.

Kinetic analysis of DNA renaturation indicates the presence of multiple copies of certain sequences in a genome and provides a means of evaluating its informational content (6-9). Based on kinetic analysis, nuclear DNA of eukaryotic cells can be divided into three classes, according to the extent of repetition: (a) a set of sequences with a high degree of reiteration, generally appearing as a satellite in CsCl density gradients, typically exemplified by the satellite found in rodent DNA (10-12); (b) moderately repeated sequences, which renature with an intermediate rate, present in all eukaryotes; and (c) those sequences which renature at a rate compatible with the genome complexity of the organism in question. These sequences are considered to be represented just once per haploid genome and are called "unique" sequences.

The function of these different fractions has been studied by hybridization with RNA. The data obtained indicate that transcription from the satellite sequences of mouse DNA is not detected (11). It is possible that the guinea pig satellite DNA is also not transcribed (13). It is likely that these sequences have a structural role, as was originally suggested by Walker (14). However, most of the reported hybridization experiments showed RNA sequences complementary to repetitive DNA (8,15).

In order to further the understanding of DNA puff formation, we have now characterized the different DNA fractions present in the *Rhynchosciara* cell genome. We have also conducted hybridization experiments using the repetitive fractions and nuclear RNA. The evidence we obtained indicates that the reiterated fractions are transcribed, but not to the same extent. It also indicates that the amplification phenomenon is related to the "intermediate" fraction.

METHODS*

Animals and Gland Dissection

Rhynchosciara angelae was cultured as previously described by Lara *et al.*

* Abbreviations: A_{260}, absorption at 260 nm; $C_0 t$, initial DNA concentration in moles of

(16). All experiments were carried out with fourth instar larvae at the time of appearance of the giant chromosomal puffs. The salivary glands were obtained by dissection in 36mM NaCl, 52mM KCl, 5mM CaCl$_2 \cdot$H$_2$O. This solution has the same molarity and Na/K ratio as the hemolymph of *Rhynchosciara* larvae in late fourth instar (17). For a definition of the periods in which the fourth instar was divided for convenience of experimentation, see ref. 18.

DNA Preparation

Rhynchosciara salivary gland DNA was obtained according to Meneghini *et al.* (19). *Escherichia coli* and *Xanthomonas campestris* DNAs were prepared according to Marmur (20). The preparations were purified by banding in CsCl gradients. For this purpose, 4.271 g of CsCl (Harshaw, optical grade) was added to 3.5 g of DNA solution in 10mM tris, *p*H 7, giving initial density of 1.700 g/cm^3 as measured by refractometry (21); centrifugation was carried out at 42,000 rpm for a minimum of 36 hr at 20° in a Spinco model L ultracentrifuge in a 50Ti rotor. About 15 fractions were collected from the bottom of the tube, which were monitored by measuring ultraviolet absorbance at 260 nm. Those fractions containing DNA were pooled, and the DNA was concentrated either by ethanol precipitation or by pelleting by centrifugation (44,000 rpm for 20 hr at 15°). The molecular weights of these preparations were around 10^8 daltons. When lesser molecular weights were desired, the samples were treated ultrasonically for 2 min at 0.3 ma in a Raytheon 10 kc oscillator.

Molecular weight determinations were obtained from the sedimentation coefficient of either denatured DNA in alkaline solutions, measured in an analytical ultracentrifuge, or native DNA in sucrose gradients, using *Rhynchosciara* rRNA as a marker and applying Studier's formula (22).

Isotopically labeled *Rhynchosciara* DNA was obtained from glands dissected from animals which had been injected with 2 μl of ^{3}H-methylthymidine (23.4 c/mM, 0.5 mc/ml, Amersham) either 2 or 24 hr previously.

Buoyant Density of Repeated DNA Sequences

The density gradients were prepared by adding 4.271 g of CsCl to 3.25 ml of 10 mM Tris buffer, *p*H 8.0, containing sheared *R. angelae* salivary gland tritiated DNA (p = 1.695 g/cm^3) and *X. campestris* DNA (p = 1.723) as a marker. After centrifugation, 0.1 ml fractions were collected by piercing the bottom of the tube. The A_{260} of each fraction was measured after dilution with 0.5 ml of

---

nucleotides per liter multiplied by the time in seconds (8,9); rRNA, ribosomal RNA; SSC, 0.15 M NaCl plus 15 mM Na-citrate, *p*H 7.2; T_m, temperature at which 50% denaturation is observed.

water. Each sample was dialyzed against water for about 20 hr, then diluted to a final concentration of 1 μg DNA/ml in 0.12 M phosphate buffer, pH 6.8. After another dialysis step against 0.12 M phosphate buffer, the DNA samples were heat denatured and fractionated by hydroxyapatite as described below, to $C_0 t$ value of 0.5.

Renaturation Kinetics

Renaturation measurements were carried out in thermostatically controlled cells, in a Zeiss PM Q II spectrophotometer. Samples of 1.8 ml of DNA solution, in 1.0 M NaCl, were denatured with 0.1 ml NaOH, at 65°. At zero time, the solution was neutralized by adding 0.2 ml of a solution made by mixing 1.0 M Tris buffer, pH 8.0, and 1.0 N HCl (1:1) preheated to the same temperature. The drop in absorbance was then followed.

Hydroxyapatite Fractionations

Hydroxyapatite was prepared according to Miyazawa and Thomas (23). DNA denaturation was obtained by adding 0.1 N NaOH solution to a final concentration of 0.05 N to sheared DNA in 0.01 M Tris buffer, pH 7-8; then water, preheated to 65°, was added to obtain the desired DNA concentration. At zero time, 1.0 M phosphate buffer, pH 6.8, was added to obtain a final phosphate concentration of 0.12 M. The renaturation was followed at 65°, and the amount of material capable of binding to hydroxyapatite at each time was measured following the procedure of Flamm et al. (11).

In order to obtain the several fractions of *Rhynchosciara* salivary gland DNA uncontaminated with each other, the following procedure was used: DNA solutions (120 μg/ml) were incubated as described above to $C_0 t$ 0.018. At this $C_0 t$, about 50% of the fast-renaturing fraction reassociated (see *Results*) and was bound to hydroxyapatite, eluted, and concentrated (fast fraction). The unbound material was concentrated by lyophilization after dialysis and refractionated to $C_0 t$ 0.042 to eliminate the rest of the highly repeated sequences, which were discarded. The remaining fraction from this step was concentrated and fractionated to $C_0 t$ 0.18, which corresponds to renaturation of 50% of the intermediate fraction (see *Results*). The reassociated material was isolated as above, yielding the intermediate fraction; the nonreassociated material was concentrated and fractionated to $C_0 t$ 1.0. The denatured fraction at this step is the "unique" DNA.

Thermal Denaturation

Melting temperature determinations were carried out in standard SSC. The absorbance increase was monitored in a Zeiss PMQ II spectrophotometer, in thermostatically controlled cells. Temperatures were measured using a thermo-electric couple, directly immersed into the blank solution. All data were corrected for thermal expansion.

Molecular Hybridization Experiments

Some of the hybridization experiments were carried out using the different fractions of the *Rhynchosciara* salivary gland DNA, isolated as described above.

For experiments where it was important to avoid decrease in DNA molecular weight, total gland DNA, after slight shearing, was alkali denatured and allowed to renature at 65°, as previously described. When the desired $C_0 t$ values were reached, the solutions were rapidly cooled in ice, the salt concentration was increased to 6X SSC, and DNA was retained on membrane filters (Millipore GS, 13 mm, presoaked overnight in 2X SSC), at 4°, under slight pressure. The initial DNA concentrations were different in each case, so that the times of incubation at 65° were short (never greater than 2 hr). For each $C_0 t$ value, four filters were prepared and annealed with different RNA concentrations. A sample of the renaturing DNA on 0.12 M phosphate buffer was taken for control optical renaturation studies.

The hybridization procedure was basically that described by Gillespie and Spiegelman (24) and was carried at 65° for 20 hr in 6X SSC. The nuclear ³H-RNA used in hybridization experiments was obtained from isolated nuclei, as described by Armelin *et al.* (25).

RESULTS

The rate of renaturation of *R. angelae* DNA was followed according to Wetmur and Davidson (7). For evaluation of the second-order rate constant (k'_2), the reciprocal of remaining hyperchromicity $(A_{260\ (t)} - A_{260\ (\infty)}$, where $A_{260\ (\infty)}$ and $A_{260\ (t)}$ are the absorption values at 260 nm of native and partially denatured DNA, respectively) is plotted against time; the second-order rate constant is then calculated from the slope. The plot is a straight line for *Escherichia coli* DNA, a kinetically homogeneous DNA, whereas that for *R. angelae* salivary gland DNA indicates that it is composed of different classes of nucleotide sequences (Fig. 1). The slowly renaturing fraction may be considered as composed of unique sequences; its apparent second-order renaturation rate constant (k'_2), calculated from Fig. 1, is 0.43 l mol⁻¹ sec⁻¹. The amount of this fraction can be calculated by determining its zero-time A_{260} value by extrapolation. The mean value obtained with several DNA preparations was 86%; therefore, the remaining 14% of the DNA must be composed of reiterated sequences distributed between at least two other classes. Thus we can recognize at least

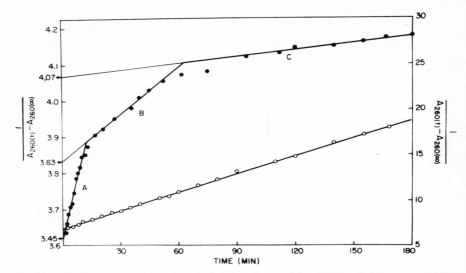

Fig. 1 Optical reassociation kinetics of Rhynchosciara *and* E. coli *DNA.* In this representation, the reciprocal of the remaining hyperchromicity $(A_{260}(t) - A_{260}(\infty)$ and $A_{260}(t)$ are the absorption values at 260 nm of native and partially denatured DNA, respectively) is plotted against time (7). •, Sheared *R. angelae* salivary gland DNA (single-strand molecular weight 1.3 × 10⁵ daltons) alkali denatured and renatured at 54 μg/ml at 65° $(T_m25°)$ in 1.0 *M* NaCl; ○, *E. coli* DNA (single-strand molecular weight 1 × 10⁶ daltons) renatured under similar conditions at 37 μg/ml. Left ordinate refers to *Rhynchosciara* values and right ordinate to *E. coli* DNA. Apparent constants for *Rhynchosciara* fractions are 1.95, 0.31, and 0.043 l mol⁻¹ sec⁻¹.

three classes of DNA sequences in *Rhynchosciara* salivary gland genome; a fast-, an intermediate-, and a slow-renaturing fraction. From the slope of the renaturation plot, it is possible to calculate an apparent k'_2 of 1.95 l mol⁻¹ sec⁻¹ for the fast fraction and of 0.33 mol⁻¹ sec⁻¹ for the intermediate fraction.

The apparent k'_2 for the slow fraction approximates closely the true second-order rate constant. A crude approximation of true k'_2 for the fast and intermediate fractions may be calculated by determining the hyperchromicity contribution of each one at each time, and replotting the reciprocal against time, according to Wells and Birnstiel (26). Using this method, the corrected rate constant for the fast fraction is 1125 l mol⁻¹ sec⁻¹ and that for the intermediate fraction is 120 l mol⁻¹ sec⁻¹. The mean contribution of each of these fractions to repetitive DNA is about 50% (53 and 47%, respectively).

Alternatively, the renaturation data can be analyzed by recording the fraction of renatured DNA $[(A_{260}(t) - A_{260}(\infty))/A_{260}(\infty)]$ against log C_0t; at the middle point of each curve, $C_0t_{1/2} \cdot k''_2 = 1$. Because of their disparate definitions, $k'_2 = 2k''_2$. In Fig. 2, the renaturation of the rapidly renaturing DNA is plotted in this way; the data were calculated from the same experiment reported in Fig. 1. The $C_0t_{1/2}$ values for each component purified from each other, calculated from the corrected values of k'_2, are 0.0017 for the fast fraction, 0.0167 for the intermediate fraction, and 45 for the slow fraction. The experimental $C_0t_{1/2}$ values for the fractions of repetitive DNA, not isolated, are approximately 0.029 for the fast fraction and 0.24 for the intermediate fraction, which corrected for their concentration in total DNA (approximately 7%), give the previous calculated values, showing that the corrected constants k'_2, are good approximations. The single-strand molecular weight of *E. coli* DNA used as standard was 1×10^6 daltons; this renatures with a rate constant k'_2 of 5 $1 \, mol^{-1} sec^{-1}$ and a $C_0t_{1/2}$ value of 0.4, in accord with reported data (7,8). Correcting this for a single-strand molecular weight of 1.3×10^5 daltons, *E. coli* DNA gives *a* k'_2 of $1.8 \, 1 \, mol^{-1} \, sec^{-1}$, which is about 48 times greater than the k'_2 for the slow fraction of *R. angelae* DNA, determined under the same conditions.

Applying the customary interpretation that there is an inverse proportionality between renaturation rate and DNA complexity and assuming a genome size

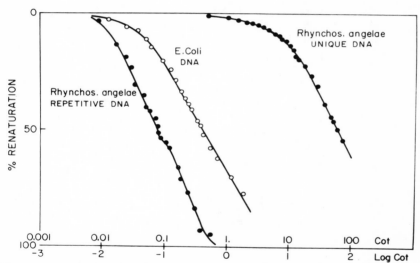

Fig. 2. Reassociation kinetics of Rhynchosciara *repeated and unique DNA and* E. coli *DNA.* The data are those presented in Fig. 1. For purposes of representation, the amounts of repetitive DNA (14%) and of unique DNA (86%) were normalized to 100% in each case. The amount of renatured DNA, expressed as a fraction of the correspondent mass, is plotted against the logarithm of total initial concentration of DNA (C_0, moles of nucleotides per liter), multiplied by the time interval in seconds (8,9). The arrows indicate the $C_0t_{1/2}$ values for the different fractions (fast 0.029, intermediate 0.24, and slow 57) and for *E. coli* DNA (0.4). The data for *E. coli* were not standardized for the same molecular weight as *Rhynchosciara* DNA.

Table I. Renaturation Data for *Rhynchosciara angelae* DNA[a]

Preparation No.	Mol wt (daltons)	k'_2 (unique fraction) (1 mol^{-1} sec^{-1})	Kinetic complexity of unique (daltons)	Genome size (daltons)	Ratio $\dfrac{k'_2 \text{(fast)}}{k'_2 \text{(unique)}}$	Ratio $\dfrac{k'_2 \text{(intermediate)}}{k'_2 \text{(unique)}}$	Fractions (% of total)		
							Fast	Intermediate	Unique
1	8.1×10^4	0.039	1.0×10^{11}	1.15×10^{11}	54.5	6.9	6.8	6.3	87.0
2	1.0×10^5	0.036	1.19×10^{11}	1.40×10^{11}	47.8	6.4	7.5	7.7	84.8
3	1.2×10^5	0.042	1.11×10^{11}	1.23×10^{11}	38.1	8.3	5.5	5.0	89.5
4	1.2×10^5	0.045	1.07×10^{11}	1.27×10^{11}	36.5	6.9	8.2	7.4	84.4
5	1.3×10^5	0.042	1.15×10^{11}	1.33×10^{11}	39.0	7.4	7.1	6.2	86.7
6	1.3×10^5	0.043	1.13×10^{11}	1.32×10^{11}	45.0	7.7	7.9	6.9	85.2
7	1.5×10^5	0.044	1.18×10^{11}	1.37×10^{11}	40.0	7.5	7.0	6.6	86.4
8	2.2×10^5	0.055	1.21×10^{11}	1.44×10^{11}	30.4	3.8	8.8	7.2	84.0
Mean	—	—	1.13×10^{11}	1.31×10^{11}	41.4	6.9	7.3	6.9	86.0

a Conditions were as detailed in the caption of Fig. 1. Single-strand molecular weights were determined as described in *Methods*. The definition of kinetic complexity used is that given by Wetmur and Davidson (7). *E. coli* was used as standard.

of 2.7×10^9 daltons for *E. coli,* it can be calculated that the kinetic complexity of the slow fraction of *R. angelae* DNA is 1.1×10^{11} daltons. Such an estimate applies to only 86% of the genome, thereby necessitating a 14% increase to obtain an estimate of total genome size. When this is done, a value of 1.3×10^{11} daltons is found. This value is similar to that found for *Sciara* by E. Rash [quoted by Gerbi (27)]. For such estimates, it would be better to take as standard a DNA with a base composition similar to that of *R. angelae* DNA (GC 33%) (5) rather than *E. coli* DNA (GC 50%). However, the effect of GC content is slight and can be neglected (7). Taking unique DNA from a rat ascites tumor as standard [data obtained from Wetmur and Davidson (7)], the genome size estimates remain unchanged.

Kinetic complexity values of 3.9×10^6 daltons were estimated for the fast fraction, which comprises about 9.5×10^9 daltons, 7.3% of the genome, and 3.3×10^7 daltons for the intermediate fraction, which comprises about 8.7×10^9 daltons, 6.7% of the genome. From these data, and using *E. coli* DNA as a standard, it can be calculated that the fast fraction is repeated 2×10^3 times, whereas the corresponding value for the intermediate fraction is 2.2×10^2. The date obtained with *Rhynchosciara* salivary gland DNA, described above, are summarized in Table I.

The heterogeneity of the salivary gland genome was also studied by hydroxy-apatite fractionation of ^{3}H-DNA, obtained at the time of appearance of the giant chromosomal puffs, and the data are presented in Fig. 3. In this figure are also shown the renaturation data for *E. coli* ^{14}C-DNA, which was used as internal standard, as well as a theoretical renaturation curve for rapidly renaturing *R. angelae* DNA (fast and intermediate fractions), calculated using the k'_2 values previously obtained. Clearly, the renaturation of only one of the fractions is apparent; its kinetic complexity and reiteration correspond to those of the intermediate fraction, observed in Figs. 1 and 2. Apparently, replication of the fast fraction is not occurring at this period of larval life. The data in Fig. 3 indicate that the amount of the intermediate fraction is 14% of total DNA, which is a higher value than that obtained by optical methods (6-7%). Although it is possible that this difference may be accounted for by the amplification occurring at this larval life period (5), we think that this is more likely due to discrepancies between the two methods used.

In some organisms, such as mouse (10,11), guinea pig (12), calf (28), and *Rhynchosciara hollenderi* (29), it has been shown that highly repetitive sequences correspond to a nuclear satellite DNA. The absorbance patterns on preparative ultracentrifugation of *R. angelae* salivary gland DNA (molecular weight 8×10^5 daltons) show (Fig. 4) that it bands symmetrically in a CsCl density gradient (1.695 g/cm^3) without visible evidence of satellite bands. The same result is obtained for this polytene tissue DNA in analytical ultracentrifugation (30). However, it is possible that the repetitive sequences have a special

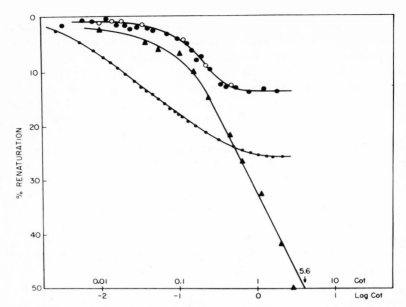

Fig. 3. Reassociation kinetics of Rhynchosciara *DNA measured by hydroxyapatite fractionation.* See *Methods* for details of the conditions and procedure
used. •, *R. angelae* salivary gland DNA after 2 hr incorporation of ^{3}H-thymidine
(C_0t of 0.33 10^{-5} moles/liter); ○ after 24 hr incorporation of ^{3}H-thymidine (C_0t
of 0.13 × 10^{-4} moles/liter); ▲, *E. coli* DNA labeled with ^{14}C; the line with small
dots represents a theoretical renaturation curve of *Rhynchosciara* repetitive DNA,
using the rate constants of fast and intermediate fractions calculated as indicated
in the text and adjusted for the present conditions ($C_0t_{1/2}$ 0.013 and 0.17,
respectively). Using the found $C_0t_{1/2}$ and the Britten and Kohne formula (8), a
complexity of about 5 × 10^7 daltons, repeated 2.7 × 10^2 times, can be calculated
for the labeled reiterated fractions.

distribution in a density gradient, but due to their special characteristics they do
not appear as a satellite band.

The fact that the fast fraction is not labeled at this larval stage allows one to
localize the position of the intermediate fraction in a density gradient. To this
end, each fraction of the density gradient was incubated under conditions that
allow for the exclusive renaturation of repetitive sequences (see *Methods* and
results described above). The renaturation percentage at each point, determined
by hydroxyapatite fractionation, is shown in Fig. 4. Clearly, this rapidly renaturing material (intermediate fraction) has a distribution different from that of the
main band; it appears as a defined peak of renaturation at the high-density zone
of the optical density band. An increase in renaturation percentage toward the
light zone is also noted.

The buoyant density of *R. angelae* DNA is 1.695 g/cm³, corresponding to a GC content of 33%. In order to calculate the mean buoyant density value of the intermediate fraction, we corrected the renaturation data for absolute DNA amounts at each point, and the values obtained are also plotted in Fig. 4. The curve obtained indicates a density value of 1.697, corresponding to a GC content of 38.7% (31). We conclude that most, if not all, of the labeled repeated sequences are heavier than the heterogeneous sequences, which comprise the vast majority of nuclear DNA.

Evidence for degree of base pairing and GC content of the rapidly renaturing families can be obtained from their thermal denaturation profiles. The data of Fig. 5 represent a thermal denaturation curve of *R. angelae* salivary gland DNA, which had been sheared, heat denatured, and incubated under conditions that led to selective renaturation of only repetitive sequences (about 20% renaturation). Two distributions of molecules are shown by the two-step transitions of the curve. A rough T_m value of each population can be estimated from the midpoint of each absorbance rise, a sharp melting transition at 74° and a more gradual increase in optical density at higher temperatures, with a midpoint at

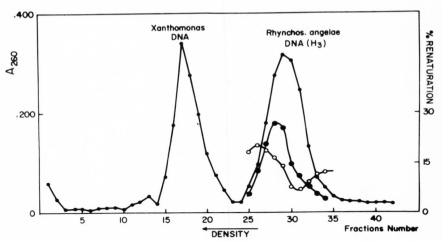

Fig. 4. Absorbance profile from a preparative CsCl gradient centrifugation and renaturation of the intermediate fraction. A mixture of *R. angelae* salivary gland ³H-DNA (ρ = 1.695) obtained after 2 hr of incorporation of ³H-thymidine and unlabeled *Xanthomonas campestris* DNA (ρ = 1.723) was centrifuged to equilibrium (conditions of centrifugation as described in *Methods*). The line with small dots represents optical density; ○, percentage of renaturation of each fraction when annealed at selective conditions, which allows for renaturation of repetitive DNA (at the C_0t used and since the fast fraction is not labeled, the renaturation refers to the intermediate fraction); ●, absolute amounts of labeled repetitive sequences at each point (mean buoyant density of 1.697 g/cm³).

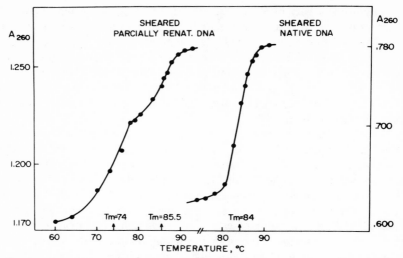

Fig. 5. Thermal denaturation of partially renatured and native Rhynchosciara *salivary gland DNA. R. angelae* DNA was sheared, heat denatured, and incubated under conditions that led to selective renaturation of only the repetitive sequences (C_0t 0.6, 20% renaturation). Two sharp-melting components with T_m 74 and 85.5° are observed. Sheared native *Rhynchosciara* salivary gland DNA shows a T_m of 84°. Both samples were melted in SSC.

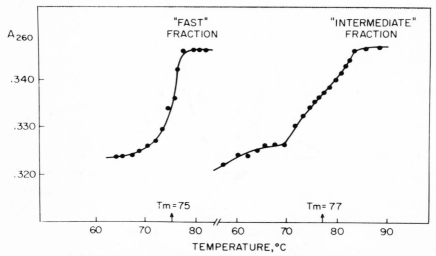

Fig. 6. Melting profile of the repeated fractions of Rhynchosciara *salivary gland DNA.* The fast-renaturing fraction and intermediate fraction of *Rhynchosciara* DNA were isolated by hydroxyapatite fractionation as described in *Methods*. Thermal denaturation in both cases was carried out in SSC (0.18 g-eq Na⁺/liter); fast fraction T_m 75°, intermediate fraction T_m 77°.

85.5°. From the shape of the melting curve, we think that this last value, 85.5°, is grossly overestimated. It is reasonable to assume that the transition steps in the melting profile could be accounted for by the melting of successive fractions of the repetitive DNA. Since the calculated GC content of the intermediate fraction is 38.7%, from which a T_m of 85.2° can be estimated (32), we conclude that the second inflection of the curve represents this fraction. Furthermore, the amount of this fraction which can be calculated from the melting profile is 40%, and this agrees with the estimates which can be obtained from the renaturation experiments. We also conclude that the T_m value of 74° corresponds to the melting of the fast fraction.

The melting-temperature curves of the fast and intermediate fractions isolated by the hydroxyapatite method are plotted in Fig. 6. The fast fraction shows a sharp profile with a T_m of 75°, similar to that shown in Fig. 5. Since this material has not been isolated as a native duplex, its native T_m is unknown. However, the shape of the curve indicates a high degree of base pairing in the renatured duplex. From its T_m, a tentative GC content for this fraction can be calculated as 15%. This is surely an underestimated value, due to a possible few percent mismatching, and because the relationship between T_m and GC% does not hold for less than 30% GC (32).

The intermediate fraction exhibits a much broader melting curve than does total native DNA. Its thermal stability (T_m value of 77°) is lower than expected [T_m 85.2°, previously calculated from its banding in CsCl (see above)]. This may arise from imprecise matching of nucleotides within the paired regions of the renatured DNA. From these data, we can calculate about 12% mismatching (33); this means that this is a family of related nucleotide sequences similar to but not identical to each other.

A good approach to the function of repetitive DNA fractions is to assay for their sequence homology with some specific RNA. For this purpose, we used RNA extracted from nuclei of salivary gland cells at the time of giant puff formation (25). Each isolated DNA fraction was immobilized in filters, and typical saturation curves are shown in Fig. 7. The data indicate that the intermediate fraction shows the highest hybridization level. The fast fraction also hybridizes significantly, but essentially no hybridization occurs with the slow fraction, as expected with the technique utilized. The hybridization level for the fast fraction is about 60% of that found for the intermediate fraction.

The isolation of DNA fractions by the hydroxyapatite technique is a very laborious procedure and cannot be assumed to yield pure fractions. Moreover, the prolonged treatment at high temperature leads to decreased molecular weights. This might affect the results, since, as pointed out by Melli and Bishop (34), differences in hybridization levels could reflect only differences in DNA molecular weight. In order to avoid this effect, the following experiment was designed. Slightly sheared DNA was allowed to renature, and at different $C_0 t$ values the DNA was fixed to membranes. For each $C_0 t$, four filters were

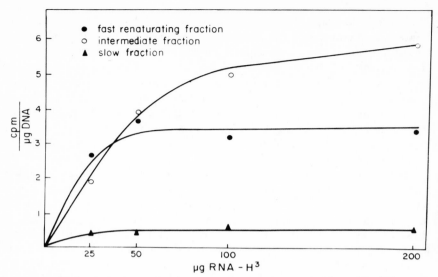

Fig. 7. Hybridization of isolated fractions of *Rhynchosciara* salivary gland DNA with nuclear[3]H-RNA. DNA fractions, isolated as described in *Methods,* were denatured, immobilized on nitrocellulose filters (approximately 20 μg per filter), and annealed with various concentrations of *Rhynchosciara* salivary gland nuclear[3]H-RNA, for 16 hr at 65°. •, fast fraction; ○, intermediate fraction; ▲, slow fraction.

prepared and these were hybridized with different concentrations of nuclear ^{3}H-RNA; we tried to approach saturation values according to Bishop *et al.* (35). The saturation values obtained were plotted against $\log C_0 t$ and are presented in Fig. 8. The curve obtained is similar to the $C_0 t$ plot of Britten and Kohne (8) and to the type (b) graph of Melli and Bishop (34). For this particular experiment, an aliquot of the DNA preparation was used for control optical renaturation experiments; these data are also plotted in Fig. 8, and from them we find $C_0 t_{1/2}$ values of 0.018 and 0.17 for the fast and intermediate fractions, respectively. Comparing these values with those obtained in the hybridization experiment, we see that, in this case, the $C_0 t_{1/2}$ for the second step, namely, 0.13, agrees quite well with the renaturation data. When a $C_0 t$ value large enough to result in renaturation of practically all repetitive DNA is attained, hybridization falls to zero, as expected under the conditions employed.

The data in Fig. 8 indicate that the hybridization of the fast fraction corresponds to 60% of that observed with the intermediate fraction. This is in good agreement with the values found in the hybridization experiment reported in Fig. 7. In Fig. 8, we also present data obtained by hybridization with *Rhynchosciara* ^{3}H-rRNA, which was used as a standard in an experiment similar to the one described. In this case, just one $C_0t_{1/2}$ value was obtained, in accord with the known complexity and reiteration values of *Rhynchosciara* rRNA cistrons (36).

In Fig. 9, we present the plot of the inverse of the hybridization values of *Rhynchosciara* DNA to nuclear ^{3}H-RNA against the inverse of RNA concentration, in the fashion suggested by Melli and Bishop (34). The data are for renaturation time equal to zero (totally denatured DNA) and for a DNA allowed to renature to a C_0t of 0.022, which corresponds to an almost total renaturation of the fast fraction. Two straight lines can be fitted to the first set of data, corresponding to hybridization of two components in the RNA fraction. In contrast, we can fit only one straight line to the second set of data, accounting for only the intermediate DNA fraction, which remained denatured and was able to hybridize under the conditions employed.

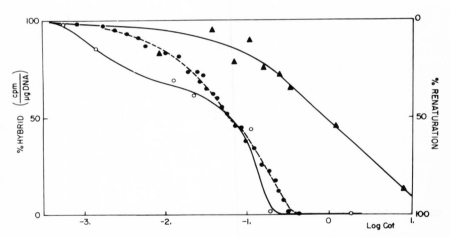

Fig. 8. Renaturation and hybridization of Rhynchosciara *salivary gland DNA with nuclear and ribosomal RNA.* Sheared, partially renatured DNA (samples of approximately 10 μg) to different C_0t values were annealed to four different concentrations of *Rhynchosciara* salivary gland nuclear ^{3}H-RNA for 16 hr at 65° or with saturation concentration of ^{3}H-rRNA for 3 hr at 65°, using the membrane method (24). Hybridization saturation value at each point is expressed as percentage of that at zero time and plotted against log C_0t. ○, Hybridization to nuclear ^{3}H-RNA; ▲, hybridization to ^{3}H-rRNA; ●, extent of renaturation of repetitive DNA, measured optically (the 14% corresponding to the repetitive sequences was normalized to 100%, as in Fig. 2). Left ordinate, percent of hybridization; right ordinate, percent of renaturation. Using the found $C_0t_{1/2}$ (0.83) for hybridization with rRNA and the Britten and Kohne formula (8), we find that the percentage of rRNA cistrons in *Rhynchosciara* DNA is 0.088 and that these cistrons are reiterated 52 times. These values are identical to those found, using a different method, for DNA from male larvae (36).

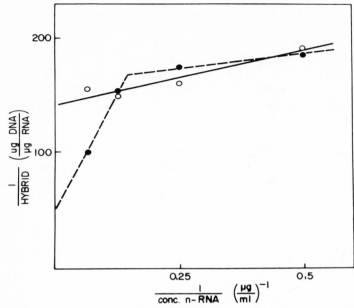

Fig. 9. Hybridization of Rhynchosciara *salivary gland nuclear RNA with total and partially denatured* Rhynchosciara *salivary gland DNA.* This is a double reciprocal plot (35) of data obtained in saturation hybridization experiments with totally denatured DNA (•) and with DNA renatured to a C_0t value of 0.022 (○). In the first case, the experiment indicates that two fractions are hybridizing, while after partial renaturation only one fraction is apparent.

CONCLUSIONS

The renaturation experiments have shown that the DNA haploid content of *R. angelae* salivary gland cells is about 48 times greater than that of *E. coli* cells. About 86% of the nucleotide sequences are not closely interrelated and renature with a k'_2 value (7) corresponding to a genome size of 1.3×10^{11} daltons. This value is remarkably similar to that reported for *Drosophila funebris* and twice as great as that for *Drosophila melanogaster* (37), which were obtained by methods similar to the ones we used; it is of the same order of magnitude as that found for *Sciara coprophila* by cytospectrophotometry [Rasch, quoted by Gerbi (27)] and for *Chironomus tentans,* calculated from Edstrom's data (38). The intra-genome homology, about 14%, is also in close agreement with what was found for other insect genomes (37) and is far lower than that found for mammalian DNA (8,9).

The *Rhynchosciara* repetitive DNA is distributed between at least two classes of sequences, namely, the fast and the intermediate fractions. The fast fraction is composed of sequences of 6.5×10^3 base pairs, repeated about 2×10^3 times, and the intermediate of 5.5×10^4 base pairs, repeated about 2.2×10^2 times. Clearly, these numbers are estimates and represent mean values. The size of the fast-renaturing family is less than that reported by Botchan *et al.* (39) for *D. melanogaster*. The complexity of each fraction and genome size have not been corrected for GC content, as contradictory evidence has been reported on its effect (7,40). The possibility of existence of another still faster renaturing fraction was tested by both optical and hydroxyapatite procedures. Negative results were obtained, even using conditions under which the velocity of renaturation was much lower. The nucleotide sequences of the intermediate fraction seem to diverge gradually; as shown in Fig. 1, the slope of the renaturation plot for this fraction decreases slowly, and no straight line can be fitted to the latter part of this curve. Moreover, the lower thermal stability of this fraction (Fig. 6) points to considerable heterogeneity in base sequence, leading to an imprecise matching of nucleotides. The situation is rather different for the fast fraction, for which the data indicate only a few percent mismatching (Fig. 6).

It is known that mismatched base pairs affect the DNA renaturation rate (13,41,42), leading to overestimates of complexity values. Clearly, in this respect, the intermediate fraction is more affected than the fast one. Using Southern's (41) relation for the intermediate fraction, which shows 12% of mismatching (see *Results*), we estimate that the k'_2 value obtained is about five times lower than expected.

The results presented in Figs. 4 and 5 indicate a striking difference in GC content between the fast and intermediate fractions. The buoyant density of the latter fraction (Fig. 4) indicates that these sequences band in CsCl density gradient in a region that includes the bands for ribosomal RNA cistrons (43) and histone messenger cistrons (44). The calculated complexity and reiteration values for these cistrons indicate that they must be contained in the intermediate fraction range (43,44).

The increased percent of renaturation found in the light regions of CsCl gradients (Fig. 4) is rather difficult to interpret. We have concluded from the melting curve of the isolated fast fraction (Fig. 6) that it has a very low GC content and should therefore band in this region. However, our data also clearly indicate that the fast fraction is not labeled at the period of larval life in which the studies were carried out. The observed increase in renaturation at the light regions of the gradient could be explained if the sequences of the fast fractions are contiguous to the intermediate or to the slow fraction, or to both (even if clustering occurs). This interpretation seems plausible, since hydroxyapatite adsorbs renatured DNA segments (in our case unlabeled) attached to single-stranded regions (in our case labeled) (8). However, it cannot be neglected that the renaturation observed might be due to the fast fraction itself. If the labeling of this fraction is very small, it would be undetected in $C_0 t$ plots such as that presented in Fig. 3. Because of the buoyant density of this fraction, its concentration is increased in the light regions of the gradient, and then its renaturation would be detected.

Our fast fraction very likely corresponds to the satellite having a T_m of 76.7° and buoyant density of 1.780 g/cm^3 which Eckhardt and Gall (29) detected with male adult DNA in *R. hollenderi,* a species very closely related to *R. angelae.*

Several different reports have shown that during the polytenization process, part of the chromosomal DNA content, corresponding to heterochromatic regions, is underreplicated (45-48). The undetected replication of fast fraction DNA at the time of giant puffs suggests that this class may represent the underreplicated heterochromatic DNA.

Satellite DNAs of many organisms, which consists of homogeneous, repetitive sequences, have been located in the centromeric heterochromatin. These include satellite DNAs of the mouse (49,50), *Plethodon* (51), *Drosophila* (52,53,39,), *R. hollenderi* (29), and *R. angelae* (54). In a recent paper, Gall *et al.* (55) have shown that satellite sequences are more abundant in diploid than polytene nuclei and suggest that this may be due to the differential synthesis in heterochromatic regions. It is plausible to assume that the fast fraction in *R. angelae* salivary gland DNA corresponds to the unreplicated centromeric α-heterochromatin (45), underrepresented in the polytene nuclei but present in a large enough amount in total adult DNA to appear as a visible satellite (29).

The replicative β-heterochromatin, which contains repetitive sequences, may be represented by at least part of the intermediate fraction. It is well known that ribosomal RNA cistrons are located in the heterochromatic regions of polytene chromosomes in *Sciara* (27) and *Rhynchosciara* (56).

At present, our understanding of the function of repetitive DNA is very poor. Some models argue for its importance in control mechanisms (57,58). There is evidence that the highly repetitive rodent satellite is not transcribed (11), suggesting a structural function for this DNA (14). Repeated sequences have been related to ribosomal RNA synthesis (59) and, in a few cases, to the synthesis of specific proteins (44,60). Our data show that the repeated DNAs have complementary sites to nuclear RNA. The $C_0 t_{1/2}$ value obtained for the intermediate fraction in the hybridization experiment (Fig. 8) is very similar to that of renaturation experiments. This may suggest that most sequences in this fraction are transcribed into nuclear RNA.

The $C_0 t_{1/2}$ value for the fast fraction in the hybridization experiments (Fig. 8) is much lower than that for renaturation. This would occur if only the most repeated sequences of this fraction are hybridizing. A further indication that this fraction is not totally transcribed is the fact that, whereas its amount is nearly equal to that of the intermediate fraction, its hybridization is only 60% of that observed with this fraction.

The intermediate fraction plays an important role in the metabolism of informational macromolecules. The calculated reiteration for rDNA (43) and histone DNA (44) indicates that these cistrons are contained in this fraction. Previous work from this laboratory indicated that the amplification occurring at the time of giant DNA puff appearance is related to repetitive DNA which is transcribed into nuclear RNA sequences (5). Since the intermediate fraction is the only repetitive fraction replicating at the time of giant puff formation, we can now conclude that this fraction is very probably involved in the amplification phenomenon.

ACKNOWLEDGMENTS

This work was supported by funds from the "Fundacão de Amparo à Pesquisa do Estado de São Paulo" and from the Multinational Biochemistry Program of the Organization of American States. J. M. H. is a Visiting Investigator from Uruguay under this Program; M. L. B. was a Visiting Professor under this Program during July-September 1969; J. B. is a predoctoral fellow of the "Fundacão de Amparo à Pesquisa do Estado de São Paulo." We thank Dr. Fernando Gallenbeck from the Chemistry Institute, University of São Paulo, for help in the analysis of the renaturation data, Dr. A. G. Gambarini from our department for preparing *Rhynchosciara* rRNA, Mr. José Reis Coelho for the maintenance of the *Rhynchosciara* cultures, and Miss Yvone de Abreu for typing the manuscript.

Preliminary accounts of this work were presented both at the Second Annual Meeting of the "Sociedade Brasileira de Bioquìmica," held jointly with the Twenty-second Annual Meeting of the "Sociedade Brasileira para o Progresso da Ciéncia," Salvador, Bahia, Brazil, July 1970, and at Session IX, Biochemistry of Differentiation and Development, Eighth International Congress of Biochemistry, Montreux, Switzerland, September 1970.

SUMMARY

Kinetic measurements indicate the existence of three DNA classes in *Rhynchosciara angelae* salivary gland DNA. The slowest-renaturing fraction, composed of unique sequences and corresponding to 86% of the genome, renatures with a second-order rate constant equivalent to a genome size of 1.3×10^{11} daltons. It was estimated that the fastest-renaturing fraction (7.3% of the genome) is composed of about 2×10^3 copies of sequences of 3.9×10^6 daltons and that the fraction renaturing with an intermediate velocity (6.7% of the genome) is composed of about 2.2×10^2 copies of sequences of 3.3×10^7 daltons.

At the time of appearance of the giant chromosomal puff, it was not possible to detect replication of the fast-renaturing fraction. It is likely that this fraction represents the centromeric a-heterochromatic sequences.

Hybridization experiments with nuclear RNA obtained at the time of giant DNA puff formation lead us to suggest that part (60%) of the fastest-renaturing fraction and most of the intermediate fraction are transcribed. Our data indicate that the sequences undergoing amplification at this stage belong to the intermediate fraction.

RESUMEN

El estudio de la cinética de renaturalización del DNA de glándulas salivares de *Rhynchosciara angelae,* muestra la existencia de tres clases de DNA. La fracción de más lenta renaturalización, compuesta de secuencias únicas, representa 86% del genomio y renaturaliza con una constante de velocidad de segundo orden equivalente a un tamaño de genomio de 1.3×10^{11} daltons.

Se ha estimado que la fracción de renaturalización más rápida (7.3% del genomio), está compuesta de aproximadamente 2.0×10^3 copias de secuencias de 3.9×10^6 daltons, y que la fracción que renaturaliza con una velocidad intermedia (6.7% del genomio), está compuesta de aproximadamente 2.2×10^2 copias de secuencias de 3.3×10^7 daltons.

En la época de la aparición de los "puffs" cromosómicos gigantes no fue posible detectar replicación de la fracción de renaturalización rápida. Es probable que esta fracción represente las secuencias de α-heterocromatina del centrómero.

Experimentos de hibridización con RNA nuclear, obtenido en el momento de la formación de los "puffs" gigantes de DNA, nos permite sugerir que se transcribe parte (60%) de la fracción de renaturalización rápida, y la mayor parte de la fracción intermedia. Nuestros datos indican que las secuencias que están sufriendo amplificación en esta etapa, pertenecen a la fracción intermedia.

REFERENCES

1. Breuer, M. E., and Pavan, C., *Chromosoma, 7,* 371 (1955).
2. Ficq, A., and Pavan, C., *Nature, 180,* 983 (1957).
3. Rudkin, G. T., and Corlette, S. L., *Proc. Natl. Acad. Sci. U.S.A., 43,* 964 (1957).
4. Crouse, H. V., and Keyl, H. G., *Chromosoma, 25,* 357 (1968).
5. Meneghini, R., Armelin, H. A., Bálsamo, J., and Lara, F. J. S., *J. Cell Biol., 49,* 913 (1971).
6. Thrower, K. J., and Peacock, A. R., *Biochem. J., 109,* 543 (1968).
7. Wetmur, J. G., and Davidson, N., *J. Mol. Biol., 31,* 349 (1968).
8. Britten, R. J., and Kohne, D. E., *Carnegie Inst. Wash. Yearbook, 65,* 78 (1967).
9. Britten, R. J., and Kohne, D. E., *Science, 161,* 529 (1968).
10. Waring, M., and Britten, R. J., *Science, 154,* 791 (1966).
11. Flamm, W. G., Walker, P. M. B., and McCallum, M., *J. Mol. Biol., 40,* 423 (1969).
12. Flamm, W. G., Walker, P. M. B., and McCallum, M., *J. Mol. Biol., 42,* 441 (1969).
13. Southern, E. M., *Nature, 227,* 794 (1970).
14. Walker, P. M. B., *Nature, 219,* 228 (1968).
15. Melli, M., and Bishop, J. O., *J. Mol. Biol., 40,* 117 (1969).
16. Lara, F. J. S., Tamaki, H., and Pavan, C., *Am. Naturalist, 99,* 189 (1965).
17. Terra, W. R., Bianchi, A. G., Gambarini, A. G., and Lara, F. J. S., manuscript in preparation.
18. Armelin, H. A., Meneghini, R., and Lara, F. J. S., *Genetics, 61,* Suppl. 1, 351 (1969).
19. Meneghini, R., and Cordeiro, M., *Cell Diff., 1,* 167 (1972).
20. Marmur, J., *J. Mol. Biol., 3,* 208 (1961).
21. Vinograd, J., and Hearst, J. E., *Fortschr. Chem. Organ. Naturstoffe, 20,* 373 (1962).
22. Studier, F. W., *J. Mol. Biol., 11,* 373 (1965).

23. Miyazawa, Y., and Thomas, C. A., Jr., *J. Mol. Biol., 11*, 223 (1965).
24. Gillespie, D., and Spiegelman, S., *J. Mol. Biol., 12*, 829 (1965).
25. Armelin, H. A., Meneghini, R., Marquez, N., and Lara, F. J. S., *Biochim. Biophys. Acta, 217*, 426 (1970).
26. Wells, R., and Birnstiel, M., *Biochem. J., 122*, 777 (1969).
27. Gerbi, S. A., *J. Mol. Biol., 58*, 499 (1971).
28. Corneo, G., Ginelli, E., and Polli, E., *Biochemistry, 9*, 1565 (1970).
29. Eckhardt, R. A., and Gall, J. G., *Chromosoma, 32*, 407 (1971).
30. Szybalski, W., personal communication.
31. Schildkraut, C. L., Marmur, J., and Doty, P., *J. Mol. Biol., 4*, 430 (1962).
32. Marmur, J., and Doty, P., *J. Mol. Biol., 5*, 109 (1962).
33. Laird, C. D., McConaughy, B. L., and McCarthy, B. J., *Nature, 224*, 149 (1969).
34. Melli, M., and Bishop, J. O., *Biochem. J., 120*, 225 (1970).
35. Bishop, J. O., Robertson, F. W., Burns, J. A., and Melli, M., *Biochem. J., 115*, 361 (1969).
36. Gambarini, A. G., Birnstiel, M. L., and Lara, F. J. S., unpublished results.
37. Laird, D. C., and McCarthy, B. J., *Genetics, 63*, 865 (1969).
38. Edstrom, J. E., *Symposium of the Society for the Study of Development and Growth*, Vol. 23, in Locke, M. (ed.), Academic Press, New York (1964).
39. Botchan, M., Kram, R., Schmid, C. W., and Hearst, J. E., *Proc. Natl. Acad. Sci. U.S.A., 68*, 1125 (1971).
40. Gillis, M., De Ley, J., and De Cleene, M., *Europ. J. Biochem., 12*, 143 (1970).
41. Southern, E. M., *Nature New Biol., 232*, 82 (1971).
42. Sutton, W. D., and McCallum, M., *Nature New Biol., 232*, 83 (1971).
43. Gambarini, A. G., and Meneghini, R., *J. Cell Biol., 54*, 421 (1972).
44. Kedes, L. H., and Birnstiel, M., *Nature New Biol., 230*, 165 (1971).
45. Heitz, E., *Biol. Zbl., 54*, 588 (1934).
46. Rudkin, G. T., *Genetics Today (Proc. XIth Internat. Congr. Genet.)*, Pergamon Press, Oxford. (1970), p. 361.
47. Berendes, H. D., and Keyl, H. G., *Genetics, 57*, 1 (1967).
48. Mulder, M. P., van Duijn, P., and Gloor, H. J., *Genetica ('s Gravenhage), 39*, 385 (1968).
49. Pardue, M. L., and Gall, J. G., *Science, 168*, 1356 (1970).
50. Jones, K. W., *Nature, 225*, 912 (1970).
51. McGregor, H. C., and Kezer, J., *Chromosoma, 33*, 167 (1971).
52. Rae, P. M. M., *Proc. Natl. Acad. Sci. U.S.A., 67*, 1018 (1970).
53. Jones, K. W., and Robertson, F. W., *Chromosoma, 31*, 331 (1970).
54. Díaz, M., unpublished results.
55. Gall, J. G., Cohen, E. H., and Lake Polan, M., *Chromosoma, 33*, 319 (1971).
56. Pardue, M. L., Gerbi, S. A., Eckhardt, R. A., and Gall, J. G., *Chromosoma, 29*, 268 (1970).
57. Britten, R. J., and Davidson, E. H., *Science, 165*, 349 (1969).
58. Georgiev, G. P., *J. Theoret. Biol., 25*, 473 (1969).
59. Birnstiel, M., Grunstein, M., Speirs, J., and Henning, W., *Nature, 223*, 1265 (1969).
60. Williamson, R., Lanyon, G., Eason, R., and Paul, J., *Biochemistry, 10*, 3014 (1971).

DISCUSSION

E. Sánchez de Jiménez (Mexico City, Mexico): What is the molecular size of the DNA used in the renaturation experiments, and how did you fix this DNA in the nitrocellulose membranes?

J. Bálsamo (São Paulo, Brazil): The DNA was about 1 million daltons.

E. Sánchez de Jiménez: ,What percentage of the DNA of 1 million molecular weight is fixed in nitrocellulose membranes?

J. Bálsamo: Ninety percent.

R. Soeiro (New York, U.S.A.): What is the source of the labeled RNA you used?

F. J. S. Lara: The RNA used for these experiments was nuclear RNA obtained from glands at the time of appearance of the giant DNA puff; what we call period V of the fourth instar. Larvae are injected with ^{3}H-uridine, and incorporation proceeds for 3 hr; then we separate nuclei and extract the RNA and structural RNA.

R. Soeiro: Was there any difference in the RNA from the time of one puff to another puff?

F. J. S. Lara: We have not tested for this as yet. We do know that RNA obtained at giant DNA puff formation is enriched for copies transcribed from the amplified regions, as compared with RNA obtained when no such puffs are present. In competition experiments, we do not see any difference within this group population.

N. O. Bianchi (Llavallol, Argentina): In mammals, there are two kinds of repetitive DNA, one type which is made up of short sequences of DNA, repeated a large number of times (for example, 1 million). Such repetitive DNA is found in mice, guinea pigs, and African green monkeys and represents 10-15% of the genome. The other type is composed of long sequences of DNA repeated a small number of times (no more than 16,000-30,000). A typical example is calf, in which 38% of the genome is represented by this type of repetitive DNA. The first type is usually not transcribed, and the second type is transcribed. My question is about your fast-renaturing type of repetitive DNA: do you have any clues about how many times it is repeated, and how long is the sequence?

F. J. S. Lara: The fast fraction is composed of sequences 6.5×10^3 base pairs long, repeated 2000 times; the intermediate fraction is composed of sequences 5.3×10^4 base pairs long, repeated 200 times. The denaturation data of isolated fractions suggest that the fast-renaturing fraction is very homogeneous, whereas the intermediate fraction is fairly heterogeneous.

The last two pieces of data show denaturation profiles of the isolated fractions; the first fraction shows a very sharp rise, which indicates that it is very homogeneous, whereas for the intermediate fraction there is a rather broad range. One of the things that we would like to do now is to fractionate the intermediate fraction by thermal chromatography; then we would like to transcribe these fractions and carry out *in situ* hybridization.

N. O. Bianchi: In *Triturus,* it is known that repetitive fractions are located in the centromere regions of the chromosome. I wonder if you have any idea if this type of repetitive fraction is also located in the centromere region?

F. J. S. Lara: Our fast fraction should correspond to the satellite found by Eckhardt and Gall. They have worked with adult flies and were able to pick this up because in the adult, and in embryonic tissues, too, the α-heterochromatin in the chromosome makes up a much greater part of the genome, as compared with polytenic tissue. We found that in the salivary gland this fraction is not replicated at the time of giant puff formation and so it gets proportionally smaller and smaller. This is why we do not pick out the satellite with the salivary gland DNA. However, direct proof of the identity of our fast fraction with Eckhardt and Gall's satellite would be obtained only by transcribing this fraction and then carrying out *in situ* hybridization. There is already evidence indicating this identity, since the T_m of this fraction indicates that its buoyant density is similar to that of the satellite.

10

Hormonal Regulation of Ovalbumin Synthesis in Chick Oviduct

R. T. Schimke, R. Palacios, R. D. Palmiter, and R. E. Rhoads

Department of Pharmacology
Stanford University School of Medicine
Stanford, California, U.S.A.

Estrogens and progesterone regulate the differentiation and function of chick oviduct (1-4). Our attention has been focused on hormonal regulation of ovalbumin synthesis, since this single polypeptide comprises 50-60% of the protein synthesized in the fully differentiated oviduct. This feature allows potentially for isolation of the molecular elements involved in specific protein synthesis, including specific polysomes, mRNA, and genes, and an analysis of various regulatory steps between transcription and translation of specific mRNAs, as affected by developmental and hormonal variables.

Figure 1 depicts schematically the effects of estrogen and progesterone on oviduct development and function. Estrogen administration to immature chicks results in cytodifferentiation of tubular gland cells, which synthesize ovalbumin. We call this primary stimulation. If its administration is stopped, the cells remain but cease ovalbumin synthesis (1,2,5). We have shown that reinitiation of ovalbumin synthesis in "inactive" cells, called secondary stimulation, can occur on pre-existing ribosomes and that both estrogen and progesterone can produce this effect (5). In contrast, concomitant administration of progesterone with estrogen prevents the typical cytodifferentiation. Rather, an abortive synthesis of ovalbumin in surface cells occurs, but such cells fail to undergo typical changes resulting in formation of tubular gland cells (4).

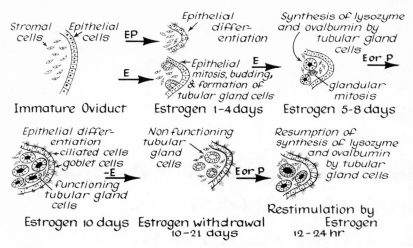

Fig. 1. *Hormone interactions in development and function of tubular gland cells of chick oviduct. E, estrogen, P, progesterone.*

In this report, we describe more recent studies on regulation of ovalbumin synthesis in this system.

MECHANISM OF "SUPERINDUCTION" OF OVALBUMIN BY ACTINOMYCIN D

Figure 2 depicts the effect of estrogen administration to chicks on the percent of protein synthesized that is ovalbumin, as measured by combined isotopic and immunological procedures (see figure caption for details) (6). As with essentially every instance of steroid hormone induction of specific protein synthesis (7), the concomitant administration of actinomycin D with estrogen prevents the increased synthesis of ovalbumin, as studied during secondary hormone stimulation (8). Figure 2 shows that once the tissue is actively synthesizing ovalbumin, administration of actinomycin D to the intact chick (or to explants in culture) increases the proportion of protein synthesized that is ovalbumin. A comparable phenomenon occurs with another egg protein, conalbumin (6). These findings are comparable to a number of examples in which the administration of actinomycin D to cells or animals actively synthesizing a specific protein (enzyme) actually increases enzyme activity. Garren *et al.* (9) coined the term "superinduction" to describe this phenomenon. It has been studied most extensively for tyrosine aminotransferase in cultured hepatoma cells. Reel and Kenney (10) have provided evidence that the actinomycin D induced accumulation of activity results from a greater effect of this drug in inhibiting degradation of the enzyme than in inhibiting its synthesis. Tomkins *et al.* (11), on the other hand, have proposed that the effect is solely on the synthesis of the enzyme. They have proposed further that the increased rate of specific enzyme synthesis results from an "unmasking" of previously inactive mRNA.

Since we are determining the rate of synthesis of ovalbumin, and this protein

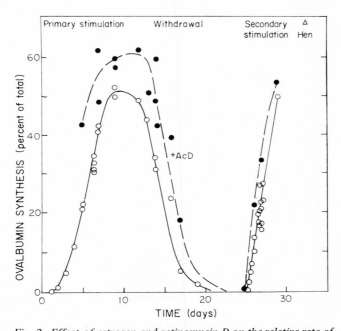

Fig. 2. *Effect of estrogen and actinomycin D on the relative rate of synthesis of ovalbumin in chick oviduct during primary stimulation, withdrawal, and secondary stimulation.* Immature chicks 4 days old were injected intramuscularly with 1 mg estradiol benzoate daily (primary stimulation), and after 10 days without estrogen admini- stration (withdrawal) administration was resumed (secondary stimu- lation). Chicks in groups of two to four were injected with actino- mycin D (5 mg/kg) for 4-5 hr prior to isolating oviducts. Fragments of oviduct were then incubated in Hanks' salt solution for 1 hr with ^{3}H amino acids (10 μc/ml). Following homogenization and centrifu- gation at $100,000 \times g$ for 1 hr, ovalbumin was precipitated from the supernatant using a specific antibody. Results are presented as percent of total acid-precipitable radioactivity in supernatant that is precipitated immunologically with antiovalbumin antibody. Details are given in Palmiter and Schimke (6). ○, Estrogen; ●, estrogen plus actinomycin D 4 hr before killing.

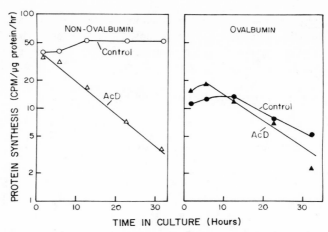

Fig. 3. The effect of actinomycin D on ovalbumin and nonovalbumin synthesis in oviduct explants. Oviduct tissue from chicks which received 25 hr of secondary estrogen stimulation was pooled and cultured in medium 199 for 32 hr. Half of the cultures contained actinomycin D at 10 μg/ml. At times indicated, to both control and actinomycin D treated cultures were added ^{3}H amino acids for 1 hr. Radioactivity incorporated into supernatant and ovalbumin was determined as described in Fig. 2, based on total supernatant protein. See Palmiter *et al.* (8) for details.

turns over slowly (8), we are dealing with an effect of actinomycin D on the rate of ovalbumin synthesis. We propose that the so-called superinduction results from two general properties of protein synthesis in this system: (a) there is differential stability of different mRNA species, and (b) the absolute rate of total protein synthesis in the system is limited by a factor common to all protein synthesis. That there is differential mRNA stability is indicated in the experiment outlined in Fig. 3, which shows that the synthesis of ovalbumin in explants is not affected by the addition of actinomycin D, whereas the synthesis of nonspecific proteins decays with a half-life of approximately 4-6 hr following actinomycin D addition. Thus the actinomycin D "superinduction" (Fig. 2) can in large part be explained by the fact that ovalbumin now constitutes a greater proportion of protein synthesized as a result of the decay of relatively unstable mRNA species. However, this alone does not explain "superinduction," since there is also an absolute increase in the rate of ovalbumin synthesis, although there is either no increase or a slight decrease in the rate of total protein synthesis following actinomycin D treatment of intact chicks (6). The absolute increase in ovalbumin symthesis is consistent with there being more mRNAs for ovalbumin. However, the observation can also be explained by a more rapid translation of the remaining mRNA species.

Our results indicate that following treatment with actinomycin D, peptide chain elongation by the polysomes that remain is more rapid. This is indicated in Fig. 4, which shows the short-term incorporation of isotope into total protein (open circles) and into total protein minus radioactivity associated with polysomes, i.e., nascent chains. The difference between these two time courses is a measure of the average transit time for protein synthesis. This time for polysomes from control tissues is approximately 20% greater than with the polysomes remaining after actinomycin D. Since the sizes of the proteins being synthesized in the two instances are similar, and the sizes of the polysomes are similar in control and actinomycin D treated tissues (6), we conclude that the increase in absolute rate of ovalbumin synthesis can be explained by an increased rate of peptide chain elongation. Thus, following actinomycin D treatment, there is an increase in the proportion of ovalbumin synthesis because of the degradation of unstable mRNAs. In addition, there is an increased rate of translation of the remaining mRNAs, since there is now less competition of such mRNAs for rate-limiting factor(s), presumably affecting peptide chain elongation.

That there is no increase in ovalbumin mRNA content following actinomycin D treatment is supported by a recent experiment indicating that there is no difference in the amount of ^{125}I-antiovalbumin bound to polysomes isolated from control and actinomycin D treated tissues (6). (See following section for discussion of this technique.)

ASSAY OF OVALBUMIN mRNA IN RABBIT RETICULOCYTE LYSATES

The desirability of a method for the assay of specific mRNA for purposes of both its isolation and its quantification in various developmental and hormonal states is obvious. We are able to synthesize ovalbumin in a rabbit reticulocyte lysate system, employing various crude and partially purified oviduct RNA fractions. The ovalbumin synthesized is isolated by immunoprecipitation (12). Figure 5A shows that no radioactivity is incorporated into immunospecific protein in the absence of added oviduct RNA. Marker ovalbumin is added to show its electrophoretic properties (open circles). Figure 5B shows radioactivity precipitated by the antibody when RNA isolated from total oviduct polysomes is added to the reticulocyte lysate. Ovalbumin can account for as much as 10% of the amino acid incorporation obtained in this system. Figure 5C shows the electrophoretic pattern of total labeled lysate protein in the absence of added oviduct RNA and shows that the vast majority of radioactivity is incorporated into globin chains and that no protein with a mobility of ovalbumin is present. The identity of the oviduct RNA-directed product as ovalbumin has been further demonstrated by the similarity of tryptic peptides of ovalbumin labeled in the reticulocyte lysate system to those of authentic ovalbumin as displayed by

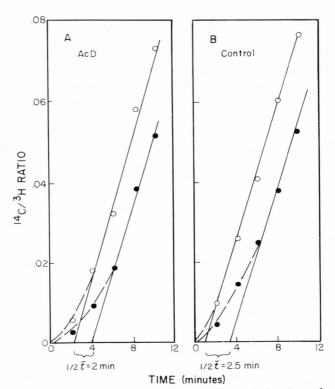

Fig. 4. Determination of the average mRNA transit time (rate of elongation) in control oviduct explants (B) and explants incubated in culture with actinomycin D (A). Explants of oviduct magnum obtained from chicks receiving 5 days of primary estrogen stimulation were incubated 5 hr in Hanks' or Hanks' plus actinomycin D (10 μg/ml). A mixture of ^{3}H amino acids (10 μc/ml) was added after 3 hr in culture. Then at 5 hr ^{14}C amino acids were added, and explants were removed at approximately 2 min intervals and placed on ice. The tissue was homogenized with detergents as in the preparation of polysomes and centrifuged 5 min at 30,000 × g. Aliquots of the supernatant, containing both soluble proteins and solubilized polysomes containing nascent chains, were precipitated with 5% TCA, collected on filters, washed with 5% TCA, dissolved in NCS, and counted. The remainder of the supernatant was centrifuged 2 hr at 105,000 × g to remove polysomes, and aliquots of that supernatant were precipitated with 5% TCA and counted as above. The ratios of ^{14}C in both the first (○) and second (⊙) supernatant to the ^{3}H radioactivity in the first supernatant are plotted. The horizontal distance between the two curves equals one half of the average mRNA transit time (19). Ratios of ^{14}C to ^{3}H were plotted to control for differences in the size of the oviduct fragments homogenized at each time point; i.e., the ^{3}H

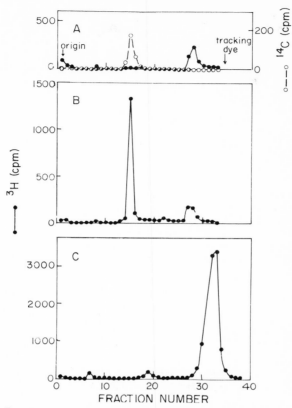

Fig. 5. SDS-acrylamide gel electrophoresis of products of protein synthesis in rabbit reticulocyte lysates. The reticulo-cyte lysate system is described by Rhoads *et al.* (12). (A) Reaction mixture contained ^{14}C-ovalbumin, prepared in ovi-duct explants (8), but no oviduct RNA. Radioactivity is that precipitated with ovalbumin antibody and electrophoresed after dissociation in SDS and dithiothreitol. (B) Reaction mixture contained 40 µg/ml of oviduct polysomal RNA, prepared by centrifugation of polysomes in a linear sucrose gradient in the presence of SDS. That fraction sedimenting between 14S and 20S was precipitated several times with ethanol. Radioactivity is that present in the ovalbumin immu-noprecipitate. (C) Radioactivity incorporated into total pro-tein in the absence of added oviduct RNA and precipitated with TCA before solution in SDS. Details are given by Rhoads *et al.* (12).

counts represent essentially a measure of total protein. Acid-insoluble ^{3}H radioactivity was between 50,000 and 70,000 cpm (35% efficiency) in all samples.

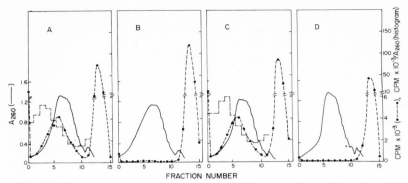

Fig. 6. Binding of [125] *I-antiovalbumin and* [125] *I-anti-BSA to hen oviduct polysomes.*
Polysomes (10 A_{260} units in 1.0 ml) were incubated at 4° with (A) 30 μg of
[125]I-antiovalbumin for 30 min, (B) 500 μg of unlabeled antiovalbumin for 30 min
followed by 30 μg of ^{125}I-antiovalbumin for 30 min more, (C) 500 μg of unlabeled
anti-BSA for 30 min followed by 30 μg of ^{125}I-antiovalbumin for 30 min, and (D)
30 μg of ^{125}I-anti-BSA for 30 min. After the incubation, the polysomes were layered
over a continuous sucrose gradient and centrifuged. Fractions (1.0 ml) were collected
to measure specific activity and radioactivity. See Palacios *et al.* (17) for details.

ion-exchange column chromatography (8). Ovalbumin is therefore the third
eukaryotic protein to be synthesized in a heterologous cell-free system (13–16).

IMMUNOLOGICAL IDENTIFICATION AND PRECIPITATION
OF OVALBUMIN-SYNTHESIZING POLYSOMES

The ability to obtain ovalbumin-synthesizing polysomes specifically will
assist in the isolation of specific mRNA and in the assessment of possible specific
regulatory proteins involved in translational control of ovalbumin synthesis. We
have developed methods that allow for specific binding of antiovalbumin antibody to oviduct polysomes and for the specific precipitation of these polysomes.
Figure 6 indicates the specificity of the binding of ^{125}I-antiovalbumin
γ-globulin to polysomes prepared in a manner that removes monosomes and a
small fraction of the small polysomes and that leaves the remaining polysomes in
an undergraded state. Figure 6A shows the binding of 30 μg of
[125]I-antiovalbumin, indicating binding particularly to the polysomes with an
estimated 12 ribosomes, the size class of polysomes which would be expected to
synthesize a protein of the molecular weight of ovalbumin (42,000). That the
sites for antibody binding can be saturated is shown in Fig. 6B, where the
polysomes are first incubated with 500 μg of unlabeled antiovalbumin antibody
before the addition of labeled antibody. In this case, no binding in the polysome
region is present. If, on the other hand, the tissue is first incubated with 500 μg

of antibody directed against bovine serum albumin, the specific binding by antiovalbum is not diminished (Fig. 6C). Figure 6D shows that labeled anti-bovine serum albumin antibody does not bind to oviduct polysomes. Likewise, the labeled antiovalbumin antibody does not bind to polysomes from hen brain or liver. In addition, the binding is not the result of adsorbed ovalbumin from supernatant, since the mixing of liver polysomes with hen oviduct supernatant,

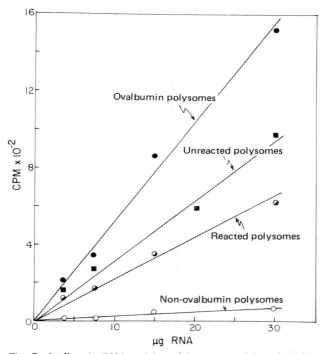

Fig. 7. *Ovalbumin RNA activity of immunoprecipitated oviduct polysomes.* Hen oviduct polysomes (80 A_{260} units) were incubated with 14 mg of antiovalbumin γ-globulin for 30 min at 4°, followed by 1.9 mg of ovalbumin for 30 min, and finally 42 mg of additional antibody for 30 min. The precipitate was collected by centrifugation through 1.0 M sucrose. RNA was extracted from the precipitated polysomes (●), from the unreacted polysomes (■), from the total reaction misture with all additions, but without precipitation (◑), and from polysomes remaining after immunoprecipitation (○). RNA was extracted using SDS at 25° with precipitation by ethanol. RNA was dissolved in 0.085 M Tris-Cl, pH 7.5, containing 0.01 M NaCl, and various amounts were added to rabbit reticulocyte lysate as described in Fig. 5 and Rhoads *et al.* (12). Details are given in Palmiter *et al.* (18).

which contains large amounts of ovalbumin, prior to polysome preparation did not result in binding of labeled antibody to liver polysomes.

By addition of antiovalbumin, then ovalbumin, and subsequently more antiovalbumin antibody, sufficient cross-linking occurs so that ovalbumin polysomes can be precipitated. In this technique, centrifugation through 1.0 M sucrose has been found necessary to ensure that nonspecific cosedimentation of polysomes does not occur. An anti-bovine serum albumin antibody reaction has served as a control in all experiments. That such immunoprecipitation enriches for mRNA activity is shown in the results of Fig. 7, in which RNAs prepared from various fractions during immunoprecipitation are compared for ability to encode for ovalbumin synthesis in the rabbit reticulocyte lysate system. From comparison of total polysomal RNA before and after incubation with antibody, i.e., reacted and nonreacted polysomes, there would appear to be some mRNA inactivation resulting from the incubation procedures. More important, however, is the finding of the twofold increase in specific activity of the RNA isolated from specifically immunoprecipitable polysomes. RNA isolated from polysomes remaining after immunoprecipitation is essentially incapable of directing ovalbumin synthesis. Inasmuch as ovalbumin constitutes 50% of the protein synthesized by this tissue, a twofold increase in specific activity is all that one can expect of this experiment. We are currently developing methods to separate the mRNA from ribosomal RNA.

CONCLUSIONS

The results presented have provided a simple explanation for the mechanism of "superinduction" by actinomycin D in this system. More importantly, our results give promise of allowing for the isolation of specific mRNA for ovalbumin, based on the existence of a suitable assay, and the ability to isolate specifically those polysomes that synthesize ovalbumin. With such an mRNA in hand, it will be possible to answer fundamental questions concerning hormonal regulation of differentiation and cell function, including, for example, effects on specific mRNA synthesis, gene amplification, and facilitation of transport of mRNA from nucleus to cytoplasm. In addition, the techniques developed should be applicable to the isolation of mRNAs that are present in smaller amounts than that for ovalbumin and hence allow for a more profound understanding of the role of specific nucleic acids in the regulation of cell development and function.

ACKNOWLEDGMENTS

This work was supported by research grant GM 14931 from the National Institutes of Health, Public Health Service International Research Fellowship

F05 TW 1601, and research grant P427c and postdoctoral fellowship PF-625 from the American Cancer Society.

SUMMARY

Estrogens and progesterone regulate the differentiation and function of chick oviduct. Our attention has been focused on hormonal regulation of ovalbumin synthesis, since this single polypeptide comprises 50-60% of protein synthesized by the fully differentiated oviduct. This feature allows for the potential isolation of molecular elements involved in specific protein synthesis, i.e., polysomes, mRNA, genes, etc. Estrogen administration to immature chicks results in cytodifferentiation of tubular gland cells, which synthesize ovalbumin. If its administration is stopped, the cells remain but cease ovalbumin synthesis. We have shown that the reinitiation of ovalbumin synthesis in such "inactive" cells can occur on pre-existing ribosomes and that both estrogen and progesterone can produce this effect (5).

We are able to label specifically those polysomes synthesizing ovalbumin with ^{125}I-labeled ovalbumin antibody, to quantitate the number of these polysomes, and to relate this to the rate of ovalbumin synthesis *in vivo*. Our studies indicate that steroid hormones affect the concentration of translatable mRNA, the rate of peptide chain initiation, and the rate of peptide elongation, depending on the hormonal state of the tissue. Actinomycin D blocks the induction of ovalbumin, but once induced (by hormone) it produces "superinduction" (an increase in ovalbumin synthesis), which can be explained on the basis of a long-lived mRNA for ovalbumin, and an accelerated rate of peptide chain elongation.

We are also able to obtain synthesis of ovalbumin in a rabbit reticulocyte lysate using RNA isolated from oviduct. With this assay, we are now quantitating the amount of mRNA present under various hormonal conditions and comparing this with the rate of ovalbumin synthesis *in vivo*.

The oviduct synthesizes various egg-white proteins in addition to ovalbumin, including conalbumin, lysozyme, and ovomucoid. Estrogen and progesterone do not regulate the synthesis of all these proteins coordinately, suggesting that their synthesis is regulated independently. This raises questions as to the number of hormone receptors and the mechanism of action of these receptors.

RESUMEN

Los estrógenos y la progesterona regulan la diferenciación y la función del oviducto de pollo. Hemos centrado nuestro interés en la regulación hormonal de la síntesis de ovoalbúmina ya que este polipéptido en particular constituye el 50-60% de la proteína sintetizada por el oviducto completamente diferenciado. Esta característica permitiría el aislamiento de los elementos moleculares que participan en la síntesis proteica específica; es decir, polisomas, RNA mensajero, genes, etc. La administración de estrógenos a gallinas inmaduras conduce a la diferenciación celular de las células de las glándulas tubulares, que sintetizan ovoalbúmina. Si esta administración cesa, las células permanecen, pero la síntesis de ovoalbúmina se detiene. Hemos demostrado que la reiniciación de la síntesis de ovoalbúmina en estas "células inactivas" puede tener lugar en ribosomas pre-existentes, y que tanto el estrógeno como la progesterona pueden producir dicho effecto (5).

Hemos conseguido marcar específicamente los polisomas que sintetizan ovoalbúmina con anticuerpos antiovoalbúmina marcados con ^{125}I, y de este modo cuantificar el número de estos polisomas y relacionar este parámetro a la velocidad de síntesis de ovoalbúmina *in vivo*. Nuestros trabajos señalan que las hormonas esteroides afectan la concentración de RNA mensajero que puede ser traducida, la velocidad de iniciación de cadenas peptídicas, y la velocidad de elongación de péptidos, en dependiendo del estado hormonal del tejido. La actinomicina D bloquea la inducción de ovoalbúmina, pero una vez inducida ésta (por la hormona), el antibiótico produce una "superinducción" (un aumento en la síntesis de ovoalbúmina), que puede ser explicada sobre la base de un RNA mensajero para ovoalbúmina, de vida media prolongada, y una velocidad aumentada de elongación de cadenas peptídicas.

Hemos podido obtener asimismo síntesis de ovoalbúmina en un lisado de reticulocitos de conejo empleando RNA aislado de oviducto. Con esta técnica, estamos obteniendo datos cuantitativos de la cantidad de RNA mensajero presente en diversas situaciones hormonales, y estamos comparando éstos con la velocidad de síntesis de ovoalbúmina *in vitro*.

Además de ovoalbúmina, el oviducto sintetiza varias proteínas de la clara de huevo, entre las cuales se encuentran conalbúmina, lisozima y ovomucoide. Estrógenos y progesterona no regulan la síntesis de todas estas proteínas en forma coordinada, lo que sugiere que la síntesis de las mismas es regulada independientemente. Esto da lugar a una serie de preguntas en cuanto al número de receptores hormonales y su mecanismo de acción.

REFERENCES

1. Oka, T., and Schimke, R. T., *J. Cell Biol., 41,* 816 (1969).
2. Oka, T., and Schimke, R. T., *J. Cell Biol., 43,* 123 (1969).
3. O'Malley, B. W., McGuire, W. L., Kohler, P. O., and Korenman, S. G., *Rec. Progr. Hormone Res., 25,* 105 (1969).
4. Palmiter, R. D., and Wrenn, J. R., *J. Cell Biol., 50,* 598 (1971).
5. Palmiter, R. D., Christensen, A. K., and Schimke, R. T., *J. Biol. Chem., 245,* 833 (1970).
6. Palmiter, R. D., and Schimke, R. T., manuscript in preparation.
7. Schimke, R. T., in Fraser, F. C., and McKusick, V. A. (eds.), *Congenital Malformations,* Excerpta Medica, Amsterdam (1969), p. 60.
8. Palmiter, R. D., Oka, T., and Schimke, R. T., *J. Biol. Chem., 246,* 724 (1971).
9. Garren, L. D., Howell, R. R., Tomkins, G. M., and Crocco, R. M., *Proc. Natl. Acad. Sci. U.S.A., 52,* 1121 (1964).
10. Reel, J. R., and Kenney, F. T., *Proc. Natl. Acad. Sci. U.S.A., 61,* 200 (1968).
11. Tomkins, G. M., Gelehrter, T. D., Granner, D., Martin, Dr., Jr., Samuels, H. H., and Thompson, E. B., *Science, 166,* 1474 (1969).
12. Rhoads, R. E., McKnight, G. S., and Schimke, R. T., *J. Biol. Chem., 246,* (1971).
13. Laycock, D. G., and Hunt, J. A., *Nature, 221,* 1118 (1969).
14. Evans, M. J., and Lingrel, J. B., *Biochemistry, 8,* 829 (1969).
15. Gurdon, J. B., Lane, C. D., Woodland, H. R., and Marbaix, G., *Nature, 233,* 177 (1971).
16. Stavnezer, J., and Huang, R. C. C., *Nature, 230,* 172 (1971).
17. Palacios, R., Palmiter, R. D., and Schimke, R. T., *J. Biol. Chem., 247,* 2316 (1972).
18. Palmiter, R. D., Palacios, R., and Schimke, R. T., *J. Biol. Chem., 247,* 3296 (1972).
19. Fan, H., and Penman, S., *J. Mol. Biol., 50,* 655 (1970).

DISCUSSION

R. P. Perry (Philadelphia, U.S.A.): Could you clarify the remark you made that you isolate this RNA by procedures which take advantage of the properties of poly A?

R. T. Schimke (Stanford, U.S.A.): We need a bulk method to get milligram quantities of messenger in order to do sequencing and to put the messengers into protein-synthesizing systems. The most successful method takes advantage of the partition of poly A between the phenol and aqueous phases at different pH values. That is, by using high salts and buffering with a large amount of Tris at pH 7, messenger primarily partitions into the phenol phase, whereas at pH 9 it partitions into the aqueous phase, while bulk (i.e., ribosomal) RNA goes the other way. This is a very simple and very bulk method that works. The other approach is based on the fact that poly A precipitates at pH around 5. This goes back to Doty's work. These are the approaches that have been most successful. We are presently testing other possibilities, such as the poly dT columns, and I have no doubt that they will work.

E. Sánchez de Jiménez (Mexico City, Mexico): Do you get preferentially ovalbumin synthesis instead of a mixture of globin and ovalbumin in the reticulocyte lysate system?

R. T. Schimke: That is an interesting problem. Incidentally, I am surprised someone really believes that we are still making ovalbumin and did not question that. We have taken that material, digested it, and made tryptic peptides of it, and those cochromatographed with authentic ovalbumin. Your question is an interesting one because the most that we have been able to get in terms of ovalbumin synthesis is roughly about 10% of total incorporation. Addition of more nucleic acid does not work. I do not know the reasons for this, although I could speculate in any number of ways. In general, what one finds in this system is no increase in the total incorporation of isotope, rather a general decrease. This is probably related to some inhibitors.

11

mRNA Synthesis in Erythropoiesis: Specific Effect of Erythropoietin on the Synthesis of DNA-like RNA

Marco Perretta, Alfonso Valenzuela, and Luis Valladares

Laboratorio de Bioquímica
Departamento de Ciencias Fisiológicas
Facultad de Ciencias Pecuarias y Medicina Veterinaria
Universidad de Chile
Santiago, Chile

The erythropoietic mechanism is a gradual process of cell differentiation and proliferation leading from primitive cells (stem cells) to highly differentiated cells (erythrocytes). This phenomenon, which occurs in bone marrow, seems to be essentially the same for different mammals (1).

The Erythropoiesis expressed in molecular terms is focused on the synthesis of hemoglobin, qualitatively and quantitatively the principal protein product. Concomitant with this synthetic pathway, the disappearances of other molecules, such as DNA, RNA, and several classes of enzymes, are other molecular characteristics of the process. These morphological and biochemical changes led us to explore the moment at which the cell differentiation process starts and what molecules are involved in it.

Erythropoietin is the central factor initiating and regulating erythropoiesis and thus may control the synthesis of hemoglobin. The first molecular action of erythropoietin known is the early stimulation of the synthesis of several RNA types (2-5). At this stage, it is natural to expect that messenger RNA synthesis occurs. Lingrel (6) has reported the presence of a high molecular weight RNA, labeled at early times in bone marrow of anemic rabbits. Fractions of this RNA have the characteristics of messenger RNA (6). Scherrer and Marcaud (7) have reported the synthesis of a rapidly labeled RNA in the nuclei of avian erythroblasts. This RNA, termed nascent messenger-like RNA, sediments predominantly in the 30-80S zone, and it is more unstable than other RNA types. These findings support the previous idea of Torelli *et al.* (8) that the information for protein synthesis must be prepared in earlier stages of the erythropoietic process. Gross and Goldwasser (3), using an *in vitro* system of rat bone marrow cells under the effect of erythropoietin, have described the synthesis of rapidly labeled RNAs with sedimentation constants of 4, 6, 9, 45, 55-65, and 150S. The 150S RNA had a half-life of about 6 min, while the other RNAs were more stable.

We have shown in previous papers (1,2) that erythropoietin stimulates the synthesis of an RNA fraction isolated by the thermal phenol method and fractionated on methylated albumin columns. The action of the hormone seems to be discriminatory, because only one RNA species is activated in the fraction extracted at 60°. This RNA exhibits an increased ability to stimulate incorporation of ^{14}C-valine into the proteins of a cell-free system obtained from rabbit reticulocytes, in comparison with the same RNA fraction isolated from rats not treated with the hormone.

In a recent paper, Gross and Goldwasser (5) have reported that erythropoietin induces the synthesis of a 9S RNA in cultured bone marrow cells from polycythemic rats and mice. Synthesis of 9S RNA starts 1 hr after addition of the hormone to the medium, while hemoglobin synthesis is initiated 8-10 hr later in cultured rat cells. In accord with the findings of other investigators (9-11), the 9S RNA has many of the properties proposed for hemoglobin messenger RNA.

In this work, we show that different RNAs obtained at different times after the hormone action support our previous suggestion that erythropoietin can induce the synthesis of a DNA-like RNA at a very early time and that the stimulated synthesis of other RNA species seems to be an indirect consequence of the previous specific action of the hormone.

A preliminary report of the present results has been presented elsewhere (12).

EXPERIMENTAL

The materials and methods were as previously described (2). The RNAs were isolated according to the thermal phenol method at 10°, 40°, and 60° (13). The three RNA fractions were chromatographed on methylated albumin kieselguhr (MAK) columns (14). The RNAs were eluted with 300 ml total volume of a linear gradient of NaCl from 0.2 to 1.6 M in 0.1 M phosphate buffer, pH 6.7. Fractions of 5 ml of eluate were collected. After this, the column was washed with 50 ml of 0.1 M Tris-HCl buffer, pH 6.7, and eluted with 180 ml total volume of a linear gradient of sodium dodecyl sulfate (SDS) from 0 to 1% in the Tris buffer. Fractions of 5 ml were collected and treated as indicated by Roberts and Quinlivan (15) to eliminate the SDS. Aliquots of each of the fractions were assayed for their optical density at 260 nm and counted in a Nuclear Chicago gas flow counter at infinite thinness.

In order to recover the RNA of each peak of the elution profiles, the tubes were pooled, the solution was dialyzed, and the RNA was precipitated as described (2). The RNA as a dry powder was stored at $-10°$ in a sealed glass tube. These RNA fractions were used in the experiments with the reticulocyte cell-free system and in sedimentation analysis.

The cell-free system was prepared from reticulocytes obtained from anemic rabbits, according to the method of Arnstein *et al.* (16).

Sedimentation analysis experiments were performed in a Beckman model L-2-65B ultracentrifuge with the SW39 rotor using a 5-20% sucrose density gradient. Other conditions are indicated in the figure captions and the footnote to Table I.

RESULTS

The experimental conditions used in this work gave good separation of the various species of bone marrow RNA, and typical and reproducible elution patterns were obtained for the $10°$, $40°$, and $60°$ RNA fractions. These RNAs, separated by means of the thermal phenol method, were chromatographed on MAK columns. The RNA fraction placed on the column was successively eluted with a NaCl gradient and then with a SDS gradient. Under these conditions, most of the RNA fixed on the column was eluted; 98% of the added radioactivity was recovered in the elution tubes. The remaining RNA was eluted with a strong ammonium hydroxide solution and discarded.

Figure 1 shows the incorporation of labeled formate into the $10°$, $40°$, and $60°$ RNA fractions isolated by MAK chromatography. In the experiment, the animals received both the hormone and the ^{14}C-formate for 30 min. As shown in Fig. 1A, the RNA species obtained from the $10°$ RNA and eluted with the NaCl gradient were slightly labeled while the RNAs eluted with SDS were strongly labeled. The stimulatory action of erythropoietin was rather weak, except on the first peak of the profile, which may correspond to transfer RNA (15). The profile obtained with the $40°$ RNA (Fig. 1B) is different, and the RNA fractions were strongly labeled. However, these RNA fractions were slightly stimulated by the hormone. The $60°$ RNA displays a very different pattern. As is shown in Figs 1C and 2A, these RNA fractions were not labeled, except for slight uptake of the precursor in the P3 peak of the profile. Erythropoietin produced a significant stimulation of labeling of these RNA species, particularly in the P3 RNA type.

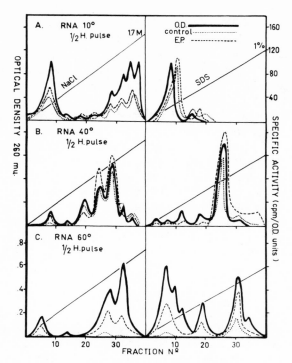

Fig. 1. Incorporation of ^{14}C-formate into the 10°, 40°, and 60° RNA fractions obtained from normal and erythropoietin-treated rat bone marrow. The three RNA fractions were chromatographed on methylated albumin-kieselguhr (MAK) columns. Normal rats were injected intravenously with 5 units of erythropoietin and 10 μc of ^{14}C-formate for 30 min. The heavy line represents optical density, the dotted line the specific activity (counts/min/optical density unit) of RNA from control animals, and the broken line the specific activity of RNA from rats treated with the hormone.

These experiments allow us to conclude that a different distribution of radioactivity in the three RNA fractions is obtained after the hormone action, the principal characteristic being the high stimulation of the 60° RNA in comparison with the low activation of the 10° and 40° RNA by erythropoietin. These findings suggest that erythropoietin has a specific action on RNA metabolism. For this reason, our attention was directed to the study of the rate of labeling of the 60° RNA fractions at different times.

When rats are simultaneously pulsed with the hormone and ^{14}C-formate for

1 hr, a similar optical density profile is obtained (Fig. 2A) but a marked difference in the radioactive profiles is observed (Fig. 2B). In control animals, all the RNA species were strongly labeled, except for P2 fraction. Erythropoietin exerted a prominent stimulation on labeling of the RNA fractions, except for the FII RNA, which was practically not stimulated.

When the rats were pulsed with the hormone and ^{14}C-formate for 2 hr, the distribution of the radioactivity was different in comparison to the other

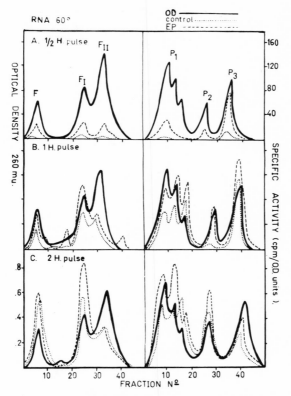

Fig. 2. Effect of erythropoietin on the incorporation of ^{14} *C-formate into 60° RNA under different time pulses of the hormone and the labeled precursor.* The 60° RNA was treated on MAK columns as indicated in the text. The animals were pulsed for 30 min (A), 60 min (B), and 120 min (C) with erythropoietin and ^{14}C-formate. The continuous line represents the optical density, the dotted line the specific activity (counts/min/optical density unit) of RNA from control animals, and the broken line the specific activity of RNA from rats treated with the hormone.

profiles, the most prominent characteristic being diminution of the specific activity of the P3 RNA while that of the other RNA fractions, except FII RNA, was enhanced (Fig. 2C).

In order to demonstrate the rate of RNA labeling, radioactivity of each RNA species was plotted against time as shown in Fig. 3A. The P3 RNA had a fairly rapid turnover, in comparison to the other RNA fractions. The data resembles a typical precursor-product curve. Figure 3B shows the rate of labeling of the RNAs stimulated by erythropoietin. The data obtained are similar to those of Fig. 3A, with the difference that the specific activities of the RNA fractions are higher than those of 3A, except for FII RNA. These findings suggest that P3 RNA may be a precursor of the FI, P1, and P2 RNA species.

We have shown that the 60° RNA promotes a higher incorporation of a labeled amino acid into the proteins of a reticulocyte cell-free system, in comparison with the 10° and 40° RNA fractions. This property of the 60° RNA disappears in polycythemic rats and appears again with the action of erythropoietin (2).

The effect of the FI and FII RNA fractions, obtained from the marrow of rats treated with erythropoietin for 4 hr, on the incorporation of ^{14}C-valine into the proteins of a cell-free system prepared from rabbit reticulocytes is shown in Table I. The FI RNA increased the incorporation of the labeled amino acid into

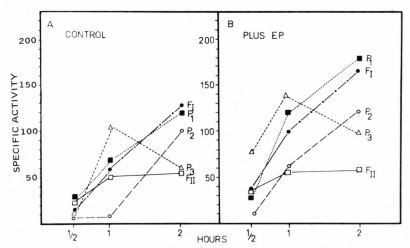

Fig. 3. Rate of labeling of the 60° RNA separated by MAK columns. The specific activities of the RNA species obtained from the peaks of the fractions FI, FII, P1, P2, and P3 are plotted against time. The values were obtained from Fig. 2. The specific activities of the RNA species obtained from control and hormone treated animals are shown in A and B, respectively.

the proteins, while the FII RNA was unable to augment the specific activity of the same proteins. The major importance of this observation is that the FI RNA activity is greater when it is obtained from animals treated with erythropoietin.

Table I. Effect of the FI and FII RNA Fractions on the
Incorporation of ^{14}C-Valine into Proteins in a Rabbit
Reticulocyte Cell-Free System[a]

Experimental conditions of the cell-free system (CFS)	Specific activity (counts/min/mg protein)
CFS without exogenous RNA	263 ± 65
CFS plus 150 μg of FI RNA obtained from	
Normal rat	459 ± 46
Normal rat treated with erythropoietin	749 ± 106
CFS plus 150 μg of FII RNA obtained from	
Normal rat	333 ± 56
Normal rat treated with erythropoietin	366 ± 91

[a] Data are the means of three samples ± standard error of the mean. One group of rats was injected intravenously with 5 units of erythropoietin for 4 hr. The FI and FII RNA fractions were isolated from bone marrow 60° RNA through the MAK column step. The samples were incubated for 1 hr at 37°. The reaction was stopped with hot trichloroacetic acid. Other conditions are indicated in the text. The results are of a typical experiment from a series of five.

Table II. Effect of the F, FI, FII, P1, P2, and P3 RNA Fractions
on the Incorporation of ^{14}C-Valine into Protein in a Rabbit
Reticulocyte Cell-Free System[a]

Experimental conditions of the cell-free system (CFS)	Specific activity (counts/min/mg protein)
CFS without exogenous RNA	229
CFS plus 150 μg of F RNA	370
CFS plus 150 μg of FI RNA	704
CFS plus 150 μg of FII RNA	247
CFS plus 150 μg of P1 RNA and P2 RNA	227
CFS plus 150 μg of P3 RNA	498
CFS plus 150 μg of Poly A[b]	416

[a] The RNA fractions were obtained from normal rats following the method indicated in the text. The results are of a typical experiment. Other conditions are similar to those described in Table I.

[b] The poly A was incubated with 0.2 μc of ^{14}C-L-lysine (U).

Table II shows the results obtained when the RNA fractions (F, FI, FII, P1-P2, and P3) obtained from the MAK column were tested in the cell-free system. It was observed that the FI RNA promotes the highest incorporation of ^{14}C-valine into the proteins while the P3 and F RNA fractions stimulate to a lesser extent incorporation of the labeled amino acid into the proteins. The other RNA fractions behaved similarly to the control sample. As a test of the *in vitro* system, the incorporation of ^{14}C-lysine into the proteins using poly A as messenger RNA is also shown.

We have performed some preliminary examinations of the sedimentation characteristics of the RNA fractions obtained from the MAK column. The F, FI, and FII RNAs were heterogeneous with sedimentation constants ranging between 4S and 100S. The FI RNA presented a large peak in the light region of the profile. The P1, P2, and P3 RNAs were also heterogeneous, but showed some differences. While the P3 fraction is composed of a heterodisperse material which sedimented in the range between 7S and 60S, the range of P2 was betwen 10S and 85S, and the sedimentation coefficients of the P1 RNA fluctuated between 30S and 110S, with a large peak at 110S.

CONCLUSIONS

Several authors have shown that various kinds of bone marrow RNA are stimulated by erythropoietin in *in vivo* and *in vitro* experiments (1-5).

We have found that erythropoietin augments the specific activity of the bone marrow RNA extracted at 10°, 40°, and 60°, but only the 60° RNA has a marked capacity to enhance amino acid incorporation into the protein in a cell-free system. According to Pavlov (4), the 10° RNA corresponds to soluble RNA and other low molecular weight RNAs, the 40° RNA to RNA with the characteristics of ribosomal RNA, and the 60° RNA to types of RNA with the properties of DNA-like base composition, including messenger RNA.

Our work reported herein shows that erythropoietin can exert a specific action on the RNA metabolism of rat bone marrow by inducing the synthesis of a particular RNA species. While the 60° RNA types are strongly activated by erythropoietin, those obtained from the 10° and 40° extractions are slightly stimulated by the hormone. These results may be interpreted as follows: erythropoietin is able to induce the synthesis of a special type of RNA extracted at 60°; the appearance of the other RNAs extracted at 10° and 40° may result from an indirect effect of the hormone.

The peculiar behavior of the 60° RNAs led us to study their rate of labeling. If we carefully examine the 60° RNA profile, it is possible to find some similarities to the profiles obtained by Roberts and Quinlivan (15) for nuclear and cytoplasmic RNA of Erlich ascites cells and to those observed by Billing and

Barbiroli (17) with RNAs from Friend cells. According to these investigators, the tenaciously bound RNA fractions eluted with SDS correspond to heterogeneous RNAs of smaller size than those eluted with NaCl. They also showed that the base composition is high in adenine or uracil, depending on the cytoplasmic or nuclear origin of the RNA. These evidences support our previous ideas (2) that the 60° RNA is DNA-like and that the several types of RNA obtained in the MAK column may correspond to the same type of molecules.

The incorporation of ^{14}C-formate in animals not treated with erythropoietin indicates that the P3 RNA is the first RNA labeled. With longer pulses of ^{14}C-formate, the specific activity of the P3 RNA reaches a peak which gradually decreases. In the P1 and FI RNA fractions, activity increases continuously. In this way, a radioactive wave is provoked starting from P3 RNA to FI RNA, the latter becoming the most labeled. If we consider that control rats have normal amounts of circulating erythropoietin, the appearance of the P3 RNA may be due to the action of the hormone. This is confirmed in that when the animals are treated with erythropoietin, the whole RNA system is activated in a similar fashion. The results of these labeling experiments suggest that the P3 RNA may be the precursor of the other RNAs and be under the control of erythropoietin.

The experiments on incorporation of labeled amino acid into protein in a cell-free system must be considered as preliminary indications of the functional properties of the different types of RNA tested. We have reported (2) that the FI RNA fraction responds specifically to the effect of erythropoietin, by the criterion that ^{14}C-formate incorporation into the macromolecule is augmented after hormonal action and by the fact that its ability to incorporate ^{14}C-valine into protein is greatly increased in comparison with the other RNA fractions. The data that we show here demonstrates that the hormone can induce the synthesis of a specific RNA of unknown nature, which may suffer metabolic transformations in order to be expressed through protein synthesis in the cytoplasm. This RNA seems to be the precursor of the FI RNA.

This assumption is supported by the following findings: (a) a high molecular weight RNA labeled at early times in bone marrow from anemic rabbits (6), (b) a 150S RNA found in rat bone marrow cells within a few minutes after the addition of erythropoietin to the *in vitro* system, and (c) the synthesis of a 9S RNA induced by erythropoietin after 1 hr in cultured bone marrow cells from polycythemic rats and mice (3,5).

If we correlate the several facts already mentioned, it is possible to suggest that the synthesis of an RNA similar to the P3 RNA we have found might be the consequence of an early and direct action of the hormone, in which stable RNA is formed. This RNA could form part of a large, metabolically unstable RNA, protecting the message until complete biochemical units for the synthesis of proteins are developed.

Whether the synthesis of the P3 RNA occurs prior to the synthesis of a large RNA or the P3 RNA forms part of the large RNA immediately after the action of the hormone, to originate the FI RNA, remains to be elucidated.

The investigations are being continued with regard to characterization of the RNA stimulated by the hormone.

ACKNOWLEDGMENTS

This work was supported in part by the Comisión Nacional de Investigación Cientifica y Tecnológica (Grant No. 204) and the Comisión Central de Investigación Cientifica de la Universidad de Chile (Grant No. 174). The competent technical assistance of Mr. Fernando Garrido and Mr. Jorge Merino is gratefully acknowledged. This work was presented in part at the Thirteenth Annual Meeting of the Sociedad de Biologia de Chile in 1970, and abstracts have been published in *Arch. Biol. Med. Exptl., 7,* R42 (1970), and *Arch. Biol. Med. Exptl., 7,* R43 (1970). A. V. is a Fellow of the Comisión Nacional de Investigación Cientifica y Tecnológica de Chile (CONICYT). Part of this work is from the thesis submitted by L. V. to the University of Chile for the degree of biochemist.

SUMMARY

It has been shown that erythropoietin is involved in the regulatory mechanism of the erythropoietic process. Its molecular action is characterized by the activation of the biosynthesis of several RNA types, at early times. RNA biosynthesis was measured by the incorporation of ^{14}C-formate into the purine bases. The RNA was isolated by the phenol method at $10°$, $40°$, and $60°$. The $10°$ RNA corresponds to transfer RNA and other low molecular weight RNA, the $40°$ RNA to ribosomal RNA, and the $60°$ RNA to types of RNA with DNA-like base composition and includes messenger RNA. Each RNA fraction was chromatographed in methylated albumin-kieselguhr (MAK) columns. The RNA fixed in the column was first eluted with a sodium chloride gradient and then with a sodium dodecyl sulfate (SDS) gradient.

Short pulses of erythropoietin stimulate the synthesis of the several types of rat bone marrow RNA in different fashions. While the RNAs obtained at $60°$ are strongly activated by the hormone, those eluted from the $10°$ and $40°$ fractions are only slightly stimulated. Some types of RNA species obtained from the $60°$ RNA fraction seem to respond specifically to the hormone action. The time course of the rate of labeled formate incorporation into the $60°$ RNA fractions eluted from the MAK column indicates that the P3 RNA is precursor of the P1, P2, and FI RNAs. FI RNA exhibits an increased ability to incorporate ^{14}C-valine into the proteins of a cell-free system prepared from rabbit reticulocytes.

These results suggest that the action of erythropoietin is selective. It activates one RNA fraction, probably with messenger properties. The activation of ribosomal and transfer RNAs reflects an indirect effect of the hormone.

RESUMEN

La eritropoyesis es un proceso gradual de diferenciación y proliferación celular que se inicia en células basales indiferenciadas (stem cells) hasta llegar a células altamente especializadas, como son los eritrocitos. Este fenómeno parece ser muy similar en los mamíferos.

La eritropoyesis, expresada en términos moleculares, está orientada hacia la síntesis de la hemoglobina, la proteína cuali y cuantitativamente más importante de este mecanismo. La desaparición de otras moléculas como el DNA, RNA y varias clases de enzimas constituye otra de las características del proceso en la médula ósea de rata.

La eritropoyetina es el factor central que inicia y regula la eritropoyesis y por ende controla la síntesis de hemoglobina. Su primera reacción bioquímica conocida es la de estimular el metabolismo del RNA, entre los cuales se encuentra el RNA mensajero. En relación con esto, una serie de autores han demostrado que la información contenida en el DNA es transferida al RNA en las etapas iniciales del proceso eritropoyético, en la forma de un RNA de gran tamaño molecular. Así, Gross y Goldwasser han demostrado que la eritropoyetina en la médula ósea de rata en sistemas *in vitro,* estimulada la síntesis de una variada gama de RNAs, siendo un RNA 150S y un RNA 9S los más característicos. Este último tiene mucho de las propiedades propuestas para el RNA mensajero de la hemoglobina.

En este trabajo se mide la síntesis del RNA mediante la incorporación de formiato C^{14} a las bases púricas de la macromolécula, las cuales son aislados por el método del fenol a $10°$, $40°$ y $60°$. Los RNA extraídos a $10°$ son de bajo peso molecular, como RNA de transferencia; los RNA aislados a $40°$ son de naturaleza ribosomal y los de $60°$ corresponden a RNA de composición de bases parecida al DNA, entre los cuales se incluyen RNA de tipo mensajero. Cada una de estas fracciones son cromatografiadas en una columna de albúmina metilada y kieselguhr (MAK) y son eluídos, primero con un gradiente salina de NaCl y luego con un gradiente de dodecil sulfato de sodio (SDS).

Pulsos cortos de la eritropoyetina estimulan la síntesis de varios tipos de RNA de una manera diferente. Mientras los RNAs obtenidos de la fracción RNA-60° son fuertemente activados por la hormona, aquellos RNA eluídos de las fracciones de $10°$ y $40°$ lo son ligeramente. Algunos tipos de RNA de la fracción RNA-60° tratada en la columna MAK parecen responder en forma específica a la acción hormonal. La velocidad de incorporación del formiato marcado a estas clases de RNA indican que el RNA P3 es precursor del P1, P2 y FI, siendo este último el más marcado con formiato y el que presenta una mayor capacidad para incorporar valina-C^{14} a las proteínas de un sistema acelular preparado de reticulocitos de conejo.

Estos resultados sugieren que la acción de la eritropoyetina sobre el metabolismo del RNA es selectiva. Activa una fracción de RNA, probablemente de tipo mensajero, mientras que la activación del RNA ribosomal y de transferencia parece ser el reflejo de una acción indirecta de la hormona.

REFERENCES

1. Perretta, M., *Arch. Biol. Med. Exptl., 6,* 89 (1969).
2. Perretta, M., Valenzuela, A., Sage, N., and Oyanguren, C., *Arch. Biol. Med. Exptl., 8,* 30 (1971).
3. Gross, M., and Goldwasser, E., *Biochemistry, 8,* 1795 (1969).
4. Pavlov, A. D., *Biochim. Biophys. Acta, 195,* 156 (1969).
5. Gross, M., and Goldwasser, E., *J. Biol. Chem., 246,* 2480 (1971).
6. Lingrel, J. B., *Biochim. Biophys. Acta, 142,* 75 (1967).
7. Scherrer, K., and Marcaud, L., *J. Cell Physiol., 72,* Suppl. 1, 181 (1968).
8. Torelli, U., Artusi, T., Grossi, G., Emilia, G., and Mauri, C., *Nature, 207,* 755 (1965).
9. Evans, M. J., and Lingrel, J. B., *Biochemistry, 8,* 829 (1969).

10. Evans, M. J., and Lingrel, J. B., *Biochemistry, 8,* 3000 (1969).
11. Hunt, J. A., and Laycock, D. G., *Cold Spring Harbor Symp. Quant. Biol., 34,* 579 (1969).
12. Valenzuela, A., Valladares, L., and Perretta, M., *Arch. Biol. Med. Exptl., 7,* R42, R43 (1970).
13. Georgiev, G. P., Samarina, O. P., Lerman, M. L., Smirnov, M. N., and Severtozov, A. N., *Nature, 200,* 1291 (1963).
14. Mandel, J. D., and Hershey, A. D., *Anal. Biochem., 1,* 66 (1960).
15. Roberts, W. K., and Quinlivan, V. D., *Biochemistry, 8,* 288 (1969).
16. Arnstein, H. R. V., Cox, R. A., and Hunt, J. A., *Biochem. J., 92,* 648 (1964).
17. Billing, J. R., and Barbiroli, B., *Biochim. Biophys. Acta, 217,* 434 (1970).

DISCUSSION

G. D. Novelli (Oak Ridge, U.S.A.): What was the source of the hormone?

M. Perretta (Santiago, Chile): We prepare the hormone from the plasma of anemic rabbits following the method of Lowy and Borsook; it is roughly the four-stage ethanol fractionation of the plasma.

G. D. Novelli: There is another glycoprotein very similar to the erythropoietin that stimulates granulocyte formation. Are you aware of that?

M. Perretta: We know that; in fact, we have a lot of experiments that show that the effect of the extract is produced by erythropoietin. If we treat with mild sulfuric acid, all the action is not reproduced.

P. Chambon (Strasbourg, France): Do you know if this RNase exhibits any specificity?

M. Perretta: This RNase resembles in action the pancreatic ribonuclease. It splits the polynucleotide at pyrimidine nucleotides but leaves the cyclic phosphate.

B. Hardesty (Austin, U.S.A.): Is it implicit in these experiments that you really have two 150S RNA species for α and β chains?

M. Perretta: No, I do not think so. The existence of the large RNA is the finding of Drs. Gross and Goldwasser and only seems to represent one RNA species.

F. J. S. Lara (São Paulo, Brazil): My question applies both to your paper and to Dr. Schimke's paper. In cases where you have rather specific proteins being produced such as in your case or Dr. Schimke's, do you think that you might have an increase of the genes that are codifying those specific proteins?

R. T. Schimke (Stanford, U.S.A.): Dr. Donald Brown isolated a messenger for silk fibroin, and he does not find gene amplification in that case, although the silk gland is making essentially only one protein. It is not really necessary to have gene amplification if you have a messenger that is extremely stable, and I certainly think that is the case with the ovalbumin messenger, which is a very stable messenger; you can accumulate a tremendous capacity to synthesize that protein if you simply continue to build up a large amount of that messenger.

E. Sánchez de Jiménez (Mexico City, Mexico): In hybridization experiments with hemoglobin messenger RNA, we did not find any amplification in the red cell; that is, the hybridization is the same if we test it with DNA from the red cells or DNA from other cells that do not synthesize hemoglobin.

12

Messenger RNA: Its Origin and Fate in Mammalian Cells

Robert P. Perry, J. R. Greenberg, D. E. Kelley, J. LaTorre, and G. Schochetman

Institute for Cancer Research
Fox Chase, Philadelphia, Pennsylvania, U.S.A.

One of the central problems of eukaryotic cell biology concerns the elucidation of the origin and fate of messenger RNA (mRNA). The mRNAs, which function in the cytoplasm as templates for protein synthesis, are synthesized in the nucleus as part of a heterogeneous population of molecules, the so-called heterogeneous nuclear RNAs (HnRNAs). The HnRNAs range in size from about 5×10^5 daltons to more than 10^7 daltons, whereas the mRNAs range from about 10^5 to 2×10^6 daltons. Only a relatively small fraction of the HnRNA (less than 20% in terms of total nucleotide) can actually be accounted for as cytoplasmic mRNA; the remainder appears to be degraded within the nucleus at a relatively rapid rate [for references, see review by Darnell (1)].

These observations have posed some interesting questions: Are all mRNAs synthesized as parts of larger precursor molecules which must be subsequently processed before transport to the cytoplasm? Are all HnRNA molecules potential mRNA precursors or do some perform an as yet unknown function? Attempts to answer these questions by examining base sequence homologies with DNA-RNA hybridization methods have not been completely successful, mainly because of the difficulty of performing competition experiments with RNA complementary to the nonreiterated portion of the genome. The majority of both classes of RNA (two thirds of the HnRNA and four fifths of the mRNA

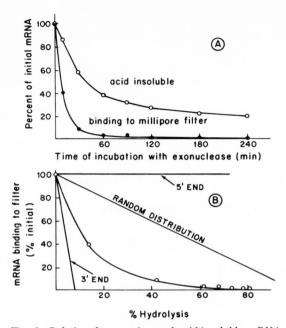

Fig. 1. *Relative decrease in total acid-insoluble mRNA and in mRNA capable of binding to Millipore filters as a function of time of incubation with exoribonuclease (A) and of percent total hydrolysis (B).* L cells, cultured as previously described (18), were labeled 22 hr with ^{32}P (2 μc/ml). Polyribosomes were purified (19), and RNA was extracted from them using phenol-chloroform (20). The ^{32}P-labeled RNA (specific activity 14,000 cpm/μg) was passed through a Millipore filter (11), and the poly A-containing mRNA, which is selectively adsorbed, was eluted from the filter with 6 × 0.5 ml of 0.01 M Tris buffer, pH 7.4, containing 0.1% SDS. NaCl was added to a final concentration of 0.1 M, the mRNA was precipitated with ethanol, redissolved, passed through Sephadex G25 equilibrated with 0.05 M NaCl and 0.001 M EDTA, and exposed to exoribonuclease. The exoribonuclease was isolated from Ehrlich ascites tumor cell nuclei as described previously (see ref. 14) and further purified by phosphocellulose and hydroxyapatite column chromatography using continuous gradient elution at pH 7.4. Peak activity of the enzyme was eluted between 0.25 and 0.30 M NaCl on phosphocellulose and between 0.25 and 0.30 M potassium phosphate on hydroxyapatite. The concentration of total RNA in the reaction mixture was estimated to be about 7 μg (20 mμmoles) per milliliter. The incubation was carried out at 37° in a 0.3 ml volume containing 1

in cultured L cells) is transcribed from rarely repeated or unique DNA sequences (2), and as yet we have not been able to ascertain the extent of base sequence homology between these fractions.

Evidence that at least some cytoplasmic mRNAs are derived from larger nuclear precursors comes from the study of viral-directed RNAs in SV40-transformed cells, (3,4) or in cells infected with herpes virus (5). It remains to be established whether all types of mRNA are processed from larger HnRNAs. The processing of RNA is, of course, not a new concept, the phenomenon having been studied in considerable detail in the case of the ribosomal RNA components [cf. review by Perry (6)] and tRNA (see Chapter 16, this volume).

A new facet to the problem of conversion of HnRNA to mRNA has been provided by the recent discovery (7-11) that both HnRNA and mRNA contain large, covalently attached sequences of polyadenylic acid (poly A) approximately 200 nucleotides long, which appear to be synthesized in a post-transcriptional (processing?) step (12,13). In order to understand more fully the implications of these findings, we have investigated the following characteristics of L cell mRNA: (a) the location of poly A sequences within the mRNA molecules, (b) the distribution of poly A among various mRNA species, (c) correlation of poly A content with certain metabolic parameters of the mRNAs such as speed of entry into polyribosomes and lifetime, and (d) whether poly A sequences are required for transport of the bulk of the mRNA to the cytoplasm and/or its incorporation into functional polyribosomes.

LOCATION OF POLY A SEQUENCES

To attack the problem of poly A location, we were fortunate to have a highly purified nuclear exoribonuclease specific for 3'-OH termini (14). This enzyme, which we had been using for studies of ribosomal RNA processing (15), attaches to the 3'-OH ends of RNA molecules (it does not recognize 3'-phosphate termini) and hydrolyzes the RNA processively, i.e., without dissociation, producing 5'-mononucleotides (14-17). Thus, if the poly A region

---

unit/ml of exoribonuclease, 40 mM Tris-chloride, pH 7.4, 4 mM $MgCl_2$, 0.3 mM dithiothreitol, 40 mM potassium phosphate, and 40 μg/ml bovine serum albumin. Exonuclease units were determined with commercial poly A as described previously (see ref. 14). At the indicated times, aliquots were withdrawn from the reaction, diluted into a buffer containing 0.01 M Tris (pH 7.4), 0.1 M NaCl, 0.001 M EDTA, and 0.1% Sarkosyl and extracted with phenol-chloroform (1:1). One half of the material was assayed for trichloroacetic acid precipitable radioactivity and the other assayed for radioactivity binding to Millipore filters. The theoretical curves in (B) are based on a poly A segment of approximately 7×10^4 daltons in an mRNA molecule of 10^6 daltons.

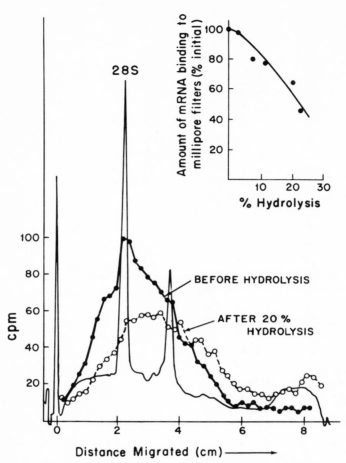

Fig. 2. *Polyacrylamide gel profiles of* ^{32} *P-labeled mRNA before and after hydrolysis*. The mRNA used in Fig. 1 was hydrolyzed with the exoribonuclease in an experiment similar to that described in Fig. 1 until 20% of the radioactivity was rendered acid soluble (inset). The reaction mixture was made 1% in sodium dodecyl sulfate and 15% in sucrose and layered directly onto 2.7% polyacrylamide gels. Electrophoresis was carried out as described previously (21). •, Initial mRNA substrate before hydrolysis; ○, partially hydrolyzed mRNA after 20% hydrolysis. All of the radioactivity in the initial substrate was accounted for by the sum of that in partially hydrolyzed RNA plus the 20% in 5'-mononucleotides.

of mRNA is located at or near the 3'-OH terminus, then incubation of mRNA with the exoribonuclease under conditions approaching enzyme excess should result in the disappearance of poly A at a rate much faster than that of total RNA.

An experiment of this type is shown in Fig. 1. In this experiment, we used as substrate an mRNA preparation from L cells steady state-labeled with ^{32}P. The mRNA was extracted from polyribosomes and further purified by adsorption and elution from Millipore filters. The latter procedure is selective for the poly A-containing mRNA molecules (11). This purified mRNA was incubated with the exoribonuclease at a relatively high enzyme/substrate ratio (50 units/μmole nucleotide), and after various periods the residual substrate was measured with respect to total acid-insoluble radioactivity and to the amount still capable of binding to Millipore filters (poly A-containing mRNA). It is seen (Fig. 1A) that the proportion of RNA which contains poly A decreases much more rapidly, especially during the initial stages of hydrolysis, than the total acid-precipitable RNA. The data replotted in terms of percent hydrolysis (Fig. 1B) clearly support the conclusion that most of the poly A sequences are near the 3'-OH terminus.

The enzyme preparation contained no detectable endonuclease contamination, as may be seen in Fig. 2, which compares the gel electrophoresis profile of the initial mRNA substrate with that of the residual substrate after 20% of the total nucleotides were rendered acid soluble. The absence of significant quantities of small RNA fragments after hydrolysis to this extent attests to the purity of the exonuclease preparation (cf. 15,22).

The 5'-mononucleotides released in such a reaction contain a preponderance (54%) of adenylic acid residues, but also some of the other nucleotides (Table I). This observation, taken together with the fact that the reduction in poly A-containing mRNA is not as rapid as one would theoretically expect if all the poly A were at the 3'-OH terminus, suggests that the enzymes may not have been working synchronously on all mRNA molecules, so that some molecules were hydrolyzed beyond their poly A regions while others were hydrolyzed to a much lesser degree. However, these observations could also mean that the poly A regions are near, but not at, the 3'-OH ends of the mRNA molecules or that some mRNA molecules have poly A regions distant from the 3'-OH end, perhaps even at the 5' end.

These two possibilities were evaluated by an experiment in which we directly determined the proportion of poly A segments which have free 3'-OH termini. We took advantage of the fact that the nuclear exoribonuclease, while effective against substrates with 3'-OH termini, does not hydrolyze molecules that contain a 3'-phosphate terminus (17) and the fact that the poly A fragments may be excised from the mRNA by treatment with pancreatic ribonuclease at an appropriate salt concentration (9,22). Thus such fragments should be hydrolyzed by the nuclear exoribonuclease if they have come from the 3'-OH terminus, whereas they should be resistant if they have come from internal regions or the 5' terminus, in which case they would have a 3'-phosphate group. In the experiments shown in Fig. 3, it was found that about 90% of the poly A was indeed susceptible to attack by the exoribonuclease. When the poly A fragments were incubated with alkaline phosphatase before being exposed to the exoribonuclease, essentially all of the poly A was susceptible to exoribonuclease hydrolysis.

These results clearly indicate that the poly A sequences are located at the 3'-OH ends of at least 90% of the poly A-containing mRNA molecules. Whether the poly A is located elsewhere in a small proportion of the mRNA molecules remains to be established. If these results are considered together with the idea that the poly A sequences of mRNA originate by a post-transcriptional addition to HnRNA (12), we can conclude that the conversion of HnRNA to mRNA must involve conservation of a piece near the 3'-OH terminus and elimination of nucleotides at the 5'-P(PP) end of the molecules.

DO ALL mRNA MOLECULES CONTAIN POLY A?

Given methods for fractionating RNA into the poly A-containing and the poly A-lacking components, it is a relatively simple matter to analyze a sample of labeled polyribosomal RNA with regard to the question of whether all mRNA

Table I. Base Composition of L Cell ^{32}P-Labeled mRNA and of 5'-Mononucleotides Released from the mRNA on Digestion with the Nuclear Exoribonuclease[a]

Nucleotide	Overall base composition of mRNA[b] (%)	Acid-soluble exonuclease product[c] (%)
GMP	28	13
UMP	29	13
AMP	25	54
CMP	18	19

[a] Base compositions were determined by thin layer chromatography on polyethyleneimine-cellulose as described elsewhere (23).

[b] Determined from a KOH hydrolysate of ^{32}P-mRNA substrate.

[c] Twenty-two percent of total radioactivity in mRNA was rendered acid soluble.

molecules contain poly A. We have used two such methods: the Millipore filter selection technique devised by Lee *et al.* (11) and a method developed in our

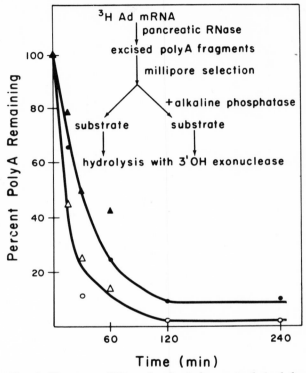

Fig. 3. The susceptibility of poly A fragments derived from mRNA to hydrolysis by nuclear exoribonuclease. L cell mRNA from cells treated 30 min with 0.08 μg/ml actinomycin D and labeled for 1 hr with ^{3}H-adenosine (10 μc/ml, 15.5 c/mmole) in the presence of the drug was extracted from polyribosomes as described in Fig. 1. Poly A fragments were prepared by treating mRNA with pancreatic RNase (2 μg/ml) for 60 min at 37° in 0.27 *M* NaCl. After phenol-chloroform (1:1) extraction, the RNA was bound and eluted from Millipore filters. The poly A fragments were incubated for 30 min at 24° in a solution containing 40 m*M* Tris (*p*H 7.4), 4 m*M* MgCl$_2$, 0.3 m*M* dithiothreitol, and 40 μg/ml bovine serum albumin with (○, △) or without (●, ▲) 50 μg/ml *Escherichia coli* alkaline phosphatase (E.C. 3.1.3.1, BAFP: Worthington Biochemical Corp.) and then for various times with 1 unit/ml ascites nuclear exoribonuclease. Circles and triangles represent separate experiments. Poly A was assayed by either adsorption to Millipore filters or acid insolubility. Both assay methods gave similar results.

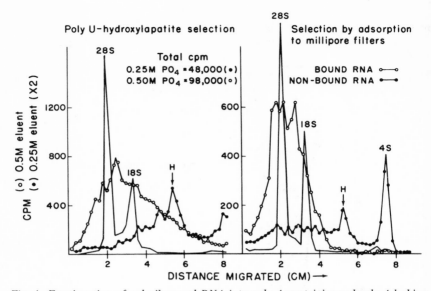

Fig. 4. Fractionation of polyribosomal RNA into poly A-containing and poly A-lacking components. L cells were treated 30 min with 0.08 μg/ml actinomycin D and labeled for 1 hr with 10 μc/ml ^{3}H-adenosine (left panel) or ^{3}H-uridine (right panel) in the presence of the drug. RNA was extracted from polyribosomes as described in Fig. 1. Left panel: The polyribosomal RNA was incubated with 100 μg poly U (Miles Laboratories) in 1 ml of 1 M NaCl, 0.01 M phosphate buffer, and 0.1% Sarkosyl for 1 hr at 25° and then diluted tenfold with 0.2 M NaCl, 0.01 M phosphate buffer, and 0.1% Sarkosyl and adsorbed to 2 g of dry hydroxylapatite-cellulose (1:1). The sample was loaded on a column, and RNA fractions were eluted at room temperature with 15 ml of 0.2 M NaCl-0.1% Sarkosyl buffer containing either 0.25 M phosphate (●) or 0.50 M phosphate (○). The unreacted RNA elutes at 0.25 M phosphate, whereas the triplex, 2 poly U : poly A-mRNA, elutes as 0.50 M phosphate. The eluted samples were dialyzed against 0.1 M (NH$_4$)HCO$_3$ buffer, lyophilized, and submitted to gel electrophoresis as described in Fig. 2. Right panel: The polyribosomal RNA was passed through a Millipore filter and the adsorbed fraction (○) eluted as described in Fig. 1. The filtrate (●) was also collected, and both fractions were precipitated with ethanol, redissolved, and submitted to gel electrophoresis as described in Fig. 2. The curves from each pair of samples were superimposed and plotted together with the A_{260nm} trace of the ribosomal RNA (———) which was present in the 0.25 M phosphate and Millipore filtrate samples. The position of the histone message is designated as "H."

own laboratory (24) which consists of reacting the RNA with an excess of polyuridylic acid (poly U) and separating the triplex structures, 2 poly U : poly A-mRNA, from the nonreactive RNA by hydroxylapatite chromatography. As will be seen, both methods have given similar results.

The mRNA of L cells consists of a group of large components, 0.5-2.0 × 10^6 daltons in size, and a fairly discrete class of components about 150,000 daltons in size, which have been tentatively identified as the histone messages (h-mRNA) (25,26). When preparations of labeled polyribosomal RNA were fractionated as described above (Fig. 4), it was observed that the h-mRNA, together with 4S RNA, failed to complex with poly U and failed to adsorb to Millipore filters, indicating therefore that it contains little or no poly A. By the same criteria,

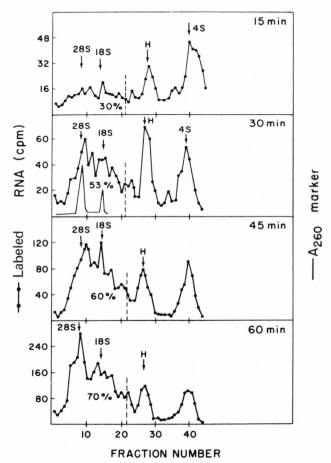

Fig. 5. Acrylamide gel profiles of polyribosomal RNA labeled for various periods of time. L cells were treated with 0.08 μg/ml actinomycin D and labeled for 15, 30, 45, and 60 min with 5 μc/ml ³H-uridine. RNA was extracted from polyribosomes as described in Fig. 1 and analyzed by polyacrylamide gel electrophoresis. The percentage of total radioactive RNA with mobility less than that of the vertical dashed line is given in each panel.

about 80% of the large polyribosomal RNA components contain poly A. As will be discussed later, the remaining 20% of the large components which do not contain poly A are probably not actually in polyribosomes, but rather in the ribonucleoprotein structures which cosediment with polyribosomes in sucrose gradients.

The observation that h-mRNA is lacking in poly A sequences was especially interesting in view of its distinctive kinetic properties. It is known from previous studies that the metabolic lifetime of h-mRNA is about one-third that of most other mRNAs (27-29) and moreover that newly synthesized h-mRNA appears in cytoplasmic polyribosomes without the lag characteristic of the other mRNA species (26,30).

To determine more precisely the correlation between the time of entry of poly A-containing mRNA and the time of entry of the large mRNA components into the cytoplasmic polyribosomes, we performed the kinetic experiment illustrated in Figs. 5 and 6. Cells were treated with low levels of actinomycin D to suppress labeling of the ribosomal RNA components and labeled for varying periods of time with ^{3}H-uridine. The polyribosomal RNA was extracted and analyzed with respect to both size (by gel electrophoresis) and poly A content by the Millipore binding assay. After brief labeling periods, the majority of the labeled RNA is composed of h-mRNA and 4S RNA components, whereas after 60 min the large mRNA components comprise about 70% of the labeled RNA. The distribution of large mRNA components labeled during a 60 min incubation resembles the "steady state" distribution. This may be seen by comparing the gel profile from 60 min-labeled cells (Fig. 5) with that from steady state-labeled cells (Fig. 2). As illustrated in Fig. 6, there is a remarkably good correlation between the proportion of labeled polyribosomal RNA which contains poly A and the proportion which comprises the large mRNA components, the latter being adjusted to account for the 20% non poly A-containing fraction discussed earlier. These results are consistent with the idea that the large mRNA components, which constitute the bulk of the mRNA population, are delayed in their entry into the cytoplasm because of a processing step involving the addition of adenylate residues. The delay due to processing, estimated by extrapolating the linear portion of a specific activity *vs.* time curve (inset, Fig. 6), is approximately 15 min. However, the fact that a small amount of poly A-containing mRNA can be detected in the polyribosomes within 5 min after labeling suggests that the lag is not uniform for all mRNAs and that 15 min represents an average of several different lag times. This average delay time is comparable to a previous estimate for mRNA processing in HeLa cells (31). The h-mRNAs, which are apparently not processed in this way, do not exhibit such a delay. These messages are apparently capable of reaching the cytoplasm and functioning as a template for protein synthesis without having any detectable poly A.

DO ALL LARGE mRNAs REQUIRE POLY A SEQUENCES FOR TRANS-PORT TO CYTOPLASM AND/OR INCORPORATION INTO FUNCTIONAL POLYRIBOSOMES?

One may ask whether the 20% of the large polyribosomal RNAs which contain no detectable poly A are similar to the histone messages in their lack of

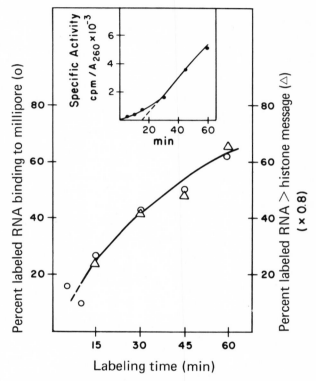

Fig. 6. Correlation between the proportion of poly A-containing polyribosomal RNA and the proportion of large RNA components at various labeling times. The polyribosomal RNA samples from the experiment of Fig. 5 were used to measure the fraction of total labeled RNA which binds to Millipore filters (○) and percent large mRNA component (△). The latter values were obtained by multiplying the percentage calculated in Fig. 5 by 0.8 to correct for the proportion of large components which do not contain poly A (*cf.* Fig. 4). The 5 and 10 min points are from a similar experiment. Inset: A plot of the overall specific activity of the polyribosomes from which these data were obtained.

poly A requirement, or whether these components represent some nonfunctional form of mRNA or "messenger-like" RNA. It is possible to distinguish the radioactive RNA which is truly bound to ribosomes, and hence part of the functional polyribosomes, from radioactive RNA in large ribonucleoprotein structures (RNP) which cosediment with polyribosomes in sucrose gradients if the polyribosome fractions are subjected to density analysis in CsCl (18,19). In these analyses, shown schematically in Fig. 7, the labeled mRNA which is part of the polyribosome structure bands at ρ 1.54 g/cm^3, coincidentally with the ribosomes, detected by their absorbance at 260 nm. On the other hand, the radioactive RNP or radioactive RNP complexed with a single monoribosome

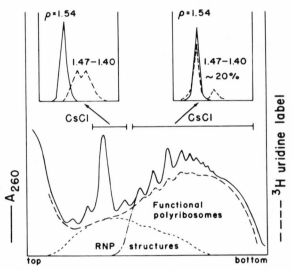

Fig. 7. Schematic diagram of the characterization of poly-ribosomal structures by CsCl buoyant density analysis. See refs. (18) and (19) for methodological details. The bottom traces depict the distribution on a sucrose gradient of ribosomes, observed by A_{260nm} absorbance, and of mRNA and free ribonucleoprotein structures, observed by radioactivity measurement. The relative proportion of radioactivity in functional mRNA and in the cosedimenting ribonucleoprotein can be readily determined by fixing the structures in formaldehyde and banding on CsCl. The insets represent CsCl gradients of the material from the polyribosome and mono-ribosome-98S regions (horizontal bars). The functional mRNA bands coincidentally with the ribosomes at ρ of 1.54 g/cm^3, whereas ribonucleoprotein and ribonucleoprotein-monoribosome complexes band at ρ 1.40 and 1.47, respectively.

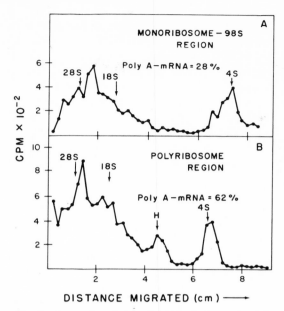

Fig. 8. Comparison by acrylamide gel electrophoresis of radioactive RNA extracted from monoribosome-98S region (A) and polyribosome region (B) of a sucrose gradient. Cells were labeled for 1 hr with ^{3}H-uridine as described in Fig. 5. The regions are defined by the horizontal bars in Fig. 7. The percentage of poly A-containing mRNA was determined by the Millipore adsorption assay.

band at ρ 1.40 or 1.47, respectively, clearly distinct from the ribosomal A_{260} peak. From such an analysis, it was found that about one fifth of the radioactive RNA in the polyribosome fractions and essentially all of the radioactive RNA in the fractions from the monoribosome to 98S region are in the form of RNP structures (*cf.* Fig. 9 and also ref. 19).

The proportion of poly A-containing RNA in the monoribosome-98S region is considerably smaller than that found in the polyribosome region, and yet a large portion of the labeled RNA is composed of components with electrophoretic mobilities indistinguishable from those of the large polyribosomal mRNA components (Fig. 8). The RNP structures thus appear to contain large RNA components lacking poly A which are not normally found in functional polyribosomes. It seems very likely, therefore, that the RNP structures are the source of the poly A-lacking large RNA components found in polyribosome fractions. From these considerations, we have deduced a distribution of the

Table II. Distribution of Radioactive RNA in Polyribosome Fractions of Control and Cordycepin-Treated Cells[a]

Structure	RNA species		Large components			
	All species	Histone plus 4S	Plus poly A		Minus poly A	
			MF	PF	MF	PF
Control cells						
Functional polyribosomes	80	20	60	60	0	0
RNP structures	20	4	5	7	11	9
Total	100	24	65	67	11	9
Cordycepin-treated cells						
Functional polyribosomes	25	7	6	17	12	1
RNP structures	16	4	1	-	11	-
Total	41	11	7	-	23	-

[a] The entries in this table are averages of three sets of data. Values are expressed as percentages of the total radioactivity in all RNA species of control cells. The relative amounts of radioactivity in functional polyribosomes and RNP structures are obtained from CsCl analyses (e.g., Fig. 9); the realtive amounts of radioactivity in histone plus 4S RNA and in large RNA components are obtained from gel electrophoretograms (e.g., Figs. 5 and 8); and the proportion of poly A-containing mRNA (plus poly A) was measured by selective adsorption to Millipore filters (MF) or by selective binding to poly U-glass fiber filters (PF). The minus poly A values were obtained by subtracting the plus poly A values from the total amount of large components. The relative RNA distributions for the RNP structures were obtained from measurements on samples from the monoribosome-98S regions of sucrose gradients (e.g. Fig. 8A).

various types of RNA in the polyribosome fractions (Table II) which is consistent with all of our experimental data.

It would appear that only those large mRNA components which contain poly A are capable of becoming engaged in functional polyribosomes. To test this idea further, we analyzed the polyribosomal RNA from cells incubated with 3'-deoxyadenosine (cordycepin). It had been shown previously (12,32) that this analogue partially suppresses the entry of newly made mRNA into cytoplasmic polyribosomes, presumably by interfering with the addition of poly A to the mRNA precursors in the nucleus. We inquired whether under these circumstances some poly A-deficient large mRNAs might be present in functioning polyribosomes. In order to detect mRNAs containing relatively short poly A sequences, we assayed for the ability of the mRNA to anneal to poly U-impregnated glass fiber filters as well as for its ability to bind to Millipore filters. The poly U annealing method (33) should in principle detect mRNAs with poly A sequences as little as 10-20 nucleotides long, whereas the Millipore method may require poly A sequences of at least 50-75 nucleotides (34).

The results of these experiments (Fig. 9 and Table II) indicate that there are indeed some large mRNA components in the functioning polyribosomes of cordycepin-treated cells which do not bind effectively to Millipore filters. These

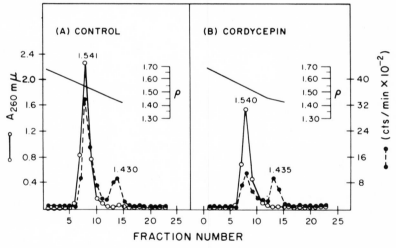

Fig. 9. *Buoyant density analysis of the polyribosome fractions of control (A) and cordycepin-treated (B) cells.* L cells were incubated for 20 min with 0.08 µg/ml actinomycin D and divided into two parts. To one part was added cordycepin (Sigma Chemical Co.) at a final concentration of 30 µg/ml; the other portion served as a control. After 10 min, ^{3}H-uridine was added, and both cultures were further incubated for 1 hr. Polyribosomes were prepared (19) and analyzed on CsCl as described in Fig. 7.

components bind to poly U filters, however, and therefore probably contain shorter than normal poly A sequences. Thus it would seem that all of the large RNA components require at least some minimal length of poly A at their 3'-OH termini in order to find their way into cytoplasmic polyribosomes. It is worth noting that under these partially inhibitory conditions we did not observe any accumulation of nonribosomal bound mRNA. This is consistent with the notion that the poly A is required for a nuclear event involving processing of the mRNA (12) rather than a cytoplasmic event involving formation of polyribosomes.

POLY A AS AN mRNA DIAGNOSTIC

In addition to throwing new light on the HnRNA to mRNA processing problem, poly A may also prove of value as an mRNA diagnostic. The low poly A content of the RNP structures and the relative insensitivity of RNP synthesis to cordycepin suggest that a large portion of the RNA of the RNP structures, although exhibiting an electrophoretic mobility which closely resembles that of true mRNA, is not, in fact, the same type of RNA. This further indicates that many of the free RNP structures normally found in the cell cytoplasm are probably not polyribosome precursors. In contrast, the "mRNP" which is released from polyribosomes on temperature shock (19) contains its normal poly A complement, indicating that mRNA can exist in the cytoplasm free of ribosomes without losing its poly A.

ACKNOWLEDGMENTS

The authors wish to dedicate this paper to the memory of the late Dr. Jack Schultz. His legacy to us: an appreciation for the harmony and beauty of nature, in all her complexity.

This research was supported by Grant GB-15397 from the National Science Foundation, U.S. Public Health Service Grants CA-06927 and RR-05539, and an appropriation from the Commonwealth of Pennsylvania. J. L. is a recipient of a fellowship from the Consejo Nacional de Investigaciones Científicas y Técnicas, Argentina. G. S. was supported by U.S. Public Health Service Training Grant 5T01-GM-00694-09 administered by the Graduate Group in Molecular Biology, University of Pennsylvania.

SUMMARY

The discovery of large polyadenylic acid (poly A) sequences in messenger RNA (mRNA) and heterogeneous nuclear RNA (HnRNA) has provided a new and valuable tool which can be used to help elucidate the relationship between these two classes of RNA. Poly A content may also be used as a means of discriminating between the cytoplasmic ribonucleoproteins (RNP) which are true precursors of polyribosomal mRNA and those which are not.

Experiments with a highly purified exoribonuclease have indicated that the poly A sequences are located at the 3'-OH termini of the mRNA molecules. This fact, when taken together with other findings, implies that the conversion of HnRNA to mRNA most probably involves conservation of a piece near the 3'-OH terminus and elimination of nucleotides at the 5'-P(PP) end.

In cultured L cells, all of the large (0.5-2.0 × 10^6 daltons) mRNA components appear to contain poly A sequences. Experiments with the analogue, 3'-deoxyadenosine (cordycepin), indicate that the poly A is necessary for the proper processing of HnRNA to mRNA in the nucleus. However, under these conditions some mRNA with shorter than normal segments of poly A can be detected in functioning polyribosomes, suggesting that the full poly A sequence may not be critically required.

The mRNAs which code for histones form a relatively discrete class with molecular weights of approximately 150,000. These h-mRNAs contain no detectable poly A and are distinguished by appearing in the cytoplasm without the lag characteristic of the large mRNA components and by having a lifetime less than a third of that of most other mRNAs.

RESUMEN

El descubrimiento de secuencias largas de ácido poliadenílico (poli A) en el RNA mensajero (mRNA) y en el RNA nuclear heterogéneo (HnRNA) ha provisto una nueva y valiosa forma la cual puede utilizarse para ayudar a elucidar las relaciones que existen entre estas dos clases de RNA. El contenido de poli A puede utilizarse además como un criterio para discriminar entre las ribonucleoproteínas (RNP) citoplásmicas, que son las verdaderas precursoras del mRNA, y aquellas que no lo son.

Experimentos utilizando una exoribonucleasa altamente purificada, indican que las secuencias de poli A están localizadas cerca del extremo 3'-OH en las moléculas de mRNA. Este hecho, cuando se considera conjuntamente con otros resultados, implica que la transformación de HnRNA→mRNA comprende probablemente la conservación de un fragmento cerca del extremo 3'-OH y la eliminación de nucleótidos en el extremo 5'-P-(PP).

En células de cultivo L todos los componentes de mRNA grandes (0.5-2.0 × 10^6 daltons) parecen contener secuencias de poli A. Experimentos con 3'-deoxiadenosina (cordicepina), indican que el poli A es necesario para la transformación adecuada del HnRNA a mRNA en el núcleo. Por otra parte, bajo estas condiciones algún mRNA con segmentos de poli A más cortos que los normales puede ser descubierto en polisomas funcionales, lo cual sugiere que la secuencia completa de poli A no debe ser necesaria.

Los mRNA que codifican para las histonas foran una clase relativamente única con pesos moleculares de aproximadamente 150,000. Estos hRNA no muestran evidencia de contener poli A y se distinguen porque aparecen en el citoplasma sin el retardo característico de los componentes grandes de mRNA y porque tienen una duración de vida menor que una tercera parte de la de la mayoría de lo otros RNAs.

REFERENCES

1. Darnell, J. E., *Bacteriol. Rev., 32,* 262 (1968).
2. Greenberg, J. R., and Perry, R. P., *J. Cell Biol., 50,* 774 (1971).
3. Lindberg, U., and Darnell, J. E., *Proc. Natl. Acad. Sci. U.S.A., 65,* 1089 (1970).
4. Tonegawa, S., Walter, G., Bernardini, A., and Dulbecco, R., *Cold Spring Harbor Symp. Quant. Biol., 35,* 823 (1970).
5. Wagner, E. K., and Roizman, B., *Proc. Natl. Acad. Sci. U.S.A., 64,* 626 (1969).

6. Perry, R. P., in Lima-de-Faria (ed.), *Handbook of Molecular Cytology*, North-Holland Publ. Co., Amsterdam (1969), p. 620.
7. Kates, J., *Cold Spring Harbor Symp. Quant. Biol., 35*, 743 (1970).
8. Lim, L., and Canellakis, E. S., *Nature, 227*, 710 (1970).
9. Darnell, J. E., Wall, R., and Tushinski, R. J., *Proc. Natl. Acad. Sci. U.S.A., 68*, 1321 (1971).
10. Edmonds, M., Vaughan, M. H., and Nakazato, H., *Proc. Natl. Acad. Sci. U.S.A., 68*, 1336 (1971).
11. Lee, S. Y., Mendecki, J., and Brawerman, G., *Proc. Natl. Acad. Sci. U.S.A., 68*, 1331 (1971).
12. Darnell, J. E., Philipson, L., Wall, R., and Adesnik, M., *Science, 174*, 507 (1971).
13. Philipson, L., Wall, R., Glickman, R., and Darnell, J. E., *Proc. Natl. Acad. Sci. U.S.A., 68*, 2806 (1971).
14. Lazarus, H. M., and Sporn, M. B., *Proc. Natl. Acad. Sci. U.S.A., 57*, 1386 (1967).
15. Perry, R. P., and Kelley, D. E., *J. Mol. Biol, 70*, 265 (1972).
16. Lazarus, H. M., Sporn, M. B., and Bradley, D. F., *Proc. Natl. Acad. Sci. U.S.A., 60*, 1503 (1968).
17. Sporn, M. B., Lazarus, H. M., Smith, J. M., and Henderson, W. R., *Biochemistry, 8*, 1698 (1968).
18. Perry, R. P., and Kelley, D. E., *J. Mol. Biol., 35*, 37 (1968).
19. Schochetman, G., and Perry, R. P., *J. Mol. Biol., 63*, 577 (1972).
20. Perry, R. P., LaTorre, J., Kelley, D. E., and Greenberg, J. R., *Biochim. Biophys. Acta, 262*, 220 (1972).
21. Perry, R. P., and Kelley, D. E., *J. Cell. Physiol., 72*, 235 (1968).
22. Molloy, G. R., Sporn, M. B., Kelley, D. E., and Perry, R. P., *Biochemistry, 11*, 3256 (1972).
23. Kelley, D. E., and Perry, R. P., *Biochim. Biophys. Acta, 238*, 357 (1971).
24. Greenberg, J. R. and Perry, R. P., *J. Mol. Biol., 72*, (1972).
25. Perry, R. P., Greenberg, J. R., and Tartof, K. D., *Cold Spring Harbor Symp. Quant. Biol., 35*, 577 (1970).
26. Schochetman, G., and Perry, R. P., *J. Mol. Biol., 63*, 591 (1972).
27. Borun, T. W., Scharff, M. D., and Robbins, E., *Proc. Natl. Acad. Sci. U.S.A., 58*, 1977 (1967).
28. Gallwitz, D., and Mueller, G. C., *J. Biol. Chem., 244*, 5947 (1969).
29. Craig, N., Kelley, D. E., and Perry, R. P., *Biochim. Biophys. Acta, 246*, 493 (1971).
30. Schochetman, G., Ph.D. dissertation, University of Pennsylvania (1970).
31. Penman, S., Vesco, C., and Penman, M., *J. Mol. Biol., 34*, 49 (1968).
32. Penman, S., Rosbash, M., and Penman, M., *Proc. Natl. Acad. Sci. U.S.A., 67*, 1678 (1970).
33. Sheldon, R., Jurale, C., and Kates, J., *Proc. Natl. Acad. Sci. U.S.A., 69*, 417 (1972).
34. Darnell, J. E., personal communication.

DISCUSSION

R. T. Schimke (Stanford, U.S.A.): Have you considered the possibility that the poly A may have something to do with the relative stability of the messenger? It is obviously a major problem, and it looks like you may have a handle on it.

R. P. Perry (Philadelphia, U.S.A.): We have looked into this by posing the following question: do the steady state-labeled mRNAs contain a different amount of poly A as compared to pulse-labeled mRNA? If poly A has something to do with messenger stability, one might expect more or less, probably less, poly A on old message than on new message. We indeed find evidence of this. The steady state-labeled mRNA, which is predominantly old message, contains shorter sequences of poly A as compared to pulse-labeled mRNA, which is predominantly new message.

R. T. Schimke: Does cordycepin affect this turnover of messenger?

R. P. Perry: I have not studied that.

E. P. Geiduschek (La Jolla, U.S.A.): Did you determine the kinetic constants of the exonuclease?

R. P. Perry: We tried to use excess amounts of the enzyme. However, since the enzyme has not been purified to homogeneity, we do not know precisely the enzyme/substrate ratio on a molecule-to-molecule basis. Although we were not able to assess stoichiometry, we did use as high an enzyme/substrate ratio as we could so that we would achieve maximum synchrony in the reaction. Moreover, we found no differences in the basic result when the enzyme/substrate ratio was varied by a factor of about 3.

J. E. Allende (Santiago, Chile): I wonder if the fact that histone messages do not have any poly A is related to the fact that histone messages already have a high A content because of the high lysine content of the proteins that they code for. Have you given this any thought?

R. P. Perry: No, I had not actually thought of relating it to the type of protein. However, I do not think that histones could have sequences of lysine residues which are long enough to account for poly A sequences of the size I have been talking about. I think a pertinent question might be: how big a stretch of adenylic acid residues would one need in order for the poly A to be detected by the Millipore assay or by the poly U-binding assay. I cannot give you hard numbers, but according to work done in Darnell's laboratory Millipore binding requires somewhere between 50 and 75 nucleotides. For poly U binding, that is, to obtain stable U:A duplexes or 2U:A triplexes, one should need only about 10-15 nucleotides. I would say in the case of the histone message, that if it has any poly A sequences, they would be less than 15 nucleotides long. This would correspond to a run of about five lysines.

F. J. S. Lara (São Paulo, Brazil): I have done some experiments using the Millipore assay with *Rhynchosciara* where there are different RNA patterns at different larval stages. We found a very interesting result: if one takes whole-cell RNA before birth and analyzes it, there is a certain radioactivity distribution, and during birth time the RNA is of a different kind, it is enriched for the puffed region of the genome, and there is much less radioactivity incorporated. If one does the poly A assay in the first case, one gets a smear that goes along with the radioactivity, but at the time of birth, there is a definite peak of poly A around one region. These are very preliminary data, but they might indicate different stabilities of messages of different types.

R. P. Perry: If I just would be permitted one comment about procedures for isolation of RNA containing poly A because this subject was mentioned by Dr. Schimke in this discussion: although it has been reported by Lee *et al.* (11) that the poly A sequences will normally go into the phenol phase in a phenol-SDS extraction at neutral pH, if one adds chloroform to the phenol (1 vol of chloroform to 1 vol of phenol) one can retain all the poly A-containing RNA in the aqueous phase. I think this is an important fact because if one is not careful, the poly A can be sheared off the mRNA during vigorous shaking of phenol-aqueous mixtures. This is especially critical when one extracts polyribosomal RNA.

F. J. S. Lara: In my particular case, I was aware of that difficulty and I extracted

Rhynchosciara RNA by a method which does not involve the phenol, and so the poly A should remain attached.

R. T. Schimke: You showed a very interesting range of distributions of your "messenger" in which looked as if in general it was relatively heavier than one would predict from the size of the proteins that the cells are making. Have you ever, in general, made the correlation between the size of your messenger and the size of the proteins? The reason I ask is that our messenger appears to be roughly 50% larger than it should be—as is also the hemoglobin messenger—so one wonders whether the extra size has to do with the overall secondary structure of the entire messenger rather than having some specific unique sequences that are involved in translation, transport, etc.

R. P. Perry: I agree completely: the messages are much too big on the basis of the size distribution of L cell proteins. As you say, in the cases of ovalbumin mRNA or hemoglobin mRNA, one sees the same thing. We have to consider that this mRNA is not pure template, but as in the case of various phage RNAs it may contain a lot of other sequence information besides that specifying protein structure.

M. Azzam (Buenos Aires, Argentina): Is it known whether the precursor mRNA from nucleus could be translated *in vitro?*

R. P. Perry: I have never done that kind of experiment myself. I believe that several workers have demonstrated so-called template activity with nuclear RNA, but without any real measure of specificity, i.e., of the types of protein being made. Someone else may have a better answer to this question, perhaps Dr. Schimke.

R. T. Schimke: We have high molecular weight RNA which certainly makes ovalbumin. However, we do not know whether the RNA is of nuclear origin. I presume that it is, although there are other explanations for it.

13

Messenger RNA Processing in Vertebrate Cells

R. Brentani, C. S. Peres, C. H. Oda, and L. Wang

Departamento de Bioquímica
Instituto de Química
Universidade de São Paulo,
São Paulo, Brasil

For some years, we have been engaged in the study of messenger RNA (mRNA) processing in metazoan cells. This line of investigation has led to the demonstration of mRNA in a purified nucleolar fraction, characterized as such by some of its biological, chemical, and biophysical properties.

Thus, rat liver nucleolar RNA has been found to stimulate amino acid incorporation *in vitro* by mRNA-depleted ribosomes (1,2), to hybridize with several times more DNA than ribosomal RNA, to present a DNA-like base composition (3), and to be only about 12% hydrogen-bonded, as shown by kinetics of reaction with formaldehyde, ultraviolet absorbance-temperature profiles, spectrophotometric titration, and hydrogen-tritium exchange kinetics (4,5).

When chromatin, nucleoplasmic, and nucleolar RNA were assayed for their template activity, the nucleolar fraction was the most active, indicating that its effect was not a consequence of contamination by material from other subnuclear sources (2).

These findings led us to state a hypothesis whereby the nucleolus might be involved in the processing of cytoplasmic mRNA (6).

Others have investigated the template activity of nuclear subfractions in the

Walker adenocarcinoma (7) and AH 130 hepatoma (8), but in these tumors the nucleolar RNA was not the most active, a discrepancy that may have biological significance.

Conclusive evidence of the informational nature of this nucleolar RNA would consist of the demonstration of its ability to direct the synthesis of a specific protein. A suitable model is collagen, which can be characterized by its unusually high content of glycine and proline, its solubility in hot trichloroacetic acid, and its sensitivity toward collagenase (9). This enzyme can split tetra-peptides of sequence Pro-X-Gly-Pro (10), so that even short collagen peptides are sufficient for identification.

In this report, we shall describe our studies of the *in vitro* synthesis of collagen by rat liver ribosomes under the direction of chick embryo nucleolar and nucleoplasmic RNA. Also, we have studied the origin of nucleolar mRNA, by performing hybridization experiments between rat liver nucleolar RNA and chromatin DNA, since a flow of mRNA from chromatin to the nucleolus has been reported (11,12).

MATERIALS AND METHODS

Animals

Male Wistar strain albino rats (200-250 g body weight) were obtained from a closed colony bred at the Faculdade de Medicina. For the preparation of labeled nucleolar RNA, 8-10 mc of carrier-free ^{32}P-orthophosphate was injected intra-peritoneally 3 hr before sacrifice (^{32}P was obtained from the Instituto de Energia Atômica). For purification of labeled ribosomal RNA, 500 μc of methyl-^{3}H-methionine (Schwarz BioResearch, specific activity 188 mc/mM) was injected daily for 5 days, intraperitoneally, into partially hepatectomized rats. The rats were killed by cervical concussion, and their livers were rapidly removed and placed on crushed ice until cell fractionation was begun. All subsequent steps were performed at 4°. Eight-day-old chick embryos were purchased at a nearby hatchery, brought to the laboratory, and decapitated, and their bodies were placed on ice.

Cell Fractionation

Rat liver and chick embryo nuclei and nucleoli were purified according to the methods of Penman *et al.* (13) and Penman *et al.* (14), respectively. Ribosomes, microsomes, and "pH 5 enzymes" were prepared as previously reported (15). Chick embryo initiation factors were purified as described by Heywood (16).

RNA and DNA Extractions and Hybridization Experiments

RNA and DNA extractions and hybridization experiments were done as described elsewhere (3).

Cesium Chloride Centrifugation

CsCl centrifugation was performed following the method of Flamm *et al.* (17).

Amino Acid Incorporation

Unless otherwise specified, rat liver ribosomes were incubated as described

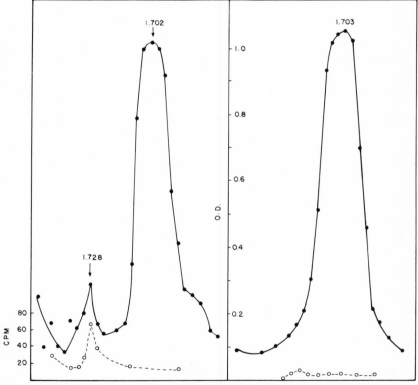

Fig. 1. CsCl centrifugation of DNA from subnuclear fractions. Chromatin and nucleolus-associated chromatin DNA were analyzed in CsCl gradients and separate fractions were hybridized with ribosomal RNA as described in *Materials and Methods.*

elsewhere (3). At fixed intervals, 0.12 ml aliquots were delivered onto Whatman 3M filter paper disks, which were dried under a hot air stream and placed in 12% ice-cold trichloroacetic acid containing 0.2% nonradioactive amino acid and washed following the procedure of Mans and Novelli (18).

Preincubation of Rat Liver Ribosomes

The same incubation mixture as above was employed for preincubation of rat liver ribosomes, omitting radioactive amino acids. After 12 min at 37°, the whole mixture was centrifuged at 105,000 × g for 120 min and the resulting pellet utilized as "preincubated ribosomes."

RESULTS

Figure 1 shows that chromatin DNA exhibits a single homogeneous peak, when analyzed in a CsCl gradient, whereas nucleolus-associated chromatin DNA presents a second smaller peak of greater density. When ribosomal RNA, specifically labeled with methyl-^{3}H-methionine (see *Materials and Methods*), was hybridized with separate fractions from the gradients, hybrid formation occurred only at the heavy nucleolar satellite region, known to contain the ribosomal

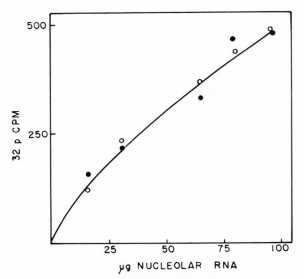

Fig. 2. Hybridization of nucleolar RNA with chromatin and whole nuclear DNA. ●, Whole nuclear DNA; ○, chromatin DNA.

Table I. Amino Acid Incorporation *in vitro*[a]

Additions	Incorporation (% of preincubated ribosomes)
Preincubated	100
+ CIF	97
+ NuRNA	98
+ NuRNA + CIF	206
+ NpRNA + CIF	166
+ NuRNA + CIF + NaF	116
Normal ribosomes	309

[a] CIF, chick embryo initiation factors; NuRNA, nucleolar RNA; NpRNA, nucleoplasmic RNA; NaF, 0.015 M sodium fluoride. Preincubated ribosomes (1.75 mg) were incubated in a final volume of 1.0 ml with 1.0 mg pH 5 enzyme, 1.75 mg CIF, 0.5 μM ATP, 0.05 μM GTP, 87.5 mM sucrose, 5.0 mM MgCl$_2$, 10 mM Tris-HCl buffer (pH 7.4), 20 mM phosphoenolpyruvate (sodium), 30 μg pyruvate kinase (E.C. 2.7.1.40), 20 mM KCl, 12.5 mM NaCl, (0.5 μc) ^{3}H-proline and glycine. After 10 min, the reaction was stopped, aliquots were taken, and their radioactivity was determined as described in *Materials and Methods*.

cistrons (19). No hybrid formation occurred with chromatin DNA, showing this material to be uncontaminated by ribosomal cistrons.

When rat liver nucleolar RNA was hybridized at 55° with either chromatin DNA or total nuclear DNA (Fig. 2), the reaction proceeded equally well with both DNAs, suggesting that nucleolar RNA participating in the reaction originated in chromatin rather than in nucleolus-associated DNA cistrons.

Table I shows some results of experiments on the effect of purified RNA from chick embryo subnuclear fractions on the amino acid incorporating activity of rat liver preincubated ribosomes. It is evident that chick embryo nucleolar RNA is able to stimulate the incorporation of glycine and proline by preincubated rat liver ribosomes when the system is supplemented with chick embryo initiation factors, which are free from cytoplasmic mRNA. That this effect of nucleolar RNA cannot be attributed to its contamination by nucleoplasmic RNA is demonstrated by the lesser stimulatory activity of the latter fraction. Finally, this incorporation occurs into newly synthesized peptides, since it is inhibited by NaF, a known initiation inhibitor (20).

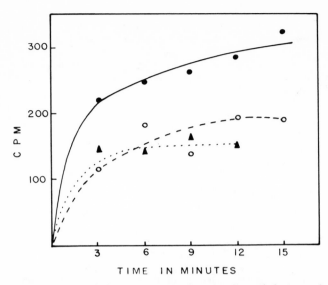

Fig. 3. Chemical characterization of the product of glycine and proline incorporation under the direction of chick embryo nucleolar RNA. Preincubated rat liver ribosomes were reincubated in the presence of 250 μg nucleolar RNA, under conditions given in Table I and *Materials and Methods.* ●, Complete, ○, complete plus 500 μg collagenase; ▲, washed as described in *Materials and Methods*, including the hot TCA step.

The chemical nature of the labeled product is clarified by the results shown in Fig. 3. The sensitivity of the labeled product to collagenase and the solubility of the product in hot trichloroacetic acid allow us to believe that the system is actually synthesizing collagen.

As would be expected, the enzyme does not hinder the incorporation of proline by normal rat liver ribosomes (Fig. 4). The considerably lesser effect of collagenase on the stimulation of leucine incorporation by nucleolar RNA (Fig. 5) can be explained by the low content of this amino acid in chick embryo collagen (9).

CONCLUSIONS

The results presented in Fig. 2 show that nucleolar RNA was able to hybridize with chromatin DNA, which was free from nucleolar satellite contamination, so that neither mature ribosomal RNAs nor their nucleolar precursors can be involved in the reaction.

As seen in Table I, chick embryo nucleolar RNA was able to stimulate amino

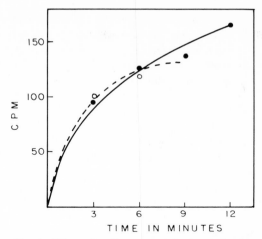

Fig. 4. Effect of collagenase on incorporation by normal rat liver ribosomes. Rat liver ribosomes were incubated under the conditions described in Fig. 3. ●, Complete; ○, complete plus 500 μg collagenase.

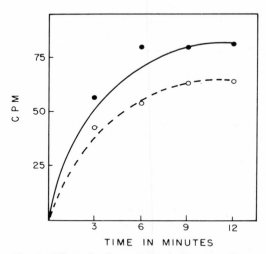

Fig. 5. Effect of collagenase on the incorporation of leucine directed by chick embryo nucleolar RNA. Details of the experiment are given in the caption of Fig. 3. ●, Complete, ○, complete plus 500 μg collagenase.

acid incorporation by preincubated rat liver ribosomes supplemented with chick embryo initiation factors. It has been reported that preincubated ribosomes become dependent on such solubilized factors when separated from the incubation mixture by centrifugation (21). Evidence has also been presented showing that these factors are organ and species specific (22,23). The sensitivity of this stimulation to NaF is also noteworthy, since many of the early results on the *in vitro* direction of protein synthesis by exogenous "mRNA" were but nonspecific stimulation of already initiated peptide elongation (24). Characterization of the incorporation product as collagen by its high content of glycine and proline, low content of leucine, solubility in hot trichloroacetic acid, and sensitivity toward collagenase permits the final identification of nucleolar RNA as messenger RNA, since it is able to direct, *in vitro,* the synthesis of a specific protein. Furthermore, as collagen is made at the polysomal level in the cytoplasm (25), it becomes evident that part of the nucleolar mRNA moves to the cytoplasm, where it becomes operative.

The concept of nucleolar participation in the processing of mRNA does not necessarily conflict with that of specific nucleoprotein particles being involved in mRNA transport (26).

ACKNOWLEDGMENTS

We are indebted to Dr. J. Carneiro for helpful discussion and for generous offers of ^{3}H-proline and purified collagenase. We are also happy to acknowledge the able technical assistance of Mr. A. M. Olmo. This work was made possible by grants from the "Fundacáo de Amparo á Pesquisa do Estado de São Paulo," Conselho Nacional de Pesquisas, and FORGE Foundation.

SUMMARY

The fate of nucleolar messenger ribonucleic acid was determined. Nucleolar RNA, labeled with ^{32}P-orthophosphate, from rat liver was shown to hybridize with purified homologous chromatin DNA, under conditions in which nucleoplasmic RNA was much less efficient in the same reaction.

Nucleolar RNA was extracted from 7-day-old chick embryos and added to an amino acid incorporating system. Under the experimental conditions used, the incorporation of glycine and proline was stimulated, but not that of leucine. The incorporation product was hot trichloroacetic acid soluble and, to a great extent, destroyed by purified collagenase. These results are taken as evidence that nucleolar RNA is able to direct the *in vitro* synthesis of collagen.

It is concluded that some messengers, after their synthesis at the chromatin level, flow to the nucleolus before reaching the cytoplasm, where they are utilized. Since mRNA has been found in both mammalian and avian nucleoli, this mechanism may be widespread in biological systems.

RESUMEN

El destino del ácido ribonucléico mensajero nucleolar fue determinado. Se demostró que el RNA nucleolar, marcado con ^{32}P-ortofosfato, del hígado de rata, hibridiza con cromatina purificade del DNA homólogo, en condiciones en las cuales el RNA nucleoplásmico es mucho menos eficiente en la misma reacción.

El RNA nucleolar fue obtenido de embriones de pollo de 7 días y agregado a un sistema de incorporación de aminoácidos. Bajo las condiciones empleadas, la incorporación de glicina y prolina es estimulada, pero no la de leucina. El producto de la incorporación es soluble en ácido tricloroacético caliente, y en gran parte destruído por colagenasa pura. Estos resultados pueden tomarse como evidencia de que el RNA nucleolar es capaz de dirigir la síntesis de colágeno.

Puede por lo tanto concluirse que algunos mensajeros, después de ser sintetizados al nivel de cromatina, se dirigen al nucleolo antes de dirigirse al citoplasma, donde son utilizados. Ya que el mRNA se ha encontrado en nucleolos de aves y mamíferos, este mecanismo puede muy bien estar presente en muchos sistemas biológicos.

REFERENCES

1. Brentani, M., Brentani, R., and Raw, I., *Nature, 201,* 1130 (1964).
2. Brentani, R., Brentani, M., and Raw, I., *Nature, 214,* 1122 (1967).
3. Brentani, R., and Brentani, M., *Genetics,* Suppl. 61, 391 (1969).
4. Brentani, M., Doctorate thesis (1971).
5. Brentani, M., Kubota, M., and Brentani, R., *Biochem. J., 130,* 11 (1972).
6. Brentani, R., *Rev. Bras. Pesquisas Med. Biol., 1,* 25 (1968).
7. Jacob, S. T., and Busch, H., *Biochim. Biophys. Acta, 138,* 249 (1967).
8. Akino, T., and Amano, M., *J. Biochem., 67,* 533 (1970).
9. Eastoe, J. E., in Ramachandran, G. N. (ed.), *Treatise on Collagen,* vol. 1, Academic Press, New York (1967), p. 1.
10. Hannig, K., and Nordwig, A., in Ramachandran, G. N. (ed.), *Treatise on Collagen,* vol. 1, Academic Press, New York (1967), p. 73.
11. Sirlin, J. L., Jacob, J., and Kato, K., *Exptl. Cell Res., 27,* 355 (1962).
12. Rho, J. H., and Bonner, J., *Proc. Natl. Acad. Sci. U.S.A., 47,* 1611 (1961).
13. Penman, S., Smith, I., and Holtzman, E., *Science, 154,* 786 (1966).
14. Penman, S., Vesco, C., and Holtzman, M., *J. Mol. Biol., 34,* 49 (1968).
15. Brentani, R., Brentani, M., Raw, I., Cunha, J. L. M., and Wrotchinsky, N., *Biochem. J., 106,* 263 (1968).
16. Heywood, S. M., *Cold Spring Harbor Symp. Quant. Biol., 34,* 799 (1969).
17. Flamm, W. G., Bond, H. E. and Burr, H. E., *Biochim. Biophys. Acta, 129,* 310 (1966).
18. Mans, R. J., and Novelli, D., *Arch. Biochem. Biophys., 94,* 48 (1961).
19. Busch, H., and Smetana, K., *The Nucleolus,* Academic Press, New York (1970).
20. Lin, S.-Y., Mosteller, R. D., and Hardesty, B., *J. Mol. Biol., 21,* 51 (1966).
21. Miller, R. L., and Schweet, R., *Arch. Biochem. Biophys., 125,* 632 (1968).
22. Heywood, S. M., *Nature, 225,* 696 (1970).
23. Naora, H., and Kodaira, K., *Biochim. Biophys. Acta, 209,* 196 (1970).
24. Chantrenne, H., Burny, A., and Marbaix, G., *Progr. Nucleic Acid Res. Mol. Biol., 7,* 173 (1967).

25. Gould, B. S., in Ramachandran, G. N. (ed.), *Treatise on Collagen*, vol. 2, Academic Press, New York (1968), p. 139.
26. Perry, R. P., and Kelley, D. E., *J. Mol. Biol.*, *35*, 37 (1968).

DISCUSSION

R. T. Schimke (Stanford, U.S.A.): Your messenger must have a very high GC content, about 67% GC, which is higher than in ribosomal RNA. I wonder if there is any relationship between the GC content of an RNA and the nuclear fraction one isolates it from?

R. Brentani (São Paulo, Brazil): I think not. The characterization work I showed was done in a rat liver system, where the GC content of the RNA was 46%. Just recently, we switched to the chick embryo to try to demonstrate that the nucleolus contains an mRNA which codes for a specific protein.

R. T. Schimke: I realize that your rat liver study was done without the characterization of what the mRNA was. It may be that all you are looking at there is messengers that have a high GC content.

R. Brentani: Yes, but the work on rat liver reveals 46% GC content for nucleolar 18S RNA.

R. T. Schimke: That may be enough for it to be associated with the nucleolus.

F. L. Sacerdote (Mendoza, Argentina): Please tell me something more about those factors in chick embryos which you have characterized or designated as CIF.

R. Brentani: I did not characterize the factor to any great extent. I was not getting any stimulation of preincubated ribosomes by chick nuclear RNA; then I came across Heywood's results on myosin synthesis, which showed quite clearly that myosin would be synthesized only in the presence of a KCl wash of myosin-synthesizing muscle polysomes. When this was added to previously washed reticulocyte ribosomes, they would synthesize myosin. I did practically the same thing—one can preincubate and centrifuge ribosomes and remove such factors. If you add back a KCl wash from chick embryo ribosomes, the system will work.

14

Effects of Neonatal Thyroidectomy on Nuclear and Microsomal RNA Synthesis in Developing Rat Brain

Carlos J. Gomez, Beatriz Duvilanski, Alicia E. R. de Guglielmone, and Ana Maria Soto

Departamento de Química Biológica
Facultad de Farmacia y Bioquímica
Universidad de Buenos Aires
Buenos Aires, Argentina

Histological (1,2) and biochemical (3-8) studies have shown that neonatal thyroid deficiency in rats produces striking alterations in developing brain, which are characterized by a marked impairment in the formation of different kinds of membranes. Although it is well known that RNA metabolism plays an important role in the regulation of the growth rate of tissues other than the brain (9,10), some contradictory results have been reported recently in relation to the effect of thyroid on cerebral RNA metabolism. Evidence from two different sources (6,7,11) suggests that at 14, 25, and 35 days after birth cerebral RNA synthesis is unaffected by neonatal thyroidectomy, which contrasts markedly with our findings (12) showing that in 10-day-old rats this condition produces a marked decrease in the synthesis of the "rapidly labeled" nuclear and microsomal RNA. In an effort to clarify this controversial problem, we studied the kinetics of labeling of brain nuclear and microsomal RNA in 10-day-old normal and cretinoid rats. The results to be reported confirm our previous finding (12) and suggest that neonatal thyroidectomy also produces alterations in nuclear post-transcriptional mechanisms of control.

EXPERIMENTAL PROCEDURE

Experiments were performed with 10-day-old normal and neonatally radio-thyroidectomized Wistar rats, prepared and kept as previously reported (3). Under light ether anesthesia, rats were injected intro-arachnoidally with a solution containing 2 μc of ^{3}H-5-orotic acid (specific activity 20 c/mmole). At different intervals after the injection, the animals were killed by decapitation. Cerebral hemispheres were rapidly excised, freed of cerebellum and cerebral peduncles, and homogenized in 5 vol of cold 0.32 M sucrose, 1 mM MgCl$_2$, 0.4 mM potassium phosphate buffer (pH 6.7) as previously reported (12). The measurement of radioactivity in the initial homogenate and in the acid-soluble fraction, as well as the isolation of purified nuclear and microsomal fractions, was done as previously described (12). RNA was extracted from nuclei by the procedure of Vesco and Guiditta (13) with some minor modifications, consisting of further purification of the isolated RNA according to Di Girolamo *et al.* (14); the final product was dissolved in a solution of 0.1 M NaCl, 10 mM sodium acetate buffer (pH 5.0). Microsomal RNA was extracted and purified according to Vesco and Guiditta (12), the final product being dissolved in a solution of 10 mM Tris-HCl buffer (pH 7.4).

Aliquots of both nuclear and microsomal RNA solutions were used to determine RNA content by measuring the absorbance at 260 nm and using as a standard a yeast RNA (Sigma) solution prepared under similar conditions, while other aliquots were transferred to counting vials containing 12 ml of Bray's (15) solution. Nuclear and microsomal RNA, extracted and purified as above, were

Table I. Changes of Radioactivity in the Brain and
its Acid-Soluble Fraction[a]

Time after injection	Initial homogenate (dpm/mg wet tissue)		Acid-soluble fraction (dpm/mg wet tissue)	
20 min	1284 ± 172	1206 ± 181	1221 ± 167	1179 ± 181
1 hr	1391 ± 201	1485 ± 299	1253 ± 164	1384 ± 290
2 hr	2430 ± 287	2203 ± 248	1976 ± 225	1821 ± 201
4 hr	1829 ± 210	2024 ± 240	1345 ± 170	1522 ± 263

[a] Results were obtained in 10-day-old normal and neonatally thyroidectomized rats, after the intra-arachnoidal injection of 2 μc ^{3}H-orotic acid; other details are in the text. Data are the mean ± S.E.M. of five experiments for each group and time interval. Comparison of results from normal and hypothyroid rats by means of the Student's t test shows that differences were not statistically significant.

used for linear sucrose gradient analysis; for the purpose of comparing results from normal and hypothyroid rats, the amount of RNA extracted from nuclei or microsomes of 1 g original wet tissue was analyzed in each experiment. Thus 150-200 μg of nuclear RNA was layered over 5 ml of a linear sucrose gradient (5-25% w/v) in 10 mM sodium acetate (pH 5.1), 100 mM NaCl, 1 mM EDTA, and 20 μg/ml of polyvinyl sulfate. A solution containing 650-800 μg of microsomal RNA was layered over a linear sucrose gradient (5-20% w/v) in 10 mM Tris-HCl (pH 7.4), 100 mM NaCl, and 20 μg/ml of polyvinyl sulfate. The gradients were centrifuged in the SW39 rotor of the Spinco ultracentrifuge, at 4° for 5 hr at 114,000 $\times$ g; at the end of the run, approximately 25 fractions of two drops each were collected from each gradient and diluted to 1 ml with distilled water. Aliquots were used to measure radioactivity and absorbance at 260 nm. All radioactivity measurements were performed in a Packard TriCarb spectrometer; all samples were counted with an efficiency of 20-26% and a background of 16 cpm. Counts were corrected to 100% efficiency by the channel's ratio method.

RESULTS AND CONCLUSIONS

The radioactivity of the brain homogenate and that of its acid-soluble fraction followed similar kinetics in normal and hypothyroid animals (Table I). The relatively high standard errors reflect the inaccuracy of the injection because of the small volume (0.01 ml) injected into each rat; in spite of this, the mean values of both groups were very similar. This leads us to suggest that the specific radioactivity of the acid-soluble pool of precursors is unaffected by the neonatal lack of thyroid, which obviates the possibility that changes of isotope incorporation into RNAs may be due to a hormonal effect on the pool of precursors.

To minimize variations due to the inaccuracy of the injection of the labeled precursor, incorporation into RNAs was expressed as relative specific radioactivities (RSR), estimated as the ratio between the specific radioactivity of RNA (dpm/mg RNA) and the total radioactivity of the initial homogenate (dpm/mg wet tissue), the latter being closely dependent on the injected precursor. The time course of incorporation into nuclear RNA was similar in brain from normal and hypothyroid rats, and was almost linear at 20 and 60 min after the injection (Table II). During the first 60 min of labeling, the RSR of nuclear RNA of hypothyroid brain was about 40% lower than that of the normal one, but with further exposure to the radioactive precursor, the values of RSR were essentially the same in both groups. In contrast to nuclear RNA, incorporation into microsomal RNA was almost linear in both groups during the 4 hr studied, the RSR of microsomal RNA of hypothyroid brain was 35-45% lower than that of normal throughout the labeling period.

Our results clearly show that neonatal thyroidectomy (at least at this stage

Table II. Changes of the Relative Specific Radioactivities
of Brain Nuclear and Microsomal RNA[a]

Time after injection	Nuclear RNA		Microsomal RNA	
	Normal	Hypothyroid	Normal	Hypothyroid
20 min	71.4 ± 2.1	43.2 ± 3.7	2.00 ± 0.12	1.09 ±0.14
	$P<0.001$		$P<0.005$	
1 hr	162.9 ± 5.4	103.7 ± 9.6	7.50 ± 0.24	4.89 ±0.34
	$P<0.001$		$P<0.001$	
2 hr	182.8 ± 10.8	175.3 ± 10.7	11.80 ± 0.7	17.20 ±0.18
			$P<0.01$	
4 hr	172.5 ± 8.9	179.9 ± 9.3	25.5 ± 1.4	17.30 ±1.8
			$P<0.02$	

[a] Experimental conditions were as in Table I, and determinations of relative specific radioactivities were as detailed in the text. Each value is the mean of five determinations for each group and time interval; results from normal and hypothyroid rats were compared as in Table I. P values are included only when the difference is statistically significant.

of development) leads to a significant decrease in the synthesis of rapidly labeled RNA. Our findings differ from those of Balazs et al. (6), who found a normal rate of nuclear RNA synthesis in 14-day-old neonatally thyroidectomized rats. This discrepancy could be due to the fact that the shortest labeling period studied by these workers was 90 min, while we found that the decreased rate of incorporation in hypothyroid rats occurs only during the first 60 min after the injection of the labeled precursor.

It is well known that one of the early effects of growth and developmental hormones is a marked stimulation of the synthesis of rapidly labeled RNA in target tissues (9,10), and this phenomenon has been interpreted in several ways. In animal cells, the major part of the transcriptional activity of nuclei consists of the formation of large RNAs which are DNA-like in base composition, character-ized by a very rapid labeling, mostly restricted to the nucleus, and potential precursors of mRNA (16-20): Other rapidly labeled species are rRNA precursors, 5S RNA, and tRNA, which are transcribed independently from different genes (17). The transformation of rRNA precursors into 28 and 18S rRNA (16,19) and that of giant and heterogeneous D-RNA into cytoplasmic mRNA (18,20) may represent important post-transcriptional regulatory controls, taking place within the nucleus.

The work of Mandel and his associates (21,22) demonstrated the existence of giant D-RNA in nuclei of brain cells and also provided evidence that this RNA may be a precursor of cytoplasmic mRNA. On this basis, we decided to study the rate of labeling and decay of the different RNA species of nuclei and microsomes.

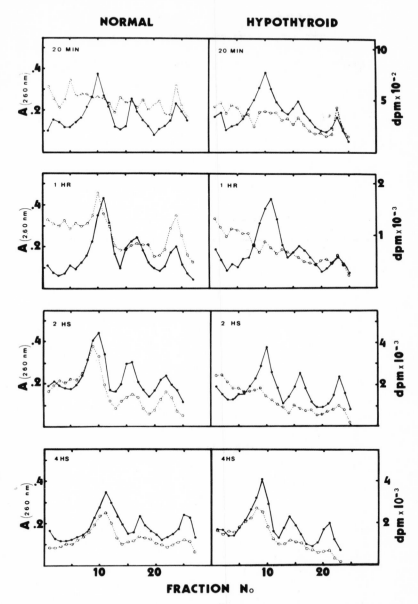

Fig. 1. *Absorbance (●) and radioactivity profiles (○) of brain nuclear RNA after different labeling periods.* Linear sucrose gradients and centrifugation conditions are detailed in the text. The radioactivity of each fraction was normalized for that present in the initial homogenate, expressed as dpm/μg wet tissue $\times 10^{-3}$.

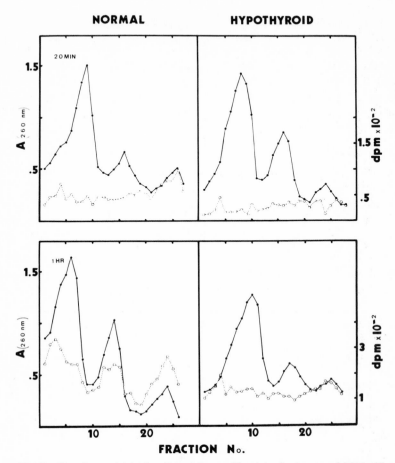

Fig. 2. Absorbance (•) and radioactivity profiles (○) of microsomal RNA, 20 and 60 min after the administration of labeled orotic acid. Radioactivity of each fraction was normalized as in Fig. 1.

Nuclear RNA analyzed on sucrose gradients (Fig. 1) shows three peaks of absorbance, which correspond (left to right) to 28S, 18S, and 4-5S, while microsomes (Figs. 2 and 3) show predominantly the peaks of 28S and 18S rRNA, and small amounts of 5S RNA. In both nuclei and microsomes, the ratio of 28S to 18S rRNA was slightly higher than 2:1, indicating that RNA degradation does not occur during isolation and gradient analysis.

In analyses of the rates of labeling, the most important differences found in nuclei from normal and hypothyroid rats were the following: (a) After short labeling periods, the radioactivity was higher in normal than in hypothyroid rats.

The radioactivity was evenly distributed along the gradient in both cases. (b) After this, nuclei of hypothyroid rats showed an increased labeling in the region heavier than 28S and a delay in the formation of labeled 28S and 18S rRNA. In microsomes (Figs. 2 and 3), the most important difference was a delay in the formation of 28S and 18S rRNA in hypothyroid as compared to normal rats. It is also worth noting that the rate of labeling of the 5S region was decreased in hypothyroid animals.

After normalization of the radioactivity for the total ^{3}H content of the

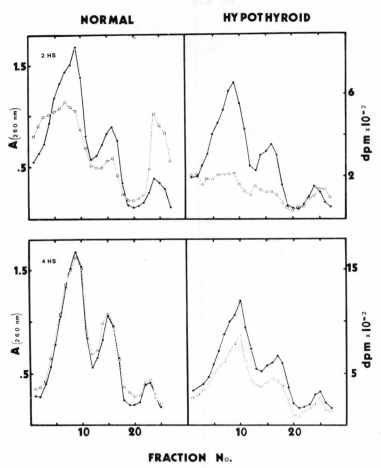

Fig. 3. *Absorbance (●) and radioactivity profiles (○) of microsomal RNA, 2 and 4 hr after exposure to labeled orotic acid.* Radioactivity of each fraction was normalized as in Fig. 1.

Table III. Relative Specific Radioactivites of Nuclear and Microsomal RNA
Species of Normal and Hypothyroid Brains[a]

Time after injection		Nuclear RNA				Microsomal RNA		
		>28S	28S	18S	4S	28S	18S	5S
20 min	N	98	43	60	60	0.69	1.91	4.07
	H	73	28	34	53	0.28	0.92	1.95
1 hr	N	355	109	92	184	3.80	6.61	18.80
	H	224	51	80	96	2.55	4.36	9.15
2 hr	N	254	187	128	156	8.83	7.64	24.80
	H	353	121	104	119	3.83	4.62	12.40
4 hr	N	171	184	168	132	23.50	25.20	25.00
	H	254	167	165	82	16.70	16.30	16.90

[a] Rats received an intra-arachnoidal injection of 2 μc ^{3}H-orotic acid and were killed after the time intervals indicated in the table. After the brain was removed, nuclear and microsomal RNAs were extracted, purified, and analyzed by linear sucrose gradients. Radioactivity of each fraction was normalized for that in the initial homogenate (dpm/μg wet tissue), and the specific radioactivites of the various species were estimated from the central region of each peak in the absorbance and radioactivity profiles, using the conversion factor of 24 absorbance units = 1 mg RNA. Results are presented as dpm/μg RNA and are the mean of three experiments for each group and time N, normal rats; H, hypothyroid rats.

homogenate, the RSR of RNA species separated on gradients was estimated. Since the centrifugation conditions used in this work did not permit a clear separation of the rRNA precursors (45S and 32S) and the giant D-RNA, the RSR of the entire region heavier than 28S was determined in nuclei. This represents a rough estimation of the average radioactivity of these different kinds of RNA. The results presented in Table III clearly demonstrate that in nuclei, RSR of the heaviest region is that showing the most striking change. While in normal rats there was a very rapid labeling and also a high rate of decay, in hypothyroid rats the incorporation was markedly decreased during the first hour and showed a markedly slower rate of decay. These findings demonstrate a decrease in the transcriptional capacity of hypothyroid nuclei. Whether this involves giant D-RNA or rRNA precursors remains to be clarified. It is also of interest that the slower rate of decay found in hypothyroid rats points toward the existence of alterations of post-transcriptional mechanism of control, brought about by the lack of thyroid. Both maturation processes might be involved.

It has been shown (13,21,23) that, in the brain, nuclear rapidly labeled RNA is DNA-like in base composition and that after short periods of labeling 70-80% of the labeled polysomal RNA has the characteristics of mRNA. The above findings, together with the results reported here, lend support to the view that one of the alterations produced by neonatal thyroidectomy might be a defective transcription and/or maturation of the giant and heterogeneous D-RNA. This agrees with recent reports on the effects of other hormones in liver and uterus (24-26). It must be noted, however, that the comparison of RSRs of rRNA in nuclei and microsomes does not rule out the possibility that neonatal thyroidectomy may also alter the regulatory mechanisms involved in the maturation and/or transport of ribosomal RNA. This kind of regulation has been suggested to occur in growing mammalian tissues (19).

SUMMARY

The time course of incorporation of precursor into brain nuclear and microsomal RNA was studied after the intro-arachnoidal injection of ^{3}H-5-orotic acid into 10-day-old normal and neonatally radiothyroidectomized rats. Neonatal thyroidectomy produces a significant decrease in the formation of "rapidly labeled" nuclear RNA. A diminished incorporation into microsomal RNA was also observed after longer labeling periods. Kinetic studies of the labeling of different RNA species separated by linear sucrose gradients confirm that neonatal thyroidectomy leads to a decreased transcriptional capacity and suggest possible alterations in post-transcriptional control mechanisms at the nuclear level.

RESUMEN

El tiempo de incorporación del precursor en el RNA microsomal y nuclear del cerebro fue estudiado después de una inyección intra-aracnoidea de ácido orótico-5-^{3}H a ratas/de 10 días, y a ratas radiotiroidectomizadas al nacer. La tiroidectomía al nacer produce una disminución significativa en la formación de RNA nuclear marcado rápidamente. Una incorporación menor fue observada en el RNA microsomal después de tiempos largos de incorporación. Estudios cinéticos del marcaje de las diferentes especies de RNA separadas en gradientes lineales de sacarosa confirman que la tiroidectomía neonatal conduce a una disminución de la capacidad transcripcional y sugiere posibles alteraciones en los mecanismos posttranscripcionales al nivel celular.

REFERENCES

1. Eayrs, J. T., in Hamburgh, M., and Barrington, E. J. W. (eds.), *Hormones in Development,* Appleton-Century-Crofts, New York (1971), p. 345.
2. LeGrand, J., in Hamburgh, M., and Barrington, E. J. W. (eds.), *Hormones in Development,* Appleton-Century-Crofts, New York (1971), p. 381.
3. Gomez, C. J., and Ramirez de Guglielmone, A. E., *J. Neurochem., 14,* 1119 (1967).
4. Pasquini, J. M., Kaplun, B., Garcia Argiz, C. A., and Gomez, C. J., *Brain Res., 6,* 621 (1967).
5. Garcia Argiz, C. A., Pasquini, J. M., Kaplun, B., and Gomez, C. J., *Brain Res., 6,* 635 (1967).

6. Balazs, R., Cocks, W. A., Eayrs, J. T., and Kovacs, S., in Hamburgh, M., and Barrington, E. J. W. (eds.), *Hormones in Development*, Appleton-Century-Crofts, New York (1971), p. 357.

7. Geel, S. E., and Timiras, P. S., in Lajtha, A. (ed.), *Protein Metabolism of the Nervous System*, Plenum Press, New York (1970), p. 335.

8. Szijan, I., Chepelinsky, A. B., and Piras, M. M., *Brain Res., 20,* 313 (1970).

9. Tata, J. R., *Nature, 219,* 331 (1968).

10. Tata, J. R., in Hamburgh, M., and Barrington, E. J. W. (eds.), *Hormones in Development*, Appleton-Century-Crofts, New York (1971), p. 19.

11. Geel, S. E., and Valcana, T., in Ford, D. R. (ed.), *Influence of Hormones on the Nervous System*, S. Karger, New York (1971), p. 165.

12. Gomez, C. J., Guglielmone, A. E. R., and Duvilansky, B., *Acta Physiol. Latinoam., 21,* 152 (1971).

13. Vesco, C., and Guiditta, A., *Biochim. Biophys. Acta, 142,* 385 (1967).

14. Di Girolamo, A., Henshaw, E. C., and Hiatt, H. H., *J. Mol. Biol., 8,* 479 (1964).

15. Bray, G. A., *Anal. Biochem., 1,* 279 (1960).

16. Darnell, J. E., *Bacteriol. Rev., 32,* 262 (1968).

17. Perry, R. P., Greenberg, J. R., and Tartoff, K. D., *Cold Spring Harbor Symp. Quant. Biol., 35,* 577 (1970).

18. Spohr, G., Grandboulan, N., Morel, C., and Scherrer, K., *Europ. J. Biochem., 17,* 268 (1970).

19. Burdon, R. H., *Progr. Nucl. Acid Res. Mol. Biol., 11,* 33 (1971).

20. Georgiev, G. P., in San Pietro, A., Lamborg, M. R., and Kenney, F. T. (eds.), *Regulatory Mechanisms for Protein Synthesis in Mammalian Cells*, Academic Press, New York (1968), p. 25.

21. Jacob, M., Stevenin, J., Jund, R., Judes, C., and Mandel, P., *J. Neurochem., 13,* 619 (1966).

22. Stevenin, J., Mandel, P., and Jacob, M., *Proc. Natl. Acad. Sci. U.S.A., 62,* 490 (1969).

23. Jacob, M., Samec, J., Stevenin, J., Garel, P., and Mandel, P., *J. Neurochem., 14,* 169 (1967).

24. Hanoune, J., and Feigelson, P., *Biochim. Biophys. Acta, 199,* 214 (1970).

25. Church, R. B., and McCarthy, B. J., *Biochim. Biophys. Acta, 199,* 103 (1970).

26. Hahn, W. E., Schjeide, O. A., and Gorbman, A., *Proc. Natl. Acad. Sci. U.S.A., 62,* 112 (1969).

15

Structure–Function Relations in tRNA

Robert M. Bock

Laboratory of Molecular Biology
University of Wisconsin
Madison, Wisconsin, U.S.A.

The transfer RNA molecule is able to recognize both specific amino acids and corresponding genetic code words. In so doing, it translates the information encoded in nucleic acid messages into protein products. Multiple discrete steps in this process include amino acid binding, transport to the ribosome, binding to one ribosomal site, peptide bond formation, translocation to another ribosomal site, and release from the ribosome. Initiation of protein synthesis requires different tRNAs as compared to those utilized for the growth of initiated protein chains. Other reactions known to involve tRNA as a reactant include cell wall synthesis, phospholipid synthesis, phosphoserine synthesis, and repression of synthesis of certain amino acid metabolizing enzymes. Knowledge of the three-dimensional structure of tRNA molecules will provide a framework for integrating our understanding of these many metabolic functions.

Excellent progress in sequence determination has given us some general rules about primary and secondary structure of tRNA. Over 30 complete tRNA sequences are known and include examples from bacterial, yeast, animal, and plant tissues. The next chapter in this volume gives the details of our knowledge of tRNA sequences, but I must here point out certain features for my discussion of three-dimensional folding. In Fig. 1, we may note that all known tRNA sequences have three sets of base pairs of fixed length 5, 5, and 7. It is very probable that these assume a double-strand helical conformation as found in double-strand viral RNA. The longest of these segments often includes one non Watson-Crick base pair. A fourth segment is found to have either three or four possible base pairs, and in some tRNAs one of these is not a Watson-Crick pair.

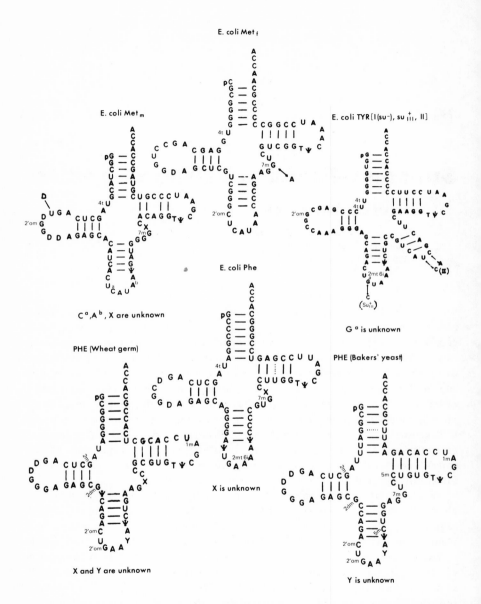

Fig. 1. Sequences of chain-initiator (upper middle) and chain-propagator tRNAs (all except upper middle). Note that there is great similarity in size, possible base-paired sections, and location of certain bases or base clusters. This holds true for plant, animal, and microbial tRNA.

A fifth segment is found to be so widely variable in length that it cannot be considered one of the general features shared by many tRNAs; it is unlikely to be involved in intimate contact with the ribosome or other enzymes which are general reactants with all tRNA. The terminus at which the bases CCA are found must be exposed to accept the amino acid, and this exposure is confirmed by its measured chemical reactivity in solution. The anticodon is found to occupy a similar locus in all tRNAs and must be exposed to form base pairs with the coded message. Again, this exposure is confirmed by its chemical and enzymatic reactivity.

Our knowledge of the functional roles of the rest of the molecule is not adequate to predict just which bases must be exposed to the surface. The presence of modified bases tells us that these areas must have been exposed at least during some stage of the maturation of the tRNA molecule. In spite of this, the ribothymidylic and pseudouridylic residues appear unavailable to chemical reagents in solution. The tetramer GTΨC inhibits binding of tRNA to ribosomes, which is in conflict with the simplest interpretation of the buried behavior of this sequence in tRNA.

The functional role of the modified bases has eluded our understanding. They seem of more use to the sequencer than to the cell. Many appear dispensable for normal protein synthesis functions. However, isopentenyl adenosine (ipA) has a measurable effect on the translation rate when measured in low Mg^{2+} buffers. Ribothymidylic absence does not block protein synthesis. Pseudouridylic residues near the anticodon appear to be needed to permit His-tRNA plus its synthetase to prevent expression of the histidine biosynthesis operon. The glycine acceptor tRNA, which does not bind to ribosomes but functions in cell wall synthesis, has neither T nor Ψ in the GTΨC loop. The science of relating tRNA functions to mutations which cause defects in base modification has just been born. Several mutants are known where a physiological function is impaired by an apparent lack of a tRNA modification, but the location of the modification and the molecular basis of the lost function are yet to be determined.

One of the minor bases in tRNA has been particularly useful in providing clearcut evidence on tRNA folding. Yaniv found that the 4-thiouracil in the eighth base position of several *Escherichia coli* tRNAs could be photochemically linked to a cytidine which is the thirteenth base in the chain. Further research by Yaniv and by my collegues has shown that all the reactivities of tRNA needed for protein synthesis are functional even though these two bases are covalently linked. Recently, Leonard *et al.* (4) determined the structure of the photochemically linked bases. We can now propose with considerable confidence the spatial relation these two bases must have to each other in native tRNA.

Ten species of tRNA have yielded X-ray-diffracting single crystals. Single crystals containing multiple species of tRNA have been grown from two different sources of tRNA. At the University of Wisconsin, we have grown over 50 different tRNA cyrstal forms differing in counter ion, pH, precipitating solvent, and tRNA species. About ten of these forms diffracted X-rays with resolution better than 10 Å. Crystals from yeast tRNA^{fMet}, $E.$ $coli$ tRNA^{Arg}, and tRNA^{Leu} have acceptable unit cells, and we are concentrating our efforts on these species. The unit cell dimensions and molecular packing have been reported earlier. Our current efforts are directed to obtaining isomorphous crystals with a heavy atom uniquely placed so that the phases of the diffraction pattern may be solved.

The strategy of these efforts includes the development of both general and species-specific heavy atom introduction. Cramer, Eckstein, and colleagues have replaced bases in the CCA terminus with iodo-CMP or with a sulfur-containing AMP which could be a binding site for mercury. The introduction of these bases is catalyzed by a specific enzyme which must be purified to remove all nucleases and must be carefully removed from the tRNA after treatment. Cramer has succeeded in growing crystals from the modified tRNA, and other workers are taking up his method. We have attempted to synthesize a reagent which could be added to pregrown crystals of any tRNA and would bind strongly to one site only. Dr. A. Yamazaki in my laboratory has synthesized a series of phenylboronic acids designed to have strong affinity to the vicinal hydroxyl group at the CCA terminus and to contain a heavy atom. An example of this series is (2-nitro,4-iodo)phenylboronic acid. A second class of rather general derivatizing agents developed in our laboratory by Hecht and Schmidt are mercury- and iodine-containing carboxylic acids suitably activated to permit specific derivatization of an a-amino acid on the CCA terminus of tRNA without interfering reaction with the heterocyclic bases. We have also been able to grow crystals of tRNA with a single mercury attached to the 4-thiouracil which is eight bases from the 5′ terminus. Numerous $E.$ $coli$ tRNAs have this base and bind a single mercury atom, but plant and animal tRNAs do not appear to contain 4-thiouracil. A number of reactions of minor bases with heavy atom reagents are known and could be of use when the tRNA contains only one or two of the particular minor base.

Protein crystallographers have solved the phases of protein diffraction patterns with the aid of heavy atoms soaked into the crystal. The specific site where they would bind was not known until after the structure was solved. In the same manner, we have been able to introduce lead and uranyl ions into tRNA crystals at specific but unidentified loci. Although at least five laboratories now have

---

$Fig.$ $2.$ $Proposed$ $models$ of $tRNA$ $structure.$ (A) Detailed model proposed by Levitt. (B) Arrangement of helical segments of tRNA proposed by Connors et $al.$ (C) Model of yeast phenylalanine tRNA folding proposed by Cramer et $al.$ (D) Model of $E.$ $coli$ tRNA folding proposed by Yaniv.

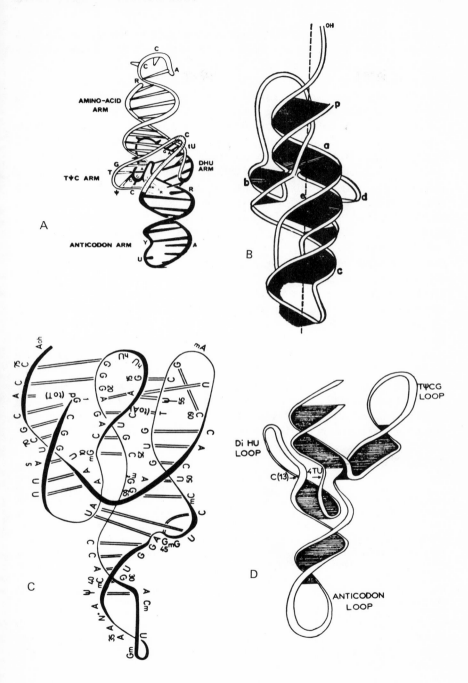

heavy atom derivatives in isomorphous crystals of tRNA, in no case have the number of clean derivatives and the simplicity of the crystal been amenable to a unique solution of the phases, and thus the three-dimensional structure. Nevertheless, the progress in the 3 years that crystalline tRNA has existed is substantial and offers every reason to expect that detailed three-dimensional structures will be known early in this decade.

The construction of tRNA models has been a most useful activity but will be even more useful as detailed rules of nucleotide dimensions are added to the models. As soon as one tRNA structure is known in detail, it is likely that the presence of short helical segments with their strongly scattering phosphate groups in known relation to each other will permit searches for such structures. Model-calculated diffraction patterns may aid in establishing provisional phases for many tRNA crystals. While this technique is much more applicable to tRNA than to proteins, the number of variables one must consider in our models makes the computation lengthy and very expensive. The knowledge of one structure in detail could provide a starting model for many tRNAs with a resultant saving of time and computing resources.

At the present time, the models proposed by Levitt, by Conners *et al.,* and by Fuller *et al.* represent our understanding of tRNA structure in general (Fig. 2). Although each of these models could be refined with better values of the nucleotide bond lengths and angles as well as the preferred stacking angles, such efforts might better await more definitive X-ray structures. There is no compelling reason to choose among these models, and they have not reached the degree of sophistication we must attain before the unique features that differentiate one amino acid acceptor activity from another or chain-initiating from chain-propagating structures can be compared. We share your impatience and are doing our best to hasten the day when such structural details will be known.

SUMMARY

Studies of tRNA structure-function relations are now under way using X-ray crystallography of tRNA and of model compounds. Chemical and physical-chemical studies in solutions, enzymic and chemical synthesis of modified tRNA, and genetic analysis of the function, maturation, and modification of tRNA contribute much to our understanding of tRNA structure. While there is detailed understanding of codon recognition, only early fragmentary information is available on the basis for amino acid recognition. In spite of many bits of information on surface exposure, general shape in solution, packing in crystals, and the sequences of many tRNAs, the details of molecular folding are almost completely unknown. At the present time, we can say with confidence that helical sections exist, that they are predominantly parallel to the long axis of the whole molecule, that the anticodon and the CCA terminus are freely exposed to the solvent, and that the gross external shape must fit well-known crystal unit cell volumes as well as hydrodynamic dimensions measured in solution. It is known that the D loop folds back close to the base of the CCA stem. However, the structure that makes each tRNA unique and the detailed folding of any loop remain unknown at this time.

RESUMEN

Los estudios de las relaciones entre la estructura y función del tRNA se llevan a cabo actualmente empleando la cristalografía con rayos X de tRNA y de compuestos modelos. Estudios químicos y químico-físicos en soluciones, síntesis enzimatica y química de tRNAs modificados, y el análisis genético de la función, la maduración, y la modificación del tRNA han contribuido grandemente a nuestro entendimiente de la estructura del tRNA. Aún cuando el reconocimiento de codones se comprende en detalle, se tiene sólo información fragmentaria de la base para el reconocimiento de los aminoácidos. A pesar de los numerosos dates sobre la exposición de la superficie, forma general en solución, empaquetamiento en cristales y secuencias de numerosos tRNAs, los detalles del plegado molecular se deconocen case totalmente. Al presente, se puede decir con seguridad que la parte helioidal existe, que son predominantemente paralelos al eje más largo de la molécula, que el anticodón y el terminal CCA están expuestos libremente al solvente, y que la forma externa general debe coincidir con la unidad del cristal del volumen celular, al igual que con las dimensiones hidrodinámicas medidas en solución. Se sabe que el lazo D se pliega hacia atrás, cerca de la base de la rama CCA. Sin embargo, la estructura que hace a cada tRNA único y los detalles del plegado de los lazes todavía no se conocen.

REFERENCES

An excellent collection of references on this subject can be found in recent review articles:

1. Arnott, S., *Progr. Biophys. Mol. Biol., 22,* 179 (1971).
2. Söll, D., *Science, 173,* 293 (1971).
3. Gauss, D. H. von der Haar, F., Maelicke, A., and Cramer, F., *Ann. Rev. Biochem., 40,* 1045 (1971).
4. Leonard, N. J., Bergström, D. E., and Tolman, G. L., *Biochem. Biophys. Res. Commun., 44,* 1524 (1971).

DISCUSSION

Speaker unidentified: Do you know whether the helical region is the 11-turn or the 12-turn RNA type?

R. M. Bock (Madison, U.S.A.): There are two types of evidence that pertain to this. One is the fitting of the C-axis projection with a variety of helices. We definitely get a better fit for both leucine-tRNA and yeast Met-F-tRNA with an 11-turn than with a 12-, or with a DNA-type helix. The other type of data is the base-stacking evidence which has been obtained by Sundaralingam, by Rich, and by Paul Sigler. The experimental details and the confidence that they have in the stacking distances have not yet been debated by them. I think that there is a possibility that there could be a 12-turn helix or that there could be both 11- and 12-turn helices in the same molecule.

H. G. Zachau (Munich, Germany): Which tRNA did your group prepare in 600 mg quantity?

R. M. Bock: Yeast formylmethionine.

H. G. Zachau: You mentioned something quite interesting with regard to 2-thio-U:A, but I did not get the story.

R. M. Bock: Nisimura has found modified 2-thio-U bases which are modified at the 5 position in addition. One type of modification appears to have extended its codon reading so that in addition to A and G it can also read a U. Another modification at 5 (still a thio-U) appears to have restricted the modification so that it can read code words ending in A. The interesting thing is that Samuel Weiss found this type of modification in one of the five leucine acceptors of T4 phage. We see that modifying enzymes could easily change the code-reading capacity of tRNA. This is very exciting and makes us want to know whether the reading of the code is an important metabolic variable which can be changed to read certain families of codes at one time. We are very excited about that because of the possible role of the cytokinin base. This base appears only in tRNAs that read code words beginning with the letter U, and we wonder whether variations on that base lead to a selectivity of reading messages.

16

Nucleotide Sequence and Function of Transfer RNA and Precursor Transfer RNA

J. D. Smith

Medical Research Council
Laboratory of Molecular Biology
Cambridge, England

At present, we have to consider the functional interactions of the tRNA molecule without knowing its three-dimensional structure. Comparison of tRNA sequences has shown that they have a common hydrogen-bonded structure defined by the cloverleaf arrangement, and in addition they have certain common sequences or correlated sequences which may also be involved in the tertiary structure. Consideration of proposed tRNA structures shows that if we knew a few additional interactions between bases in the sequence the number of types of possible models would be severely restricted (for review, see ref. 1). Until the structure of tRNA comes from X-ray diffraction analysis, less direct methods are useful both in understanding tRNA structure and in locating regions of the sequence involved in specific interactions, although it is clear that the latter problem cannot be properly solved without knowing the structure. In trying to locate regions of the tRNA sequence involved in specific interactions with the aminoacyl-tRNA synthetase, several approaches have been valuable: dissection of the tRNA molecule by recombination of fragments obtained by limited nuclease digestion, comparison of sequences of isoaccepting tRNAs, and location of inactivation targets by chemical modification of bases (for review, see ref. 2).

This communication discusses results pertinent to tRNA sequence-function relations which my colleagues and I have obtained by genetic methods. The aim is to change specific bases in the tRNA by mutation and see what effect these changes have on tRNA structure and function. One of the most interesting results concerns the role of a precursor molecule in the biosynthesis of tRNA; this is discussed in the section headed *Precursor tRNA*.

The tRNAs which can be studied genetically are suppressor tRNAs whose coding properties have been altered by mutation. Mutations resulting in missense or nonsense codons in the messenger RNA can be corrected by specific suppressor tRNAs which translate the mutant codon as an acceptable amino acid (see ref. 3). The amber suppressor su^+_{III} results from a mutation in one of the two genes specifying $Escherichia\ coli$ tRNA$_I^{Tyr}$. The mutation changes the tRNA anticodon from $\overset{*}{G}$UA ($\overset{*}{G}$ is a modified G residue) to CUA so that the suppressor tRNA translates the terminator triplet UAG as tyrosine (4,5). From su^+_{III}, we have selected mutants with defective or altered suppressor activity. Many of these mutants specify tRNAs with single base substitutions at various positions in the tRNA sequence. We have also isolated second-site revertants from some of the suppressor-defective, single base substitution mutants by selecting for partial or complete restoration of suppressor activity. In these, the original base substitution is compensated by a second base substitution. These double mutants are interesting in showing how pairs of bases may interact in tRNA structure or function. (For simplicity in nomenclature, su^+_{III} is considered the *wild type,* the suppressor-defective mutants derived from this as *mutants,* and the second-site revertants of these as *revertants.*)

METHODS

To overcome the difficulty that the su_{III} tRNA constitutes only a fraction of the total *E. coli* tyrosine tRNA, we isolated the nondefective $\phi 80\ psu^+_{III}$ transducing phage (6). This carries a segment of the bacterial chromosome equivalent to about 5% of the phage genome and contains a single copy of the su^+_{III} tRNA gene. In cells infected with this phage, synthesis of su_{III} tyrosine tRNA is greatly increased because of the large number of copies of the tRNA gene. Each su_{III} mutant was obtained as a $\phi 80\ psu$ derivative, and all isolations of tRNA or precursor tRNA are from cells infected with phage carrying the appropriate mutant tRNA gene. The su_{III} mutants were selected on the basis of their efficiency in suppressing amber mutations in the β-galactosidase, galactokinase, or tryptophan genes. They were isolated after mutagenesis, either in $\phi 80$ psu^+_{III} or in *E. coli* MB93 ara^-_{amber} lac^-_{125} $gal^-_{U42\ kinase\ amber}$ $gal^-_{epimerase}$ $tryp^-_{amber}$ su^+_{III} (singlet) / F8 $gal^-_{U42\ kinase\ amber}$ $gal^-_{epimerase}$. All the genetic and biochemical procedures have been described in detail elsewhere (5-8).

RESULTS

Mutant tRNAs

Many of the mutants selected as defective or partially defective in suppressor activity specify tRNAs differing from su^+_{III} by single base substitutions at different positions in the tRNA. The sequence changes of these are shown in Fig. 1. (They will be designated by the base present at the mutant site and its residue number from the 5′ end. The stems of the cloverleaf are lettered counterclockwise a-e from the amino acid acceptor stem, the loops from I → IV from the "dihydrouracil" loop.)

All the completely or partially suppressor-defective mutants result in diminished su_{III} tRNA synthesis (0-20% of normal) (7-8). Pulse-label experiments show that this is not due to normal synthesis of an unstable mature tRNA (9). Most of these changes in the tRNA sequence result in defective maturation of a larger tRNA precursor molecule which is an intermediate in tRNA biosynthesis; this is discussed in the next section.

Both the reduced tRNA synthesis and altered properties of the mutant tRNA can contribute to the weak suppressor phenotype of these mutants. In several, the tRNA itself is defective or altered in function. The change in stem c of A31 tRNA results in altered kinetics of aminoacylation with tyrosine tRNA synthetase; the K_m is ten to 20 times greater than that of su^+_{III} tRNA (7). A15 tRNA is defective in a step in protein synthesis subsequent to its binding to the ribosome. Although the tRNA functions normally in aminoacylation and in ribosome binding in response to the triplet UAG, it functions inefficiently in protein synthesis (7). A46 tRNA has similar properties but also shows altered kinetics of aminoacylation (10), and in both these mutant tRNAs the functional defect while on the ribosome may be related to the similar conformational changes in these tRNAs, which are discussed below. Two su_{III} mutations, A2 and A81, which result in mispaired bases in stem a of the tRNA, are temperature sensitive in their *in vivo* suppressor activity (8). We have also shown that a change in the anticodon from CUA to UUA results in an ochre suppressing tRNA (11).

Many of the base substitutions shown in Fig. 1 might be expected to change the tRNA structure, particularly those resulting in unpaired bases in the stems of the cloverleaf arrangement. It is more informative to know how base changes in the loops may alter the structure. Only two such single mutants have been isolated: A15 and A17 in loop I. Cashmore (12) has shown that the G → A change at residue 15 results in increased reactivity to methoxyamine of specific cytosine residues both in loop I and in stem d. This result implies that in the tRNA structure there is normally an interaction between these two regions

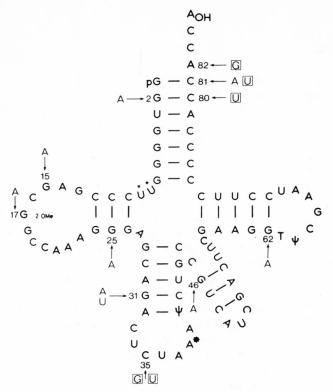

Fig. 1. *The nucleotide sequence of* E. coli su⁺$_{III}$ I *tyrosine tRNA,*
showing the positions of single base changes in individual mutants.
The sequence changes *not* enclosed in boxes are those of mutants
selected for defective suppressor activity and whose tRNA synthesis
is defective.

which is altered by the mutation A15. This is in agreement with the postulated
hydrogen bonding between G15 and C57 based on comparison of tRNA sequences (13,14). Similar studies on A46 mutant tRNA confirm the interaction
between loop I and stem d (Hooper and Cashmore, unpublished observations).
This approach offers a useful method for studying interactions between different
regions of the tRNA structure.

In the double mutants (Table I) a second base change has partly or
completely compensated for the defect of the original mutation. In A2U80,
A25U11, A31U41, U31A41, and A46U54, the second mutation restores base
pairing in stems a, b, c, and d, respectively, of the cloverleaf, resulting in each
case in a different pair from that in su⁺$_{III}$. The *in vivo* suppressor activities and

Table I. Base Substitutions in Second-Site Revertants Restoring Suppressor Activity[a]

First sequence change	Phenotype of suppressor mutant	Second-sequence change in the double mutant			
		Partial revertant to su^+	References	Strong revertant (*in vivo*) suppression > 50% that of su^+_{III}	References
G → A2 (stem a)	Temperature-sensitive weak su^+			C → U80 (restores base pair in stem a)	8,9
G → A15 (loop 1)	Weak su^+	C → D19 (loop I) C → D20 (loopl)	8,9 8,9		
G → A25 (stem b)	su^-	C → U19 (loop I)	8,9	C → U11 (restores base pair in stem b)	8,9
G → A46 (stem d)	Weak su^+			C → U54 (restores base pair in stem d)	10
G → A31 (stem c)	Weak su^+	C → D19 (loop I)	15	C → U41 (restores base pair in stem c)	15
		C → U51 (loop III)	15	C → U45 (stem d) C → U16 (loop I)	15 15
G → U31 (stem c)	Weak su^+			C → A41 (restores base pair in stem c)	15
				C → U45 (stem d) C → U16 (loop I)	15 15

[a] The sequence changes can be located in Fig. 1. D is dihydrouracil; the C → D changes presumably result from C → U changes in loop I followed by modification of U → D.

amounts of tRNA synthesized in these revertants are approximately the same as in su^+_{III}. The tRNAs are aminoacylated with tyrosine; the kinetics of aminoacylation of A2U80 and A25U11 have been determined and are the same as that of su^+_{III} tRNA. Evidently, at these positions the identity of the base pair is unimportant (8,9).

In several of the revertants in Table I, the second change is in a base unrelated to the original mutant base in the cloverleaf arrangement. Some of these revertants have only weak suppressor activity, and their significance is difficult to assess. Revertants of A31 and U31 with strong suppressor activity (50-70% of su^+_{III}) have been isolated in our laboratory by Dr. K. Anderson (15). In both A31 and U31, a normal base pair cannot be made at this position in stem c of the tRNA. A31 and U31 suppress the lac^-_{125} amber (measured by the rate of β-galactosidase synthesis in strains carrying the suppressors) with 19 and 7% the efficiency of su^+_{III}. This is closely correlated with the level of su_{III} tyrosine tRNA synthesized by these mutants. Both of these mutants can revert to almost normal suppressor phenotype by either of three second base changes: (a) by a substitution at residue 41 which allows a normal base pair at this position in stem c, (b) by the change C16 → U in loop I, or (c) by the change C45 → U in stem d. In each revertant, the increase in suppressor activity is quantitatively paralleled by an increase in the level of tRNA synthesized (15). From this, we conclude that the mutant tRNAs, A31 and U31, and their revertants can function *in the cell* as suppressor tRNAs about as efficiently as su^+_{III}. The suppressor phenotypes of these mutants can be explained by differences in the amounts of tRNA synthesized.

The studies on the double mutants show that (a) tRNAs with certain pairs of altered bases are functional and (b) the second base change restores the level of tRNA synthesis. We will now discuss how this effect probably results from alteration in the structure of a precursor tRNA molecule.

Precursor tRNA

Ribosomal RNAs are transcribed as large precursor molecules which go through a maturation process during which those sequences which do not appear in the final product are removed. In eukaryotic cells, there is evidence that tRNAs are also transcribed as longer sequences. An RNA fraction which behaves kinetically as a precursor to 4S RNA has been described in Krebs ascites tumor cells (16) and HeLa cells (17,18). Its properties suggest that it is ten to 20 nucleotides longer than the average tRNA (19). We have found that tyrosine tRNA$_I$ of *E. coli* is transcribed as a longer precursor molecule. The isolation of a *single* tRNA precursor species has allowed determination of its nucleotide sequence and a detailed examination of this step in tRNA biosynthesis. The results we now discuss have been reported (Altman (20); Altman and Smith (21)].

[32]P pulse labeling of cells infected with ϕ80 *psu* phages carrying the mutant tRNA genes A15, A17, A25, A31, or A62 shows that during synthesis of these tRNAs a transient precursor molecule accumulates. On polyacrylamide gel electrophoresis, this migrates just behind 5S RNA. It consists of the entire tyrosine tRNA sequence, but without the usual base modifications, joined at the 5' end of a sequence of 41 additional nucleotides and at the 3' end to two or three additional nucleotides. The sequence determination of the 5' segment is summarized in Fig. 2, and Fig. 3 shows possible secondary structures whose role in tRNA biosynthesis we discuss later. A tyrosine tRNA precursor has also been isolated from cells infected with ϕ80 psu_o^- which are synthesizing normal $tRNA_I^{Tyr}$. This turns over much more rapidly than the mutant tRNA precursors and can only be detected in short label pulses at 25°. While the sequence of this has not been determined, analysis of T1 and pancreatic ribonuclease digestion products indicates that the additional 5' segments of both normal and the mutant tRNA precursors are the same, but that the additional 3' terminal segment of the "wild-type" precursor is longer by six to ten residues. The tyrosine tRNA gene is thus normally transcribed as a longer precursor; the mutant tRNAs differ in that their precursors are processed less efficiently and so transiently accumulate.

Since the sequence of the precursor begins with pppG, we conclude that the initial transcript is intact at this end. The 3' terminus of the initially transcribed RNA may, however, be longer than the isolated su_0^- tRNA precursor, and evidently the mutant tRNA precursors have undergone some degradation at this end. Accurate *in vitro* transcription of the tRNA gene should determine whether

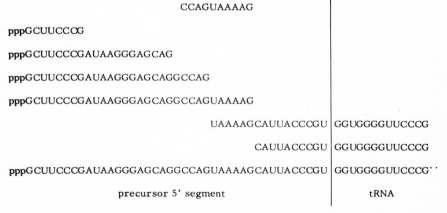

Fig. 2. *Nucleotide sequences.* Sequence of the 5' segment of A25 precursor tRNA and the sequences of isolated products of T1 ribonuclease digestion from which the complete sequence was deduced.

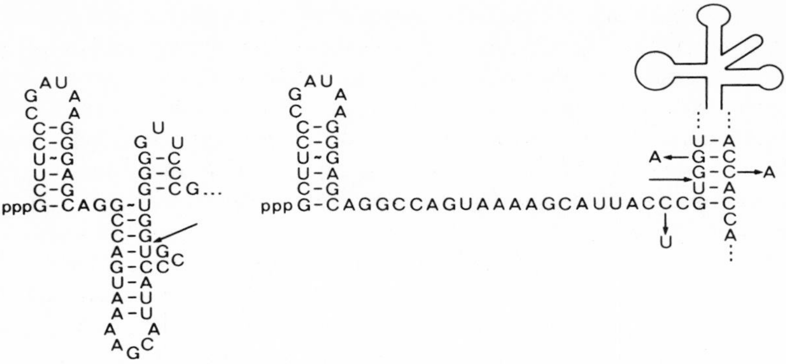

STRUCTURE I   STRUCTURE II

Fig. 3. Two possible configurations for tyrosine tRNA precursor. The arrows pointing toward the sequence indicate the beginning of the 5' end of the tRNA sequence and the point of cleavage by the 5' cleavage enzyme. The arrows pointing outward indicate the positions of mutants mentioned in the text: P(C → U), A2(G → A), and A81(C → A).

a still longer sequence is transcribed at the 3' terminus. In the *in vitro* transcription of $\phi80$ psu^+_{III} which has been reported, the tRNA sequences are in molecules larger than expected and heterogeneous in size, perhaps due to incorrect initiation or termination (22).

The mutant precursor contains the common tRNA terminal CCA sequence, and this is joined at the 3' end to the additional sequence UC(U); the last residue has not been conclusively identified. This implies that in this tRNA the CCA sequence is encoded in the gene.

In the secondary structure of A25 precursor, the tRNA sequence has probably assumed the configuration of mature tRNA as shown in structure II of Fig. 3. This conclusion is based on analysis of the products of partial digestion with T1 ribonuclease in 0.02 M Mg^{2+} at 0°. Isolation in good yield of the partial products in lines 2, 3, and 4 in Fig. 2 is consistent with the loop structure at the 5' terminus. Analysis of products containing portions of the tRNA sequence shows that the predominant enzymatic splits are at the same G residues in similar digests of mature tRNA.

Processing of the Precursor

Maturation of the precursor involves removal of the 5' and 3' segments. Crude extracts (30,000 × *g* supernatant) of *E. coli* contain an endonuclease which splits off the 5' segment of A25 precursor tRNA at the pGG-- terminus of the mature tRNA. The released 5' precursor fragment is not recovered intact but is further degraded to a fragment comprising the first 23-24 nucleotides at the 5' end, 5'-mononucleotides, and some dinucleotides. Further purification of the endonuclease has shown that these additional splits are caused by other nucleases in the crude extract [H. D. Robertson, S. Altman, and J. D. Smith, (23)]. The purified enzyme splits A25 precursor at the 3'-phosphodiester linkage of the 5'-terminal phosphate of the tRNA sequence releasing the complete additional 5' segment and generating the correct 5' terminus of mature tRNA.

A separate enzyme system appears to be involved in processing of the 3' terminus. The *E. coli* 30,000 × *g* supernatant fraction contains an activity which removes at least the first two nucleotides from A25 precursor; this has not been further studied. We also note that the processing does not require or involve modification of the tRNA bases.

Why are many of the mutant tRNAs defective in their maturation? The mutants defective in tRNA synthesis are those expected to give an altered tRNA conformation. These are A2, A25, A31, U31, A46, A62, and A81, which have non hydrogen-bonded pairs in stems a, b, c, d, or e; A15, which has an altered tRNA conformation; and A17, in which a common tRNA sequence possibly involved in the tertiary structure has been changed. Except for A2 and A81, these mutants all accumulate precursor. Mutants with base substitutions not expected to alter the tRNA conformation include U80 and U81 (which allow G:U pairs in stem a), G82, and the double mutants in which base pairing is restored in stems a, b, c, and d. These synthesize tRNA at about the normal level, and those which have been examined (U81, G82, and A2U80) do not accumulate precursor. These findings show that ability of the tRNA part of the precursor to assume a correct tRNA conformation is important in processing. However, it is not obvious how the precursor structure would be altered in the double mutants such as A31 U16, which also synthesize tRNA normally and where the base changes are unrelated to each other in the cloverleaf.

In structure II (Fig. 3), recognition of the conformation of the tRNA sequence could be necessary for efficient action of the cleavage enzymes, and although *in vitro* A25 precursor is split by the 5' cleavage enzyme, the rate of this reaction may be much faster with the wild-type precursor. Another possibility is that the mutant precursor has an alternative configuration which cannot be processed. We have suggested that the partly transcribed precursor could have the secondary structure I (Fig. 3), which on completion of transcription would be expected to be converted to structure II, where the tRNA sequence has assumed its tertiary structure. If only structure II can be cleaved, a change in kinetics of transition between the two structures could result in a decrease in the rate of processing. Whichever the mechanism, an alternative nonproductive degradation of mutant tRNA precursor has to be postulated to explain the low level of tRNA synthesized.

All the mutations so far considered are in the tRNA sequence itself. One would expect that mutations altering the rate of tRNA synthesis could also occur in the precursor segments. One such mutant (P) has been isolated as a second-site revertant of the temperature-sensitive suppressor mutant A2. In the mutant A2, the tRNA with the base substitution $G \rightarrow A2$ is synthesized at about 5-10% of the normal rate. The effect of the second mutation P is to increase the level of synthesis of A2 tRNA three to five times. We have shown that the P mutation results in a $C \rightarrow U$ change in the precursor $5'$ segment at a position four residues from the beginning of the tRNA sequence (Fig. 3). Since it is located near the cleavage point in processing, it is quite possible that this mutation affects the rate of tRNA maturation and may be part of a sequence recognition site for the $5'$ cleavage enzyme.

The significance of the extra sequences, in particular the long additional $5'$ sequence, raises the question of whether these are transcribed portions of transcription signals on the DNA, or whether they are of importance during transcription, possibly by protecting the $5'$ end of the partly transcribed tRNA from degradation. These questions may be answered by comparing sequences of other tRNA precursors or by isolating other mutants affecting the rate of tRNA synthesis and in which the precursor sequence is altered.

SUMMARY

This communication discusses how mutations in a transfer RNA gene may alter the structure, function, and synthesis of tRNA. The *E. coli* amber suppressor gene su_{III} specifies a tyrosine tRNA$_I$ in which the anticodon is changed to CUA. Several su_{III} mutants having defective or altered suppressor activity have been isolated. These specify mutant tyrosine tRNAs with single base substitutions at different positions in the tRNA sequence. The properties of some of these are discussed. From several of the mutants, second-site revertants to normal suppressor activity have been isolated. They result in a second base substitution in the tRNA. In some of the double mutants, a G:C base pair in the cloverleaf structure has been changed to an A:U pair. This can occur at several positions without apparently changing tRNA function. Base substitutions expected to alter the tRNA structure result in decreased tRNA synthesis. This is due to defective maturation of a tRNA precursor. *E. coli* tyrosine tRNA$_I$ is transcribed *in vivo* as a longer precursor which is processed to give mature tRNA. The nucleotide sequence of the precursor, its *in vitro* cleavage by a specific endonuclease from *E. coli,* and the significance of the additional sequences in the precursor are discussed.

RESUMEN

Esta comunicación discute cómo mutaciones en el gene para el RNA de transferencia pueden alterar la estructura, función y síntesis del tRNA. El gene supresor ámbar su_{III} de *E. coli* especifica un tRNA$_I$ para tirosina en el cual el anticodón es cambiado a CUA. Se han aislado diversas mutantes su_{III} las cuales tienen una actividad de supresor modificada. Estas especifican mutantes del tRNA para tirosina con la substitución de una sola base en diferentes posiciones en la secuencia del tRNA. Las propiedades de algunas de estas mutantes son discutidas. De algunas de estas mutantes se han aislado revertantes de segundo sitio las cuales revierten a la actividad del supresor normal. Estas resultan en una sustitución de una segunda base en el tRNA. En algunas de las mutantes dobles un par de bases, G·C, ha sido sustituido por un par A·U en la estructura en hoja de trébol. Esto puede ocurrir en varias posiciones sin que aparentemente cambie la función del tRNA. Sustituciones de bases las cuales se espera alteren la estructura del tRNA resultan en una disminución de la síntesis de tRNA. Esto se debe a la maduración defectuosa del precursor del tRNA. El tRNA para tirosina de *E. coli* es transcrito *in vivo* como un precursor grande, el cual es procesado para producir el tRNA maduro. La secuencia nucleótida del precursor, su rompimiento *in vitro* por las endonucleasas y el significado de secuencias adicionales en el precursor, son discutidas.

REFERENCES

1. Cramer, F., *Progr. Nucleic Acid Res., 11,* 391 (1971).
2. Chambers, R. W., *Progr. Nucleic Acid Res., 11,* 489 (1971).
3. Gorini, L., *Ann. Rev. Genet., 4,* 107 (1970).
4. Goodman, H. M., Abelson, J., Landy, A., Brenner, S., and Smith, J. D., *Nature, 217,* 1019 (1968).
5. Goodman, H. M., Abelson, J. N., Landy, A., Zadrazil, S., and Smith, J. D., *Europ. J. Biochem., 13,* 461 (1970).
6. Russell, R. L., Abelson, J. N., Landy, A., Gefter, M. L., Brenner, S., and Smith, J. D., *J. Mol. Biol., 47,* 1 (1970).
7. Abelson, J. N., Gefter, M. L., Barnett, L., Landy, A., Russell, R. L., and Smith, J. D., *J. Mol. Biol., 47,* 15 (1970).
8. Smith, J. D., Barnett, L., Brenner, S., and Russell, R. L., *J. Mol. Biol., 54,* 1 (1970).
9. Smith, J. D., Anderson, K., Cashmore, A., Hooper, M. L., and Russell, R. L., *Cold Spring Harbor Symp. Quant. Biol., 35,* 21 (1970).
10. Hooper, M. L., unpublished observations.
11. Altman, S., Brenner, S., and Smith, J. D., *J. Mol. Biol., 56,* 195 (1971).
12. Cashmore, A., *Nature New Biol., 230,* 236 (1971).
13. Hirsh, D., *Nature, 228,* 57 (1970).
14. Levitt, M., *Nature, 224,* 759 (1969).
15. Anderson, K., and Smith, J. D., *J. Mol. Biol., 69,* 349 (1972).
16. Burdon, R. H., Martin, B. T., and Lal, B. M., *J. Mol. Biol., 28,* 357 (1967).
17. Bernhardt, D., and Darnell, J. E., *J. Mol. Biol., 42,* 43 (1969).
18. Mowshowitz, D. B., *J. Mol. Biol., 50,* 143 (1970).
19. Burdon, R. H., and Clason, A. E., *J. Mol. Biol., 39,* 113 (1969).
20. Altman, S., *Nature New Biol., 229,* 19 (1971).
21. Altman, S., and Smith, J. D., *Nature New Biol., 233,* 35 (1971).
22. Daniel, V., Sarid, S., Beckmann, J. S., and Littauer, U. Z., *Proc. Natl. Acad. Sci. U.S.A., 66,* 1260 (1970).
23. Robertson, H. D., Altman, S., and Smith, J. D., *J. Biol. Chem., 247,* 5243 (1972).

DISCUSSION

J. T. August (New York, U.S.A.): Could you tell us why the precursor forms have been retained during the evolutionary development of *E. coli?*

J. D. Smith (Cambridge, England): I do not know the answer to that. However, there is one portion of the 5′ additional segment which is interesting because it contains a sequence of nine nucleotides which is identical to a sequence within the tRNA. I think this may be of interest in considering the evolution of its precursor sequences.

R. P. Perry (Philadelphia, U.S.A.): Is there any evidence that there might be any other enzymes involved in the final processing of the 5′ segment? That is, once you make an endonucleolytic clip, have you any idea how the final piece is removed? The reason I ask is because in mammalian cells there is some evidence that ribosomal RNA may be processed by a combination of both endo- and exonucleases.

J. D. Smith: It is certain that the initial split is endonucleolytic, breaking only one bond. But if you look in the infected cells, you should be able to see the split-off segments if they are there, and since they cannot be found I would assume you are right, that there is another enzyme, possibly an exonuclease, which breaks them down.

Unidentified speaker: Is there any evidence that the maturation nucleases that function in *E. coli* also function for the maturation of phage tRNAs?

J. D. Smith: Yes, Dr. W. McClain has shown that the precursors to T4-specified tRNAs are specifically cleaved by the crude enzyme preparation from *E. coli*. We do not yet know whether the purified endonuclease is active in this reaction.

E. P. Geiduschek (La Jolla, U.S.A.): Are any of the endonucleases that you have mentioned known to split next to the 5′-terminal G?

J. D. Smith: Yes, the 5′ processing endonuclease I have discussed.

E. P. Geiduschek: Do you know whether perhaps this endonuclease might be able to process messenger precursor transcripts into messenger that lacks the 5′ terminus?

J. D. Smith: The crude enzyme appears to split the small $\phi 80$ transcription product known as "minimessenger." However, it is not known whether this RNA is a true messenger.

H. G. Zachau (Munich, Germany): I have a question which relates to your very first remarks on chain specificity. As probably all of us are aware, if one finds the mutation and bond position which changes the amino acid acceptance activity from, let's say, tyrosine to alanine or something that could be very close to get in this recognition site, what is your indication or evidence that amino acids really are accepted. I am clear that you do not know which ones, but what are the indications that there are others?

J. D. Smith: This is a question that will be discussed next by Alain Ghysen.

H. G. Zachau: But it is your evidence.

J. D. Smith: Yes, we started with certain amber mutations which cannot be suppressed by su^+_{III}, presumably because tyrosine inserted at this position would not give a functional product. One of these mutations is *E. coli* 1000B, lac^-_{amber}, the amber mutation being in the β-galactosidase gene. Drs. M. L. Hooper and R. Russell in our laboratory found four su_{III} mutants which will suppress certain of these amber mutations including 1000B. The sequence changes associated with these four mutations are A2, A81, U81, and G82, all base substitutions in the amino acid acceptor stem. We do not yet have direct biochemical evidence that these mutants insert a different amino acid. However, we can exclude the only other likely explanation. This would be that su^+_{III} tRNA cannot translate these amber codons because of their position in the messenger RNA, and the su_{III} mutant tRNAs simply allow such translation. Dr. M. L. Hooper has shown that su^+_{III} will relieve the polar effects on transacetylase synthesis resulting from the 1000B lac^-_{amber} mutation. Furthermore, since we have several amber mutations in $\phi 80$ which behave the same way toward su^+_{III} and the four su_{III} mutants, we think the "codon environment" explanation most unlikely.

17

Changes in Specificity of Suppression in Transfer Ribonucleic Acid Mutants

Alain Ghysen, Oscar Reyes, Catherine C. Allende, and Jorge E. Allende

Departamento de Biología
Facultad de Ciencias
Universidad de Chile
Santiago, Chile

The majority of the aminoacyl-tRNA synthetases recognize two or more tRNA species. The extraordinary specificity of the various synthetases for their substrate tRNAs (for a recent review, see ref. 4) could be related to the base sequence of the tRNA, to its overall geometry, or to both features. It is of interest, therefore, to study changes in the tRNA sequence and the effect of such changes in biosynthetic systems.

This approach has been used in the case of a particular species of tRNA, the *sup3* tyrosine tRNA (1,5). Many mutants of *sup3* were isolated, which alter to different extents the activity of the tRNA and therefore the efficiency of suppression. However, none of those mutants has been reported to alter the specificity of the charging reaction.

We have approached this problem by looking for a change in the specificity of suppression. The system we used is based on the existence of bacterial amber (nonsense) mutations which are not suppressed by some of the amber suppressors. The most obvious difference between the different amber suppressors is the amino acid which they charge. Therefore, one can interpret the failure of a given suppressor to correct an amber mutation as meaning that the amino acid introduced by that suppressor is not convenient and that the resulting protein is not functional. Then a change in the specificity of suppression would be a consequence of a change in the specificity of charging.

In the present communication, we describe the isolation and characterization of mutants of *sup3* which suppress a bacterial mutation not suppressed by *sup3* itself.

MATERIALS AND METHODS

Strains

All bacterial strains were *Escherichia coli* K12. SC172 (Hfr H *lys⁻gal⁻ₐₘ*) has been constructed by transduction of the *galₐₘ* mutation of RH303 (*cysₐₘ galₐₘ* 80ʳ, obtained from Dr. R. Thomas) into L4 (Hfr H *lys⁻glt* A⁻, obtained from Dr. P. Starlinger).

SC175 (F⁻*leu⁻ₐₘ*) is a *tyr⁺ lys⁺* 80ˢ λˢ recombinant obtained from a cross between WU36.10 (F⁻*tyr⁻_oc leu⁻ₐₘ* λʳ 80ʳ, obtained from Dr. S. Person) and L4.

275B (Hfr *lac* Z1000ₐₘ *trpₐₘ str* A) was obtained from Dr. D. Zipser.

SC54 is a λˢ F⁻derivative of CA244 [Hfr H *lacₐₘ trpₐₘ* (λ), obtained from Dr. S. Brenner].

The set of λ*sus* mutants which we used to characterize the suppression was obtained from Dr. R. Thomas; the phage φ80 *p sup3* was obtained from Dr. Ozeki.

Isolation and Purification of Missuppressing Mutants of φ80 *p sup 3*

Stocks of φ80 *p sup3* were mutagenized according to Adelberg *et al.* (2). The resulting lysates were used to infect a culture of SC172 at a multiplicity of infection of 0.2. After 15 min of adsorption at 37°, the cells were plated on minimal galactose-lysine agar and incubated 3 days at 37°. At that time, clones of different sizes appeared; one or more clone of each size was purified by at least two single-clone isolations on selective medium. The purified lysogens were induced, and the resulting phages were purified by at least two single-plaque isolations before characterization.

RESULTS

Isolation of φ80 *p sup3* Mutants

The *galₐₘ* mutation of strain SC172 is suppressible by *sup2* but not by *sup1* or *sup3* (R. Thomas, personal communication). Infection of this strain by φ80 *p sup3* followed by plating on selective medium permits one to select rare phenotypically *gal⁺* derivatives. The number of these derivatives is clearly related to the efficiency of mutagenesis of the phage (Table I). Different *gal⁺* derivatives

Table I. Isolation of Missuppressing Mutants from $\phi80\ p\ sup3^a$

Plaque-forming units/ml	gal_{am}-suppressing phages among the plaque-forming units	Stock No.	Mutants studied			
			Class I	Class II	Class III	Class IV
1×10^{10}	3×10^{-9}	6^b	A,B	—	—	—
4×10^9	1×10^{-7}	8	A,B,$^cC^c$	D	F	—
1.7×10^9	3×10^{-7}	7	A	B,C	E	D
1×10^8	3×10^{-6}	1	A,B	—	—	—
1.9×10^7	1×10^{-4}	2	B,C	E	—	—
1.2×10^7	1×10^{-4}	3	—	A,C	—	—
3×10^5	3×10^{-4}	5	A	B	—	—
2.6×10^5	5×10^{-4}	4	A,B,E,F, G,H,I,K^c	D,L,$^cp^c$	0	J

[a] The different stocks used are arranged according to the efficiency of nitrosoguanidine treatment. Two to 13 mutants of each stock were analyzed and classified according to the data of Table II. Each mutant is identified by the number of the starting stock and by an isolation letter.

[b] Stock No. 6 was not submitted to mutagenesis.

[c] These mutants are defective and were characterized only by the λsus assay of Table II.

Table II. Characterization of Missuppressing Mutants of φ80 p $sup3^a$

	λsus 213	λsus7	λsus 216	λsus 221	λsus 337	λsus 3	gal_{am}	leu_{am}	lac_{am}
sup1	+	+	−	−	−	+	−	NT^b	NT
sup2	+	+	+	+	−	+	+	NT	NT
φ80 p $sup3$	+	+	−	±	+	−	−	±	−
Class I	+	+	+	+	+	+	+	+	+
Class II	+	+	+	+	+	±	±	+	·
Class III	+	+	+	+	−	+	±	+	±
Class IV	+	−	+	+	−	±	±	+	±

^{a} Ability to suppress the λsus mutants was observed by putting drops of a diluted stock of phages (16^6 /ml) on a lawn of SC54 lysogen for the mutant of φ80 p $sup3$ to be tested. Ability to suppress the bacterial mutations gal_{am} from SC172, leu_{am} from SC175, and lac_{am} from 275B was observed by spot test of the φ80 p $sup3$ mutant on a lawn of the bacteria plated on selective medium.
^{b} NT, not tested.

from each infection were purified as explained in *Materials and Methods*. In most cases, the purified phages are still able to suppress the gal_{am} mutation of SC172.

Characterization of the Mutants

The mutant phages were characterized in two ways. First, we tested whether or not they are able to correct three bacterial amber mutations which are not, or not fully, suppressed by *sup3*. Second, we lysogenized SC54 with the mutants and observed the pattern of suppression of those lysogens by using a set of λ*sus* (amber) mutations which are differentially corrected by the known amber suppressors. The results of those experiments are given in Table II.

The patterns of suppression of the λ*sus* by the normal φ80 *p sup3* and by our mutants are clearly different. Furthermore, this test allows us to distinguish four classes among the missuppressing mutants. It should be noted that among the four classes, two (I and II) are still able to suppress λ*sus* 227, which is specific for *sup3*, while the two others are not (classes III and IV).

The suppression of the bacterial amber mutations also demonstrates the differences between the mutants and the original φ80 *p sup3*, and in some cases confirms the differences between the four classes detected by the λ*sus* assay.

Studies on the thermosensitivity of suppression (Table III) further distinguish classes III and IV, which no longer suppress at 42°, from classes I and II, which do.

Table III. Thermosensitivity of Suppression by
φ80 *p sup3* Mutants[a]

	lac_{am}			trp_{am}		
	32°	37°	42°	32°	37°	42°
φ 80 *sup3*	+	+	+	+	+	+
Class I	+	+	+	+	+	+
Class II	+	+	+	+	+	+
Class III	±	±	−	±	±	−
Class IV	±	±	−	±	±	−

[a] Strain SC54 was plated on minimal glucose or minimal tryptophan-lactose agar. Drops of the different phages were added, and the plates were incubated 48 hr at the indicated temperature. One representative of each mutant class has been used, namely, 1A, 3A, 7E, and 7D for classes I, II, III, and IV, respectively.

Quantitation of the Missuppression

The lac_{am} mutation of strain 275B is well corrected by the class I mutants but not by $\phi80\ p\ sup3$ (Table II). Since that mutation affects the β-galactosidase gene, we were able to quantitate the missuppression. We lysogenized 275B with $\phi80$, $\phi80\ p\ sup3$, $\phi80\ p\ sup3$ 1A (class I), and $\phi80\ p\ sup3$ 3A (class II) and assayed the level of β-galactosidase activity in IPTG-induced standing cultures. The results (Table IV) confirm the different specificities of suppression of $sup3$, class I and class II mutants.

Do the Mutations Affect the $sup3$ Gene?

Some phages code for proteins which interfere with the bacterial translational machinery or with some bacterial transfer RNA. In one case, an effect of this interference on the interaction between the ribosome and the $sup3$ tRNA has been noted (6). There is no evidence suggesting that $\phi80$ could code for such a protein. However, we wanted to eliminate the possibility that our mutations would affect the phage moiety of $\phi80\ p\ sup3$ and alter suppression in an indirect way. Therefore, we used the property of $\phi80\ p\ sup3$ to segregate the $sup3$ character with a frequency of 2-5% (3). We started with $\phi80\ p\ sup3$, $\phi80\ p\ sup3$ 1A (class I), and $\phi80\ p\ sup3$ 3A (class II) and isolated five derivatives of each of those phages which have lost the sup character. Those derivatives were used to lysogenize SC54. The lysogens were made $sup3$ by transduction, and spot tested with the set of λsus mutants. In all cases, the pattern of suppression was

Table IV. Missuppression of the lac_{am} Mutations of 275B[a]

Bacterial strain	β-Galactosidase activity (% of the wild type)
Wild type	100
275B ($\phi80$)	<0.2
175B ($\phi80\ p\ sup3$)	<0.2
275B ($\phi80\ p\ sup\ 3$ class I)	10.3
175B ($\phi80\ p\ sup3$ class II)	0.7

[a] The phage mutants used were 1A and 3A for classes I and II. Overnight cultures in presence of IPTG were assayed by the standard ONPG assay.

identical to that of *sup3*. We can conclude that the phage moiety of the mutants does not carry the ability of modifying the specificity of suppression.

CONCLUSIONS

Thirty-four mutants of ϕ80 *p sup3* have been studied, which differ from the original phage by their pattern of suppression. These mutants fall into four well-defined classes. For two of them, we have shown that the mutation carried by ϕ80 *p sup3* disappears when the phage loses its *sup3* gene. For the two other classes, we observed that the missuppression phenotype is accompanied by a loss of suppressor activity at 42°, which strongly suggests that the mutation leading to missuppression affects the tRNA itself. Those results allow us to assume that all four classes of mutants most probably directly affect the *sup3* tRNA gene.

The frequency of appearance of the missuppresion mutation is obviously related to the efficiency of the nitrosoguanidine treatment, which is known not to cause addition-deletion mutations. Then we can conclude that single base substitutions are enough to modify seriously the specificity of suppression. This conclusion is reinforced by the fact that there exist spontaneous mutations leading to the same missuppression behavior, and the ones we studied are identical to one important class of nitrosoguanidine-induced mutations.

The interpretation of the alterations in the specificity of suppression that we observed with our mutants is not obvious. The most evident explanation would be that missuppression involves mischarging, i.e., charging of the mutant tRNA by amino acids other than tyrosine, the one which is normally charged. If this were so, then the amino acids charged by the mutants of groups III and IV should be similar to glutamine, and the others probably to basic amino acids. The amino acid charged by the class I and class II mutants should be similar to both tyrosine and glutamine, or more probably there could be an ambiguity leading to the incorporation of both tyrosine and a basic amino acid. However, in the case of class I mutants, attempts to find *in vitro* competition of charge of tyrosine in the presence of large excesses of the 19 other amino acids were unsuccessful. Equally negative was an *in vivo* experiment where we tried to decrease the missuppression by increasing the tyrosine concentration.

The second interpretation of our results would be that the mutated tRNAs still charge tyrosine uniquely and that the alteration in the specificity of suppression is not related to mischarging effects.

Biochemical experiments are in progress to determine which one of the two hypotheses is correct.

ACKNOWLEDGMENTS

We thank Dr. Raúl Goldschmidt for interesting discussions and for his help in performing the β-galactosidase assay. This work was supported by the International Institute of Education (A.G.), CONICYT Chile, and the Comisión de Investigación Científica, Universidad de Chile.

SUMMARY

Bacteriophage φ80 *sup3* was mutagenized, and mutants were selected for their ability to suppress a bacterial amber mutation (*gal⁻*) which is not suppressed by *sup3*. Four mutants isolated in this fashion also show an altered pattern of suppression with a set of specific phage λ *sus* mutants. Work is now in progress to characterize the effect of the mutations on the tRNA function.

RESUMEN

Se mutagenizó el bacteriófago φ 80 *sup 3* y se seleccionaron mutantes por su capacidad para suprimir la mutación bacteriana ámbar (gal⁻) que no es suprimible por *sup 3*. Cuatro mutantes seleccionados en esta forma mostran también un esquema alterado de supresión con un conjunto de mutantes de fago λ *sus* específicas. Se está investigando los efectos de la mutación sobre la función del tRNA.

REFERENCES

1. Abelson, J. N., Gefter, M. L., Barnett, L., Landy, A., Russell, R. L., and Smith, J. D., *J. Mol. Biol., 47,* 15 (1970).
2. Adelberg, E. A., Mandel, M., and Chein Ching Chen, G., *Biochem. Biophys. Res. Commun., 18,* 788 (1965).
3. Andoh, T., and Ozeki, H., *Proc. Natl. Acad. Sci. U.S.A., 59,* 792 (1968).
4. Gauss, D. H., von der Haar, F., Maelicke, A., and Cramer, F., *Ann. Rev. Biochem., 40,* 1045 (1971).
5. Smith, J. D., Barnett, L., Brenner, S., and Russell, R. L., *J. Mol. Biol., 54,* 1 (1970).
6. Strigini, P., and Corini, L., *J. Mol. Biol., 47,* 517 (1970).

DISCUSSION

C. Weissmann (Zurich, Switzerland): If you think in terms of a neighboring effect to explain the lack of suppression by the *sup3* tRNA, then you would have to imagine that there are positions where the wild-type tyrosine tRNA cannot insert its tyrosine either.

A. Ghysen (Santiago, Chile): Yes, but there are two different species of tyrosine tRNA which have the same anticodon. It is then possible that one of them is not acceptable at some places where the other can work. This kind of situation could happen in the case of some amber mutations in the coat protein of RNA phage MS2. Those mutations make UAG a codon for glutamine; however, they are not suppressed by *sup7*, a suppressor which inserts glutamine with an efficiency of almost 70%. In this case, it is difficult to imagine any other explanation than a context effect.

J. D. Smith (Cambridge, England): I note that certain of the mutants you have discussed also have thermosensitive suppressor activity. It is interesting that when we selected for temperature-sensitive suppressor mutants, we obtained two; both gave base substitutions in the amino-acid acceptor arm and both showed anomalous suppression, being able to suppress amber mutants not suppressed by *sup 3*.

18

Conformational States
of Transfer Ribonucleic Acids

H. G. Zachau, R. E. Streeck, and U. J. Hänggi

*Institut für Physiologische Chemie und Physikalische
  Biochemie der Universität München*
German Federal Republic

The occurrence of different conformations of tRNAs is described or postulated in many recent publications. No review of the topic is attempted here, but rather a discussion of a few selected experiments. Although the figures are taken from our work, the main body of this article will include discussion of publications from various laboratories. For more general information, the reader may turn to one or the other of the numerous review articles on tRNA (e.g., refs. 1-5).

EXPERIMENTS AND RESULTS

Conformational Differences Between Uncharged tRNA, Aminoacyl-tRNA, and Peptidyl-tRNA

During protein synthesis, a molecule of aminoacyl-tRNA is attached to the mRNA-ribosome complex; it receives a peptidyl residue from peptidyl-tRNA, is translocated from one binding site on the ribosome to another one, and finally, after a second translation step, is released as uncharged tRNA (e.g., reviews 6-8). It was postulated that binding and release as well as the translocation are related to conformational differences among uncharged tRNA, aminoacyl-tRNA, and peptidyl-tRNA or may even be induced by changes of the tRNA conformation.

Several methods were employed in the search for conformational differences among the different functional states of tRNA. Differences between the rotatory dispersion spectra of charged and uncharged tRNAs, which had been reported some time ago (9), were not confirmed in later experiments (10). No differences were found in circular dichroism (11,12) except for the region of the s^4U absorption in tRNA^{fMet} and fMet-tRNA^{fMet} (13). In sedimentation velocity experiments (14), in studies on complexing with Mn^{2+} (15), poly C (16), and steroids (17), and in column chromatogrpahy (18), certain differences between charged and uncharged tRNAs were observed. In other chromatography experiments (19), the elution profiles of uncharged and charged tRNAs overlapped fully. Slight differences were detected in the ^{3}H-exchange kinetics of the two forms of tRNA (20). The fact that uncharged tRNA^{fMet} (*Escherichia coli*) did not compete with the charged form in the transformylase reaction was interpreted as being the result of a conformational difference (21).

With partial nuclease digestion, no differences were detected among the three functional states of some tRNAs (22). Charged and uncharged tRNA^{Ser} and tRNA^{Phe} from yeast, tRNA^{Phe} from *E. coli*, and acetyl-Phe-tRNA^{Phe} from yeast were treated with a number of endo- and exonucleases. The kinetics of the partial digestions were followed by disc electrophoresis and densitometry, as seen in Figs. 1 and 2. From the results, we concluded that at least in the two tRNAs from yeast no gross conformational changes occur on aminoacylation. Differences which do not alter the accessibility of the various regions of tRNA to nucleases could of course not be detected with this method. But any major change of conformation should result in such a difference of accessibility; for instance, native and denatured tRNAs behaved quite differently toward nucleases (see below).

It remains open to question whether the small conformational differences among uncharged tRNA, aminoacyl-tRNA, and peptidyl-tRNA which have been detected in a number of tRNAs with some methods but not with others occur in all tRNAs. With respect to the functional meaning of the conformational differences, one has to keep in mind that during protein synthesis not tRNA but tRNA-protein complexes are bound to and translocated on the mRNA-ribosome complex. The presence (or absence) of an aminoacyl or peptidyl group at the 3′ terminus of the tRNA may constitute a difference big enough to be detected by the protein factors; these differences are perhaps "magnified" by or during the complexing with the proteins. If this is the case, the conformational differences among the three forms of tRNA which have been found may not have the postulated functional meaning in the process of protein synthesis. If the sites of the conformational differences could be exactly localized within the tRNA molecules, we might be in a better position to answer this question.

Differences between aminoacyl- and peptidyl-tRNAs in the conformation of their anticodon loops, as they were postulated by Woese (23) and by Ghosh and

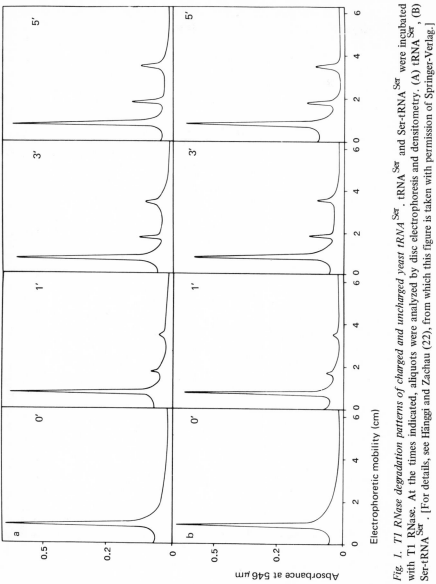

Fig. 1. *T1 RNase degradation patterns of charged and uncharged yeast tRNA*^{Ser}. *tRNA*^{Ser} *and Ser-tRNA*^{Ser} were incubated with T1 RNase. At the times indicated, aliquots were analyzed by disc electrophoresis and densitometry. (A) tRNA^{Ser}, (B) Ser-tRNA^{Ser}. [For details, see Hänggi and Zachau (22), from which this figure is taken with permission of Springer-Verlag.]

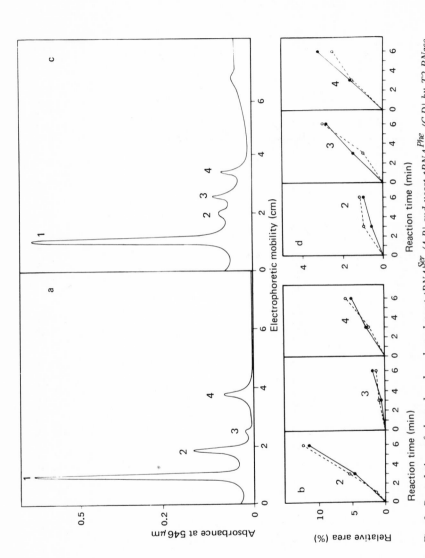

Fig. 2. Degradation of charged and uncharged yeast tRNA^{Ser} (A,B) and yeast tRNA^{Phe} (C,D) by T2 RNase. Charged and uncharged tRNA^{Ser} and tRNA^{Phe} were incubated with T2 RNase. Aliquots of the incubation mixtures were used for disc electrophoresis (e.g., A,C). The increase of bands 2-4 relative to band 1 is shown in B and D as a function of the time of degradation. ●, Charged tRNA; ○, uncharged tRNA. [For details, see Hänggi

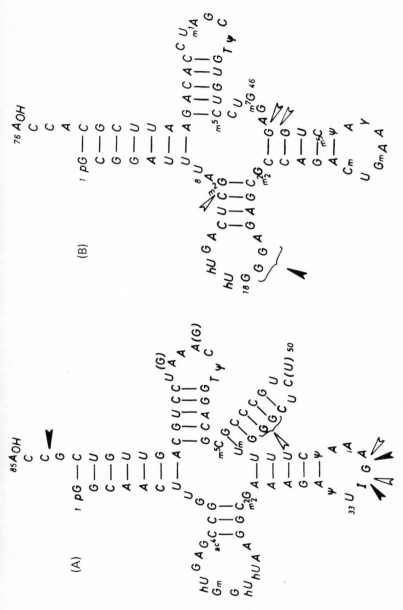

Fig. 3. Cloverleaf models of yeast tRNA^Ser I(II) (A) and tRNA^Phe (B). Filled arrows indicate positions of preferential T1 RNase splitting of native tRNAs, open arrows splits in the denatured tRNAs. [Figure is taken from Streeck and Zachau (31), with permission of North-Holland Publishing Company.]

Ghosh (24), are neither proved yet nor excluded by the experimental evidence. Some doubt has been cast on the Fuller-Hodgson model of the anticodon loop (25), which was the basis of these hypotheses, by recent experiments (26) and theoretical considerations (27). Experiments have been done in which the strongly fluorescent compounds proflavine or ethidium bromide were covalently inserted in place of the Y base next to the anticodon of yeast tRNA^{Phe} (28). A detailed investigation of the optical properties of these tRNA derivatives in the various functional states of the tRNA may help to elucidate the conformational changes in the anticodon loop.

Different Conformations of Uncharged tRNAs

A number of tRNAs can be reversibly denatured, as was first found by Lindahl *et al.* (29) and by Gartland and Sueoka (30). Heating of native tRNAs in the presence of EDTA renders them inactive with respect to amino acid acceptance and other activities. The denatured tRNAs can be completely renatured by heating in the presence of Mg^{2+}. Conformational differences between the native and denatured forms of yeast tRNA^{Ser} and tRNA^{Phe} have been recently localized by partial T1 RNase digestion experiments (Fig. 3) (31). With several other nucleases, similar results were obtained (32).

In addition to the native and denatured conformations of tRNA, as defined by the just-mentioned heating steps, other forms of tRNA can be detected in aminoacylation experiments. When native yeast tRNA^{Phe} was preincubated with large amounts of phenylalanyl-tRNA synthetase, its acceptor activity for phenylalanine in the standard assay system was significantly increased (33). The interpretation given is that native tRNA^{Phe} contains a certain percentage of inactive molecules which can be converted into active ones by complex formation with the synthetase. More closely related to the heat-denatured form of tRNAs may be an inactive form of yeast tRNA^{Lys}, which was prepared from an active one by prolonged dialysis against water and which could be converted back to the active form by incubation in the presence of salts prior to the acceptance assay (34).

Two conformations were postulated, at least for some tRNAs, on the basis of phosphorylation experiments with polynucleotide kinase (32,35) and dephosphorylation experiments with phosphomonoesterase (32). Only 20-30% of dephosphorylated yeast tRNA^{Ser} could be phosphorylated under standard conditions (Fig. 4); for full phosphorylation, a large excess of kinase was required. The existence of two conformations of tRNA which must differ at or near the 5′ terminus of the molecule was most clearly demonstrated in experiments with half molecules (Fig. 5). In a series of experiments, it was shown (35) that these two conformations cannot be explained by the native and denatured forms of tRNA in their usual definition.

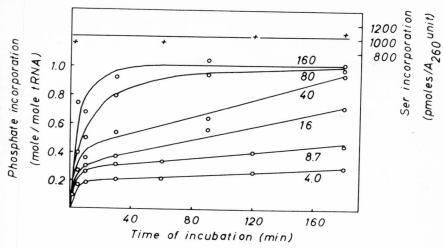

Fig. 4. *Phosphorylation of dephosphorylated yeast tRNA^{Ser}*. ○, Dephosphorylated tRNA^{Ser} was incubated with increasing amounts of polynucleotide kinase (4-160 units/ nmol tRNA^{Ser}, as indicated on the curves). +, Serine acceptance was determined in aliquots of the incubation mixtures containing the highest amount of polynucleotide kinase. [For details, see Hänggi *et al.* (35), from which this figure is taken with permission of Elsevier Publishing Company.]

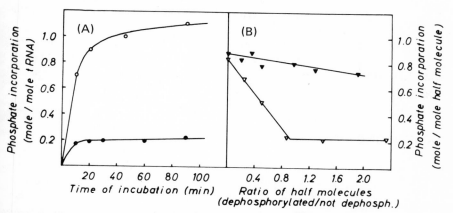

Fig. 5. *Phosphorylation of dephosphorylated yeast tRNA^{Phe} and half molecules from yeast tRNA^{Phe}*. (A) Dephosphorylated tRNA^{Phe} (●) and an equimolar mixture of dephosphorylated tRNA^{Phe} half molecules (○) were incubated with polynucleotide kinase. (B) Dephosphorylated 3'-half (▲) and dephosphorylated 5'-half (△) were incubated with polynucleotide kinase and increasing amounts of the not dephosphorylated 5'- and 3'-halves, respectively. [For details, see Hänggi *et al.* (35), from which this figure is taken with permission of Elsevier Publishing Company.]

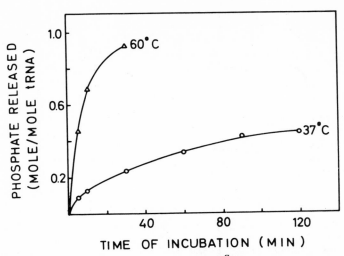

Fig. 6. Dephosphorylation of yeast tRNA^{Ser} at 37° and 60°. For each time point, 4.4 A_{260} units of tRNA^{Ser} was incubated with 0.016 units of bacterial alkaline phosphatase in 0.1 ml of 0.1 M Tris-HCl, pH 8.3.

The dephosphorylation of tRNA with phosphomonoesterase was investigated in less detail (32) but gave results (Fig. 6) rather analogous to those of the phosphorylation reaction.

Similar effects as with phosphorylation and dephosphorylation were observed in experiments on the degradation of tRNA from its 3' end with polynucleotide phosphorylase (36-38). Only a certain percentage of tRNA was degradable at room temperature. Additional tRNA was converted from the resistant to the degradable form at elevated temperatures.

CONCLUDING REMARKS

It may be the same two conformations which were detected by preincubation with synthetase, by phosphorylation and dephosphorylation, and by degradation with polynucleotide phosphorylase. The characteristics of the four reactions are somewhat different with respect to temperature and salt and enzyme concentrations. But this may be due to the fact that the two conformations can be detected in these cases only in enzymatic reactions. It is difficult to evaluate which of the differences are related to the different enzymes and which to the conformations of the tRNAs. In this respect, the problems concerning the native and denatured tRNAs are somewhat easier; here the two conformations can be characterized not only by an enzymatic assay but also by physicochemical measurements. As was pointed out before, the existence of native and denatured tRNAs seems to have little direct relation to the other effects.

The physical characteristics and the possible biological significance of the conformational differences among uncharged tRNA, aminoacyl-tRNA, and peptidyl-tRNA have been discussed above. It may be interesting to search for relations between these differences and those found among the various forms of uncharged tRNAs.

The coexistence of different conformations in mixtures of tRNA fragments has recently been proved, and details are given in Thiebe *et al.* (39). The finding of plateaus lower than 100% in the aminoacylation reaction and other biochemical assays, when modified tRNAs or synthetases from another organism were investigated (1-5), may at least in some cases be due to the coexistence of different conformations in the tRNA preparations.

The various results described in this article demonstrate that the definition of a certain conformational state of tRNA can only be operational. Native tRNA, for instance, which is prepared by a defined heating procedure, contains a mixture of molecules, some of which are reactive in a particular reaction while others are not. Also, denatured tRNA seems to consist of several closely related structures (19). The same may be true for other conformational states of tRNA.

SUMMARY

Twenty-four primary sequences of tRNAs are known by now. With respect to secondary structure, it is agreed that the cloverleaf model is the best two-dimensional representation of the truly three-dimensional structure. The three-dimensional structure itself, however, is unknown. The functions of tRNAs are described in terms of their interactions with the various components of the protein-synthesizing system. The interaction between tRNAs and mRNA, i.e., the anticodon-codon interaction, is fairly well understood. Little is known, however, about the interactions of tRNAs with proteins. Work is going on in many laboratories particularly on the interactions of specific tRNAs with the aminoacyl-tRNA synthetases. This work will be briefly reviewed. The two unknown topics, three-dimensional structure and protein recognition, are closely related, both experimentally and with respect to the results.

Recent work in our laboratory is discussed: (a) tRNA fragments were prepared by endonuclease treatment (40), by treatment with spleen exonuclease (41), and by specific chemical chain scissions (42). The study of the interactions of such fragments with aminoacyl-tRNA synthetases and CCA transferase permits some conclusions on the synthetase recognition site of tRNAs. (b) Pertaining to the same topic are studies on structural differences between native and denatured tRNAs (32). (c) The mechanism of tRNA synthetase interaction was investigated by fluorescence methods (43). In this context also, experiments on the convalent insertion of fluorescent dyes into tRNAs (42) are discussed.

RESUMEN

Se conocen actualmente 24 secuencias primarias de tRNAs. Con respecto a la estructura secundaria, existe acuerdo en que el modelo en hoja de trébol es la mejor representación bidimensional de la estructura verdaderamente tridimensional, que aún se desconoce. Se describirán las funciones de los tRNA en términos de sus interacciones con los diversos componentes del sistema de síntesis de proteínas. Las interacciones entre los tRNAs y el mRNA, es decir, la interacción codón-anticodón, son entendidas bastante bien. En cambio, se sabe poco acerca de las interacciones de tRNAs con proteínas. En muchos laboratorios se está trabajando en particular sobre las interacciones de tRNA específicos con sus aminoacil-tRNA sintetasas. Se resumirán brevemente estos trabajos. Los dos tópicos que se desconocen, la estructura tridimensional y el reconocimiento de proteínas, están estrechamente vinculados, tanto experimentalmente como en lo que respecta a los resultados.

En la parte principal de la presentación se hará referencia a trabajos realizados recientemente en nuestros laboratorios.

1. Se prepararon fragmentos de tRNA por tratamiento con endonucleasa (R. Thiebe, K. Harbens y H. G. Zachau, en preparación), por tratamiento con exonucleasa de bazo (P. Philippsen, Tesis, Munich, 1971) y por escisión química de la cadena (W. Wintermeyer, Tesis, Munich, 1971). El estudio de las interacciones de los antedichos fragmentos con aminocil-tRNA sintetasas y CCA-transferasa permite obtener algunas conclusiones sobre los sitios de reconocimiento de la sintetasa en los tRNAs.

2. Al mismo tema pertenecen estudios sobre diferencias estructurales entre tRNAs nativos y desnaturalizados (R. E. Streeck, Tesis, Munich, 1971).

3. El mecanismo de la interacción tRNA-sintetasa fue investigado mediante el empleo de métodos de fluorescencia (R. Rigler, M. Ehrenberg, E. Cronvall, R. Hirsch, U. Pachmann, y H. G. Zachau, en preparación). En este contexto se tratarán asimismo experimentos sobre la inserción covalente de colorantes fluorescentes en tRNAs (W. Wintermeyer, Tesis, Munich, 1971).

REFERENCES

1. Yarus, M., *Ann. Rev. Biochem., 38,* 841, (1969).
2. Zachau, H. G., *Angew. Chem., 81,* 645 (1969); Internat. Ed. *8,* 711 (1969); updated version in Bosch, L. (ed.), *"The Mechanism of Protein Synthesis and Its Regulation,"* North-Holland Publ. Co., Amsterdam, (1972), p. 173.
3. Chambers, R. W., *Progr. Nucleic Acid Res. Mol. Biol., 11,* 489 (1971).
4. Gauss, D. H., von der Haar, F., Maelicke, A., and Cramer, F., *Ann. Rev. Biochem., 40,* 1045 (1971).
5. Zachau, H. G., Symposium on Functional Units of Protein Biosynthesis, Seventh FEBS Meeting, Varna (1971).
6. The Mechanism of Protein Biosynthesis *Cold Spring Harbor Symp. Quant. Biol., 34,* (1969).
7. Lengyel, P., and Söll, D., *Bacteriol. Rev., 33,* 264 (1969).
8. McConkey, E. (ed.), *Protein Synthesis,* Vol. I, M. Dekker Publ. (1971) (articles, e.g., by Loftfield, R. B.).
9. Sarin, P. S., and Zamecnik, P. C., *Biochem. Biophys. Res. Commun., 20,* 400 (1965).
10. Bernardi, A., and Cantoni, G. L., *J. Biol. Chem., 244,* 1468 (1969).
11. Hashizume, H., and Imahori, K., *J. Biochem. Tokyo, 61,* 738 (1967).
12. Adler, A. J., and Fasman, G. D., *Biochim. Biophys. Acta, 204,* 183 (1970).
13. Watanabe, K., and Imahori, K., *Biochem. Biophys. Res. Commun., 45,* 488 (1971).
14. Kaji, H., and Tanaka, Y., *Biochim. Biophys. Acta, 138,* 642 (1967).
15. Cohn, M., Danchin, A., and Grunberg-Manago, M., *J. Mol. Biol., 39,* 199 (1969).
16. Danchin, A., and Grunberg-Manago, M., *FEBS Letters, 9,* 327 (1970).
17. Chin, R.-C., and Kidson, C., *Proc. Natl. Acad. Sci. U.S.A., 68,* 2448 (1971).
18. Stern, R., Zutra, L. E., and Littauer, U. Z., *Biochemistry, 8,* 313 (1969).

19. Adams, A., and Zachau, H. G., *Europ. J. Biochem. 5,* 556 (1968).
20. Gantt, R. R., Englander, S. W., and Simpsen, M. V., *Biochemistry, 8,* 475 (1969).
21. Schofield, P., *Biochemistry, 9,* 1694 (1970).
22. Hänggi, U. J., and Zachau, H. G., *Europ. J. Biochem., 18,* 496 (1971).
23. Woese, C., *Nature, 226,* 817 (1970).
24. Ghosh, K., and Ghosh, H. P., *Biochem. Biophys. Res. Commun., 40,* 135 (1970).
25. Fuller, W., and Hodgson, A., *Nature, 215,* 817 (1967).
26. Uhlenbeck, O. C., Baller, J., and Doty, P., *Nature, 225,* 508 (1970).
27. Ninio, J., *J. Mol. Biol., 56,* 63 (1971).
28. Wintermeyer, W., and Zachau, H. G., *FEBS Letters, 18,* 214 (1971).
29. Lindahl, T., Adams, A., and Fresco, J. R., *Proc. Natl. Acad. Sci. U.S.A., 55,* 941 (1966).
30. Gartland, W. J., and Sueoka, N., *Proc. Natl. Acad. Sci. U.S.A., 55,* 948 (1966).
31. Streeck, R. E., and Zachau, H. G., *FEBS Letters, 13,* 329 (1971).
32. Streeck, R. E., thesis, München (1971).
33. Renaud, M., Bollack, C., Befort, N., and Ebel, J. P., abst., Symposium on tRNA, Strasbourg (1971).
34. Mitra, S. K., and Smith, C. J., *J. Biol. Chem., 247,* 925 (1972).
35. Hänggi, U. J., Streeck, R. E., Voigt, H. P., and Zachau, H. G., *Biochim. Biophys. Acta, 217,* 278 (1970).
36. Thang, M. N., Guschlbauer, W., Zachau, H. G., and Grunberg-Manago, M., *J. Mol. Biol., 26,* 403 (1967).
37. Thang, M. N., Beltchev, B., and Grunberg-Manago, M., *Europ. J. Biochem., 19,* 184 (1971).
38. Beltchev, B., Thang, M. N., and Portier, C., *Europ. J. Biochem., 19,* 194 (1971).
39. Thiebe, R., Harbers, K., and Zachau, H. G., *Europ. J. Biochem., 26,* 144 (1972).
40. Harbers, K., Thiebe, R., and Zachau, H. G., *Europ. J. Biochem., 26,* 132, (1972).
41. Philippsen, P., thesis, München (1971).
42. Wintermeyer, W., thesis, München (1971).
43. Rigler, R., Cronvall, E., Ehrenberg, M., Pachmann, U., Hirsch, R., and Zachau, H. G., *FEBS Letters, 18,* 193 (1971).

DISCUSSION

K. Moldave (Irvine, U.S.A.): Have you looked, in addition to the acceptance assay, at the interaction of your fragments with a synthetase? I am thinking of the possibility that you may be getting an interaction, a recognition of the fragments, but that the conformation or the structure is not proper for acceptance of the amino acid itself.

H. G. Zachau (Munich, Germany): Yes. In a collaboration between our group and that of R. Rigler, Stockholm, the changes of fluorescence intensity and polarization of seryl-tRNA synthetase on addition of tRNA fragments and fragment combinations have been investigated (43). Interactions of the synthetase with homologous and heterologous fragment combinations have been observed also in some cases where no aminoacylation was achieved.

G. D. Novelli (Oak Ridge, U.S.A.): Dr. Stulberg in my laboratory investigated interactions between synthetase and tRNA fragments by studying the inhibition of tRNA charging on addition of the fragment. Have you done something similar?

H. G. Zachau: We have found inhibition only with a few fragment combinations (39). Therefore, inhibition by fragments seems not to be a generally applicable method.

G. D. Novelli: Have you comments on the method of tRNA charging by heterologous synthetases as a means to investigate recognition sites?

H. G. Zachau: This is a valuable method. The interpretation of the results is sometimes rather difficult (5). We have applied the method only in a few cases.

B. Hardesty (Austin, U.S.A.): Could you comment on the spectral shifts on insertion of proflavine or ethidium bromide in tRNA^{Phe}?

H. G. Zachau: The spectral shifts are very similar to the ones observed in intercalations of dyes into DNA. Our data support one of the intercalation models (28).

F. Lipmann (New York, U.S.A.): I wonder, have you tried to use the tRNA dye compounds on ribosomes? Did you get some shift of fluorescence during the binding or after the binding?

H. G. Zachau: Up to now, the binding of the compounds to poly U ribosomes has been studied only with radioactivity, not yet with fluorescence. In fact, it was in the beginning of Mr. Wintermeyer's work several years ago that he studied the interactions using the fluorescence of the Y base of tRNA^{Phe}. The results were not very conclusive at the time. We plan to take them up again with the new tRNA^{Phe} dye compounds.

J. D. Smith (Cambridge, England): Have you compared binding to UUU and UUC?

H. G. Zachau: Not yet.

19

Modification of Leucine tRNA of *Escherichia coli* After Bacteriophage T4 Infection

Arturo Yudelevich

Unidad de Virología
Facultad de Medicina
Universidad de Chile
and
Laboratorio de Bioquímica
Departamento de Biología Celular
Universidad Católica
Santiago, Chile

A number of metabolic alterations occur when *Escherichia coli* is infected with T-even bacteriophages. Among them, several alterations involving tRNA have been reported. Sueoka and Kano-Sueoka (1) and Kano-Sueoka and Sueoka (2) found that one of the five species of leucine tRNA (Leu_1-tRNA) normally present in *E. coli* is altered following T-even bacteriophage infection. Waters and Novelli (3) confirmed this observation using reversed-phase column chromatography and also demonstrated the appearance of two new peaks late after infection. These tRNA species are not detectable in normal cells.

We have determined the nucleotide sequence of Leu_1-tRNA (4) isolated from *E. coli* B and studied the nature of the alteration affecting this tRNA after T4 infection (5). The alteration is a specific cleavage of the tRNA molecule, giving rise to two fragments of similar size.

Our efforts are now directed toward determining whether this alteration of Leu_1-tRNA has any biological significance in the process of infection. We have recently isolated a T4 strain that will not induce cleavage of Leu_1-tRNA after infection and which may help us to answer this question.

MATERIALS AND METHODS

Materials

Radioactive chemicals were obtained from the Radiochemical Centre, Amersham, Bucks., England, or from NEN, Boston, Mass., U.S.A.

In all experiments involving ^{32}P labeling, the low phosphate medium as described by Landy et al. (6) was used.

Preparation of ^{32}P-labeled tRNA and tRNA Fragments

Labeled leucine tRNA and tRNA fragments were prepared as previously described (5).

Polyacrylamide Gel Electrophoresis

Slabs of 10% polyacrylamide gel (40 by 20 by 0.3 cm) were prepared as described by Adams et al. (7). Sucrose (final concentration 10%) and Bromophenol Blue were added to the samples. Electrophoresis was carried out for 16-20 hr at 30 ma at $4°$.

The RNA was extracted from the gels by cutting out the appropriate band and grinding in a glass homogenizer with 0.5 M sodium acetate, 0.01 M Tris-HCl (pH 9.0), and 0.001 M EDTA. After centrifugation at low speed, the gel was again extracted, and the combined supernatants were then passed through a millipore filter. Carrier tRNA was added to a final concentration of 50 μg/ml. The tRNA was finally precipitated with ethanol.

Nucleotide Sequence Determinations

The methods described by Sanger et al. (8) and Brownlee and Sanger (9) were used.

Preparation of Cell-free Extracts

Crude extracts from uninfected and T4-infected *E. coli* Q13 were prepared by grinding 1 g of cells with 2.5 g of alumina, 3 ml of 0.01 M Tris-HCl (pH 7.4) containing 0.001 M $MgCl_2$ and 0.002 M mercaptoethanol was added to the paste. The mixture was centrifuged at 10,000 rpm in a Sorvall centrifuge for 20 min, and the supernatant was used as a source of cleaving enzyme.

RESULTS

Examination of ^{32}P-labeled RNA by electrophoresis on slabs of polyacrylamide gels revealed that two new bands were present in samples obtained from T4-infected cultures. *E. coli* was grown in the presence of carrier-free ^{32}P-phosphate, half of the culture was infected with T4, and the rest was used as control. The RNA fraction isolated by phenol extraction was fractionated by electrophoresis on polyacrylamide gels, and the different fractions were detected by radioautography. As shown in Fig. 1, two new bands moving ahead of 4S RNA can be seen only in samples from infected cultures. The two bands are

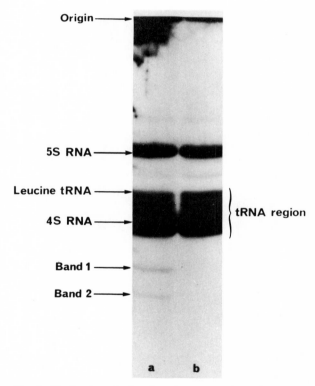

Fig. 1. *Electrophoretic fractionation on a polyacrylamide gel of ^{32}P-labeled RNA samples prepared from uninfected and T4-infected* E. coli *B. The gel (9.5% acrylamide, 0.5% bisacrylamide) was prepared as described in Materials and Methods. (a) RNA prepared from 2 min T4-infected* E. coli *B. (b) RNA prepared from uninfected* E. coli *B.*

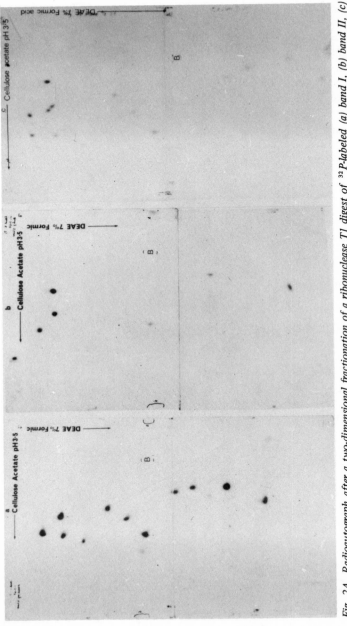

Fig. 2A. Radioautograph after a two-dimensional fractionation of a ribonuclease T1 digest of ^{32}P-labeled (a) band I, (b) band II, (c) Leu$_1$-tRNA.

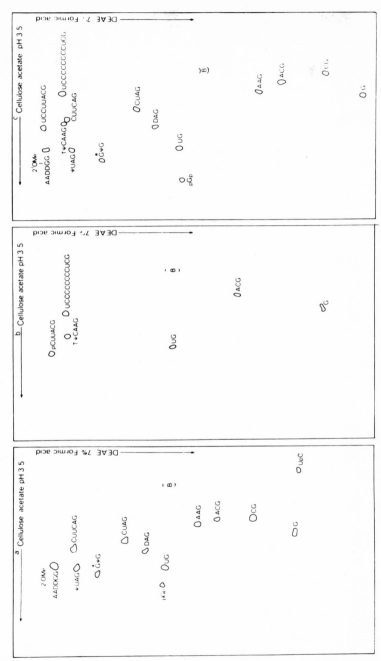

Fig. 2B. Diagram showing position and sequences of the nucleotides obtained in Fig. 2A.

observed only if labeling with ^{32}P-phosphate is done before infection, and they will not appear if chloramphenicol (50 μg/ml) is added prior to infection.

The nature of the two bands appearing after phage infection was established by determining their nucleotide sequences. Both ^{32}P-labeled bands were eluted from the gel and digested with ribonuclease T1 and pancreatic ribonuclease. The oligonucleotides thus obtained were fractionated and analyzed using the two-dimensional system described by Sanger et al. (8) and Brownlee and Sanger (9). The method involves ionophoresis on cellulose acetate in the first dimension and ionophoresis on DEAE paper in the second. Figures 2A and 2B show a two-dimensional fractionation of ribonuclease T1 digests and a diagram of the position and sequences of the resulting oligonucleotides of each of the two bands appearing after bacteriophage infection and of purified Leu_1-tRNA. The sequences of the nucleotides obtained by T1 digestion of both bands were obtained using alkaline digestion, pancreatic ribonuclease, ribonuclease U_2, venom phosphodiesterase or pancreatic ribonuclease after treatment with carbodiimide, or a combination of these procedures.

Examination of the fingerprints (Fig. 2) shows clearly that band 1 and band 2 are closely related to Leu_1-tRNA in terms of their nucleotide sequence. Complete characterization of the oligonucleotides obtained from band 1 reveals that this band is a fragment of the Leu_1-tRNA molecule corresponding to the 5′ end of the molecule extending up to residue C48 (see Fig. 3). T1 digestion of band I yielded in addition a new spot not present in T1 digests from Leu_1-tRNA. This spot was identified as UpC.

The oligonucleotides originating from band 2 after T1 digestion were characterized in a similar way. The results obtained (see Fig. 2) indicated that band 2 corresponds to the 3′ end of the Leu_1-tRNA molecule and has 39 nucleotide residues. All the expected oligonucleotides from such a fragment are present with the exception of one oligonucleotide (UCCUUACG) which is replaced by another oligonucleotide whose sequence was determined as being pCUUACG. The appearance of a spot having the sequence pCUUACG in fragment II and the appearance of UpC in T1 digests obtained from fragment I permit us to establish the exact position where Leu_1-tRNA is cleaved after T4 infection (see Fig. 3). This was confirmed by the appearance of pCp in a fingerprint of a pancreatic ribonuclease digest of fragment II. pCp is not present in fingerprints of a pancreatic ribonuclease digest of Leu_1-tRNA.

The cleavage of Leu_1-tRNA following T4 infection occurs very early; fragments can be observed by 1 min after infection and begin to disappear by 5 min after infection. After 7-8 min, one can detect only traces of fragments.

We have tried to obtain in vitro cleavage of Leu_1-tRNA using subcellular extracts prepared from an RNase-less and polynucleotide phosphorylase-less mutant of E. coli (strain Q13) infected with T4. It should be pointed out that

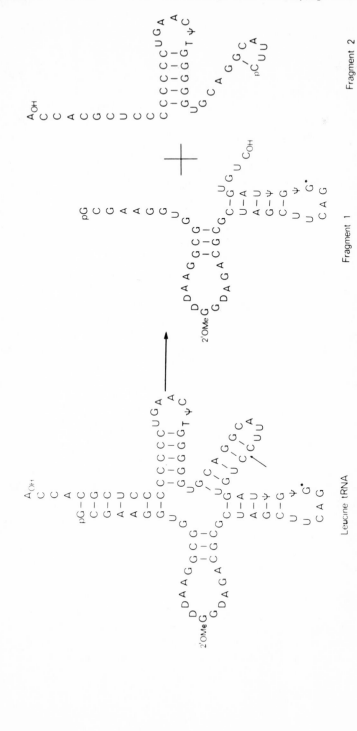

Fig. 3. Nucleotide sequence of Leu₁-tRNA and of both fragments produced after infection with T4. The arrow indicates the point where cleavage occurs.

when strain Q13 is used as a host for T4 infection, normal cleavage of
Leu_1-tRNA is observed.

^{32}P-labeled Leu_1-tRNA, purified by acrylamide gel electrophoresis, was
incubated with a crude extract of T4-infected Q13 prepared by grinding with
alumina. As a control, incubation was done with uninfected extracts of Q13. In
both cases, we observed the appearance of fragments of a size similar to those
produced *in vivo*, when the reaction mixtures were analyzed by electrophoresis
in polyacrylamide gels. Both fragments were analyzed by T1 ribonuclease
digestion. The oligonucleotides obtained were separated using the techniques
described by Sanger *et al.* (8). The fragments obtained by incubation with Q13
extracts are not equivalent to the fragments obtained *in vivo*. One fragment
corresponds to the 5' end of the molecule and extends up to residue G46, and
the second fragment corresponds to the rest of the molecule. Therefore, they
must originate by cleavage of a single phosphodiester bond between residues
G46 and U47. The fragments produced by incubation with extracts from
uninfected Q13 and infected Q13 proved to be identical, and we have been
unable up to now to obtain *in vitro* fragments similar to those produced *in vivo*
after T4 infection.

In order to establish the biological significance of the T4-induced cleavage of
Leu_1-tRNA, we have isolated a T4 strain that will not produce this cleavage
after infection. Wild-type T4 was treated with hydroxylamine, and among the
survivors about 50 plaques were picked randomly and examined for Leu_1-tRNA
cleavage after infection. Only one of the isolates, though able to infect and
produce plaques on *E. coli*, did not produce cleavage of Leu_1-tRNA on infection
(see Fig. 4).

CONCLUSIONS

Infection of *E. coli* with bacteriophage T4 results in the cleavage of
Leu_1-tRNA; two fragments of roughly equal size are produced. Protein synthesis
is needed for this cleavage to occur, since chloramphenicol blocks the appearance of fragments. It seems likely that the break in the tRNA is caused by a
T4-induced nuclease. We have tried to detect this activity *in vitro* without
success as yet. However, we have detected a different type of cleavage, produced
by incubation of ^{32}P-labeled Leu_1-tRNA with extracts from infected and uninfected *E. coli* Q13. This cleavage occurs in a region very near to the point where
this tRNA is cleaved after T4 infection. This may indicate that this is a very
exposed region in the Leu_1-tRNA molecule.

A problem which remains to be answered is whether or not this alteration
has any physiological significance. Kano-Sueoka and Sueoka (10) have suggested
a mechanism by which alteration of Leu_1-tRNA may inhibit host mRNA
translation. We have isolated a T4 strain that will not induce this alteration, and

this should allow us to test this proposal. It must be kept in mind that the problem of control of host protein synthesis may be a rather complex one. Hsu

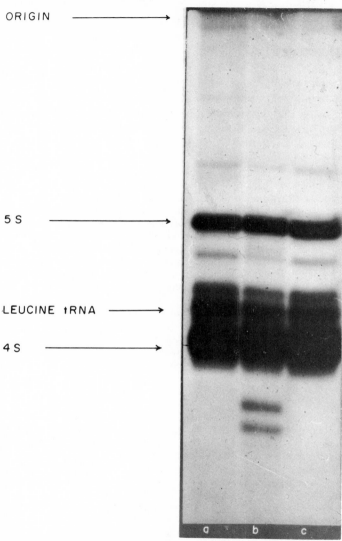

ORIGIN

5 S

LEUCINE tRNA

4 S

Fig. 4. Electrophoretic fractionation on a polyacrylamide gel of ^{32}P-labeled RNA samples prepared from(a) uninfected E. coli *B., (b) T4 wild-type infected* E. coli *B. (c)* E. coli *B infected with a T4 strain isolated after hydroxylamine treatment.*

and Weiss (11) have reported that a factor prepared from ribosomes from T4-infected *E. coli* will inhibit the formation of initiation complexes of *E. coli* mRNA with uninfected ribosomes. These results have been confirmed and extended by Klem *et al.* (12), Schedl *et al.* (13), Dube and Rudland (14), and Steitz *et al.* (15).

ACKNOWLEDGMENTS

This work was partially supported by a grant from CIC, Universidad de Chile, and Fondo de Investigaciones de la Universidad Católica. Part of this work was done while the author was at the Medical Research Council, Cambridge, England, supported by a fellowship from the Anna Fuller Fund.

SUMMARY

Infection of *E. coli* B with bacteriophage T4 leads to an alteration of one of the five species of leucine tRNA present in this strain. Examination by polyacrylamide gel electrophoresis and ribonuclease T1 fingerprints of ^{32}P-labeled RNA isolated from T4-infected *E. coli* reveals that leucine tRNA is fragmented into two pieces of roughly equal size. The fragments can be observed 1 min after infection, and they begin to disappear 4 min later.

Sequence studies show that the fragmentation results from the cleavage of a single phosphodiester bond in the leucine tRNA molecule, giving rise to two fragments. Fragment I contains 39 nucleotides corresponding to the 3' end of the molecule and begins with a pC residue. Fragment II contains 48 residues corresponding to the 5' end of the molecule and is terminated with a C_{OH} residue.

Incubation of ^{32}P-labeled leucine tRNA with cell-free extracts prepared from uninfected or T4-infected *E. coli* Q13 results in the appearance of two fragments of similar size. These fragments are different from those obtained *in vivo* after T4 infection.

A T4 strain unable to produce fragmentation of leucine tRNA after infection has been isolated.

RESUMEN

La infección de *Escherichia coli B* con el bacteriófago T_4 conduce a una alteración de una de las cinco especies de tRNA de leucina presentes en esta cepa. El examen por electroforesis en gel de poliacrilamida y el mapeo nucleototídico con ribonucleasa T_1 del RNA marcado con ^{32}P aislado de *E. coli* infectado por T_4, revela que el tRNA de leucina se halla fragmentado en dos trozos de approximadamente del mismo tamaño. Los fragmentos pueden observarse un minuto después de la infección y comienzan a desaparecer cuatro minutos más tarde.

Estudios de secuencia demuestran que la fragmentación tiene lugar por ruptura de un único enlace fosfodiéster en la molécula del tRNA de leucina, lo que da lugar a la formación de dos fragmentos. El fragmento I contiene 39 nucleótidos que corresponden al extremo 3' de la molécula y comienza con un risiduo pC. El fragmento II contiene 48 residuos que corresponden al extremo 5' de la molécula y finaliza con un residuo C_{OH}.

La incubación de ^{32}P-tRNA de leucina con homogeneizados de células de *E. coli* Q13, infectadas con T_4, resulta en la aparición de dos fragmentos de igual tamaño. Estos dos fragmentos son distintos de los que se obtienen *in vivo* después de la infección con T_4.

Una cepa de T_4 que no produce la fragmentación del tRNA de leucina después de la infección ha sido aislada.

REFERENCES

1. Sueoka, N., and Kano-Sueoka, T., *Proc. Natl. Acad. Sci. U.S.A., 52,* 1535 (1964).
2. Kano-Sueoka, T., and Sueoka, N., *J. Mol. Biol., 20,* 183 (1966).
3. Waters, L. C., and Novelli, G. D., *Proc. Natl. Acad. Sci. U.S.A., 57,* 979 (1967).
4. Dube, S. K., Marcker, K. A., and Yudelevich, A., *FEBS Letters, 9,* 168 (1970).
5. Yudelevich, A., *J. Mol. Biol., 60,* 21 (1971).
6. Landy, A., Abelson, J., Goodman, H. M., and Smith, S. D., *J. Mol. Biol., 29,* 457 (1967).
7. Adams, J. M., Jeppesen, P. G. N., Sanger, F., and Barrell, B. G., *Nature, 233,* 1009 (1969).
8. Sanger, F., Brownlee, G. G., and Barrell, B. G., *J. Mol. Biol. 13,* 373 (1965).
9. Brownlee, G. G., and Sanger, F., *J. Mol. Biol., 23,* 337 (1967).
10. Kano-Sueoka, T., and Sueoka, N., *Proc. Natl. Acad. Sci. U.S.A., 62,* 1229 (1969).
11. Hsu, W., and Weiss, S. B., *Proc. Natl. Acad. Sci. U.S.A., 64,* 345 (1965).
12. Klem, E. B., Hsu, W., and Weiss, S. B., *Proc. Natl. Acad. Sci. U.S.A., 67,* 696 (1970).
13. Schedl, P. D., Singer, R. E., and Conway, T. W., *Biochem. Biophys. Res. Commun., 38,* 631 (1970).
14. Dube, S. K., and Rudland, P. S., *Nature, 226,* 824 (1970).
15. Steitz, J. A., Dube, S. K., and Rudland, P. S., *Nature, 226,* 824 (1970).

DISCUSSION

R. M. Bock (Madison, U.S.A.): In relation to Dr. S. Weiss's findings that new tRNAs are made after T4 infection, it seems that this could be a very fascinating metabolic relationship. One tRNA, which is recognizing the CUG codon, is destroyed and could be replaced by a very selective codon-recognizing tRNA.

A. Yudelevich (Santiago, Chile): You may be right. There are reports that there are two leucine tRNAs coded by T4. One of them has been characterized as recognizing the UUG codon. I do not know the codon specificity of the second one.

G. D. Novelli (Oak Ridge, U.S.A.): We found that later on in infection two new leucine tRNAs appear that are coded for by the phage genome. I wonder if the mutant you have isolated, that no longer cleaves leucine tRNA, still codes for the late leucine-tRNAs.

A. Yudelevich: I do not know, but it would be interesting to look into that.

20

Reconstitution of 50S Ribosomal Subunits and the Role of 5S RNA

M. Nomura and S. Fahnestock

Institute for Enzyme Research
and
Departments of Biochemistry and Genetics
University of Wisconsin
Madison, Wisconsin, U.S.A.

Bacterial 30S ribosomal subunits can be reconstituted from 16S ribosomal RNA and about 21 30S ribosomal proteins (1,2). The reconstituted 30S subunits have physical properties, protein composition, and functional capability almost identical to those of the original 30S subunits. This indicates that the information for the correct assembly of 30S ribosomal subunits is contained in the structure of their molecular components and not in some other nonribosomal factors.

The 30S ribosome reconstitution system has provided a useful system in which the mechanism of assembly of the ribosome can be studied. For example, the binding of each of the purified proteins to 16S ribosomal RNA has been studied, and the order of addition of proteins during the *in vitro* assembly reaction has been elucidated (3). We have found that under the conditions of reconstitution, only certain proteins bind to the 16S RNA and some other proteins bind only when some of the first proteins are bound. An assembly map has been constructed from these experimental data (3).

The 30S reconstitution system has also provided a means by which the functional role of each of the molecular components can be studied. For example, molecular components responsible for the mutational alteration of 30S subunits can be identified using the reconstitution technique. Mutants resistant to streptomycin are known to affect the 30S ribosomal subunits (4,5). Using the reconstitution technique, the mutational change in the properties of 30S sub-units could be definitely correlated to a change in one of the 30S ribosomal proteins, P10 (6,7). [P10 is S12 according to the nomenclature of Wittmann (8).]

Another approach used for the functional analysis of 30S ribosomal compo-nents is to perform reconstitution in the presence of 16S RNA and a mixture of all the purified proteins with one component omitted. The information obtained from this type of experiment has been described in previous papers (2,9). Chemical modification of 30S subunits is another approach for analysis of the functional role of ribosomal components. The available reconstitution system has been useful in the identification of the altered component responsible for the ribosomal functions altered by chemical modification (10).

Finally, the *in vitro* assembly system may also be useful for the study of three-dimensional organization of the 30S ribosomal proteins. It has been suggested that the assembly map mentioned above reflects the topological relationships among ribosomal proteins in the ribosome structure (3). Studies using several other approaches, such as modifying reagents or enzymes, are just beginning, and results obtained so far tend to support the above suggestion (11-15).

From this brief survey of the studies related to the assembly of 30S subunits, it is clear that availability of a similar *in vitro* reconstitution system for the 50S ribosomal subunits should be very useful. Although we encountered great difficulty in reconstituting *Escherichia coli* 50S subunits, we have recently achieved our aim, the reconstitution of 50S subunits, using a thermophilic organism, *Bacillus stearothermophilus* (16).

IN VITRO RECONSTITUTION OF 50S SUBUNITS

It was originally reasoned that the difficulty with 50S reconstitution might reflect the greater complexity of the assembly of 50S subunits compared to the assembly of 30S subunits, as well as higher kinetic energy barriers which would be overcome only by a longer incubation time at higher temperatures. *E. coli* 50S ribosomal components or partially assembled intermediate particles might be too unstable to permit higher incubation temperatures, and therefore the *B. stearothermophilus* system was selected as a possible reconstitution system. Using this system, reconstitution of functionally active 50S ribosomal subunits has succeeded (16). In fact, it was observed that the reconstitution of 50S subunits in this system is much slower than that of 30S subunits even at the optimum temperature (60°).

Figure 1 shows the procedure originally used for the reconstitution. The RNA fraction ("RNA50") was shown to contain one protein still tightly bound to 23S rRNA. This protein (called L3) was not present in the "total" 50S

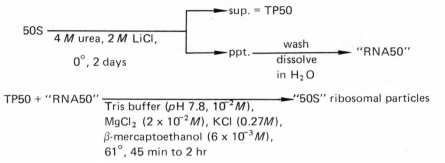

Fig. 1. *The procedure for reconstitution of 50S ribosomal subunits from* B. stearothermophilus.

protein fraction. Thus this original reconstitution is *not* from a completely protein-free RNA preparation. L3 can be removed from 23S rRNA by treatment with acetic acid (66%) or with HCl at pH 2. The protein-free RNA preparation can be obtained either by exhaustive phenol treatments of 50S subunits or by redissolving the precipitate after pH 2 treatment of the RNA50 fraction (Fig. 2). It has been demonstrated that functional 50S subunits can be reconstituted from a mixture of protein-free RNA fraction, TP50, and the extracted protein L3. Presence of L3 is essential for the reconstitution (ref. 17; Fahnestock and Nomura, manuscript in preparation).

The above reconstitution reactions were done using purified 50S ribosomal subunits as starting materials. However, several reconstitution experiments were done using 70S ribosomes as starting materials. Figure 3 summarizes the procedure used in this case. The biological activity of the reconstituted 50S particles in this case was originally found to be consistently higher than the activity of the 50S particles obtained by the first procedure, namely, that using purified 50S subunits as starting materials. From genetic studies on ribosome assembly in *E. coli,* some crucial role of 30S subunits (or their precursors or components) in the

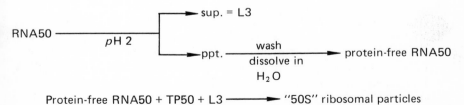

Fig. 2. *Reconstitution of 50S ribosomal subunits from a mixture of protein-free RNAs and proteins.*

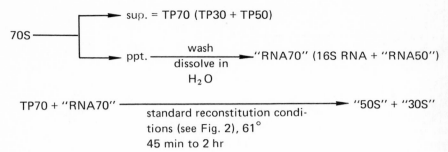

Fig. 3. *Simultaneous reconstitution of 50S and 30S ribosomal subunits.*

assembly of 50S subunits has been previously proposed as a general principle of the *in vivo* ribosome assembly reaction (18). Thus the above *in vitro* observation was thought to give some support to this proposal. Furthermore, addition of 30S ribosomal subunits to the 50S reconstitution system (such as shown in Fig. 1) caused occasional stimulation of reconstitution (mentioned in ref. 16). However, by repeating experiments, the stimulatory effect of 30S subunits has been found *not* to be reproducible. It was also found that the procedure described in Fig. 3 does not give any significantly higher reconstitution activity than that obtained according to the procedure described in Fig. 2, if freshly prepared 50S subunits are used to make RNA and protein components for the reconstitution (S. Fahnestock, unpublished experiments). Thus the reconstitution of 50S subunits *in vitro* under the present conditions does not require the presence of 30S subunits (or their components). The role of 30S subunits in the *in vivo* 50S assembly suggested from *in vivo* experiments remains unknown.

THE ROLE OF 5S RNA

The 50S ribosome assembly system just described now provides a system which we can use to study many questions similar to those regarding the 30S assembly described in the Introduction of this article. Here, we shall summarize our recent experiments on one of these problems, namely, the role of 5S RNA in the 50S ribosomal subunits.

The function of 5S RNA is unknown, although the primary sequence of 5S RNAs from various sources has been elucidated (19-21). It has been assumed that 5S RNA has some important function. No experimental proof has been available for this assumption. In addition, recent studies failed to find 5S RNA in *Neurospora* mitochondrial ribosomes (22). It was thus necessary first to test whether 5S RNA is essential for the assembly of functional 50S subunits (23).

5S RNA is present both in the RNA50 fraction and in the TP50 fraction obtained according to the procedure shown in Fig. 1. 5S RNA was removed

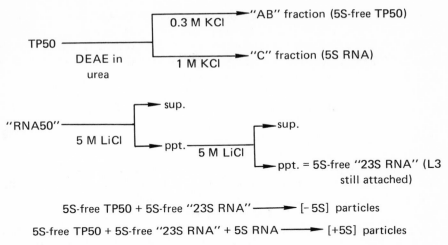

Fig. 4. *Reconstitution of "50S" particles in the presence and absence of 5S RNA.*

from these fractions by the procedure shown in Fig. 4. Reconstitution was then performed using the 5S-free TP50 and 5S-free RNA50, with and without further addition of 5S RNA. The particles reconstituted in the absence of 5S RNA were found to have no, or greatly reduced, activity in poly U-dependent polyphenyl-alanine synthesis. The activity increased linearly with increasing amount of 5S RNA added to the system, up to the molar equivalent to that of 23S RNA (23). The particles reconstituted in the absence of 5S RNA ($-$5S particles) were then examined in more detail. In addition to the poly U-dependent polyphenylalanine synthesis described above, $-$5S particles were found to have greatly reduced activity in the following reactions: (a) polypeptide synthesis directed by natural messenger RNA, (b) peptidyl transferase assay, (c) peptide chain termination factor (R1) dependent ^{3}H-UAA binding, (d) G-factor-dependent ^{3}H-GTP binding, and (e) codon-directed tRNA binding (assayed in the presence of 30S subunits). Thus 5S RNA is an essential 50S ribosomal component.

The $-$5S particles were found to be deficient in several proteins. The question was then asked whether the absence of some proteins in the $-$5S particles is related to the inactivity of the particles. It was found that restoration of activity to the inactive $-$5S particles depends on further addition of the missing proteins as well as 5S RNA. Thus some, or all, of the proteins which are absent in $-$5S particles are important for activity in polypeptide synthesis. In this sense, 5S RNA has a structural role, that is, a role in the binding of some functionally important proteins. Whether 5S RNA has any direct function in protein synthesis in the completed ribosome structure cannot be answered from the above experiments.

There have been several speculations on the role of 5S RNA. Most recently, Raacke (24) has proposed a model for protein synthesis in which the nascent polypeptide becomes esterified to the 3'-hydroxyl group of the terminal nucleoside of 5S RNA by transfer from peptidyl-tRNA, then is transferred to aminoacyl-tRNA. Thus the proposed reactions are as follows:

$$A_1 A_2 \ldots A_n\text{-tRNA} + 5S\ RNA \xrightarrow{\text{transferase I}} A_1 A_2 \ldots A_n\text{-5S} + \text{tRNA}$$

$$A_1 A_2 \ldots A_n\text{-5S RNA} + A_{n+1}\text{-tRNA} \xrightarrow{\text{transferase II}} A_1 A_2 \ldots A_{n+1}\text{-tRNA} + 5S\ RNA$$

We have tested this proposal by making use of the 50S reconstitution system which is dependent on added 5S RNA (25). First, we have treated 5S RNA with periodate and used the oxidized 5S RNA directly for the reconstitution. Periodate oxidizes the terminal ribose of 5S RNA. Analyses indicated that the periodate oxidation is complete and that the oxidized 5S RNA exists in the reconstituted "50S" particles in a form devoid of the 3'-terminal nucleoside residue and presumably retaining a phosphate at the $3'(2')$ position of the original penultimate nucleoside. It is expected that such a modified 5S RNA would not retain full activity if the peptidyl-5S RNA model were correct. The experimental results showed that biological activities of the reconstituted particles containing such modified 5S RNA are the same as those of the reconstituted 50S particles containing intact 5S RNA. Thus the peptidyl-5S RNA model appears to be unlikely.

A more convincing test of the proposal was performed using 5S RNA with a stable modification (25). This was accomplished by treatment of periodate oxidized 5S RNA with methylamine, followed by reduction with LiBH$_4$. The resultant 5S RNA has a terminal ribose converted to a 5-hydroxy-4-methyl-2-hydroxymethylphosphate morpholine derivative in which the 3'-hydroxyl involved in the Raacke model is missing and the stereochemical structure of the terminal residue is considerably altered (Fig. 5). The reconstitution experiments showed that there is no significant difference between the activity of ribosomes which contain untreated 5S RNA and those with periodate-methylamine-borohydride treated 5S RNA, in either poly U-dependent polyphenylalanine

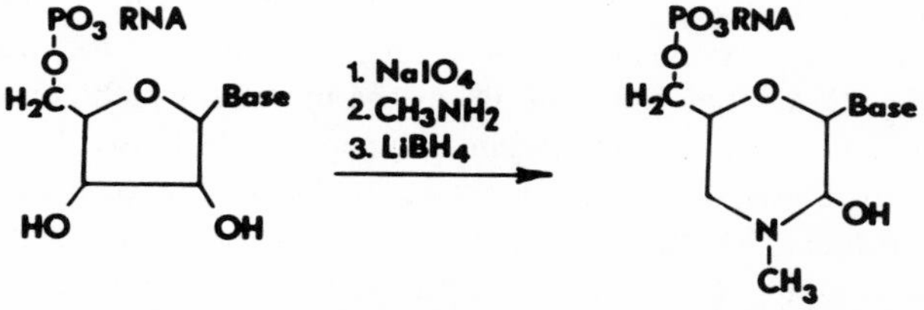

Fig. 5. Chemical modification of the terminal residue of 5S RNA.

synthesis or in the peptidyl transferase assay. These results are inconsistent with the model proposed by Raacke. It is highly unlikely that peptidyl-5S RNA is involved as an obligatory intermediate in protein synthesis.

There are some other suggestions on the functional role of 5S RNA. For example, 5S RNA from *E. coli* has a sequence (-CGAAC-, sequence from 43rd to 47th residue) which is complementary to the -GTΨC$_G^A$ sequence found in all tRNAs sequenced so far. It was hypothesized that 5S RNA has a function in tRNA binding by virtue of this complementary base pairing (26). This hypothesis could be tested specifically by using, in the present reconstitution system, 5S RNA which is chemically modified in the appropriate region. In fact, the sequence of 5S RNA from *B. stearothermophilus* has not been elucidated. It would be interesting to see whether 5S RNA from *B. stearothermophilus* also has the same sequence (-CGAAC-) at the same position. In this connection, it should also be pointed out that comparison of the sequence of *B. stearothermophilus* 5S RNA with that of *E. coli* 5S RNA would be very informative. *E. coli* 5S RNA is fully active in the present reconstitution system (Fahnestock and Nomura, unpublished experiments; see also ref. 16). For example, it is expected that the regions of 5S RNA which interact with ribosomal proteins during the assembly would have common base sequences.

CONCLUSION

A 30S ribosome reconstitution system has been useful for our experimental analyses of structure, function, and assembly of the 30S subunits. We have now developed a 50S ribosome reconstitution system in which the mechanism of assembly of 50S as well as the functional role of its molecular components can be studied. Since the 50S subunits are more complex than the 30S subunits, studies on the 50S assembly reaction as well as the functional analyses in this system would be correspondingly more difficult. Yet such studies are both rewarding and necessary for comprehensive understanding of the important organelle, the ribosome.

ACKNOWLEDGMENTS

The work described in this article was supported by the College of Agriculture and Life Sciences, University of Wisconsin, and by grants from the National Institute of General Medical Sciences (GM-15422) and National Science Foundation (GB-31086X). This is Paper No. 1536 of the Laboratory of Genetics.

SUMMARY

50S ribosomal subunits from *B. stearothermophilus* can be reconstituted from their dissociated molecular components. The reconstitution can be done using 5S RNA-free protein fraction, 5S RNA-free 23S ribosomal RNA fraction, and purified 5S RNA. The biological activity of reconstituted particles in polypeptide synthesis is dependent on the presence of 5S RNA in the system. In the absence of 5S RNA, particles (-5S particles) are produced which have greatly reduced activity in (a) polypeptide synthesis directed by synthetic as well as natural messenger RNA, (b) peptidyl transferase assay, (c) peptide chain termination factor (R1)-dependent ^{3}H-UAA binding, (d) G-factor-dependent ^{3}H-GTP binding, and (e) codon-directed tRNA binding assayed in the presence of 30S subunits. Thus 5S RNA is an essential 50S ribosomal component.

In the presence of 0.01 M Mg^{2+}, -5S RNA particles sediment with S values (47S) identical to those of the control +5S RNA particles. In the presence of 3 × 10^{-4} M Mg^{2+}, however, -5S RNA particles sediment definitely slower (44S) than the control +5S RNA particles. It appears that -5S RNA particles have a "loose" structure in low Mg^{2+}, but take a more compact structure in high Mg^{2+}.

The -5S RNA particles lack about four out of 39 possible 50S ribosomal proteins. Restoration of activity to the inactive -5S RNA particles depends on further addition of the missing proteins as well as 5S RNA. Thus 5S RNA has a structural role in the sense that some functionally important proteins fail to join the particle in the absence of 5S RNA.

RESUMEN

Las subunidades 50S de *b.B. sterothermophilus* pueden ser reconstituidas a partir de sus componentes moleculares disociados. La reconstitución puede efectuarse empleando la fracción proteica libre de RNA 5S, la fracción de RNA ribosomal 23S libre de RNA 5S, y RNA 5S purificado. La actividad biológica de las partículas reconstituidas en la síntesis polipeptídica depende de la presencia de RNA 5S en el sistema. En ausencia de RNA 5S, se producen partículas ([partículas -5S]) que tienen actividad fuertemente reducida en a)la síntesis de polipéptidos dirigida tanto por RNA mensajeros naturales como sintéticos; b) ensayo de peptidil transferasa; c) unión de ^{3}H-UAA dependiente del factor R$_1$ de terminación de cadena peptídica; d) unión de ^{3}H-GTP dependiente del factor G; y e) unión de 3H-GTP dependiente del factor G; y e) unión de tRNA dirigida por codón ensayada en presencia de subunidades 30S. Por lo tanto el RNA 5S es un componente ribosómico esencial de subunidades 50S.

En presencia de Mg^{++} 0.01 M las partículas [-RNA 5S] sedimentan con valores de S (47S) idénticos a los de las partículas control [+ RNA 5S]. Sin embargo, en presencia de Mg^{++} 3× 10^{-4} M, las partículas [-RNA 5S] sedimentan netamente en forma más lenta (44S) que las partículas control [+RNA 5S]. Parece ser que las partículas [-RNA 5S] tienen una estructura "laxa" en bajo Mg^{++} pero adquieren una estructura más compacta en alto Mg^{++}.

Las partículas [-RNA 5S] carecen de alrededor de 4 de las posibles 39 proteínas ribosomales 50S. El restablecimiento de la actividad de las partículas [-RNA 5S] depende de la adición de las proteínas que faltan, como asimismo del RNA 5S. Por lo tanto el RNA 5S tiene un papel estructural en el sentido que algunas proteínas funcionalmente importantes no pueden unirse a la partícula en ausencia de RNA 5S.

REFERENCES

1. Traub, P., and Nomura, M., *Proc. Natl. Acad. Sci. U.S.A.*, *59*, 777 (1968).
2. Nomura, M., Mizushima, S., Ozaki, M., Traub, P., and Lowry, C. V., *Cold Spring Harbor Symp. Quant. Biol.*, *34*, 49 (1969).
3. Mizushima, S., and Nomura, M., *Nature*, *226*, 1214 (1970).
4. Cox, E. C., White, J. R., and Flaks, J. G., *Proc. Natl. Acad. Sci. U.S.A.*, *51*, 703 (1964).

5. Davies, J. E., *Proc. Natl. Acad. Sci. U.S.A., 51,* 659 (1964).
6. Traub, P., and Nomura, M., *Science, 160,* 198 (1968).
7. Ozaki, M., Mizushima, S., and Nomura, M., *Nature, 222,* 333 (1969).
8. Wittmann, H. G., Stöffler, G., Hindennach, I., Kurland, C. G., Randall-Hazelbauer, L., Birge, E. A., Nomura, M., Kaltschmidt, E., Mizushima, S., Traut, R. R., and Bickle, T. A., *Mol. Gen. Genet., 111,* 327 (1971).
9. Nomura, M., *Bacteriol. Rev., 34,* 228 (1970).
10. Craven, G. R., Gavin, R., and Fanning, T., *Cold Spring Harbor Symp. Quant. Biol., 34,* 129 (1969).
11. Craven, G. R., and Gupta, V., *Proc. Natl. Acad. Sci. U.S.A., 67,* 1329 (1970).
12. Chang, F. N., and Flaks, J. G., *Proc. Natl. Acad. Sci. U.S.A., 67,* 1321 (1970).
13. Kahan, L., and Kaltschmidt, E., *Biochemistry, 11,* 2691 (1972).
14. Chang, F. N., and Flaks, J. G., *J. Mol. Biol., 68,* 177 (1972).
15. Schendel, P., Maeba, P., and Craven, G. R., *Proc. Natl. Acad. Sci. U.S.A., 69,* 544 (1972).
16. Nomura, M., and Erdmann, V. A., *Nature, 228,* 744 (1970).
17. Erdmann, V. A., Fahnestock, S., and Nomura, M., *Fed. Proc., 30,* (3, part II), 1203 (1971).
18. Nashimoto, H., and Nomura, M., *Proc. Natl. Acad. Sci. U.S.A., 67,* 1440 (1970).
19. Brownlee, G. G., Sanger, F., and Barrell, B. G., *Nature, 215,* 735 (1967).
20. Forget, B. G., and Weissman, S. M., *Science, 158,* 1695 (1967).
21. DuBuy, B., and Weissman, S. M., *J. Biol. Chem., 246,* 747 (1971).
22. Lizardi, P. M., and Luck, D. J. L., *Nature, 229,* 140 (1971).
23. Erdmann, V. A., Fahnestock, S., Higo, K., and Nomura, M., *Proc. Natl. Acad. Sci. U.S.A., 68,* 2932 (1971).
24. Raacke, I. D., *Proc. Natl. Acad. Sci. U.S.A., 68,* 2357 (1971).
25. Fahnestock, S., and Nomura, M., *Proc. Natl. Acad. Sci. U.S.A., 69,* 363 (1972).
26. Jordan, B. R., *J. Mol. Biol., 55,* 423 (1971).

DISCUSSION

D. Vazquez (Madrid, Spain): Dr. Raake has been testing her model in Wittmann's laboratory. Using the 5S RNA after removing the 3'-OH end, she found that the 5S RNA was still active, so the results are completely in agreement with your results and against her own model. Regarding the nomenclature you use for the proteins of the 50S, I note that you said L36 and L37. Are these from Wittmann's laboratory?

M. Nomura (Madison, U.S.A.): This is *Bacillus stearothermophilus*. No one has isolated and purified all of the proteins from this organism, and no other group has given names yet to them. L36 and L37 are based on our own nomenclature.

D. Vazquez: Does it mean that you find 37 proteins in the 50S?

M. Nomura: Yes, about 37, but we have not separated and characterized these proteins. Therefore, we really do not know exactly. We can do the same sort of thing as we did with the 30S in order to define the proteins.

D. Vazquez: Wittmann is also calling them L proteins, meaning larger subunit proteins, and he finds only 34 proteins so far.

M. Nomura: Yes, but Wittmann's group isolated and characterized 34 proteins from *E. coli* 50S; we are using *B. stearothermophilus*.

J. T. August (New York, U.S.A.): I am not suggesting this happens, but I wondered whether or not you have considered that there may be a turnover of the 5S RNA, in the process of this putative peptidyl transferase experiment.

M. Nomura: That is possible, but is very unlikely. The specific proposal made by Dr. Raake has been excluded by the present experiments. I also believe that this modified morpholine derivative is stable under the assay condition used.

J. T. August: We analyzed the distribution of basic proteins in *E. coli* with respect to the concentrations of DNA and RNA, and we found an apparent correlation between the distribution of these proteins and total nucleic acid concentration in the several fractions that we separated from one another.

M. Nomura: In which fractions?

J. T. August: In several fractions in the detergent lysate of *E. coli,* where a supernatant fraction contains most of the polyribosomes and then the precipitate. This suggested to us the two alternative possibilities, either that the basic proteins of *E. coli* were not specific in their binding and thus were distributed in proportion to total nucleic acid concentration, or that if, for example, the ribosomal basic proteins were specific in their binding to ribosomal RNA, there then would be another fraction, basic proteins which were binding to the other nucleic acids. We did not try to prove either of these possibilities, and I wonder if you would care to comment on what you feel would be the subcellular distribution of the ribosomal basic proteins and do they bind specifically to ribosomal RNA after they are synthesized?

M. Nomura: When Dr. Kurland analyzed the 30S ribosomal proteins, he found about ten or so proteins, which he called unit proteins, which exist in stoichiometric amounts, that is, 1 mole per mole of 16S RNA, and some other proteins which exist in less than stoichiometric amounts. People have agreed with these analytical data, but the question is whether or not we are losing ribosomal protein while isolating and purifying the ribosomes from *E. coli* cells. Although he showed that he does not lose proteins during purification of ribosomes, no one has analyzed membrane or wall fractions. Some of these fractions may contain DNA and may correspond to your DNA fraction. We have analyzed the ribosomal proteins, using radioactive *E. coli* cells. In fact, we could detect some ribosomal proteins even in the soluble fraction as well as in the membrane-containing fraction. For the identification, we used two-dimensional electrophoresis, as well as immunochemical methods. But I do not remember the quantitative data, and also which proteins are present in these fractions.

J. T. August: Do you think there is a free pool of ribosomal proteins?

M. Nomura: Yes, though in small amounts.

J. T. August: And so in *E. coli* then, as far as you are concerned, there might be the possibility that ribosomal proteins will engage in other cellular activities in addition to their function in the ribosome?

M. Nomura: I cannot answer that. I myself would like to know the answer. All I can say is that in other fractions we can find some ribosomal proteins. Whether this is due to nonspecific interaction with acidic polymers such as DNA during disruption of cells or has some physiological significance, I do not know. I think the problem has to be studied.

I. D. Algranati (Buenos Aires, Argentina): Do you use high temperature for the isolation and purification of 50S subunits or is it not necessary?

M. Nomura: No.

21

Electron Microscopic Studies
of *Escherichia coli*
Ribosomal Subunits

C. Vâsquez and A. K. Kleinschmidt

Instituto de Anatomia Gral.
and
Embriologia-Facultad de Medicina
Buenos Aires, Argentina
and
A. K. Kleinschmidt
Department of Biochemistry
New York University School of Medicine
New York, New York, U.S.A.

The ribosomes of *Escherichia coli* are composed of two distinct ribonucleoprotein subunits. The 30S subunit has a particle weight of 8×10^5 daltons (1) and consists of one 16S RNA strand (5.5×10^5 daltons) (2) and about 21 different polypeptide chains (3) having unique amino acid compositions, tryptic peptides, and molecular weights (4). The 50S subunit is larger; it has a particle weight of 1.8×10^6 daltons (1) and about 34 different polypeptide chains (3). Two distinct RNA strands are part of this subunit, a large one with a 23S value (1.1×10^6 daltons) (2) and a small one with a 5S value (4×10^4 daltons) (5). Each 30S subunit contains only one copy of each different polypeptide (6-8), and the same is assumed for the 50S subunit (7).

Little is known about the interaction between the RNA and the ribosomal protein. Several experiments have shown that inside the subunits the RNA is predominantly held in a nonhelical configuration of single strands associated with specific proteins (9-11). It also appears that RNA loops cover much of the ribosomal surface (9,12-14).

In studying *in vivo* ribosome maturation, using labeled ribosomal precursors (15) it has been observed that the biosynthesis and formation of the 30S is completed gradually. On the other hand, in reconstituting functionally active 30S subunits (16,17), it was recognized that self-assembly proceeds stepwise as a sequential and cooperative phenomenon, strongly suggesting that the mature subunits are regularly layered. From all these data, it can be assumed that the chemically and functionally heterogeneous components of the ribosomal subunits are not assembled into structures of regular symmetry comparable to that of the small isometric viruses.

The present study was started to throw light on the fine structure of the ribosome, comparing both unstained and stained subunits. Electron microscopic studies were carried out to observe a stepwise degradation of isolated and purified subunits by surface denaturation. By spreading of ribosomal subunits on a protein monolayer deposited over an aqueous denaturing hypophase containing urea, progressive conformational changes were observed. In the 30S and 50S subunits, the RNA appeared to be heavily bound to a residual protein, which when released from the RNA by further denaturation led to collapse of the ribosomal RNA filaments. The stripped RNA may coil and then disappear from the electron micrographs.

PREPARATION OF RIBOSOMES FOR ELECTRON MICROSCOPY

Ribosomal Subunit Purification

E. coli Q13 ribosomes were washed with 1 N ammonium chloride and chromatographed on DEAE-cellulose as previously described (18). Ribosomal 50S and 30S subunits were prepared by sucrose density gradient centrifugation; eight OD_{260} units of purified ribosomes, suspended in 0.1 ml of buffer a [containing 0.5 M NH_4Cl, 20 mM Tris-HCl (pH 7.8), 2 mM $MgCl_2$, 1 mM dithiothreitol], was layered onto 5 ml linear 5-30% sucrose gradients in buffer a. The gradients were centrifuged for 180 min at 38,000 rpm at 3° in a Spinco rotor SW39, and 160 μl fractions collected dropwise. The OD_{260} of each fraction was determined, and the 50S peak and the maxima of the 30S peak were chosen for examination with the electron microscope.

Spreading and One-Step Release

Purified ribosomal subunits, diluted to 5-10 μg of ribosomal RNA per milliliter in 20 mM Tris-HCl buffer (pH 7.8), 10 mM Mg^{2+}, and 100 μg/ml diisopropyl fluorophosphate (DFP) - chymotrypsin (Worthington), were spread from a wet glass ramp onto double-distilled water hypophase or urea hypophases, pH 8, the concentration of which varied from 0.1 to 8 M (19). In separate experiments, the hypophases were mixed with different concentrations of Mg^{2+} (10-100 mM). The 50S and the 30S fractions were spread at 4° or room temperature.

Film Transfer

Carbon supports reinforced with a collodion layer were mounted on platinum grids (Siemens type). At various periods of time after spreading, the resulting monolayers on top of the hypophases were transferred to the platinum grids by touching the film surface.

Incubation and RNA Streaking

In order to release the single-stranded RNA, the ribosomal subunits were incubated *in vitro* for different periods of time in mixtures of urea, pH 8 (2-8 M), and 10 mM EDTA at 4°. Aliquots of the urea-treated subunits were deposited on carbon supports by the droplet technique and dried by blotting the grid surface with filter paper.

Unstained Preparations

Ribosomal samples were applied to the grid surface by the droplet technique; usually, high concentrations (about 100 μl/ml of ribosomal RNA) were used. After blotting with filter paper, the collodion was removed by heating the preparation specimen at 180° for 10 min.

Stained Preparations

Uranyl acetate (10^{-4} M) in acetone and 2% methanol was used (20) to positively stain the ribosomal subunits. After rinsing in water (60 sec), the stain solution was applied for 1 min, and the grids were briefly rinsed with ethanol. After the grids were dried, the collodion was removed in an oven at 180° for about 10 min.

Electron Microscopy

All preparations were examined in a high resolution microscope (Siemens Elmiskop IA, single-crystal oriented cathode, decontamination device, short focal length) at low magnification (10,000X) and high magnification (55,000X) at which focal series of six or more exposures were usually taken.

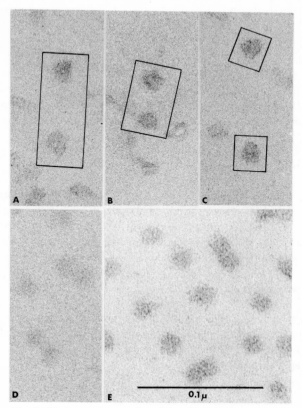

Fig. 1. Electron micrographs of E. coli *50S ribosomal subunits.* Droplet technique. (A,B,C) From various preparations of impure 30S ribosomal particles, mounted unstained onto *thin* carbon supporting films (20) and selected from focus series micrographs. The 50S particles of varied shape and contrast (in rectangles) are of higher mean contrast than the 30S particles (outside the rectangles). (D) The same as (A-C) but mounted unstained on a thicker carbon supporting film. (E) Uranyl-stained 50S ribosomal subunits from the sucrose-density peak of 50S particles. The stain deposition forming ridges is quite irregular; however, the contours often indicate more regular polygonal forms.

OBSERVATIONS ON THE RIBOSOMAL STRUCTURE

Structure of the 50S Subunit

Intact 50S subunits were prepared by the droplet technique. The particles adsorbed to the carbon support were either positively stained with uranyl acetate or observed unstained. The unstained 50S subunits were found to have round forms with an approximate diameter of 190 Å. These particles often showed one or two spikes extruding from the particle body; irregularities were also found in their internal contrast, giving the particles a light polar area at one end and a dark spike on the other (Fig. 1A,B,C). The uranyl-stained 50S subunits appeared more regular in shape than the unstained ones (Fig. 1E). Their mean diameter was about 180 Å, and some of the contours were close to the shape of a polyhedron (Fig. 1B,C,D).

Spreading of the 50S Subunits

Diluted 50S ribosomal subunits were mixed with 0.01% DFP-chymotrypsin and spread. Samples were transferred to grids at various periods of time. When double-distilled water or 0.1 *M* urea was used as a hypophase, the ribosomal

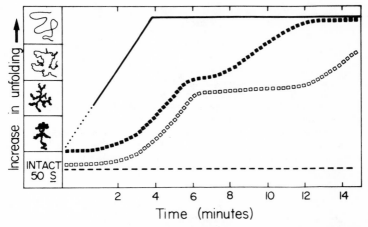

Fig. 2. *Scheme of averaged morphological changes of spread 50S E. coli ribosomal subunits, using various hypophases.* The ordinate indicates the type of morphological changes (see text), visualized by film transfer in minutes (abscissa) after spreading. Types of spreading: water, 0.1 *M* urea, or 4 *M* urea plus 100 m*M* Mg²⁺ (–––); 0.5-2 *M* urea (□□□); 4-5 *M* urea (■■■); 8 *M* urea (——).

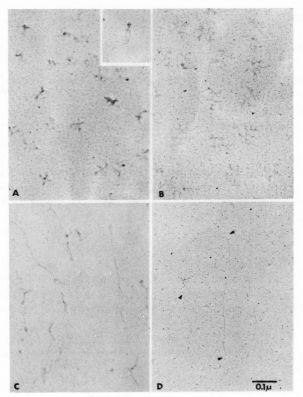

Fig. 3. Electron micrographs of spread 50S ribosomal sub-
units positively stained with uranyl acetate. (A,B) Spread
with DFP-chymotrypsin on 5 *M* urea. At (A), transfer at 4
min of the ribosomal protein film to grid. (Inset A) Intermediate configuration of more extruded material. (B) Transfer at 4-7 min. Multiple branches appear. (C) Streaking of
50S particles pretreated less than 5 min in 6 *M* urea and 10
m*M* EDTA at 4°. The filament length is plotted in Fig. 4,
bottom.

subunits were observed more or less intact in the surface of the monolayer. No
morphological changes were observed up to 16 min. With increasing urea
concentration, the 50S subunits unfolded as described in Fig. 2. When 5 *M* urea
at 4° was used, with 4 min a partial disruption of the subunits occurred (Fig.
3A). This was followed by the appearance of aggregated coarse filaments
extruding from the particles (Fig. 3A inset). Between the fourth and the seventh
minutes, complexes of protein and looped RNA, having four to six main

branches and approximately 600 Å in diameter, were observed (Fig. 3B). At the end of this period, the size of the protein monolayer on the surface of the hypophase increased to more than 50% of its original area. The increased size of the monolayer presumably resulted from the spreading of the denatured ribosomal protein into the preexisting DFP-chymotrypsin film. After 10 min, the nucleoprotein complexes were no longer visible and no ribosomal RNA was observed (which is indicated by the naked filament on the top of the vertical column of Fig. 2). Similar decomposition of the ribosomal subunits was observed using different molarities of urea, the concentration of which varied from 1 to 8 M. As expected, low molarities delayed and high molarities accelerated the ribosomal disruption. On the other hand, when magnesium ions were present in the urea hypophase, the ribosomal decay was retarded (25-50 mM Mg^{2+}) or completely stopped (100 mM Mg^{2+}) (Fig. 2).

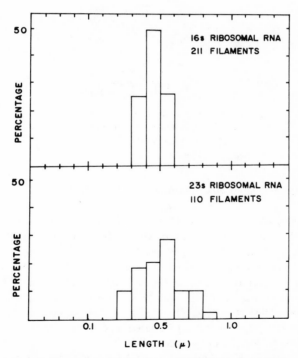

Fig. 4. Histogram of 16S ribosomal RNA (top) and 23S ribosomal RNA (bottom), prepared by streaking naked RNA filaments.

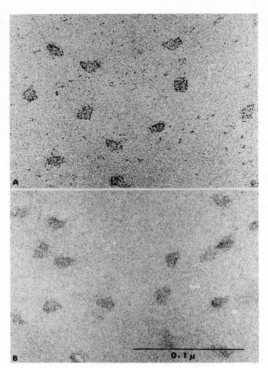

Fig. 5. Electron micrographs of 30S ribosomal sub-units. (A) Uranyl-stained sample prepared by the droplet technique. (B) Unstained sample prepared by the droplet technique.

Streaking of Urea-Treated 50S Subunits

50S subunits were incubated *in vitro* for 5 min at 4° with 6 M urea and 10 mM EDTA. By this treatment, the ribosomal RNA was released from most of the ribosomal proteins. The samples were then transferred in droplets to the carbon support. Streaking of part of the 23S ribosomal RNA occurred through blotting of the droplet at the edge of the grid with a filter paper. Within 5 min of incubation, coarse nucleoprotein complexes were observed, with a variable number of budding extrusions (Fig. 3C). Within 9 min of incubation, the ribosomal protein was progressively released, and after 12 min the naked RNA, either collapsed into tight coils or streched into long filaments, was observed (Fig. 3D). The streched, single-stranded RNA was found to have a large variation in length, with a maximum of 0.9 μ (Fig. 4, bottom). Filaments corresponding to the 5S ribosomal RNA, which would be about 0.03 μ maximum length, were not visible in these preparations.

Structure of the 30S Subunits

Droplets of the 30S subunits were deposited on the carbon-coated grids and observed unstained or stained, following the same procedure used with the 50S subunits. In the stained preparations (Fig. 5A), most of the contrast arose from the granular deposition of uranyl aggregates around the periphery of the subunits. Triangular (180 by 100 Å), elongated (180 by 90 Å), and irregular forms were observed. The same shapes and dimensions were found in the unstained preparations (Fig. 5B). The ratios of triangular, elongated, and irregular forms were, for the stained preparations, as follows: 36, 41, and 23%. For the unstained preparations, the ratios were 41, 45, and 14%.

Spreading of the 30S Subunits

Diluted 30S ribosomal subunits were spread in a DFP-chymotrypsin film on different types of hypophases. Here again, water or 0.1 M urea did not change the ribosomal structure (Fig. 6). When 3 M urea at 4° was used as hypophase, immediately after spreading a fast disruption of the 30S occurred and the subunits unfolded as shown in Fig. 7A. After 3 min, all the subunits were transformed into short nucleoprotein strands, which stained heavily with the uranyl acetate (Fig. 7B). Strand lengths ranged from 0.15 to 0.5 μ, showing variable degrees of indentation and some short branching. "Split" ribosomal

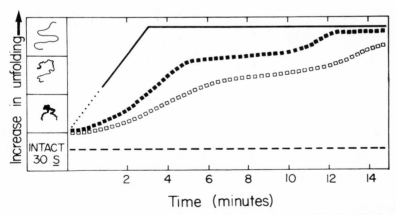

Fig. 6. Scheme of averaged morphological changes of spread 30S E. coli ribosomal subunits, using various hypophases. The ordinate indicates the type of morphological changes in minutes (abscissa), as in Fig. 2. Types of spreading: water, 0.1 M urea, or 4 M urea plus 100 mM Mg^{2+} (– – –); 0.5-2 M urea (□□□); 3-5 M urea (■■■); 8 M urea (——).

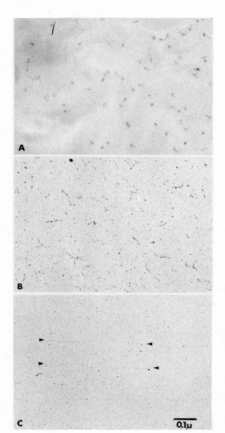

Fig. 7. Electron micrographs of spread 30S ribosomal subunits. Uranyl-stained. (A,B) Spread with DFP-chymotrypsin on 3 M urea at 4°. (A) Configurational changes immediately after spreading. (B) After 3 min transfer to grids. Stiff strands with bead-like structures (up to eight per filament). (C) Streaked naked 16S ribosomal RNA pretreated with 6 M urea and 10 mM EDTA at 4°. The filament length is plotted in Fig. 4, top.

protein concurrently spread with the chymotrypsin, slightly increasing the size of the monolayer film.

After 10 min, these strands disappeared. Probably due to the stripping of the residual ribosomal protein, the naked RNA strands collapsed, and the coiled RNA was no longer discernible. A faster pattern of disruption was observed when the spreading was made at room temperature or when higher concentrations of urea were used as hypophases. When Mg^{2+} was present in the urea hypophase, the ribosomal decay was retarded (25-50 mM Mg^{2+}) or completely stopped (100 mM Mg^{2+}) (Fig. 6).

Streaking of Urea-Treated 30S Subunits

To visualize the extended filaments of 16S ribosomal RNA, the 30S subunits were incubated *in vitro* in 6 M urea and 10 mM EDTA at 4°. After various periods of time, samples were deposited on the grids and blotted. Stretched RNA filaments were observed (Fig. 7C) having a maximum length of 0.6 μ (Fig. 4, top) and a diameter comparable to that of naked RNA. When 10-50 mM Mg^{2+} was added to the 6 M urea, release of the ribosomal RNA was retarded, and after 5 min of incubation, only incompletely disrupted 30S particles were found. At 100 mM Mg^{2+}, the ribosomal decay was completely prevented.

CONCLUSIONS

Several electron microscopic studies have been carried out on intact 50S (21-28) and 30S (21,23,28) ribosomal subunits, and different sizes and shapes have been described for both types of subunits. This was probably due to the fact that ribosomes must have an intrinsic plasticity and can easily be disrupted during the various steps used in preparation for electron microscopy. Also, the purification steps, such as addition of sucrose and ammonium chloride in various concentrations to the ribosomal solution, may influence the morphology. Thus deformation during the preparative steps and configurational changes due to contrast enhancement limited the reconstruction of suitable models.

In the present investigation, differences were observed between stained and unstained 50S subunits, the stained subunits having a more regular shape and contrast than the unstained ones. The imperfect polygonal shapes observed in the stained preparations may be a consequence of the uranyl acetate in acetone employed for the positive straining. The irregular shape and contrast found in the unstained preparations of the 50S subunits agree on the other hand with Lubin's conclusions (26) of an asymmetrical 50S particle, having a crescent and a protuberance. In the groove of the 50S particle, the smaller 30S subunit should be loosely adaptable, forming together a complete 70S ribosome. From our results on the structure of the 30S particles, it would also appear that two main populations form the bulk of the 30S subunits. We cannot yet exclude that the elongated forms are a different view of the triangular particles (see Fig. 3). The irregular forms which proportionally increase in the stained preparations must be the product of disrupted or deformed 30S subunits.

In order to follow the progressive release of ribosomal proteins and the unfolding of the polynucleotide chain, which finally collapsed under our experimental conditions, intact ribosomal subunits were spread in a DFP-chymotrypsin film on different denaturing hypophases. Figure 8 shows diagramatically the stepwise degradation of both 50S and 30S subunits. The sequence of events shows that the morphological appearance of disruption of the more complex 50S subunits in a denaturing surface is also more complex than that followed by the 30S subunits.

As indicated schematically, the 50S subunits go through different morpho-

50s RIBOSOMAL SUBUNITS   30s RIBOSOMAL SUBUNITS

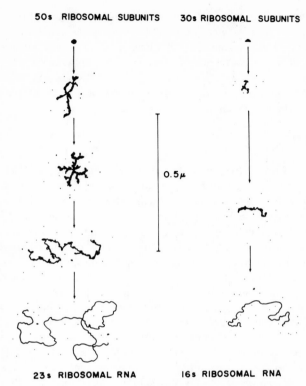

23s RIBOSOMAL RNA   16s RIBOSOMAL RNA

Fig. 8. Schematic outline of 50S and 30S ribosomal subunit degradation in denaturing surface films. The arrows should be related to the time of degradation as indicated in Fig. 2 (50S particles) and Fig. 6 (30S particles). The filaments (naked RNA at the bottom of each vertical row, as 23S ribosomal RNA and 16S ribosomal RNA, respectively) are hypothetical, and only visualized by streaking from solutions, Figs. 3D and 7C. For explanation, see text.

logical stages of disintegration. First, tightly folded nucleoprotein complexes extrude from the decaying 50S subunits. In a second stage, the subunits show four to six digitated branches coming out from the loosened center. Simultaneously, split-off proteins rapidly contribute in this stage to a further increase of the protein monolayer size at the surface of the hypophase. After the stripping of all the proteins, the RNA collapses and cannot be recognized. Only after *in vitro* incubation of the 50S subunits in urea and EDTA and the streaking of these materials over the surface of a grid was it possible to observe the stretched single-stranded RNA, but of shorter mean length than expected from naked 23S RNA.

Disintegration of the 30S subunits in a denaturing surface gave rise to short, unbranched thick rods, with some length variation (first stage). The complex, extensively branched forms observed in the 50S particle denaturation were never found in the urea-treated 30S subunits. In a second stage, the protein monolayer slowly increased in size, indicating that more protein of 30S particles was split off. The 16S RNA became depleted of protein and collapsed. Here again, this RNA was only visualized in naked stretched form after *in vitro* incubation of the 30S subunits in urea and EDTA and streaking of the samples on a grid surface.

The fact that these regular configurations occur at finite stages permits us to assume that the uncoating of protein in the surface film on urea proceeds stepwise under proper conditions of denaturation. It is tempting to correlate these steps with the well-characterized precursors described in the assembly processes of the 50S and 30S ribosomal subunits (30). However, our approach is a destructive one, and thus it has a limited value. In the 50S and 30S subunits, the RNA appears to be heavily bound to residual proteins, after a more peripheral protein moiety is taken from the particles. Recent studies (31,32) have explained the cooperative nature of the assembly reaction in the 30S subunit and have shown that the number of sites per RNA molecule which can firmly bind ribosomal protein is quite small. In our experiments, a large quantity of the ribosomal proteins are split in the early stage under urea denaturation; therefore, they must correspond to proteins which do not bind tightly to the respective ribosomal RNA or have not RNA-binding capacity at all.

The mean length of the 16S ribosomal RNA, derived from the 30S subunits, is 0.48 μ. Assuming a linear density of 1.1×10^6 daltons per micron of single-stranded RNA, the mean molecular weight of these filaments can be estimated at 0.5×10^6 daltons. On the other hand, 50S ribosomal subunits yield a 23S ribosomal RNA with a molecular weight on the order of 1.1×10^6 daltons; hence their average length should be about 1.0 μ. However, as seen in Fig. 4, the 23S ribosomal RNA shows a large variation of shorter filament length. Several authors have suggested that the 23S ribosomal RNA is formed by dimerization of two 16S RNA halves (33-35). If this is the case, the length of the 23S RNA should give a peak similar to that obtained with the 16S RNA derived from the 30S subunits (see Fig. 4). On the one hand, the large variation in filament length observed in the 23S ribosomal RNA may indicate different length combinations of RNA, i.e., random fragments with molecular weights ranging between 0.2×10^6 and 0.8×10^6 daltons. These results can be explained well by Rilley's suggestion (36) that the 23S RNA consists of one RNA chain of 0.5×10^6 daltons bonded to two others of about half this weight. On the other hand, the fragmentation of this 23S RNA may be due to the action of a latent endonuclease in the 50S subunits, which becomes active at more or less specific RNA strand sites on disintegration of the ribosomal particles (37).

ACKNOWLEDGMENTS

This work was supported by a grant from the J. A. Hartford Foundation, Inc., New York, N.Y.

SUMMARY

The fine structure of ribosomal subunits was studied using bright- and dark-field electron microscopy of both unstained and stained subunits. These techniques were also employed to observe the stepwise degradation of the subunits. Intact 50S subunits, mixed with 0.01% DFP-chymotrypsin, were spread onto a denaturing hypophase of $4 M$ urea, pH 7.3, at 4° and after various periods of time the resulting film was sampled for electron microscopy. During the first 2 min, the subunits were progressively disintegrated. Between a period of 4-8 min, complexes of RNA and protein were clearly observed. After 10 min or more, the protein was no longer visible and the RNA was seen as collapsed filaments. Incubation of the subunits in urea-EDTA for the same period of time resulted in their degradation and the appearance of 23S ribosomal RNA bound to protein. By blotting, it was possible to stretch these complexes and to follow the progressive release of the single-stranded RNA, which was observed as filaments of different lengths. The 30S subunits were studied in the same way, with essentially the same results. On the other hand, the 16S ribosomal RNA was observed as a whole piece with an average length of about 0.45 μ.

RESUMEN

Se estudió la ultraestructura de subunidades ribosómicas de *E. coli* utilizando técnicas de camp claro y oscuro en el microscopio electrónico, tanto de subunidades teñidas como no teñidas. Las mismas técnicas fueron empleadas para observar la degradación progresiva de las subunidades. Subunidades intactas 50S, mezcladas con DFP-quimotripsina al 0.01% fueron extendidas sobre una hipofase desnaturalizante de urea 4 M, pH 7.3 a 4° y se tomaron muestras de film ribosoma-proteína a distintos tiempos para ser examinados al microscopio electrónico. Durante los primeros dos minutos se observó la progresiva desintegración de las subunidades. Entre los cuatro y ocho minutos se pudieron evidenciar complejos de RNA y proteína. Después de diez minutos no se observó más proteína ribosomal y el RNA fue visto como filamentos colapsados. Al incubar las subunidades 50S en urea-EDTA por períodos similares, se evidenció su degradación ya la aparición de RNA ribosomal ligado a la proteína. Dichos complejos pudieron ser estirados observándose la liberación progresiva de un RNA monocatenario de longitud variable. Las subunidades 30S fueron estudiadas de una forma análoga, observándose una desnaturalización semejante a la ocurrida con las subunidades 50S. El RNA ribosomal 16S fue observado como filamentos monocatenarios estirados, con una longitud media de 0.45 μ.

REFERENCES

1. Tissières, A., Watson, J. D., Schlessinger, D., and Hollingsworth, B. R., *J. Mol. Biol.*, *1*, 221 (1959).

2. Kurland, C. G., *J. Mol..Biol.*, *2*, 83 (1960).
3. Kaltschmidt, E., and Wittmann, H. G., *Proc. Natl. Acad. Sci. U.S.A.*, *67*, 1276 (1970).
4. Hardy, S. J. S., Kurland, C. G., Voynow, P., and Mora, G., *Biochemistry*, *8*, 2898 (1969).
5. Rosset, R., Monier, R., and Julian, J., *Bull. Soc. Chim. Biol.*, *46*, 87 (1964).
6. Moore, P. P., Traut, R. R., Noller, H., Pearson, P., and Delius, H., *J. Mol. Biol.*, *31*, 441 (1968).
7. Traut, R., Delius, H., Ahmad-Zadeh, C., Bickle, T. A., Pearson, P., and Tissières, A., *Cold Spring Harbor Symp. Quant. Biol.*, *34*, 25 (1969).
8. Sypherd, P. S., O'Neil, D. M., and Taylor, M. M., *Cold Spring Harbor Symp. Quant. Biol.*, *34*, 77 (1969).
9. Furano, A. V., Bradley, D. F., and Childers, L. G., *Biochemistry*, *5*, 3044 (1966).
10. Cotter, R. I., McPhie, P., and Gratzer, W. B., *Nature*, *216*, 864 (1967).
11. Cotter, R. I., and Gratzer, W. B., *Nature*, *221*, 154 (1969).
12. Shakulov, R. S., Aojtkhozhin, M. A., and Spirin, A. S., *Biokhimika*, *27*, 744 (1962).
13. Santer, M., and Smith, J. R., *J. Bacteriol.*, *92*, 1099 (1966).
14. Fenwick, M. L., *Biochem. J.*, *107*, 481 (1968).
15. Gierer, L., and Gierer, A., *J. Mol. Biol.*, *34*, 293 (1968).
16. Traub, P., and Nomura, M., *Proc. Natl. Acad. Sci. U.S.A.*, *59*, 777 (1968).
17. Traub, P., and Nomura, M., *J. Mol. Biol.*, *40*, 391 (1969).
18. Iwasaki, K., Sabol, S., Wahba, A. J., and Ochoa, S., *Arch. Biochem. Biophys.*, *125*, 542 (1958).
19. Vásquez, C., and Kleinschmidt, A. K., *J. Mol. Biol.*, *34*, 134 (1968).
20. Gordon, C. N., and Kleinschmidt, A. K., *Biochim. Biophys. Acta*, *155*, 305 (1968).
21. Hall, C. E., and Slayter, H. S., *J. Mol. Biol.*, *1*, 329 (1959).
22. Huxley, H. E., and Zubay, G., *J. Mol. Biol.*, *2*, 10 (1960).
23. Spirin, A. S., Kiselev, N. A., Shakulov, R. S., and Bodganov, A. A., *Biokhimika*, *28*, 920 (1963).
24. Hart, R. G., *Proc. Natl. Acad. Sci. U.S.A.*, *53*, 1415 (1965).
25. Nanninga, N., *J. Cell Biol.*, *33*, 61 (1967).
26. Bruskov, V. I., and Kiselev, N. A., *J. Mol. Biol.*, *37*, 367 (1968).
27. Nanninga, N., *Proc. Natl. Acad. Sci. U.S.A.*, *61*, 614 (1968).
28. Lubin, M., *Proc. Natl. Acad. Sci. U.S.A.*, *61*, 1454 (1968).
29. Bassel, A., and Campbell, L. L., *J. Bacteriol.*, *98*, 811 (1969).
30. Nomura, M., *Bacteriol. Rev.*, *34*, 228 (1970).
31. Nomura, M., Traub, P., Guthrie, C., and Nashimoto, H., *J. Cell Physiol.*, *74*, 241 (1969).
32. Mizushima, S., and Nomura, M., *Nature*, *226*, 1214 (1970).
33. Mangiarotti, G., Apirion, D., Schlessinger, D., and Silengo, L., *Biochemistry*, *7*, 456 (1968).
34. Adesnik, M., and Levinthal, C., *J. Mol. Biol.*, *46*, 281 (1969).
35. Fellner, P., and Sanger, F., *Nature*, *219*, 236 (1969).
36. Rilley, W. T., *Nature*, *222*, 446 (1969).
37. Szer, W., *Biochem. Biophys. Res. Communs.*, *35*, 653 (1969).

DISCUSSION

H. N. Torres (Buenos Aires, Argentina): Is there ribosomal crystallization in *E. coli* at low temperature? It seems that the first step in ribosomal crystallization observed in eggs is preceded by a step of formation of tetramers between ribosomal particles; is there some structure of this type in *E. coli*?

C. Vásquez: Our experiments cannot answer this question.

E. De Robertis (Buenos Aires, Argentina): I think that the technique that Dr. Vásquez is using could be applied to experiments like those of Dr. Nomura on the reconstitution of the ribosomal particles. If one could extract the RNA and then add the proteins, provided that the proteins were labeled in some way for the electron microscope, it might be possible to observe the position of these proteins on the RNA molecule. I think this could be a very interesting project.

C. Vásquez: I agree with you. However, our method is a destructive one, hence just the opposite of what you are proposing.

E. De Robertis: Of course. I was suggesting a reconstruction experiment.

W. Colli (São Paulo, Brazil): When you said that the 23S molecule was made of a 16S molecule and two other short pieces, did you mean an actual molecule of 16S ribosomal RNA or some other molecule with a 16S sedimentation coefficient?

C. Vásquez: I said that the 23S RNA may consist of one RNA chain of about 0.5×10^6 daltons bound to two others of about half this weight.

Speaker unidentified: Could you clarify the curve in some of the figures you showed? Time in minutes is in the abscissa, but I could not get what you have in ordinates.

C. Vásquez: The different patterns of denaturation are in the ordinates.

Same as above: How do you express quantitatively the change of shape?

C. Vásquez: By counting the number of particles found in a given shape at different times.

Same as above: That is a sort of discrete curve?

C. Vásquez: Yes, it is a discrete curve. The pattern was always the same; a stepwise degradation was obtained with different concentrations of urea at different times. If magnesium was present in the reaction, this was retarded. All these experiments were done at 4°, but if experiments were done at room temperature or higher temperature, the degradation was accelerated, although the same denaturation patterns were obtained.

22

Aggregation Properties
of Rat Liver Ribosomes

Mario Castañeda and Ricardo Santiago

Departamento de Biología Molecular
Instituto de Investigaciones Biomedicas, U.N.A.M.
Mexico D.F., Mexico

Ribosomes are cell organelles whose function and structure have received a great deal of attention. Most of the initial studies have made use of ribosomes from bacterial cells and have implicitly carried over two assumptions: (a) the ribosomal population of a cell is homogeneous, and (b) populations from different cells present very similar properties. Although evidence has been appearing about heterogeneity in a given ribosomal cell population (1,2), information on specific characteristics of ribosomes from different cells is scarce except for size and biosynthetic data.

Studies on ribosomal solubility and effect of cations have given a general picture. Bacterial and sea urchin egg ribosomes remain in solution for several weeks. Bacterial ribosomes are converted to smaller species (3), and sea urchin ribosomes are dissociated (4) by treatment with monovalent cations. Here we report that rat liver ribosomes are rapidly precipitated out of solution by the effects of ribosomal preparation contaminants, and by K^+.

MATERIALS AND METHODS
Biological Materials and Chemical Reagents

Random-bred Wistar rats, fasted overnight, were used. After decapitation, the livers were excised and cooled to $4°$ in homogenization medium. Subsequent operations were conducted at $4°$. All chemicals were checked for iron content.

Preparation of Ribosomes

Livers were homogenized in 2.5 vol of 0.03 M Tris-HCl (pH 7.4), 0.3 M sucrose, 0.025 M KCl, 0.005 M magnesium acetate, 0.006 M 2-mercaptoethanol. The homogenate was centrifuged at 12,000 × g for 10 min, and the supernatant was used for either of the following two ribosome sucrose washings: (a) 0.4 M sucrose wash—the supernatant was brought to 0.5 M KCl, 0.01 M magnesium acetate, 0.5% DOC and centrifuged at 20,000 × g for 10 min, the resulting supernatant was layered on 20 ml of 0.4 M sucrose in the last buffer and centrifuged at 78,000 × g for 2 hr, and the pellet was rinsed with distilled water and resuspended in 0.01 M Tris-HCl (pH 7.4), 0.1 M KCl, 0.003 M magnesium acetate, 0.006 M 2-mercaptoethanol; (b) 1.5 M sucrose wash—the supernatant was made 0.5% DOC, centrifuged at 20,000 × g for 10 min, layered on 10 ml 0.5 M and 10 ml of 1.5 M sucrose solutions in homogenization buffer, and centrifuged at 78,000 × g for 4 hr, and the pellet was rinsed with distilled water and resuspended in 0.01 M Tris-HCl (pH 7.4). Both ribosomal suspensions were cleared at 20,000 × g for 10 min. The supernatant from the 0.4 M sucrose wash was stored at $-20°$ in aliquots of 150-200 μg of RNA as measured by acid digestion (5). That from the 1.5 M sucrose wash was stored as above or dialyzed against various cation concentrations.

Sucrose Gradients

Linear nonisokinetic gradients (15-30% sucrose) in sets of three were formed at 4° on a 2 ml 60% sucrose cushion and run at 60,000 × g for 6 hr in the Spinco 25.1 rotor. Sucrose solutions had the same salt concentrations as the layered ribosomal suspensions. Contents were fractionated by volume and read at 260 nm.

Other Methods of Analysis

Protein concentrations were estimated by the Lowry method (6). Nonheme iron was determined by a previous protein precipitation (7), followed by assay by the o-phenanthroline reaction.

RESULTS

Precipitation of 0.4 M Sucrose Washed Ribosomes

Ribosomes obtained from the 0.4 M sucrose wash and stored frozen form a heavy precipitate in 1-8 days, depending on the concentration of the original ribosomal suspension. The precipitate has been separated by centrifugation at

Table I. Distribution of RNA and Protein from 0.4 M Sucrose Washed Ribosomal Suspensions[a]

Fractions	RNA (%)	Protein (%)
Supernatant	0	7-20
Pellet	100	80-90

[a] Samples were stored an average of 4 days. Centrifugation is described in the text.

2000 $\times$ g for 5 min, forming a well-packed pellet. The appearance of the resuspended pellet is green and crystalline under the microscope, and when it is aerated it turns brownish and amorphous. The addition of 2-mercaptoethanol restores the original characteristics. Table I shows that all the original RNA is contained in the pellet. The amount of protein (not necessarily ribosomal) found in the pellet and in the supernatant has been variable.

Qualitative analyses for metals in the ribosomal suspension were positive for iron (K_4 [Fe(CN)$_6$], K_3 [Fe(CN)$_6$]), whereas solutions and glassware utilized for purification were negative. Of all the liver homogenate fractions, including the pellet from the clearing centrifugation, the ribosomal suspension was the only fraction to present this problem. High salt (K^+ and ammonium) and sucrose concentrations have been used to separate ribosomes from adsorbed molecules. Variations of K^+ concentration in purification buffers, from 0.001 to 0.5 M, were without effect. The use of ammonium at 0.5 M in preliminary experiments showed loss of ribosomes. On the other hand, sucrose was found useful for avoiding this precipitation, in concentrations of 1.0, 1.5, and 2.0 M. Table II shows the findings and relative purity of ribosomes purified through 0.4 and 1.5 M sucrose solutions. High absorbance ratios, lower protein content, and no green precipitate were obtained with 1.5 M sucrose. The results were about the same with 1.0 and 2.0 M sucrose in the lower cushion.

Having obtained ribosomes with no green precipitate, we have estimated the amounts of nonheme iron present in the above two ribosomal preparations. Table III shows measured iron in the suspensions as absolute values and as relative to the amount of RNA in the same sample. The difference in the values for the two types of samples, although evident, seems small. Nevertheless, if one takes into account the lower yield of ribosomes obtained by the use of the more concentrated sucrose solution, the difference is real. By normalizing against the content of ferritin in normal livers (1 mg per gram of tissue) and taking an

Table II. Some Properties of 0.4 and 1.5 M Sucrose Washed
Ribosomal Suspensions[a]

| | | Absorbance ratio (range) | | |
Sucrose wash	RNA/protein	260/230	260/280	Green
0.4 M	0.29-0.66	0.85-1.2	1.15-1.7	+
1.5 M	0.9 -1.2	1.3 -1.5	1.75-1.85	−

[a] Resuspension buffer of 1.5 M sucrose washed ribosomes was the same buffer used for 0.4 M sucrose washed ribosomes (see *Materials and Methods*).

average content of 23% of iron in ferritin, we found the difference to be considerable (Table III).

On electron microscopy, the green or brown precipitate (0.4 M sucrose wash) appeared as large clumps of a granular material, membrane-line structures, and ribosomes of general normal appearance. The clumps are almost always surrounded by ribosomes, and on all these structures there are abundant tiny points of dense material. This electron-dense material is often seen forming tetramers (Fig. 1) which resemble ferritin. Ribosomal samples prepared through the 1.5 M sucrose cushion show much less granular material and many fewer membrane-like structures. The dense material, although in smaller quantities, is still clearly present.

Precipitation of 1.5 M Sucrose Washed Ribosomes

Precipitation has been easily monitored by storing several aliquots of the ribosomal suspension at $-20°$ for different times, after which the aliquots were thawed and centrifuged at 2000 $\times$ g for 10 min. The resulting supernatants and pellets were used for estimations of RNA and protein.

Table III. Nonheme Iron in 0.4 and 1.5 M Sucrose
Washed Ribosomal Suspensions

Sucrose Wash	Actual measure (μg)	μg/μg RNA	Ferritin/g liver (%)
0.4 M	60-100	0.04-0.06	20-40
1.5 M	5-7	0.01-0.015	1-2

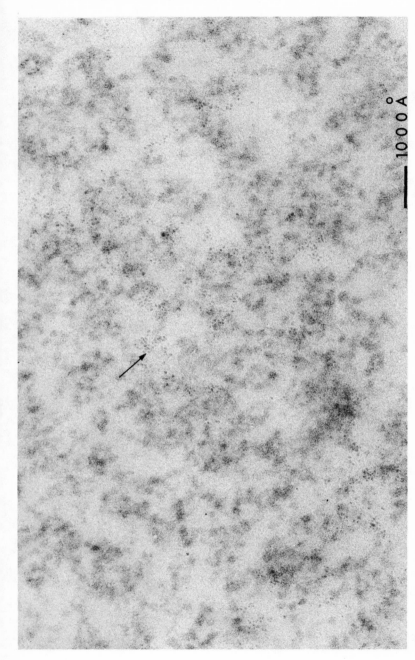

Fig. 1. Thin section of the precipitate from 0.4 M sucrose washed ribosomes. Conventional osmium tetroxide and glutaraldehyde fixation, Araldite embedding, and uranyl acetate staining. Magnification 119,000×.

1000 Å

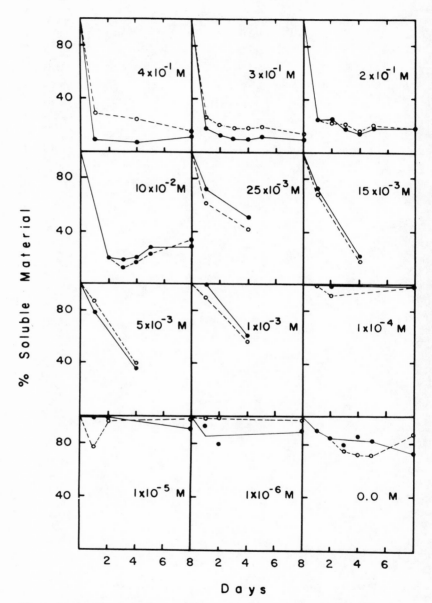

Fig. 2. *Precipitation of 1.5 M sucrose washed ribosomes by various K⁺ concentra-tions.* Conditions are described in the text.

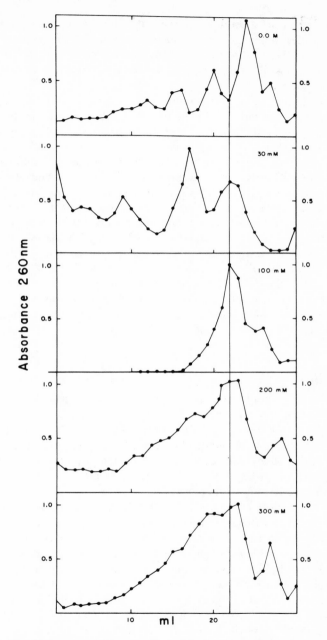

Fig. 3. Sucrose gradient profiles of fresh ribosomal samples treated and centrifuged with various K⁺ concentrations. Conditions are described in *Materials and Methods*. Sucrose solutions contained only 0.01 *M* Tris-HCl (*p*H 7.4) and K⁺.

Ribosomes prepared through the sucrose cushion retain, in the water-rinsed pellet, easily measurable amounts of sucrose, and the experiments with cations are erratic. For this reason, the ribosomal suspensions were dialyzed overnight against 0.01 M Tris-HCL (pH 7.4), with various concentrations of cations, for a good equilibration with these buffers.

We were initially testing the ability of a combination of Mg^{2+} and K^+ to precipitate ribosomes, but the finding that these ribosomes are aggregated with very minute amounts (0.0005 M) of Mg^{2+}, in the absence and in the presence (up to 0.4 M) of K^+, led us to try to find out first the picture for K^+ alone. This cation has also been found to be very efficient in precipitating these ribosomes. Figure 2 shows that K^+, at concentrations of 0.001 M and above, causes aggregation of nearly all the originally soluble ribosomal material. This result forced us to reconsider ribosomal profiles in sucrose gradients. Gradient runs of previously frozen ribosomal samples gave results similar to those found in Fig. 2. When ribosomal aliquots were layered immediately after dialysis, the gradient patterns showed a maximum of monosomal structures at 0.1 M K^+ (Fig. 3). Above or below this K^+ concentration, the monosomal peak diminishes and structures heavier than monosomes are present. The peak behind the monosomes corresponds to a species sedimenting around 40S, and has apparently shown the least modifications with these K^+ concentrations. In Tris buffer alone, the monosomal peak looks lighter and there exist heavier aggregates in either fresh or stored samples.

CONCLUSIONS

Rat liver ribosomes have been used for some time in many laboratories. The lack of information about the properties described here could be due to the fact that most people use fresh preparations of ribosomes.

The coprecipitation of ferritin-like material during purification of ribosomes could be explained by (a) adsorption to ribosomes and/or (b) independent pelleting by the centrifugal force. We have no reasons to propose a specific binding to ribosomes of ferritin-like molecules or nonspecific binding by electric charge since ferritin has an acidic pK (4.7). Nevertheless, if one thinks about a very weak negative net charge in the ribosomes (larger proportion of ribosomal proteins than in bacterial ribosomes), there could be enough non-neutralized positive charges available for the binding of negatively charged molecules. On the other hand, the molecular weight of ferritin may be adequate for centrifugal precipitation. The electron micrographs of the 0.4 M sucrose wash precipitate do not strongly support either possibility. The result is most likely due to both effects, since dense material is seen in individual ribosomes as well as in the abundant granular material, which on precipitation could entrap soluble ribosomes. The identification of this ferritin-like material by immunological means is under way.

The effect of K^+ on these ribosomes is more difficult to visualize at these early stages of study. Monovalent cations compete with ribosomal proteins very effectively, although their effects vary (3,8), possibly because of their different sizes and electronegativities in interplay with the different sites of proteins in the ribosome. We have not yet done any experiments looking for stripped ribosomal proteins, nor have we estimated the proportion of resistant derived ribosomes (8,9). These experiments are to be done, with higher K^+ concentrations. If K^+ aggregates rat liver peptidyl-tRNA-free ribosomes, it is possible that K^+ is unable to reach competition sites and only neutralizes negative charges. This neutralization of charges would bring about ribosomes with no charge and hence their precipitation. Reticulocyte and erythrocyte ribosomes seem to be also precipitated by K^+ (10). Precipitation occurs with such small amounts of K^+ that the ribosomal free negative charge must be less than the present in bacterial ribosomes.

ACKNOWLEDGMENTS

We wish to thank Miss E. Márquez and Dr. K. Kretschmer for the electron micrographs.

SUMMARY

Rat liver ribosomes prepared through a 0.4 M sucrose cushion and with low or high K^+ (0.001-0.5 M) precipitate in heavy aggregates after storage. The ribosomal suspension and the precipitate contain high amounts of nonheme iron, and electron micrographs show abundant ferritin-like dense material. This kind of precipitate can be avoided by preparing ribosomes through sucrose at 1.0 M and above.

Ribosomes purified through 1.5 M sucrose are precipitated by K^+ at concentrations from 0.001 to 0.4 M. It is thought that the structure and net charge of these ribosomes are different from those of *Escherichia coli* ribosomes.

RESUMEN

Los ribosomas de hígado de rat a preparados a través de un colchón de sacarosa 0.4 M y bajas o altas concentraciones de K^+ (o.001-0.5 M) precipitan en forma de grandes agregados después de guardados. La suspensión ribosomal y el precipitado contienen grades cantidades de hierro no-heme y las microfotografías electrónicas muestran material denso muy abundante y semejante a la ferritina. Esta clase de precipitado puede evitarse si los ribosomas se preparan como se ha descrito anteriormente, pero utilizando un colchón de sacarosa 1.0 M.

Ribosomas purificados a través de sacarosa 1.5 M, son precipitados por K^+ a concentraciones de desde 0.001 hasta 0.4 M. Se piensa que la estructura y la carga neta de estos ribosomas son diferentes a las de los ribosomas de *Escherichia coli*.

REFERENCES

1. Kurland, C. G., Voynow, P., Hardy, S. J. S., Randall, L., and Lutter, L., *Cold Spring Harbor Symp. Quant. Biol., 34,* 17 (1969).

2. Khabat, D., *Biochemistry 9,* 4160 (1970).
3. Dijoseph, C. G., Pon, C., Rapaport, N. D., and Kaji, A., *Biochim. Biophys. Acta, 240,* 407 (1971).
4. Infante, A. A., and Krauss, M., *Biochim. Biophys. Acta, 246,* 81 (1971).
5. Spirin, A. S., *Biokhimiya, 23,* 617 (1958).
6. Lowry, O. H., Rosebrough, N. J., Farr, A. L., and Randall, R. J., *J. Biol. Chem., 193,* 265 (1951).
7. Elke, S., and Schüser, I., *Separatum Experientia, 26,* 669 (1970).
8. Infante, A. A., and Graves, P. N., *Biochim. Biophys. Acta, 246,* 100 (1971).
9. Zylber, E. A., and Penman, S., *Biochim. Biophys. Acta, 204,* 221 (1970).
10. Román, R., and Sánchez, E., personal communication.

DISCUSSION

K. L. Manchester (Kingston, Jamaica): There have been some pictures published of rosettes of ribosomes from some chick material produced under cold conditions by Kerry in Britain. I do not know whether you are familiar with these, but how would they relate to the precipitation patterns that you are seeing here?

M. Castañeda (Mexico City, Mexico): There are several reports from Byers and others, and we thought at first we had those ribosomal crystals in our preparations. But our conditions are somewhat different, and we have not been able to see any tetramers or characteristic arrangements. Nevertheless, our preparations have always shown coarse precipitation by these ions even in reduced amounts of the dense iron-containing material identified as ferritin, as I showed, by electron microscopy and immunodiffusion. Apparently, ribosomes from reticulocytes and erythrocytes also show these properties of being precipitated by very low concentrations of cations.

23

Studies on HeLa Cell Nucleoli

Ruy Soeiro

Departments of Medicine and Cell Biology
Albert Einstein College of Medicine
Bronx, New York, U.S.A.

A primary role for the nucleolus in ribosome biogenesis has been well established and documented (1,2). It has been shown that the nucleolus, a well-characterized but variable nuclear morphological entity, represents the chromosomal location for the genes coding for ribosomal precursor RNA. In addition, the derivatives of this product, mature ribosomal RNA, and much of the enzymatic machinery for its synthesis, processing, and assembly with proteins are located within this nuclear organelle. While it is clear that the nucleolus functions as a site of ribosomal RNA synthesis, the capacity for other synthetic functions has not been shown. Despite a large pool of proteins, at least 80% of which are ribosomal, available evidence (3) now suggests that they are cytoplasmic in origin. Recently, several workers have shown that interruption of ribosomal RNA synthesis for even a few minutes stops the nucleolar appearance of ribosomal proteins (4-6). This implies yet another function for nucleoli, that of protein accumulation, requiring continued RNA synthesis.

Morphologically, nucleoli usually are comprised of a central fibrous core and a surrounding granular cortex. The elegant studies of Miller and his collaborators (7) have shown that the central core is comprised of tightly condensed DNA fibrils associated with growing strands of RNA, appropriate in size for ribosomal precursor RNA. This RNA is immediately associated with protein on synthesis, and probably forms, after further ribosome maturation, the RNP particles (150-200 Å) seen in the granular cortex.

While some reports have suggested trace amounts of lipid in nucleolar fractions (8), this may represent membrane contamination. No organized membrane surrounds this organelle; therefore, the forces maintaining its structure remain to be elucidated. Furthermore, while a great deal of information is available for nucleolar DNA, RNA, and its ribosomal protein complement, few data pertain to those proteins which are truly "nucleolar."

This paper will stress studies designed (a) to reveal chemical forces maintaining cortical granules in association with nucleoli and (b) to attempt to designate proteins (nonribosomal) which may be specifically nucleolar.

MATERIALS AND METHODS

Cell Culture

HeLa S-3 cells were grown in spinner culture at $3\text{-}6 \times 10^5$/ml in Eagle's minimal essential medium supplemented with 5% fetal calf serum (9).

Cell Fractionation, RNA and Protein Extraction, and Protein Electrophoresis

Cell fractions denoted cytoplasm, nuclei, nuclear supernatant, and nuclear pellet (nucleolar) were obtained by methods previously described in detail (10). The nucleoli were prepared for isolation of nascent ribonucleoprotein particles by the method of Penman (11). Nucleoli purified for protein analysis were further prepared by washing successively through (a) 15-30% sucrose (HSB) gradient, 18K for 15 min, (b) 2.2 M sucrose for 60 min at 25K, and (c) finally 0.88 M sucrose containing Triton X100 at 0.2% for 10 min at 10K, before banding on Renographin. The details of this last technique will be presented elsewhere (De Angelo and Soeiro, in preparation).

Preparation and acrylamide gel analysis of nucleolar and ribosomal subunits proteins have been described elsewhere (10). Extraction of ^{32}P-phosphoproteins was by the method of Hardy *et al.* (12).

Solutions

Solutions used were as follows: RSB, HSB, NEB, NEC, DOC, SDS [see Warner and Soeiro (10)]; NEC: NEB plus Cleland's reagent (0.01 M dithiothreitol); NPOPC: 0.01 M NaCl, 0.01 M Na pyrophosphate, 0.01 M Cleland's reagent; 0.4 M NPOPC as above with 0.4 M NaCl; NC: 0.01 M NaCl plus 0.01 M Cleland's reagent.

RESULTS

Physicochemical Study of Nucleolar Structure

The intramolecular forces involved in maintaining the nucleolar structure have not been systematically investigated. The nascent ribonucleoprotein particles of the cortex appear enmeshed in the periphery of this organelle. Accordingly, a study of the chemical forces necessary to extract these "nascent ribosomes" was undertaken. It was anticipated that more complete information regarding these extraction conditions would increase understanding of the chemical forces maintaining the nucleolus as an organelle.

Cells were labeled with uridine for 3 hr, a time sufficient to achieve an equilibrium level of the label in nucleoli. Since ribosomal RNA represents virtually all (more than 90%) of the nucleolar fraction, a simple calculation of percent of total counts extracted allows a comparison of varying conditions for extraction.

Chelators

Prior studies had utilized EDTA as a chelator. A survey of several chelating agents—EDTA, citrate, borate, and pyrophosphate—revealed pyrophosphate as markedly more efficient (see Fig. 1A). An absolute requirement for the presence of a chelator was found.

Detergents

No effects of nonionic detergents such as Nonidet NP 40, Triton X100, or Brij 58 on extraction efficiency were found. Although DOC did increase the RNA counts released, examination of the ribonucleoprotein particles revealed considerable degradation of RNA.

pH

A range of pH consistent with maintaining the integrity of both RNA and protein was explored. A clear pH dependency was determined, with an increasing fraction of the nascent ribosomes extracted with an increase in pH. This pH dependency was independent of the chelator used (see Fig. 1B) but was always more efficient with pyrophosphate.

Reducing Agent

The absence of a reducing agent markedly decreased the yield of extracted particles (see Fig. 1C) at neutral pH. However, at elevated pH (8.5) its presence was not absolutely essential.

Ionic Strength and Temperature

Higher ionic strengths (0.4 M NaCl) allowed very inefficient particle extrac-

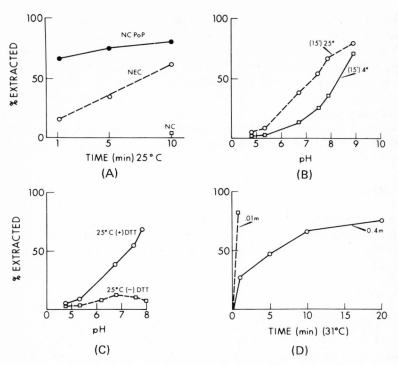

Fig. 1. *The nucleolar fraction of cells labeled 3 hr with* ^{14}C-uridine, subjected to nucleolar nascent ribosome extraction. CPM remaining in 10K supernatant after extraction is expressed at percent of particles extracted. For explanation of abbreviations, see *Materials and Methods*. (A) Kinetics of extraction at 25° with different chelators. (B) Effect of pH at 25° on extraction. (C) Effect of reducing agent on extraction at 25°. (D) Kinetics of extraction at 25° varying ionic strength.

tion at 4°. However, low ionic strength (0.01 M NaCl) and elevated pH allowed almost instantaneous particle extraction even at 4°. At pH 8.0, by increasing both the temperature and the time of extraction, an equivalent particle extraction could be attained even at higher ionic strength (see Fig. 1D). Sucrose gradient comparison (at 0.01 M NaCl) of these particles extracted at 0.4 M NaCl showed them to be quite similar to those extracted at 0.01 M NaCl.

Summary of Physicochemical Extraction Studies

Although these studies do not totally define the forces maintaining the nucleolar organelle, they suggest the following features: (a) Divalent cations probably maintain protein-protein or protein-RNA bridges as seen by the chelator requirement for efficient particle extraction. (b) Electrostatic interactions, either protein-protein or protein-RNA in nature, are important, as manifested by the effects of ionic strength. At high ionic strength, elevated temperatures are required for extraction, whereas at low ionic strength, no temperature elevation is required. This is consistent with electrostatic repulsive forces being exposed at low ionic strength that are "clouded" at higher ionic strengths. It is suggested that removal of divalent cations exposes these repulsive electrostatic forces, which may be neutralized with 0.4 M NaCl but overcome by elevated temperature. (c) Although it is tempting to speculate on the role of disulfide bonds in maintaining nucleolar structure, the potential for random disulfide linkages on cell fractionation and the lack of an absolute requirement for reducing substances prevent any final conclusion. (d) Which bonds are being titrated in this obvious pH effect are at this point unknown. (e) The lack of effect of nonionic detergents on extraction efficiency is consistent with the absence of a surrounding membrane.

Nucleolar Specific Proteins

Prior studies in this laboratory revealed that nucleoli are enriched for ribosomal peptides (10). However, the crudity of the nucleolar preparation prevented any attempt at studying "nucleolar"-specific proteins which might be either structural or enzymatic. Accordingly, a method for further purification of our crude fraction by successive washes, detergent treatment, and finally isopycnic banding was elaborated. In Fig. 2, we see an example of banded "nucleoli" labeled in its proteins. Electron micrographs of these preparations suggest that mainly the "core" fraction of the nucleolus has been preserved.

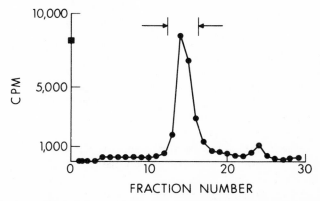

Fig. 2. The nucleolar fraction of cells labeled for 60 min isolated by isopycnic banding on Renographin.

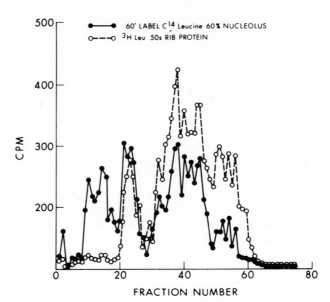

Fig. 3. ^{14}C-leucine-labeled proteins isolated from nucleoli banded as in Fig. 2 analyzed on 10% polyacrylamide gels. ^{3}H-leucine-labeled 50S ribosomal subunit proteins were used as marker peptides.

As a first approximation, it had been found by amino acid "pulse-chase" studies (13) that ribosomal proteins continued to appear in mature cytoplasmic ribosomes for 90-120 min after "chase." This fact implies a pool of ribosomal proteins, extant in the nucleolus, sufficient for cell growth over a period of one twelfth of a generation.

A significant fraction of a pulse label remains within the nucleolus after the chase. In Fig. 3, a polyacrylamide gel analysis of proteins isolated from banded nucleoli after a 60 min labeling period is shown. It can be seen that many of the bands are superimposed on marker peptides isolated from cytoplasmic 50S ribosomal subunits. However, after 90 min of chase, a similar analysis reveals that most of the comigrating peptides are now absent, and only the large peptides remain. Furthermore, after a "chase" period of 16 hr, these same peptides can still be seen (Fig. 4).

Molecular weight estimations of this group of peptides can be made by coelectrophoresis of these peptides with known markers (14). In Fig. 5, coelectrophoresis of overnight-labeled "nucleolar" peptides with heavy and light chains of γ- globulin,* 55,000 and 22,000 mol wt, respectively, reveals molecular

* Kindly supplied by Dr. Matthew Scharff.

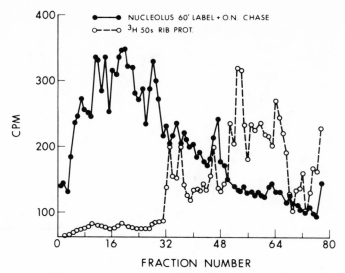

Fig. 4. ¹⁴C-leucine-labeled proteins from nucleoli analyzed on 10% polyacrylamide gels. Conditions were the same as in Fig. 3; however, nucleoli were isolated after 60 min label and overnight chase period.

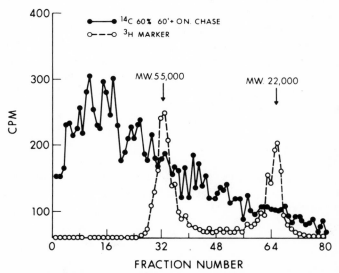

Fig. 5. Acrylamide gel analysis of "nucleolar" proteins from cells labeled for one generation. Heavy and light chains from γ-globulin served as molecular weight markers.

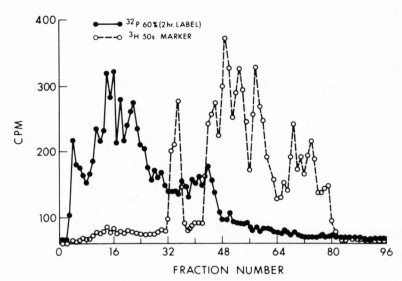

Fig. 6. Acrylamide gel analysis of "nucleolar" proteins labeled 2 hr with ^{32}P-orthophosphate. ^{3}H-50S ribosomal proteins served as marker peptides.

weights ranging from 55,000 to 100,000. Virtually all mature ribosomal proteins are smaller than this, with an average of 25,000 (13).

Finally, some interest in phosphoproteins has recently arisen by the finding of a protein kinase associated with cytoplasmic ribosomes. It was of interest to determine, therefore, whether similar phosphoproteins existed in nucleoli. Figure 6 reveals the pattern of phosphoproteins isolated from nucleoli labeled for 2 hr with ^{32}P-orthophosphate. Acrylamide gel analysis reveals a pattern quite different from that of the 50S ribosomal marker, similar to that of the "nucleolar" proteins observed above.

ACKNOWLEDGMENTS

This work was supported by a grant from the National Institutes of Health (CA 10993-03). The author is a Career Research Scientist of the Health Research Council, City of New York (I-581).

SUMMARY

Systematic extraction of nucleolar "nascent ribosomes" has been explored in terms of *p*H, detergent, salt, reducing agents, and chelators to attempt to understand the forces maintaining the nucleolus as an organelle. Amino acid pulse-chase studies of highly purified nucleoli have been done by means of polyacrylamide gels. Highly specific peptides are found which appear to be stable and phosphorylated, and which may be considered specifically nucleolar.

RESUMEN

La extracción sistemática de "ribosomas nacientes" nucleolares se ha estudiado en términos de pH, detergente, sal, agentes reductores y quelantes, con el propósito de tratar de entender las fuerzas que mantienen al nucleolo como un organito.

Estudios de desplazamiento de pulso ("pulse-chase") con amino ácidos utilizando nucleolos altamente purificados se han investigado utilizando gels de poliacrilamida. Se encontraron péptidos muy específicos, los cuales parecen ser estables, fosforilados y específicamente nucleolares.

REFERENCES

1. Birnsteil, M. L., *Ann. Rev. Plant Physiol., 18,* 25 (1967).
2. Perry, R. P., in Lima-de-Faria, A. (ed.), *Handbook of Molecular Cytology,* North-Holland Publishing Co., Amsterdam (1969), p. 620.
3. Wu, R., and Warner, J., personal communication.
4. Maisel, J. C., and McConkey, E. H., *J. Mol. Biol., 61,* 251 (1971).
5. Craig, N. C., and Perry, R. P., *Nature New Biol.* 229, 75 (1971).
6. Wu, R. S., Kumar, A., and Warner, J. R., *Proc. Natl. Acad. Sci. U.S.A., 68,* 3009 (1971).
7. Miller, O. L., and Beatty, B. R., in Lima-de-Faria, A. (ed.), *Handbook of Molecular Cytology,* North-Holland Publishing Co., Amsterdam (1969), p. 606.
8. Finamore, R. J., *Quart. Rev. Biol., 36,* 117 (1961).
9. Eagle, H., *Science, 130,* 432 (1959).
10. Warner, J. R., and Soeiro, R., *Proc. Natl. Acad. Sci. U.S.A., 58,* 1984 (1967).
11. Penman, S., Smith, I., Holtzman, E., and Greenberg, H., *Natl. Cancer Inst. Monograph, 23,* 489 (1966).
12. Hardy, S. J. S., Kurland, C. E., Voynow, P., and Mora, G., *Biochemistry, 8,* 2897 (1969).
13. Warner, J. R., *J. Mol. Biol., 19,* 383 (1966).
14. Shapiro, A. L., Vinuela, E., and Maisel, J. U., Jr., *Biochem. Biophys. Res. Commun., 28,* 815 (1967).

DISCUSSION

R. P. Perry (Philadelphia, U.S.A.): In the schematic diagram that you showed, there was 5S RNA in the 80S particle. How hard are the data supporting that point?

R. Soeiro (New York, U.S.A.): I apologize for that; the data are very weak and it really should not be in that diagram.

R. P. Perry: I was a bit confused about the last two pieces of data that you showed. What was the label, was it ^{14}C amino acids?

R. Soeiro: That was [14]C. I have not yet coelectrophoresed ^{32}P-labeled peptides with those from the particles.

R. P. Perry: But you showed earlier slides on which you had a coincidence.

R. Soeiro: Right, I meant to come back to that. There is a coincidence with the particles that we isolated from the former method using neutral pH and high temperature. With the methods that I now use (low temperature, using an elevated pH), we now get not only these extra peptides which are noncoincident, but we get also a density of the particles which is significantly lower than the formerly reported densities, which were coincidental with mature ribonucleoprotein particles from the cytoplasm.

R. P. Perry: These last two slides really represent core material in which the bulk of the granular portion of the nucleolus has been lost. That is why you lose a lot of the proteins which comigrate coincidentally with the 50S ribosomal proteins. Is that right?

R. Soeiro: You are trying to say that these are nonspecifically adsorbed?

R. P. Perry: No, simply that the particles isolated by your newer technique are more like nucleolar core material.

R. Soeiro: No, the last two slides are ribonucleoprotein particles isolated on sucrose density gradients, precisely the way the original ones were; however, they are now taken from cells labeled with a short pulse and a long chase. Under these conditions, we get these peptides which we could not see with the short pulse and the former method of isolating them.

R. P. Perry: I was worrying about the loss of the peptides which comigrated with 50S.

R. Soeiro: In the chase? It is quite clear from doing pulse-chase studies that after approximately 90 min there are no longer any labeled ribosomal, that is, mature ribosomal, proteins seen in the nucleolus. They can chase out in 90 min, and therefore the only thing left is that which is not turning over and which is very well associated, tightly associated, with these isolated nucleoli.

R. P. Perry: But are there still an 80S particle and a 50S particle?

R. Soeiro: This is simply a labeling problem. These noncoincident peptides are present in isolated 80S and 50S particles after a pulse chase, while the other ones come from a straight pulse.

P. Chambon (Strasbourg, France): Do you have any evidence that some of these peptides turn over very fast? I am asking this because if you inject animals with α-amanitin, then the nucleolus disappears very fast. It is a rather unexpected result, and one hypothesis is that one protein is required in order to prevent the nucleolus from falling apart.

R. Soeiro: One of the experiments that is in progress is an attempt to see whether these large proteins can be labeled in the presence of actinomycin, unlike ribosomal proteins. But, obviously, these peptides are not chased out, because they are stable to chase for a generation time in the cell, so they are quite stable.

24

On the Movement of the Ribosome Along the Messenger Ribonucleic Acid and on Apparent Changes in Ribosome Conformation During Protein Synthesis

Peter Lengyel, Sohan L. Gupta, Mohan L. Sopori, John Waterson, and Sherman Weissman

Department of Molecular Biophysics and Biochemistry
and
Department of Medicine
Yale University
New Haven, Connecticut, U.S.A.

During the translation of mRNA into polypeptide, the ribosome moves along the mRNA in the $5'$ to $3'$ direction (1). Each aminoacyl residue in the polypeptide is specified by three adjacent nucleotides (codon) in mRNA (2). Consequently, it is expected that the ribosome should move the length of three

---

* Abbreviations: mRNA, messenger RNA; tRNA, transfer RNA; AA-tRNA, aminoacyl-tRNA; fMet-tRNA$_f^{Met}$, formylmethionyl-tRNA$_f^{Met}$; Ala-tRNA, alanyl-tRNA; fMet-Ala-tRNA, formylmethionyl-alanyl-tRNA; GMPPCP, $5'$-guanylyl-methylenediphosphonate; INIT., initiation complex; PRE., pretranslocation complex; POST., post-translocation complex; RCF, relative centrifugal force.

nucleotides when adding one aminoacyl residue to the growing polypeptide. In this communication, we present experiments bearing out this expectation.

The addition of each aminoacyl residue to the polypeptide is a cyclic process (chain elongation cycle). Three peptide chain elongation factors (EF T_s, EF G, and EF T_u) and GTP are known to be involved in this cycle, in addition to mRNA, ribosomes, and AA-tRNA (1,3). The factors used in our studies were purified from *Bacillus stearothermophilus* (4). EF T_u was designated in earlier publications as S_3, EF T_s as S_1, and EF G as S_2. In the first phase of the cycle (AA-tRNA binding), an EF T_u-GTP-AA-tRNA complex is bound to the AA-tRNA binding site (or A site) of the ribosome-mRNA complex which has peptidyl-tRNA bound at the peptidyl-tRNA binding site (or P site) (5-12). In the second phase (peptide bond formation), the GTP from the EF T_u-GTP-AA-tRNA complex is cleaved, an EF T_u-GDP complex and P_i are released from the ribosome (7,12-17), and the peptidyl residue of the peptidyl-tRNA is released from its linkage to tRNA and forms a peptide bond with the *a*-amino group of the AA-tRNA in the A site (5,18). In the third phase (peptidyl-tRNA translocation), EF G (bound to the ribosome) triggers the cleavage of further GTP, the discharged tRNA is released from the P site, and the peptidyl-tRNA (which has just been extended by one aminoacyl residue) is shifted from the A site to the P site (19-26). Finally, EF T_s promotes the release of GDP from the EF T_u-GDP complex and a new EF T_u-GTP-AA-tRNA complex is formed (17,27-29). This finishes the process, and the stage is set for attaching another AA-tRNA (30) to the peptide chain by repeating the cycle.

During some phase of the cycle, the ribosome moves along the mRNA. The energy required for this movement is presumably obtained by GTP cleavage. For some time, peptidyl-tRNA translocation triggered by EF G was the only phase of the cycle in the cell-free system from *Escherichia coli* in which GTP cleavage was known to occur (31-33). It was assumed, therefore, that ribosome movement must also be triggered by EF G and must take place in the peptidyl-tRNA translocation phase (31-33). This assumption became less safe with the recent finding that apparently GTP is also cleaved after the binding of the EF T_u-GTP-AA-tRNA complex to the ribosome, but preceding peptide bond formation (7,13-16,34). It became conceivable that ribosome movement is triggered by the cleavage of the GTP from the EF T_u-GTP-AA-tRNA complex and takes place prior to EF G action. We attempted, therefore, to establish experimentally in which phase of the cycle the ribosome movement takes place.

STUDIES ON RIBOSOME MOVEMENT

Sequencing of a Ribosome-Binding Site of f2 Bacteriophage RNA in an Initiation Complex

The RNA of the RNA bacteriophage f2 serves as a messenger which directs the synthesis of three proteins (phage coat protein, replicase enzyme, and maturation protein) in infected *E. coli* or in an *E. coli* cell-free system (35-37). We established earlier that a ribosome binds to f2 RNA, forming a 70S initiation complex in the presence of fMet-tRNA$_f^{Met}$, GTP, and peptide chain initiation factors (38). Ribosomes are known to protect the mRNA region to which they are bound against cleavage by nucleases (39). In a previous study, we obtained the 70S initiation complex with f2 RNA, treated it with T_1 ribonuclease, and isolated the f2 RNA fragment which was protected against ribonuclease cleavage by the attached ribosome (40). The protected f2 RNA fragment was a unique RNA segment 61 nucleotides long. Its nucleotide sequence was determined (41). The 21 nucleotides adjacent to its 3′ end were found to specify the first seven amino acids of f2 coat protein (42) (fMet-Ala-Ser-Asn-Phe-Thr-Gln).

The availability of purified peptide chain elongation factors (EF T_u, EF T_s, and EF G) enabled us to extend the above study to an examination of ribosome movement (see Fig. 1).

Sequencing the 3′ Ends of Ribosome-Binding Sites on Bacteriophage f2 RNA in Initiation, Pretranslocation, and Post-translocation Complexes

As in the previous study, we first prepared an initiation complex on f2 RNA (41). This complex contains fMet-tRNA$_f^{Met}$ in the P site, and the A site is vacant. An aliquot of this was converted into a pretranslocation complex in a reaction with the appropriate factors (EF T_s and EF T_u), GTP, and Ala-tRNA (alanine is the second amino acid in the coat protein). This complex contains fMet-Ala-tRNA in the A site and discharged tRNA in the P site. Part of the pretranslocation complex was converted into a post-translocation complex in a reaction with the appropriate factor (EF G) and GTP (15) (Fig. 1). This complex contains fMet-Ala-tRNA in the P site, and the A site is vacant.

Each of the three complexes was treated with pancreatic ribonuclease to cleave those parts of the f2 RNA which were not protected by the ribosome (39). Thereafter, each was centrifuged in order to separate the ribosomes with the bound protected f2 RNA fragments from other components of the reaction mixtures (41). Each of the three isolated f2 RNA fragment-ribosome complexes was examined in two ways: (a) the f2 RNA fragments were isolated from each, and the nucleotide sequences at the 3′-terminal regions of the fragments were determined; (b) each was suspended in a reaction mixture containing labeled amino acids and other necessary ingredients, and the f2 RNA fragments in it were translated into oligopeptides which were characterized (43) (Fig. 1).

The idea prompting these experiments was the following: In initiation complexes (digested with T_1 ribonuclease), the protected f2 RNA fragment extends to the codon specifying the seventh amino acid of the coat protein (41). When the ribosome moves along the f2 RNA toward its 3′ end, then the 3′

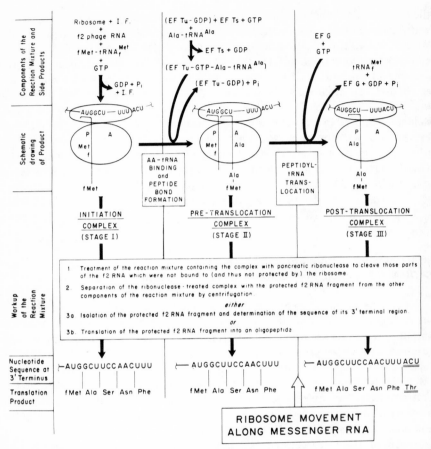

Fig. 1. *Schematic outline of experiment indicating that ribosome movement is triggered by EF G factor and GTP and occurs in the same phase as peptidyl-tRNA translocation.* The small oval shape represents the 30S ribosomal subunit, the large oval shape the 50S ribosomal subunit. P and A indicated in the 50S subunit stand for hypothetical tRNA-binding sites. The gallows shape represents tRNA. The curved line bisecting the 30S subunit represents a segment of f2 RNA; only some of the codons are shown. Details are discussed in the text.

end of the protected fragment should also be shifted toward the 3′ end of f2 RNA. Since each amino acid is specified by three adjacent nucleotides, it is presumed that the shift toward the 3′ end should be three nucleotides long when one amino acid is added to the peptide chain. Thus it would be expected that the cutoff point of the protected f2 RNA fragment should be three nucleotides further toward the 3' end in the post-translocation complex than in the initiation complex. In order to find out if the ribosome movement occurs in the course of AA-tRNA binding and peptide bond formation or in the next phase of the chain elongation cycle, i.e., translocation, one has to determine the cutoff point at the 3' end of the protected f2 fragment in the pretranslocation complex.

Results Obtained in Outline and Conclusions Derived (Fig. 1)

Identical f2 RNA fragments were found to be protected against cleavage by ribonuclease in the initiation and the pretranslocation complexes. However, the main f2 RNA fragment protected against cleavage by ribonuclease extended three nucleotides further toward the 3' end in the post-translocation complex (---UUUACU) than in either the initiation complex or the pretranslocation complex (---UUU).

These results indicate that (a) as expected, the ribosome moves the length of three nucleotides when adding one aminoacyl residue to the peptide chain, and (b) the ribosome movement takes place in the same phase in which peptidyl-tRNA is translocated, and this movement is triggered by EF G factor and GTP.

The nature of the oligopeptides translated from the various protected f2 RNA fragments provides further support for these conclusions. Thus, for example, the oligopeptides translated from the main f2 RNA fragment in the ribonuclease-treated initiation and pretranslocation complexes had a C-terminal phenylalanine residue (corresponding to ---UUU), whereas the oligopeptides translated from the main f2 RNA fragment from the ribonuclease-treated post-translocation complex had a C-terminal threonine residue (corresponding to ---UUUACU). Further details of these and other experiments were presented elsewhere (44).

It should be noted that the above conclusions about ribosome movement are based on the difference among the 3' ends of the mRNA fragments protected against ribonuclease cleavage in initiation, pretranslocation, and post-translocation complexes. Thus they reflect the movement along the mRNA of those parts of the ribosome which are protecting the mRNA. The results provide no solution of the problem of the relative positions of the two ribosomal subunits in the various phases of peptide chain elongation (1,45,46).

STUDIES ON THE SEDIMENTATION OF PRE. AND POST.
THROUGH SUCROSE GRADIENTS DURING
CENTRIFUGATION AT LOW SPEED AND HIGH SPEED

As part of the above study, each complex was sedimented through a linear sucrose gradient (5-20% w/v) at high speed (180,000 × g). It was noted that the

PRE. sedimented faster than either the INIT. or the POST. (44). Similar differences in sedimentation velocities among PRE., POST., and INIT. containing a synthetic mRNA (poly U) were reported by Schreier and Noll (47) and Chuang and Simpson (48). These differences were attributed to differences in conformation among the various ribosome complexes.

Recent publications reveal the need for caution in interpreting sedimentation patterns of ribosomes with sedimentation coefficients between 70S and 50S. According to Spirin (49), such patterns may not necessarily reflect a real class of ribosomal particles with an unusual conformation but may result from the incomplete separation of an equilibrium mixture of ribosomes and subunits, dissociating and reassociating during centrifugation. Furthermore, Infante and his associates (50-52) established that large hydrostatic pressure prevailing during high-speed centrifugation induces dissociation of free ribosomes.

We studied the following aspects of these phenomena: (a) the correlation of the requirements for the conversion of the faster-sedimenting PRE. to a slower-sedimenting complex with those needed for its conversion to the POST. and (2) the causes of the difference in sedimentation velocities between the complexes.

The curves in Fig. 2A demonstrate that treatment of the faster-sedimenting PRE. with EF G and GTP, which converts it into a POST., also converts it into a slower-sedimenting form (Fig. 2A). Under several conditions in which PRE. is not converted to POST., the faster-sedimenting form is not converted to the slower-sedimenting form (Fig. 2B), e.g., when treated with GTP in the absence of EF G or with EF G in the absence of GTP, or if the GTP analogue GMPPCP is substituted for GTP, or in the presence of an inhibitor of translocation [either fusidic acid (53) or thiostrepton (54)], or if the incubation of the reaction mixture with EF G and GTP is at $0°$ instead of $37°$ (14). One of the definitions of a PRE. is that its peptidyl residue is not released by puromycin, whereas that in a POST. is (19). The curves in Fig. 2C demonstrate that indeed most of our POST. preparation (over 92%) was reactive with puromycin, whereas little of the PRE. preparation (less than 20%) was.

ON THE POSSIBLE CAUSES OF THE DIFFERENCE IN SEDIMENTATION VELOCITY

The PRE. contains one more tRNA than either the INIT. or the POST. The difference in sedimentation velocity between the complexes ($\Delta S/S > 4/70 > 5\%$) is, however, too large to be accounted for by the difference in particle weight (Δ particle weight/particle weight $\sim 3 \times 10^4/3.6 \times 10^6 \sim 1\%$) caused by a tRNA molecule. The experiments presented in the subsequent sections on the possible causes of the difference in sedimentation velocities were performed only with the PRE. and the POST.

According to Infante and Baierlein (50), large hydrostatic pressure prevailing

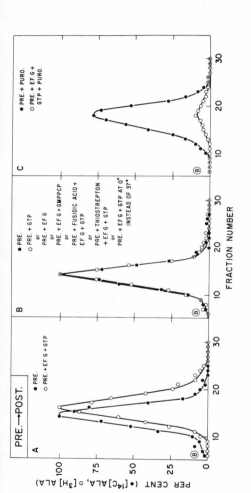

Fig. 2. Difference between the sedimentation velocities of PRE. and POST. centrifuged at high speed. The conversion of the faster-sedimenting form to the slower-sedimenting form requires the same treatment as the conversion of PRE. to POST. "Marker PRE." contained ^{14}C-Ala. (A) POST. was prepared by reacting PRE. (labeled with ^{3}H-Ala) with GTP and EF G, at 37° (PRE EF G + GTP). The POST. was mixed with "marker PRE." (PRE) prior to applying the reaction mixture to a sucrose gradient. (B) The samples PRE + GTP and PRE + EF G were prepared as in A except for the omission of EF G from the first and GTP from the second. In the sample PRE + EF G + GMPPCP, GMPPCP was substituted for GTP in the reaction mixture containing PRE + EF G. In the sample PRE. + FUSIDIC ACID + EF G + GTP, 10^{-3} M fusidic acid was present in the reaction mixtures in which the INIT. was converted to PRE. and in which the PRE. was treated with EF G and GTP. In the sample PRE. + THIOSTREPTON + EF G + GTP, 10^{-5} M thiostrepton was substituted for the fusidic acid. In the sample PRE. + EF G + GTP AT 0° INSTEAD OF 37°, the PRE. was incubated with EF G and GTP at 0°. Each of the samples was mixed with an equal volume of "marker PRE." prior to application to a linear sucrose gradient. The patterns of sedimentation of the samples excepting "marker PRE." were indistinguishable. (C) The samples were prepared as in A except that before centrifugation through a 5-20% linear sucrose gradient the reaction mixture was made 2 mM in puromycin and incubated at 0° for 10 min. Each sucrose gradient was centrifuged at 40,000 rpm, average RCF 180,000 × g, at 2° for 3.6 hr. (For further details, see ref. 60.)

during centrifugation at high speed induces dissociation of free ribosomes (i.e., couples of a small and a large subunit not complexed to mRNA and/or tRNA). The dissociation in turn may result in a peculiar sedimentation pattern: the ribosome couples are not always well separated from the subunits, and consequently one may deal with an unseparable equilibrium mixture of components dissociating and reassociating during sedimentation. This may give a false impression of the existence of ribosome couples which sediment slower than expected (49). Two of the criteria of such pressure-induced dissociation phenomena are that the apparent sedimentation velocities depend on (a) the hydrostatic pressure and (b) the concentration of ribosomes in the gradient.

Although we were dealing with ribosome-mRNA-tRNA complexes (and pressure-induced dissociation was reported not to affect such complexes), we tested them for both of these criteria:

(a) We centrifuged one aliquot of a reaction mixture containing both PRE. and POST. through an isokinetic sucrose gradient (5-30.8% w/v) (see ref. 55) at low speed (20,000 rpm, average RCF 45,000 × g) for 16.8 hr and a second aliquot at high speed (40,000 rpm, average RCF 180,000 × g) for 4.2 hr. The time of centrifugation at low speed was increased to such an extent that the complex sedimented to the same position in the gradients as in the experiments at high speed. (At this position, the hydrostatic pressure was 1200 atmospheres in high-speed centrifugations and 300 atmospheres in low-speed centrifugations.) As was done in the case of high-speed centrifugations, we verified that most of the POST. (73%) and little of the PRE. (12%) were reactive with puromycin after sedimentation at low speed. Under these conditions, no difference was detected between the sedimentation velocities of PRE. and POST. (data not shown).

It could be argued that as a consequence of the longer centrifugation time the extent of diffusion increased and obscured the difference in sedimentation velocities between PRE. and POST. However, the width of the peaks in the gradients was only 15% greater in the long runs at low speed than in the short ones at high speed. This increase cannot account for the disappearance of the difference in sedimentation velocities. These results reveal that a difference between the sedimentation velocities of PRE. and POST. is manifested at high-speed centrifugation but not at low-speed centrifugation.

(b) To test the effect or ribosome concentration on the sedimentation pattern, we applied to sucrose gradients various amounts of PRE. and POST., the maximum amount was that tested in Fig. 2. Other aliquots containing one third, one sixth, and one ninth as much were applied (in equal volumes) to other gradients. All of these were centrifuged at high speed in the conditions of Fig. 2. We found that the recovery of each complex in the peak fraction was independent of the amount of complex applied. (Recovery equals the ratio of the amount of complex found in the peak fraction to the amount applied to the gradient.) Moreover, the peaks of PRE. and POST. sedimented in the same fractions in all cases as in the experiment shown in Fig. 2 (data not shown). The width of the peak (plotted as in Fig. 2) was approximately the same in all cases (it varied between 5 and 5.5 mm).

These results do not support the idea that the difference in sedimentation velocities between PRE. and POST. is due to a different extent of reversible dissociation of the two complexes.

The results presented so far could be accounted for by one of the following two hypotheses: Large hydrostatic pressure may distort the PRE. and the POST. to a different extent. The difference in sedimentation velocity manifested during centrifugation at high speed (but not at low speed) may be due entirely or in part either (a) to such a differential distortion (i.e., change in conformation) itself, or (b) to a (larger) decrease in particle weight of the POST. (as compared to the PRE.) resulting from the irreversible loss of components triggered by the distortion.

To distinguish between hypotheses (a) and (b), we performed the following experiments: First we centrifuged a mixture of PRE. and POST. through a sucrose gradient at high speed. This resulted in a partial resolution of the two complexes as in Fig. 2A. Thereafter, we mixed the fractions containing either or both of the two complexes, concentrated the resulting solution, and applied one aliquot to a sucrose gradient which was centrifuged at low speed and another aliquot to a sucrose gradient which was centrifuged at high speed.

No difference was detected between the sedimentation patterns of the PRE. and the POST. in the gradient centrifuged at low speed. In the gradient centrifuged at high speed the PRE. sedimented faster than the POST. (data not shown). (In this case, there was a slight asymmetry in the sedimentation pattern of the POST., probably in consequence of a minor loss of components occurring during the long experiment.) These results suggest that the centrifugation of the complexes through a sucrose gradient at high speed does not cause an irreversible change in their sedimentation characteristics; i.e., the difference in sedimentation velocities between the two complexes under these conditions is not a consequence of irreversible loss of components. Consequently, our findings are inconsistent with hypothesis (b) and are in line with hypothesis (a).

CONCLUSIONS

Our studies involving high- (and low-) speed centrifugations of ribosome complexes through sucrose gradients lead to the following results: (a) As tested in a gradient centrifuged at high speed, the conversion of the slower-sedimenting INIT. to the more rapidly sedimenting complex was found to require the same treatment as its conversion to a PRE., and the conversion of the more rapidly sedimenting PRE. to the more slowly sedimenting complex was found to require the same treatment as its conversion to the POST. (b) The sedimentation patterns (including the percent recovery in the peak fractions) of PRE. and POST. (centrifuged at high speed) were apparently not altered when the concentration of the ribosome complexes in the gradients was decreased ninefold. (c) No difference was detected between the sedimentation velocities of PRE. and POST. centrifuged through a sucrose gradient at low speed. (d) No difference was detected between the sedimentation velocities of PRE. and POST. centrifuged through a sucrose gradient at low speed even if the mixture of the two complexes analyzed was one which had been partially resolved earlier by centrifugation through a sucrose gradient at high speed.

We believe that result (b) makes it improbable that the difference in sedimentation velocities between the PRE. and the POST. could be due to a difference in the pressure-induced reversible dissociation of the two complexes into subunits. Actually, Infante and Baierlein (50), who discovered the pressure effect on free ribosomes, also noted that complexed ribosomes may not be dissociated by pressure.

We propose that our results may be explained by a differential distortion (i.e., change in conformation) of the two complexes caused by the large hydrostatic pressure prevailing during centrifugation at high speed. The fact that large hydrostatic pressure blocks protein synthesis *in vivo* (56) as well as *in vitro* by causing a decrease in the stability of the AA-tRNA-ribosome-mRNA complex in the cell-free system (57) is in line with this hypothesis.

Changes in ribosome conformation in the course of the conversion of the pretranslocation complex to the post-translocation complex have been predicted (32,46). Indirect support for such a change was provided by the findings of differences in the rate of tritium exchange between the two ribosome complexes (58). Our results are in line with those of Spirin (49) and Infante and Baierlein (50) indicating that a difference in sedimentation velocity between PRE. and POST. in sucrose gradients centrifuged at high speed and large hydrostatic pressure is not a sufficient proof for a difference in conformation between the complexes.

It should be noted that we know now about the following events occurring during the translocation phase of peptide chain elongation: (a) release of discharged tRNA (23,26); (b) peptidyl-tRNA translocation (19,25); (c) GTP cleavage (20,22); (d) ribosome movement along the messenger RNA (44); and (e) change in the sedimentation velocity of the ribosome complexes centrifuged at high speed (46,47,59,60, and this paper). One can assay for each of the above events selectively.

It will be revealing to establish the temporal order of these events and the components of the translating machinery involved in each.

ACKNOWLEDGMENTS

We thank Professor F. Egami for U_2 ribonuclease and Drs. D. Crothers and

R. C. Williams, Jr., for their advice. This work was supported by research grants from the National Institutes of Health (GM 13707 and CA 10137), the National Science Founcation (GB 30700X), and the American Cancer Society (ACS E 456).

SUMMARY

Studies are presented demonstrating the following: (a) The movement of the ribosome along the messenger ribonucleic acid during protein synthesis is triggered by elongation factor G (designated previously as S_2 factor or translocase) and guanosine-5'-triphosphate. (b) One step of the ribosome along the messenger ribonucleic acid is, as expected, three nucleotides long. (c) The pretranslocation complex (i.e., the messenger-ribosome complex with peptidyl-tRNA in the A site and discharged tRNA in the P site) sediments faster than the post-translocation complex (i.e., the messenger-ribosome complex with peptidyl-tRNA in the P site and a vacant A site) during centrifugation through a sucrose gradient at high speed. This is, however, no proof for the existence of a difference in conformation between the two complexes under physiological conditions, because large hydrostatic pressure, prevailing during centrifugation at high speed, distorts (i.e., changes the conformation of) the two complexes to a different extent.

RESUMEN

Se presentan estudios que demuestran que: (a) El movimiento del ribosoma a lo largo del acido ribonucleic durante la síntesis de proteína es iniciado por el factor de elongación G (anteriormente designado factor S_2 o translocasa) y guanosina-5-trifosfato. (b) Un solo paso del ribosoma a lo largo del ácido ribonucléico mensajero es, como era de esperarse, tres nucleótidos de largo. (c) El complejo de translocación (el ribosoma mensajero se une al peptidil-RNA de transferencia en el sitio A y descarga el RNA de transferencia en el sitio P) sedimenta mas rápidamente que el complejo de post-translocación (el ribosoma mensajero se une al peptidil-RNA de transferencia en el sitio P y un sitio A libre) durante la centrifugación a velocidad alta a través de un gradiente de sacarosa. No obstante, esto no es prueba de que existe algua diferencia en la conformación de los dos compuestos bajo condiciones fisiológicas, debido a que la alta presión hidrostática prevaleciente durante la centrifugación a velocidad alta, altera (cambia la conformación) hasta cierto grado de los dos compuestos.

REFERENCES

1. Lengyel, P., and Söll, D., *Bacteriol. Rev., 33,* 264. (1969).
2. Speyer, J. F., in Taylor, J. H. (ed.), *Molecular Genetics,* Part II, Academic Press, New York, p. 137.
3. Lucas-Lenard, J., and Lipmann, F., *Ann. Rev. Biochem., 40,* 409 (1971).
4. Skoultchi, A., Ono, Y., Moon, H. M., and Lengyel, P., *Proc. Natl. Acad. Sci. U.S.A., 60,* 675 (1968).
5. Skoultchi, A., Ono, Y., Waterson, J., and Lengyel, P., *Cold Spring Harbor Symp. Quant. Biol., 34,* 437 (1969).
6. Lucas-Lenard, J., Tao, P., and Haenni, A., *Cold Spring Harbor Symp. Quant. Biol., 34,* 455 (1969).
7. Skoultchi, A., Ono, Y., Waterson, J., and Lengyel, P., *Biochemistry, 9,* 508 (1970).
8. Brot, N., Redfield, B., and Weissbach, H., *Biochem. Biophys. Res. Commun., 41,* 1388 (1970).

9. Ravel, J. M., *Proc. Natl. Acad. Sci. U.S.A., 57,* 1181 (1967).
10. Gordon, J., *Proc. Natl. Acad. Sci. U.S.A., 59,* 179 (1968).
11. Ertel, R., Brot, N., Redfield, B., Allende, J. E., and Weissbach, H., *Proc. Natl. Acad. Sci. U.S.A., 59,* 861 (1968).
12. Shorey, R., Ravel, J., Garner, G. W., and Shive, W., *J. Biol. Chem., 244,* 4555 (1969).
13. Haenni, A., Lucas-Lenard, J., and Gordon, J., *Fed. Proc., 27,* 397 (1968).
14. Ono, Y., Skoultchi, A., Waterson, J., and Lengyel, P., *Nature, 222,* 645 (1969).
15. Ono, Y., Skoultchi, A., Waterson, J., and Lengyel, P., *Nature, 223,* 697 (1969).
16. Gordon, J., *J. Biol. Chem., 244,* 5680 (1969).
17. Waterson, J., Beaud, G., and Lengyel, P., *Nature, 227,* 34 (1970).
18. Monro, R. E., Staehelin, T., Celma, M. L., and Vazquez, D., *Cold Spring Harbor Symp. Quant. Biol., 34,* 357 (1969).
19. Traut, R., and Monro, R., *J. Mol. Biol., 10, 63 (1964).*
20. Brot, N., Ertel, R., and Weissbach, H., *Biochem. Biophys. Res. Commun., 31,* 563 (1968).
21. Ertel, R., Redfield, B., Brot, N., and Weissbach, H., *Arch. Biochem. Biophys., 128,* 331 (1968).
22. Haenni, A., and Lucas-Lenard, J., *Proc. Natl. Acad. Sci. U.S.A., 61,* 1363 (1968).
23. Kuriki, Y., and Kaji, A., *Proc. Natl. Acad. Sci. U.S.A., 61,* 1399 (1968).
24. Pestka, S., *Proc. Natl. Acad. Sci. U.S.A., 61,* 726 (1968).
25. Erbe, R., Nau, M., and Leder, P., *J. Mol. Biol., 39,* 441 (1969).
26. Lucas-Lenard, J., and Haenni, A., *Proc. Natl. Acad. Sci. U.S.A., 63,* 93 (1969).
27. Miller, D. L., and Weissbach, H., *Biochem. Biophys. Res. Commun., 38,* 1016 (1970).
28. Weissbach, H., Miller, D., and Hachmann, J., *Arch. Biochem. Biophys., 137,* 262 (1970).
29. Weissbach, H., Redfield, B., and Hachmann, J., *Arch. Biochem. Biophys., 141,* 384 (1970).
30. Skogerson, L., Roufa, D., and Leder, P., *Proc. Natl. Acad. Sci. U.S.A., 68,* 276 (1971).
31. Conway, T. W., and Lipmann, F., *Proc. Natl. Acad. Sci. U.S.A., 52,* 1462 (1964).
32. Nishizuka, Y.; and Lipmann, F., *Arch. Biochem. Biophys., 116,* 344 (1966).
33. Nishizuka, Y., and Lipmann, F., *Proc. Natl. Acad. Sci. U.S.A., 55,* 212 (1966).
34. Arlinghaus, R., Schaeffer, J., and Schweet, R., *Proc. Natl. Acad. Sci. U.S.A., 51,* 1291 (1964).
35. Vinuela, E., Algranati, I. D., and Ochoa, S., *Europ. J. Biochem., 1,* 3 (1967).
36. Eggen, K., Oeschger, M. P., and Nathans, D., *Biochem. Biophys. Res. Commun., 28,* 587 (1967).
37. Lodish, H. F., *Nature, 220,* 345 (1968).
38. Kondo, M., Eggertsson, G., Eisenstadt, J., and Lengyel, P., *Nature, 220,* 368 (1968).
39. Takanami, M., Yan, Y., and Jukes, T. H., *J. Mol. Biol., 12,* 761 (1965).
40. Gupta, S. L., Chen, J., Schaefer, L., Weissman, S. M., and Lengyel, P., *Cold Spring Harbor Symp. Quant. Biol., 34,* 630 (1969).
41. Gupta, S. L., Chen, J., Schaefer, L., Lengyel, P., and Weissman, S. M., *Biochem. Biophys. Res. Commun., 39,* 883 (1970).
42. Weber, K., and Konigsberg, W., *J. Biol. Chem., 242,* 3563 (1967).
43. Kuechler, E., and Rich, A., *Nature, 225,* 920 (1970).
44. Gupta, S. L., Waterson, J., Sopori, M. L., Weissman, S. M., and Lengyel, P., *Biochemistry, 10,* 4410 (1971).
45. Bretscher, M. S., *Nature, 218,* 675 (1968).
46. Spirin, A. S., *Cold Spring Harbor Symp. Quant. Biol., 34,* 197 (1969).
47. Schreier, M. H., and Noll, H., *Proc. Natl. Acad. Sci. U.S.A., 68,* 805 (1971).
48. Chuang, D. M., and Simpson, M. V., *Proc. Natl. Acad. Sci. U.S.A., 68,* 1474 (1971).

49. Spirin, A. S., *FEBS Letters, 14,* 349 (1971).
50. Infante, A. A., and Baierlein, R., *Proc. Natl. Acad. Sci. U.S.A., 68,* 1780 (1971).
51. Infante, A. A., and Graves, P. N., *Biochim. Biophys. Acta, 246,* 100 (1971).
52. Infante, A. A., and Krauss, M., *Biochim. Biophys. Acta, 246,* 81 (1971).
53. Tanaka, N., Kinoshita, T., and Masukawa, H., *J. Biochem., 65,* 459 (1969).
54. Pestka, S., *Biochem. Biophys. Res. Commun., 40,* 667 (1970).
55. Noll, H., in Sargent, J., and Campbell, P. M. (eds.), *Techniques in Protein Synthesis,* Vol. 2, Academic Press, London (1969), p. 101.
56. Landau, J. V., *Biochim. Biophys. Acta, 149,* 506 (1967).
57. Arnold, R. M., and Albright, L. J., *Biochim. Biophys. Acta, 238,* 347 (1971).
58. Chuang, D. M., Silberstein, H. A., and Simpson, M. V., *Arch. Biochem. Biophys., 144,* 778 (1971).
59. Schreier, M. H., and Noll, H., *Nature, 227,* 128 (1970).
60. Waterson, J., Sopori, M. L., Gupta, S. L., and Lengyel, P., *Biochemistry, 11,* 1377 (1972).

25

Initiation of DNA Synthesis by Oligoribonucleotides

G. Feix

Institute of Genetics
University of Freiburg
Freiburg, Germany

The known DNA polymerases are unable to initiate the synthesis of new DNA chains without a primer (1). DNA synthesis begins by the addition of nucleotide residues to the 3'-OH terminus of a pre-existing chain which has always been of the deoxy type. Recently, however, it was discovered that oligoribonucleotides also can be used for the priming of DNA synthesis. Verma *et al.* (2) found that DNA synthesis by reverse transcriptase from avian myeloblastosis virus is initiated by an oligoribonucleotide, and, further, it has been suggested that an oligoribonucleotide might be involved in the initiation of DNA synthesis by *Escherichia coli* polymerase (3).

Oligoribonucleotides, if needed, can be produced easily by transcription and might exert a kind of positive control in initiation of DNA synthesis by virtue of their specific priming capacity. Therefore, it is of interest to study the various DNA-synthesizing enzymes with respect to their behavior toward an oligoribonucleotide primer.

I would like to give a short account on some experiments done in this connection with terminal deoxynucleotidyl transferase from calf thymus. This rather small enzyme (mol wt 32,000), which displays primer dependency, has been extensively purified by Chang and Bollum (4). It is suggested that this enzyme might be part of a larger DNA-synthesizing enzyme complex which disintegrates during enzyme purification (5).

So far, the enzyme always has been primed by either oligodeoxynucleotides or DNA (6,7). If an oligoribonucleotide such as (A-A-A-A)$_r$ is offered as primer

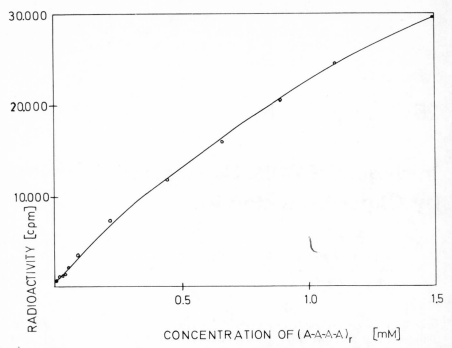

Fig. 1. Stimulation of DNA synthesis. Enzyme assays (30 μl) containing 6 μmoles potassium cacodylate (*p*H 7.0), 30 nmoles CoCl$_2$, 0.6 μmoles KCl, 30 nmoles mercaptoethanol, 30 nmoles ^{3}H-dCTP (specific activity 11,000 cpm/nmole), 7 μg enzyme [9000 units per milligram protein as measured with dCTP and CoCl$_2$ (4)], and (A-A-A-A)$_r$ as primer in the amounts indicated in the figure were incubated at 37° for 30 min. Then 15 μl aliquots were taken, diluted into a mixture of 0.05 ml 8% Na$_4$P$_2$O$_7$ (*p*H 7.0) and 0.1% bovine serum albumin, and acid precipitated with 6% TCA. The acid-precipitated radioactivity was collected on membrane filters, and after washing of the filters with 6% TCA and drying, the radioactivity was measured in a Beckman liquid scintillation spectrometer using a toluene-based scintillator.

for the polymerization of dCTP at a concentration of 10 μM (sufficient for substantial synthesis if primed by a oligodeoxynucleotide), no detectable polymerization takes place as tested by the incorporation of radioactive substrate into acid-insoluble material (8). If, however, the concentration of (A-A-A-A)$_r$ is considerably increased, DNA synthesis is stimulated as shown in Fig. 1, which illustrates the concentration dependency of (A-A-A-A)$_r$ as primer for the polymerization of dCTP.

Since a considerable primer concentration is needed for a significant incorporation of deoxynucleotides into acid-insoluble polymers, it is necessary to exclude the possibility that the oligoribonucleotides merely stimulate the reaction without being incorporated into the growing chain.

In order to show conclusively that the synthesized product is covalently linked to the 3' end of the primer, a nearest-neighbor analysis was carried out according to the following reaction:

$$(A\text{-}A\text{-}A\text{-}A\text{-}A\text{-}A)_r + (ppp^*C_d)_n \xrightarrow{\text{enzyme}} (A\text{-}A\text{-}A\text{-}A\text{-}A\text{-}A)_r\text{-}p^*C_d\text{-}(p^*C)_{n-1} + nPP_i$$

$$(A\text{-}A\text{-}A\text{-}A\text{-}A\text{-}A)_r\text{-}p^*C_d\text{-}(p^*C)_{n-1} \xrightarrow{\text{alkali}} 5A_p + Ap^* + C_d\text{-}(p^*C_d)_{n-1}$$

The use of a-^{32}P-dCTP as substrate in the enzymatic reaction followed by alkaline hydrolysis of the product and purification of Ap* from the other radioactive products by various chromatographic procedures shows that the oligoribonucleotide is indeed used as primer.

Figure 2 shows the final paper electrophoretic distribution of radioactivity which coincides with Ap (open circles). The other line in the figure (closed circles) is the result of an identical enzyme assay without the addition of $(A\text{-}A\text{-}A\text{-}A\text{-}A\text{-}A)_r$. This finding may be of some significance in the study of oligoribonucleotide-primed DNA synthesis. Therefore, it would be desirable to

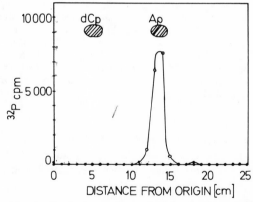

Fig. 2. Final paper electrophoretic distribution of radioactivity coinciding with Ap. An assay mixture (120 μl) containing 24 μmoles potassium cacodylate (pH 7.0), 120 nmoles CoCl, 2.2 μmoles KCl, 120 nmoles mercaptoethanol, 120 nmoles a-^{32}P-dCTP (specific activity 16,000 cpm/nmole), 100 μg enzyme, and 60 nmoles (A-A-A-A-A-A)$_r$ was incubated for 30 min at 20° and afterward for 3 hr at 31°. One-hundred microliters of the enzyme mixture was then processed (as detailed in ref. 3).

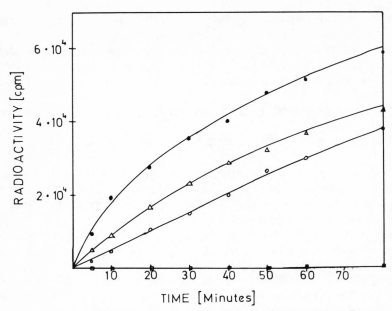

Fig. 3. Priming of terminal deoxynucleotidyl transferase reaction. Enzyme assays (100 μl) contained 20 μmoles potassium cacodylate (pH 7.0), 100 nmoles CoCl$_2$, 1.8 μmoles KCl, 100 nmoles mercaptoethanol, 100 nmoles ^{3}H-dCTP (specific activity 11,000 cpm/nmole), 21 μg enzyme, and 0.85 nmoles (pT-T-T)$_d$ (●) or 0.65 nmoles (A-A-A-A-A-A)$_r$-(T-T)$_d$* (△) or 0.8 nmoles (A-A-A-A-A-A)$_r$-T$_d$* (○) or 0.8 nmoles (A-A-A-A-A-A)$_r$ (□), respectively. The assay mixtures were incubated at 37°, and at different times 10 μl aliquots were taken and processed as detailed in Fig. 1. (Oligoribonucleotides marked with an asterisk were prepared as described in ref. 11.)

increase the priming capacity of oligoribonucleotides for the polymerization of deoxynucleotides. This could be achieved by modifying the 3′ end of the oligoribonucleotides by adding one or two deoxynucleotides using primer-dependent polynucleotide phosphorylase (9,10):

$$2(A\text{-}A\text{-}A\text{-}A\text{-}A\text{-}A)_r + 3ppT_d \xrightarrow{\text{enzyme}} \begin{array}{c} (A\text{-}A\text{-}A\text{-}A\text{-}A\text{-}A)_r\text{-}T_d \\ \\ (A\text{-}A\text{-}A\text{-}A\text{-}A\text{-}A)_r\text{-}(T\text{-}T)_d \end{array} + 3P_i$$

These oligoribonucleotides terminated with deoxynucleotides at the 3′ end can then be used as very efficient primers for the terminal deoxynucleotidyl transferase reaction (Fig. 3). It is evident from the kinetics of incorporation that the diaddition product (A-A-A-A-A-A)$_r$-(T-T)$_d$ behaves much like (pT-T-T-T)$_d$

(used as standard primer at similar concentrations) with respect to its priming activity. The monoaddition product $(A-A-A-A-A-A)_r-T_d$ shows a slightly lower priming activity. Under these conditions, the use of $(A-A-A-A-A-A)_r$ as primer shows a negligible activity.

If the oligoribonucleotides terminated with deoxynucleotides are treated with alkali, they are no longer able to initiate the polymerization of dCTP (Table I). This finding suggests strongly that this enzymatic synthesis is mediated by these oligoribonucleotides and that a contaminating oligodeoxynucleotide is not responsible for the priming of the reaction.

Further evidence that the polymerization of dCMP residues takes place at the thymidylic acid $3'$ end of $(A-A-A-A-A-A)_r-(T-T)_d$ and $(A-A-A-A-A-A)_r-T_d$ was again revealed by a nearest-neighbor analysis of the enzymatic products obtained by using $\alpha-^{32}P$-dCTP as substrate. After enzymatic digestion of the products with spleen phosphodiesterase and after purification and separation of the generated mononucleotides as described in Fig. 2, it was found that ^{32}P radioactivity had been transferred to the thymidine nucleotide which stands at the $3'$ end of the primers.

The products of the enzymatic reactions were further analyzed by poly-acrylamide gel electrophoresis (Fig. 4). The electrophoretic mobility profile of

Table I. Incorporation of ^{3}H-dCTP into TCA-Insoluble Material in the Presence of Untreated or Alkali-Treated Primers[a]

Primer (concentrations)		Incorporation (cpm)	
		30 min	60 min
No primer		450	621
$(pT-T-T-T)_d$	(36 μM)	100,560	134,732
$(pT-T-T-T)_d$ alkali-treated	(36 μM)	98,750	130,610
$(A-A-A-A-A-A)_r-(T-T)_d$	(35 μM)	75,098	106,698
$(A-A-A-A-A-A)_r-(T-T)_d$ alkali-treated	(35 μM)	467	510
$(A-A-A-A-A-A)_r-T_d$	(37 μM)	47,052	79,152
$(A-A-A-A-A-A)_r T_d$ alkali-treated	(37 μM)	513	613

[a] The enzyme assays (60 μl) containing 12 μmoles potassium caco-dylate (pH 7.0), 60 nmoles $CoCl_2$, 1.1 μmoles KCl, 60 nmoles mercaptoethanol, 60 nmoles ^{3}H-dCTP (specific activity 11,000 cpm/nmole), 14 μg enzyme, and primers in 30 min and 60 min of incubation, 20 μl aliquots were taken and processed as detailed in Fig. 1. The alkali treatment of the primers was done by incubating samples for 18 hr in 0.3N KOH at 37°, neutralizing the solutions with Dowex-50x8 resin, evaporating the samples in a Evapo-Mix (Buchler Instruments), and readjusting the concentrations by adding water.

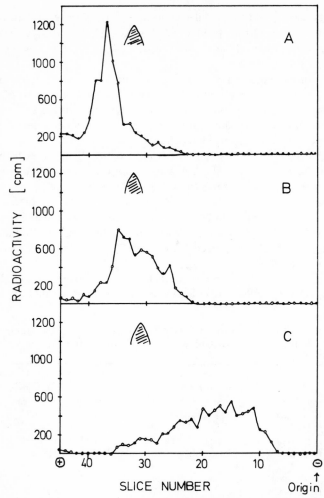

Fig. 4. *Analysis by polyacrylamide gel electrophoresis.* Assay mixtures (120 μl) containing 24 μmoles potassium cacodylate (pH 7.0), 120 nmoles $CoCl_2$, 2.2 μmoles KCl, 120 nmoles mercaptoethanol, 120 nmoles α-^{32}P-dCTP (specific activity 3,000 cpm/nmole), 50 μg enzyme, and 10.6 nmoles (pT-T-T-T)$_d$ (A) or 10.4 nmoles (A-A-A-A-A-A)$_r$-(T-T)$_d$ (B) or 11.2 nmoles (A-A-A-A-A)$_r$-T$_d$, respectively, were incubated for 30 min at 20° and afterward for 3 hr at 31°. The assay mixtures were adjusted to 0.5% SDS, heated for 1 min at 100°, and cooled rapidly. Twenty-microliter aliquots were taken and submitted to polyacrylamide electrophoresis in 5% polyacrylamide gels (as detailed in ref. 11). The hatched areas indicate the position of tRNA added as an internal marker and determined by densitometer tracing.

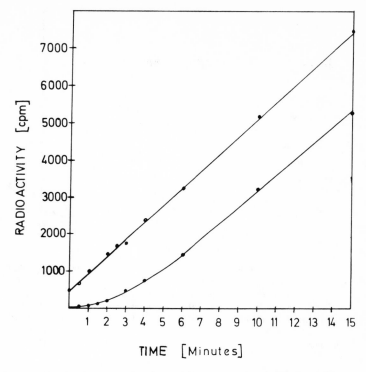

Fig. 5. *Short-time kinetics.* Enzyme assays (200 μl) containing 40 μmoles potassium cacodylate (pH 7.0), 200 nmoles $CoCl_2$, 3.6 μmoles KCl, 200 nmoles mercaptoethanol, 200 nmoles ^{3}H-dCTP (specific activity 11,000 cpm/nmole), 21 μg enzyme, and 0.16 nmoles (A-A-A-A-A-A)$_r$-T$_d$ were incubated at 37°. (○), assay mixture was preincubated for 1 hr at 0°; (●), assay mixture was not preincubated. At the times indicated in the figure, 10 μl aliquots were taken and processed as detailed in Fig. 1.

the incorporated radioactivity shows that the product of the (A-A-A-A-A-A)$_r$-(T-T)$_d$ primed reaction displays a similar size distribution as that obtained using (pT-T-T)$_d$ as primer. The product of the (A-A-A-A-A-A)$_r$-T$_d$ primed reaction is more heterogeneous, indicating that in this case the reaction is started less synchronously. This conclusion is supported by short-time kinetics (Fig. 5). The (A-A-A-A-A-A)$_r$-T$_d$ primed reaction begins slowly, with a lag of about 2 min if incubated at 37° from time zero. However, after a preincubation of the enzyme mixture for 1 hr at 0°, the reaction proceeds with linear kinetics from the beginning. There is some synthesis occurring even at 0°, which was also observed with oligodeoxynucleotide primers.

The product of such a preincubated enzyme reaction shows a more homogeneous size distribution by polyacrylamide electrophoresis (Fig. 6).

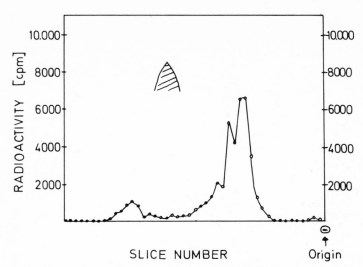

Fig. 6. Analysis by polyacrylamide gel electrophoresis. An enzyme assay
(30 µl) containing 6 µmole potassium cacodylate (pH 7.0), 30 nmoles
$CoCl_2$, 0.6 µmoles KCl, 30 nmoles mercaptoethanol, 30 nmoles
^{32}P-dCTP (specific activity 11,000 cpm/nmole), 14 µg enzyme, and 1.1
nmoles $(A-A-A-A-A-A)_r-T_d$ was incubated for 120 min at 0° and then for
150 min at 37°. A 15 µl aliquot was taken and submitted to polyacrylamide electrophoresis in 5% polyacrylamide gel (as detailed in ref. 11).

In summary, it has been shown that oligoribonucleotides are accepted by
terminal deoxynucleotidyl transferase, giving rise to the synthesis of polydeoxy-
nucleotides covalently linked to the oligoribonucleotide. The recognition of a
oligoribonucleotide as primer by the enzyme is greatly facilitated by first adding
one or two deoxynucleotides to the 3′ end of the primer.

The sequential use of two different enzymes for the initiation of DNA
synthesis might have some relevance to the *in vivo* situation. It certainly would
be of advantage for regulatory purposes if the oligoribonucleotide had to be
modified by a separate enzymatic activity before it could be used as an efficient
primer.

SUMMARY

Interest in the initiation step of DNA synthesis has been stimulated by the recent
finding that oligoribonucleotides are used as primer for DNA synthesis by reverse transcriptase of avian myeloblastosis virus and possibly by *E. coli* DNA polymerase.

Recent experiments with terminal deoxynucleotidyl transferase from calf thymus revealed that this DNA-polymerizing enzyme will also accept oligoribonucleotides as primer.
It is shown that this oligoribonucleotide-primed reaction can be greatly enhanced by first
adding one or two deoxynucleotides to the 3′ end of the primer.

The initiation of DNA synthesis by an oligoribonucleotide primer may proceed in a two-step reaction as indicated by the observations described.

RESUMEN

Interés en el primer paso de la iniciación de la síntesis de DNA ha sido estimulado como consecuencia de los recientes hallazgos, los cuales indican que oligoribonucleótidos son utilizados como modelo inicial ("primer") para la síntesis de DNA por la transcriptasa reversible del virus de la mioblastosis de las aves y posiblemente por la polimerasa del DNA de *E. coli.*

Experimentos con la transferasa deoxinucleotidil terminal del timo de ternero revelaron que esta enzima polimerizante del DNA acepta también oligoribonucleótidos como modelos iniciales. Se demostrará también que ésta última reacción puede ser aumentada grandemente si se añaden al comienzo uno o dos deoxiribonculeótidos en el extremo 3′ del modelo iniciador.

La iniciación de la síntesis de DNA por un oligoribonucleótido iniciador puede que suceda en dos pasos como lo indican las observaciones discutidas.

REFERENCES

1. Goulian, M., *Ann. Rev. Biochem., 40,* 775 (1971).
2. Verma, J. M., Meuth, N. L., Bromfeld, E., Manly, K. F., and Baltimore, D., *Nature, 233,* 131 (1971).
3. Kornberg, A., K. A. Forster Lecture, Mainz, Germany (October 1971).
4. Chang, L. M. S., and Bollum, F. J., *J. Biol. Chem., 246,* 909 (1971).
5. Chang, L. M. S., *Biochem. Biophys. Res. Commun., 44,* 124 (1971).
6. Chang, L. M. S., and Bollum, F. J., *Biochemistry, 10,* 536 (1971).
7. Jensen, R. H., Wodzinski, R. J., and Rogoff, M. H., *Biochem. Biophys. Res. Commun., 43,* 384 (1971).
8. Feix, G., *FEBS Letters, 18,* 280 (1971).
9. Kaufmann, G., and Littauer, O. Z., *FEBS Letters, 4,* 79 (1969).
10. Bon, S., Godefroy, Th., and Grunberg-Manago, M., *Europ. J. Biochem., 16,* 363 (1970).
11. Feix, G., *Biochem. Biophys. Res. Commun., 46,* 2141 (1972).

DISCUSSION

R. T. Schimke (Stanford, U.S.A.): Do you feel then that this is a system that may occur in both eukaryotes and prokaryotes?

G. Feix (Freiburg, Germany): One can think on this line because of the finding in Kornberg's laboratory with a bacterial system and the results of Baltimore's group with the tumor virus. In the case of the *E. coli* system, it has not been shown yet that an oligoribonucleotide is covalently bound to the DNA—so far, it has only been shown that a transcription product is important for the initiation of DNA synthesis. In the case of the tumor virus, it has conclusively been demonstrated that the oligoribonucleotide primer is really linked up to the growing chain. So it is quite possible that it is a more common reaction, and this certainly would be of advantage—it would be a kind of positive control of the initiation step.

26

"Enzymatic" and "Nonenzymatic" Translation

A. S. Spirin

Institute of Protein Research
Academy of Sciences of the USSR
Poustchino, Moscow Region
and
A. N. Bakh Institute of Biochemistry
Academy of Sciences of the USSR
Moscow, USSR

According to modern concepts, the translating ribosome is a cyclically working molecular machine. Each elementary working cycle of the ribosome in the process of translation (elongation) results in the reading out of one template triplet and the formation of one peptide bond. It is now known that in addition to the ribosome, the bound template, the bound peptidyl-tRNA, and the aminoacyl-tRNA, the participants of each cycle include the soluble proteins T and G (or TF1 and TF2 in the case of animal ribosomes), acting as enzymatic factors, and GTP,* which is cleaved into GDP and orthophosphate in the course of translation.

The elementary working cycle of the ribosome can be subdivided into at least five consecutive steps (Fig. 1): Step 1 is the codon-directed binding of the aminoacyl-tRNA-T factor (TF1)-GTP complex with the ribosome. This is the

---

* Abbreviations: tRNA, transfer ribonucleic acid; phe-tRNA, phenylalanyl-tRNA; poly U, polyuridylic acid; TCA, trichloroacetic acid; PCMB, *para*-chloromercuribenzoate; ME, 2-mercaptoethanol; DTT, dithiothreitol; GTP, guanosine-5'-triphosphate; GDP, guanosine-5'-diphosphate; GMP-PCP, guanylyl-5'-methylene diphosphonate.

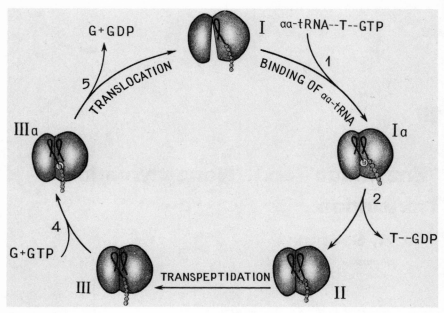

Fig. 1. The working cycle of the elongating ribosome in the process of "enzymatic" translation.

so-called enzymatic binding of aminoacyl-tRNA. First of all, the aminoacyl-tRNA complexes with the T factor and GTP outside the ribosome, and then this complex efficiently interacts with the ribosome. It is assumed that the specific (codon-directed) binding of aminoacyl-tRNA is "catalyzed" in this way by the T factor preactivated by GTP. Step 2 is the cleavage of GTP and release of the T factor (TF1) with GDP and orthophosphate. The GTPase activity of the ribosome is induced only after the attachment to it of the T factor. After GTP cleavage, the T factor seems to lose its affinity for aminoacyl-tRNA and is released from the ribosome. Step 3 is transpeptidation. The aminoacyl-tRNA that has just been bound and the peptidyl-tRNA retained on the ribosome are substrates of the reaction; the peptidyl residue is transferred to the aminoacyl-tRNA amino group, resulting in a new peptidyl-tRNA elongated by one aminoacyl residue and deacylated tRNA as products of the reaction.

$$\text{Peptidyl}(n)\text{-tRNA}' + \text{aminoacyl-tRNA}'' \rightarrow \text{peptidyl}(n+1)\text{-tRNA}'' + \text{tRNA}'$$

A new peptide bond is thus formed. The reaction is catalyzed by the ribosome itself and does not require additional enzymes. Step 4 is the binding of the G factor (TF2) and GTP with the ribosome. It appears that GTP interacts with the

G factor and activates it for binding with the ribosome. Step 5 is the cleavage of GTP, the release of the G factor (TF2), and the conjugated translocation. The GTPase activity is induced in the ribosome as a result of the attachment of the G factor. It is assumed that the G factor is an "enzyme" catalyzing the energy-dependent act of translocation. Translocation consists of the newly formed peptidyl-tRNA being displaced from the site of the ribosome which it occupies (A site) to the other site on the ribosome (P site), where it will be retained until the following act of transpeptidation; simultaneously and in conjunction with the displacement of peptidyl-tRNA, the template is shifted by one triplet, while the deacylated tRNA is pushed out (from the P site) and leaves the ribosome.

After step 5, the ribosome is again competent to bind aminoacyl-tRNA. The cycle can be repeated again. It is the manifold repetition of such cycles that forms the process of translation (elongation).

The "enzymatic," i.e., the T(TF1)-GTP dependent binding of aminoacyl-tRNA was discovered by R. Schweet's group, first in an animal ribosome system (1-4) and later also in bacterial systems (5,6). The T factor (T_u, TF1) catalyzing binding was shown to be a large SH-containing protein which is comparatively easily inactivated by heating and oxidation (7-10). This protein joins into a complex with the GTP molecule and as a result of this acquires an affinity for the aminoacyl-tRNA molecule, forming a triple aminoacyl-tRNA-T-GTP complex; the latter is the form in which aminoacyl-tRNA enters the ribosome (5,6,10-14). At first, the whole complex associates with the ribosome, and then cleavage in it of GTP to GDP and orthophosphate occurs, as a result of which the aminoacyl-tRNA is left in the ribosome while the T-GDP complex and orthophosphate are released.

It was found that codon-directed binding of aminoacyl-tRNA with the ribosome can also be achieved in the absence of the T factor and GTP (15-21). This "nonenzymatic" binding of aminoacyl-tRNA only requires Mg^{2+} concentrations higher than that optimal for "enzymatic" binding and for the working of the complete cell-free system as a whole. For example, while a high level of "enzymatic" binding is observed at 8-12 mM Mg^{2+}, a good "nonenzymatic" binding requires 20 mM Mg^{2+}. The "nonenzymatic" binding results in a correct, functional binding of the aminoacyl-tRNA molecule in the ribosome: the bound aminoacyl-tRNA is then capable of participating in the ribosome-catalyzed transpeptidation reaction (22-24). Consequently, at somewhat higher Mg^{2+} concentrations than those considered as physiological, state Ia in the working cycle of the ribosome (Fig. 1) can be sidestepped. Thus the "nonenzymatic" binding creates a kind of bypass permitting translation to proceed without an "enzyme" and energy in the first stages of the cycle.

If there is peptidyl-tRNA (in the P site) and codon-bound aminoacyl-tRNA (in the A site) in the ribosome, then they interact with each other in a reaction catalyzed by a special peptidyl transferase center of the ribosome. It was earlier believed that for such a transpeptidation reaction a soluble enzyme was required, and, in particular, the T factor (TF1) was suspected to be such an enzyme (2,3,7,8,17). This did not happen to be the case: it was established that the T factor must leave the ribosome before the transpeptidation reaction occurs (13,14), and the "peptidyl transferase" was shown to be an integral part of the large (50S and 60S) subparticle of the ribosome (25-28). The peptidyl transferase center of the ribosome seems to be formed by structural ribosomal proteins (29), is not sensitive to such oxidizing agents as PCMB (25.26), and maintains full activity in a very wide range of Mg^{2+} and K^+ or NH_4^+ concentrations (30). The reaction of transpeptidation does not require any supplementary enzymatic or energetic additions.

After the transpeptidation reaction, the peptidyl residue is bound to the tRNA residue occupying the A site of the ribosome, i.e., the codon-directed aminoacyl-tRNA binding site. The P site, i.e., the peptidyl-tRNA retaining site, is now occupied by deacylated tRNA. Hence, before the cycle begins again and the next aminoacyl-tRNA is bound, the tRNA residue of the newly formed peptidyl-tRNA has to be carried over (translocated) from the A site to the P site, and simultaneously the template (mRNA) must be also shifted (translocated) by one triplet (codon). Consequently, the transfer of rather large molecular masses within the ribosome is needed, and thus the translocation is a mechanical function. Translocation appears to be the most characteristic event in the functioning ribosome; it is translocation that makes the ribosome a molecular machine and not a simple analogue of a large enzyme. It can be asserted that elucidation of the basic mechanism of translocation would mean the elucidation of the main principle of the working of the ribosome.

It seemed established that translocation as a mechanical function necessarily requires GTP energy and the participation of a corresponding "enzyme," the G factor, responsible for involving GTP in the process of translocation and for the conjugated cleavage of GTP in the ribosome (25,31-38). Indeed, in the absence of the G factor and GTP, the ribosome can bind aminoacyl-tRNA and form a peptide bond, but at this point the cycle is interrupted and no following translation occurs; thus the matter is limited to the formation of one peptide bond (34-39). The G factor (TF2) catalyzing translocation is a rather large protein very sensitive to oxidation of its SH groups (1-3,32,40-43). For binding with an untranslocated (pretranslocated) ribosome, it must interact with a GTP molecule. After association of the pretranslocated ribosome with the G factor and GTP, the GTPase activity is induced in the ribosome with the participation of the G factor. Translocation seems to proceed in conjunction with GTP cleavage or, more likely, with the subsequent release of the G factor (TF2) from the ribosome (44,45). The molecular mechanism of translocation is not known.

It was quite unexpected to find that, in certain conditions, translocation in the ribosome can be achieved without participation of the G factor and GTP. The possibility of "nonenzymatic" translocation was first discovered and definitely enunciated by Pestka (46,47) and later confirmed in our laboratory (48,49). It was shown that under conditions of "nonenzymatic" binding of Phe-tRNA with thoroughly washed *Escherichia coli* ribosomes charged with poly U, at 20 mM Mg^{2+}, the formation of oligophenylalanines (as well as TCA-insoluble polyphenylalanines after prolonged incubation) can be observed in the absence of G factor and GTP (46-48). However, purely conceptually, the possibility of mechanical functions being performed "without energy" was difficult to comprehend, and doubt on the purity of ribosomal preparations from G factor served as a shield for many serious investigators against the necessity of accepting these data as a fact.

The main evidence in favor of translocation taking place spontaneously, in a system without addition of the G factor and GTP, and not as a result of the presence of admixtures of the transfer factor, was based on the following: In the first place, the energy of activation measured for the usual "enzymatic" cell-free system strongly differs from that of the newly discovered "nonenzymatic" system (47). Secondly, the GTPase-resistant analogue of GTP, guanylyl-methylene diphosphonate (GMP-PCP), a competitive inhibitor of G-GTP dependent translocation, did not appear to have any influence on the "nonenzymatic" translocation (46-48). In the third place, powerful SH inhibitors, such as *para*-chloromercuribenzyl sulfonate and PCMB, which completely inactivate the G factor, did not inhibit the "nonenzymatic" translocation (46-48). It was also shown that fusidic acid, a specific inhibitor of the G factor, does not affect the "nonenzymatic" translocation (47).

Table I is presented as a demonstration of the fact that both GMP-PCP and

Table I. Effect of GMP-PCP and PCMB on Polyphenylalanine Synthesis in the Complete ("Enzymatic") Poly U-Directed Cell-Free System[a]

Inhibitor	Concentration of inhibitor (M)	TCA-insoluble ^{14}C-polyphenylalanine (cpm)
− GMP-PCP	−	6360
+ GMP-PCP	10^{-3}	160
− PCMB	−	7500
+ PCMB	3×10^{-4}	60

[a] The reaction mixture was prepared in a 20 mM MgCl$_2$, 100 mM KCl, 10 mM Tris-HCl buffer; 0.3 ml contained about 50 μg ribosomes, 20 μg poly U, about 70 μg ^{14}C-Phe-labeled total aminoacyl-tRNA, about 50 μg protein fraction containing transfer factors, 30 μg GTP, 250 μg phosphoenolpyruvate, 1 μg phosphoenolpyruvate kinase. Incubation time was 30 min at 25°.

Table II. Effect of GMP-PCP and PCMB on the "Nonenzymatic" Poly U-Directed Cell-Free System[a]

Inhibitor	Concentration of inhibitor (M)	Total binding of ^{14}C-Phe (cpm)	$Phe_2 + Phe_{>2}$[b] (chromatographically) (cpm)
– GMP-PCP	–	1610	720
+ GMP-PCP	10^{-3}	2060	720
– PCMB	–	2620	846
+ PCMB	3×10^{-4}	3040	1420

[a] Conditions and ingredient concentrations were the same as in Table I, with the exception that the protein fraction containing transfer factors, GTP, phosphoenolpyruvate, and phosphoenolpyruvate kinase were omitted.
[b] In the chromatograms, 50-65% of the label migrated as ^{14}C-Phe$_2$; the rest of the label was represented by ^{14}C-Phe$_{\geqslant 3}$.

PCMB do totally inhibit the complete ("enzymatic") cell-free system. Table II represents data showing the result of introduction of the same inhibitors into a system where transfer factors, GTP, and GTP-generating additions have been omitted but all the other components, ionic conditions, and incubation time have been preserved. It is seen that neither GMP-PCP nor PCMB inhibits the binding of Phe-tRNA and the formation of di- and oligo-phenylalanines in this "nonenzymatic" system.

Under "nonenzymatic" conditions, short oligo-phenylalanines were mainly formed during the first 30 min at 25°. Further incubation of the system, up to a few hours, led to an accumulation of long TCA-insoluble ^{14}C-polyphenyla-lanines. It was noticed, however, that in repeated experiments the rate of polyphenylalanine synthesis could vary greatly, even when the same original preparations were used. Occasionally, the "nonenzymatic" system was even practically inactive in the synthesis of long TCA-insoluble polyphenyla-lanines. This roused suspicion and again fed suppositions concerning some kind of "enzymatic" contaminations.

These doubts were conclusively decided by the unexpected discovery of the fact that the capability for "nonenzymatic" translocation may be latent and is abruptly stimulated by the oxidation or blocking of some SH groups of the ribosome, in particular under the action of PCMB (49). Thus the oxidation-reduction level of the ribosome appeared to be the factor determining its activity in the "nonenzymatic" system.

Figure 2 shows that the system consisting of thoroughly washed ribosomes, poly U, and ^{14}C-Phe-tRNA, without the addition of any enzymatic factors and GTP, carries out poly U-directed synthesis of TCA-insoluble ^{14}C-poly-phenylalanine in the presence of PCMB and practically does not do so in the presence of DTT. Figure 3 shows that if DTT or ME is added to the already working PCMB-activated system, the rate of "nonenzymatic" translation decreases. On the contrary, as seen in Figure 4, if the system was incubated for a few hours with DTT and did not display noticeable polymerizing activity, the subsequent addition of PCMB activated it. Separate experiments confirmed that

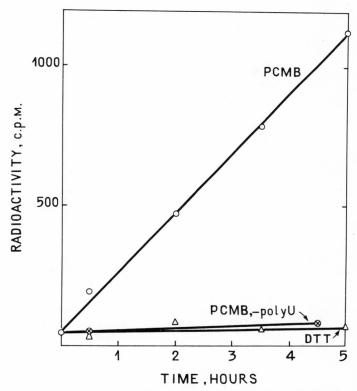

Fig. 2. *Effect of PCMB and DTT on the poly U-directed synthesis of polyphenylalanine in the "nonenzymatic" (devoid of transfer factors and GTP) cell-free system.* PCMB was present in 10^{-4} M concentration, DTT in 10^{-3} M concentration. The concentrations of ingredients of the system, ionic conditions, and incubation temperature were the same as in Table II. The amount of TCA-insoluble ^{14} C-polyphenylalanine (cpm) is plotted *vs.* incubation time. ○, with PCMB; △, with DTT; ⊕, with PCMB, without poly U. [The figure is reproduced from Gavrilova and Spirin (49) by permission of North-Holland Publ. Co.]

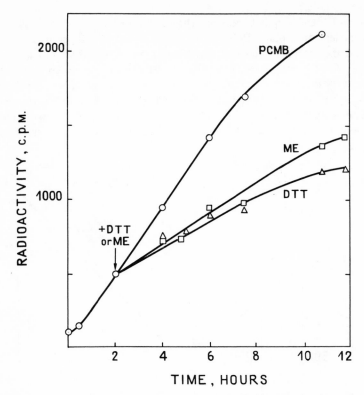

Fig. 3. Effect of adding DTT and ME to the PCMB-stimulated "non-enzymatic" system. PCMB was initially present in 10^{-4} *M* concentration; after 2 hr incubation, DTT or ME was added to a concentration of 10^{-3} *M* or 2×10^{-3} *M*, respectively, to the experimental sample, while the control sample was further incubated without the additions (in the presence of PCMB). Other conditions were the same as in Fig. 2. ○, with PCMB; △, plus DTT; □, plus ME. [The figure is reproduced from Gavrilova and Spirin (49) by permission of North-Holland Publ. Co.]

DTT and ME inhibit neither "nonenzymatic" binding of ^{14}C-Phe-tRNA to the ribosome nor peptidyl transferase activity of the ribosomes. It follows that the inhibitory action of DTT and ME and the activating effect of PCMB in the "nonenzymatic" system are most likely related to the capability of ribosomes for spontaneous translocation: in the presence of SH compounds it is suppressed, whereas it is activated as a result of oxidation or blocking of some SH groups of the ribosome by PCMB.

It is interesting that ribosomes washed in buffers without SH compounds can also exhibit a capability for spontaneous ("nonenzymatic") translocation (46,47), possibly due to oxidation by the air dissolved in the buffers.

In any case, the possibility of translocation taking place without the participation of transfer "enzymatic" proteins and GTP definitely demonstrates that the principal mechanism of translocation is an intrinsic feature of the structural organization of the ribosome itself and is not prescribed by external factors. In normal conditions, this principal ability of the ribosome is realized "enzymatically," by the G factor and GTP, with a high efficiency. However, conditions can be created when the same ability is realized without the "enzyme" and energy, although naturally at much lower rates. Consequently, a bypass can be made at this point of the working cycle of the ribosome as well, omitting the stages of binding and release of the G factor and GTP.

The complete (three-step) working cycle of the "nonenzymatic" translation is represented in Fig. 5. In contrast to the working cycle of normal "enzymatic" translation (Fig. 1), two steps of which can be blocked by GMP-PCP and PCMB, none of the steps of the "nonenzymatic" translation are inhibited by these

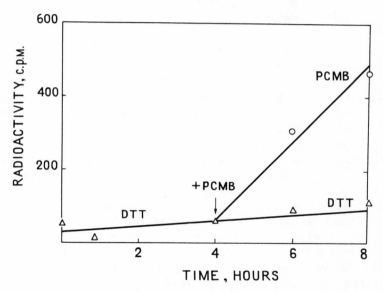

Fig. 4. *Effect of adding PCMB to the DTT-inhibited "nonenzymatic" system.* DTT was initially present in 10^{-4} M concentration. After 4 hr incubation, PCMB was added to 5×10^{-4} M concentration to the experimental sample, while the control sample was further incubated without the addition (in the presence of DTT). Other conditions were the same as in Fig. 2. △, with DTT; ○, plus PCMB. [The figure is reproduced from Gavrilova and Spirin (49) by permission of North-Holland Publ. Co.]

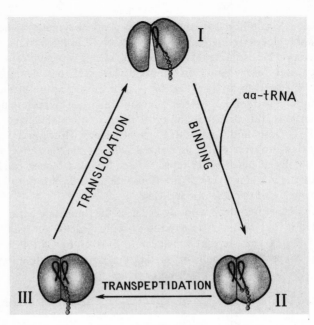

Fig. 5. The working cycle of the ribosome in the process of "nonenzymatic" translation.

agents. That is why the introduction of PCMB into the system or use of PCMB-treated ribosomes presents the best way of discriminating the "nonenzymatic" from the "enzymatic" translation.

The most interesting and promising result of the discovery of "nonenzymatic" translation seems to be a new approach to the problem of the functional role of the transfer factors and GTP and to the ribosomal mechanism of translocation. Three years ago, a hypothetical model of translocation was suggested according to which the driving mechanism of all spatial shifts of tRNA and mRNA was the periodical movement of the two ribosomal subparticles in a locking and unlocking manner (50-52). The model, as can be seen, presumed that the mechanism of translocation is inherent in the structural organization of the ribosome itself and, in particular, is laid down by its two-subparticle construction. The data showing that translocation can be produced by the ribosome itself, without the participation of additional factors, are in full agreement with this main idea. Moreover, the system of "nonenzymatic" translation, since it is not complicated by the participation of the transfer factors and GTP, permits, in its turn, a check on the suggested hypothesis of the molecular mechanism of translocation (50-52). The role of the G factor and GTP can be regarded as that of catalyzers, both kinetically and thermodynamically (at the expense of GTP cleavage) promoting the ribosome-inherent mechanism of translocation.

The experimental data demonstrating the role of the lability of ribosomal subparticle association in performing translocation will be presented elsewhere.

SUMMARY

The elementary working cycle of the translating (elongating) ribosome can be subdivided into the following five consecutive steps: step 1, binding of aminoacyl-tRNA with T factor and GTP; step 2, hydrolysis of GTP and release of the T factor; step 3, transpeptidation (peptide bond formation); step 4, binding of G factor with GTP; step 5, hydrolysis of GTP, release of the G factor, and the conjugated translocation. Repetition of these cycles creates the process of translation.

Besides the T-GTP dependent ("enzymatic") binding of aminoacyl-tRNA, the so-called nonenzymatic binding, in the absence of the T factor and GTP, can be observed in a cell-free system. The "nonenzymatic" binding requires a higher Mg^{2+} concentration than the "enzymatic" binding and seems to be less efficient. Nonetheless, the "nonenzymatically" bound aminoacyl-tRNA may occupy the normal functional site of the ribosome and can then participate in peptide bond formation.

Transpeptidation, i.e., the reaction of peptide bond formation, is catalyzed by the ribosome itself. The peptidyl transferase center is an integral part of the large (50S or 60S) ribosomal subparticle. No additional "enzymatic" or energetic factors are required for the transpeptidation reaction.

Translocation is a mechanical transfer of tRNA residues and mRNA chain in the ribosome after transpeptidation. The absolute requirement for the "enzymatic" G factor and GTP energy in the translocation process is usually presumed. However, "nonenzymatic" translocation in the absence of the G factor and GTP can be observed in a cell-free system as well. It has been shown that while p-chloromercuribenzoate completely inhibits "enzymatic" translocation through inactivation of the G factor, it stimulates "nonenzymatic" translocation in the ribosome. Hence, the capability for translocation is found to be an intrinsic feature of the structural organization of the ribosome itself. A kinematic model of translocation based on the assumption of mutual mobility (locking-unlocking) of the two ribosomal subparticles is suggested.

Thus, in the absence of transfer factors (T and G) and GTP, the ribosome is capable of (a) "nonenzymatically" binding aminoacyl-tRNA, (b) catalyzing peptide bond formation, and (c) "nonenzymatically" performing translocation. Repetition of this three-step cycle creates the process of "nonenzymatic" translation. The system of "nonenzymatic" translation, though less efficient than the "enzymatic" one, was shown to synthesize long polyphenylalanine chains in the presence of poly U as a template. In contrast to the usual "enzymatic" cell-free system, the "nonenzymatic" system works well in the presence of p-chloromercuribenzoate. The discovery of "nonenzymatic" translation seems to generate a new approach to the study of the mechanism of translocation and the role of transfer factors and GTP in translation.

RESUMEN

El ciclo de trabajo elemental del ribosoma traductor (elongador) puede ser dividido en las cinco etapas consecutivas siguientes: 1) unión del aminoacil-tRNA con el factor T y GTP; 2) hidrólisis del GTP y liberación del factor T; 3) transpeptidación (formación del enlace peptídico); 4) unión del factor G con GTP; 5) hidrólisis del GTP, liberación del factor G y la translocación conjugadaLa repetición de estos ciclos crea el proceso de la traducción.

Además de la unión del aminoacil-tRNA T-GTP-dependiente (enzimática), puede observarse en el sistema acelular la llamada unión no enzimática, en ausencia del factor T y GTP. La unión no enzimática requiere una concentración de Mg^{2+} mayor que la unión enzimática, y parece ser menos eficiente. Sin embargo, el aminoacil-tRNA unido en forma no enzimática ocupa el sitio funcional normal del ribosoma y puede tomar parte por lo tanto en la formación de la unión peptídica.

La transpeptidación, es decir, la reacción de formación del enlace peptídico, es catalizada por el ribosoma mismo. El centro de peptidil transferasa es una parte integral de la subparticula ribosómica mayor (50S o 60S). No se requieren factores adicionales "enzimáticos" o energéticos para la reacción de transpeptidación.

La translocación es una función de la transferencia mecánica de los residuos de tRNA y de la cadena de mRNA en el ribosoma después de la transpeptidación. Se supone generalmente un requerimiento absoluto de factor G y energía de GTP en el proceso "enzimático" de translocación. Sin embargo, la translocación "no enzimática" en ausencia de factor G y GTP puede ser también observada en el sistema acelular. Se ha demostrado que el p-cloromercuribenzoato inhibe completamente la translocación enzimática por inactivación del factor G pero estimula la translocación no enzimática en el ribosoma. Por lo tanto, se encuentra que la translocación es una característica intrínseca de la organización estructural del ribosoma propiamente dicho. Se sugiere un modelo cinemático de la translocación basado en la suposición de la movilidad mutua (cierreapertura) de las dos subpartículas ribosomales.

Es así como, en ausencia de factores de transferencia (T y G) y GTP, el ribosoma es capaz de 1) unir en forma no enzimática aminoacil-tRNA; 2) catalizar la formación de la unión peptídica; 3) llevar a cabo la translocación no enzimática. La repetición de este ciclo de tres pasos crea el proceso de traducción "no enzimática". Se ha demostrado que el sistema de traducción "no enzimático", si bien es menos eficiente que el "enzimático", sintetiza largas cadenas de polifenilalanina en presencia de poliU como molde.

En contraposición con el sistema acelular "enzimático" usual, el sistema no enzimático funciona bien en presencia de p-cloromercuribenzoato. El descubrimiento de la traducción no enzimática parece abrir un nuevo enfoque para el estudio del mecanismo de la translocación y del papel de los factores de transferencia y el GTP en la traducción.

REFERENCES

1. Arlinghaus, R., Favelukes, G., and Schweet, R., *Biochem. Biophys. Res. Commun., 11*, 92 (1963).
2. Hardesty, B., Arlinghaus, R., Shaeffer, J., and Schweet, R., *Cold Spring Harbor Symp. Quant. Biol., 28*, 215 (1963).
3. Arlinghaus, R., Shaeffer, J., and Schweet, R., *Proc. Natl. Acad. Sci. U.S.A., 51*, 1291 (1964).
4. Ravel, J. M., Mosteller, R. D., and Hardesty, B., *Proc. Natl. Acad. Sci. U.S.A., 56*, 701 (1966).
5. Ravel, J. M., *Proc. Natl. Acad. Sci. U.S.A., 57*, 1811 (1967).
6. Ravel, J. M., Shorey, R. L., and Shive, W., *Biochem. Biophys. Res. Commun., 29*, 68 (1967).
7. Allende, J., Monro, R., and Lipmann, F., *Proc. Natl. Acad. Sci. U.S.A., 51*, 1211 (1964).
8. Nishizuka, Y., and Lipmann, F., *Proc. Natl. Acad. Sci. U.S.A., 55*, 212 (1966).
9. Lucas-Lenard, J., and Lipmann, F., *Proc. Natl. Acad. Sci. U.S.A., 55*, 1562 (1966).

10. Hardesty, B., Culp, W., and McKeehan, W., *Cold Spring Harbor Symp. Quant. Biol., 34,* 331 (1969).
11. Ravel, J. M., Shorey, R. L., Garner, C. W., Dawkins, R. C., and Shive, W., *Cold Spring Harbor Symp. Quant. Biol., 34,* 321 (1969).
12. Weissbach, H., Brot, N., Miller, D., Rosman, M., and Ertel, R., *Cold Spring Harbor Symp. Quant. Biol., 34,* 419 (1969).
13. Skoultchi, A., Ono, Y., Waterson, J., and Lengyel, P., *Cold Spring Harbor Symp. Quant. Biol., 34,* 437 (1969).
14. Lucas-Lenard, J., Tao, P., and Haenni, A.-L., *Cold Spring Harbor Symp. Quant. Biol., 34,* 455 (1969).
15. Kaji, A., and Kaji, H., *Biochem. Biophys. Res. Commun., 13,* 186 (1963).
16. Kaji, A., and Kaji, H., *Proc. Natl. Acad. Sci. U.S.A., 52,* 1541 (1964).
17. Nakamoto, T., Conway, T. W., Allende, J. E., Spyrides, G. J., and Lipmann, F., *Cold Spring Harbor Symp. Quant. Biol., 28,* 227 (1963).
18. Spyrides, G. J., *Proc. Natl. Acad. Sci. U.S.A., 51,* 1220 (1964).
19. Nirenberg, M. W., and Leder, P., *Science, 145,* 1399 (1964).
20. Leder, P., and Nirenberg, M. W., *Proc. Natl. Acad. Sci. U.S.A., 52,* 420 (1964).
21. Leder, P., and Nirenberg, M. W., *Proc. Natl. Acad. Sci. U.S.A., 52,* 1521 (1964).
22. Gottesman, M. E., *J. Biol. Chem., 242,* 5564 (1967).
23. Pestka, S., *J. Biol. Chem., 242,* 4939 (1967).
24. Pulkrábek, P., and Rychlík, I., *Biochim. Biophys. Acta, 155,* 219 (1968).
25. Traut, R. R., and Monro, R. E., *J. Mol. Biol., 10,* 63 (1964).
26. Monro, R. E., *J. Mol. Biol., 26,* 147 (1967).
27. Maden, B. E. H., Traut, R. R., and Monro, R. F., *J. Mol. Biol., 35,* 333 (1968).
28. Vazquez, D., Battaner, E., Neth, R., Heller, G., and Monro, R. E., *Cold Spring Harbor Symp. Quant. Biol., 34,* 369 (1969).
29. Staehelin, T., Maglott, D., and Monro, R. E., *Cold Spring Harbor Symp. Quant. Biol., 34,* 39 (1969).
30. Maden, B. E. H., and Monro, R. E., *Europ. J. Biochem., 6,* 309 (1968).
31. Conway, T. W., and Lipmann, F., *Proc. Natl. Acad. Sci. U.S.A., 52,* 1462 (1964).
32. Nishizuka, Y., and Lipmann, F., *Arch. Biochem. Biophys., 116,* 344 (1966).
33. Haenni, A.-L., and Lucas-Lenard, J., *Proc. Natl. Acad. Sci. U.S.A., 61,* 1363 (1968).
34. Lucas-Lenard, J., and Haenni, A.-L., *Proc. Natl. Acad. Sci. U.S.A., 59,* 554 (1968).
35. Lucas-Lenard, J., and Haenni, A.-L., *Proc. Natl. Acad. Sci. U.S.A., 63,* 93 (1969).
36. Erbe, R. W., and Leder, P., *Biochem. Biophys. Res. Commun., 31,* 798 (1968).
37. Erbe, R. W., Nau, M. M., and Leder, P., *J. Mol. Biol., 39,* 441 (1969).
38. Brot, N., Ertel, R., and Weissbach, H., *Biochem. Biophys. Res. Commun., 31,* 563 (1968).
39. Pestka, S., *Proc. Natl. Acad. Sci. U.S.A., 61,* 726 (1968).
40. Lucas-Lenard, J., and Lipmann, F., *Proc. Natl. Acad. Sci. U.S.A., 55,* 1562 (1966).
41. Parmeggiani, A., and Gottschalk, E. M., *Cold Spring Harbor Symp. Quant. Biol., 34,* 377 (1969).
42. Kaziro, Y., Inoue, N., Kuriki, Y., Mizumato, K., Tanaka, M., and Kawakita, M., *Cold Spring Harbor Symp. Quant. Biol., 34,* 385 (1969).
43. Moldave, K., Galasinki, W., Rao, P., and Siler, J., *Cold Spring Harbor Symp. Quant. Biol., 34,* 347 (1969).
44. Bodley, J. W., Zieve, F. J., Lin, L., and Zieve, S. T., *Biochem. Biophys. Res. Commun., 37,* 437 (1969).
45. McKeehan, W., and Hardesty, B., *Biochem. Biophys. Res. Commun., 36,* 625 (1969).
46. Pestka, S., *J. Biol. Chem., 243,* 2810 (1968).

47. Pestka, S., *J. Biol. Chem., 244,* 1533 (1969).
48. Gavrilova, L. P., and Smolyaninov, V. V., *Molekul. Biol. (USSR), 5,* 883 (1971).
49. Gavrilova, L. P., and Spirin, A. S., *FEBS Letters, 17,* 324 (1971).
50. Spirin, A. S., *Dokl. Akad. Nauk SSSR, 179,* 1467 (1968).
51. Spirin, A. S., *Currents Mod. Biol., 2,* 115 (1968).
52. Spirin, A. S., *Cold Spring Harbor Symp. Quant. Biol., 34,* 197 (1969).

DISCUSSION

R. Brentani (São Paulo, Brazil): You said that the activity of the ribosomes in your system can increase with repeated washing. Did you check whether there was modification in the size of these ribosomes through washing?

A. S. Spirin (Poustchino, USSR): We didn't find any definite changes in size or in other physical properties during washing. The appearance or increase of the activity of the nonenzymatic system as a result of washing is not reproducible from time to time. This may be the effect of some oxidation of the SH groups of ribosomes by oxygen of the air.

R. Bock (Madison, U.S.A.): Have you checked to see whether the nonhydrolyzable analogues of GTP inhibit this process and whether organic solvents enhance it?

A. S. Spirin: Is your question about using GMP-PCP? GMP-PCP does not inhibit the process of nonenzymatic translation. I can say that we can have both results with organic solvents, activation and suppression, because introduction of organic solvents into the reaction medium shifts the magnesium optimum of the process.

R. Bock: It would be interesting to check whether messengers that are not monotonic will also participate in the translocation, because it is possible that you are not translocating a triplet at a time, but since the base of the message is monotonic, there could be a series of discrete one-base steps.

A. S. Spirin: Dr. S. Pestka has carried out experiments with UUUG, UUUUUUG, and UUUUUUUUUG, and he found for the nonenzymatic system that no formation of peptides occurred in the first case, just diphenylalanine was formed in the case of the heptanucleotide, and the formation of triphenylalanine required the decanucleotide. It means that the system looks like real translation of poly U.

H. R. Mahler (Bloomington, U.S.A.): Have you checked whether more than one ribosome is capable of participating in this nonenzymatic cycle on any one messenger molecule? In other words, do you form nonenzymatic polysomes?

A. S. Spirin: No, we have not checked it.

F. Lipmann (New York, U.S.A.): Have you used other messenger RNAs besides poly U?

A. S. Spirin: This is exactly what we plan to do now.

E. P. Geiduschek (La Jolla, U.S.A.): Do you have any information on the efficiency of nonenzymatic synthesis?

A. S. Spirin: No, we just know that the whole process requires hours instead of minutes in the case of enzymatic translocation. It seems that the whole enzymatic system is about two orders of magnitude more efficient than the nonenzymatic system.

E. P. Geiduschek: Have you tried to use just single 30S subunits in the nonenzymatic system to see whether each one can serve many 50S subunits?

A. S. Spirin: No, we have not. It is unlikely because we know that the association of the subunits within translating ribosome is completely irreversible. If translating ribosome is dissociated by some artificial way, for example, by very low magnesium concentration, then the reassociation does not occur. If you precharge 30S with Phe-tRNA and poly U and take polyphenylalanine-charged 50S, they cannot associate with each other at all. This means that they cannot continue the synthesis of the same polypeptide if it was just once interrupted by dissociation.

F. Lipmann: What electrolytes do you use in your medium? Do you use potassium and magnesium? At what concentrations?

A. S. Spirin: We used 20 mM magnesium chloride with 100 mM potassium chloride and 10 mM Tris buffer, pH 7, 25°. In more recent experiments, we used 13 mM magnesium because the system works better under these conditions.

Unidentified speaker: Did you check whether the nonenzymatic synthesis can proceed without mRNA?

A. S. Spirin: No formation of oligophenylalanine or polyphenylalanine or even diphenylalanine occurs in the absence of poly U.

27

The Ribosome Cycle in Bacteria

I. D. Algranati, N. S. González, M. García-Patrone, C. A. Perazzolo, and M. E. Azzam

Instituto de Investigaciones Bioquímicas "Fundación Campomar"
and
Facultad de Ciencias Exactas
Buenos Aires, Argentina

A growing bacterial cell contains 10,000 to 30,000 ribosomes, most or perhaps all of which are involved in protein synthesis during the exponential phase.

Many studies have shown that ribosomal subunits, once formed, are quite stable, at least for several generations under normal physiological conditions (1-3).

A simple calculation based on the average *in vivo* rates of protein synthesis and of the formation of functional ribosomes indicates that at any time during cell growth only a small proportion of the ribosomes engaged in translation (no more than 1-5%) are newly made particles. All the others have been used previously for many rounds of polypeptide synthesis (4). Therefore, the ribosomes participate periodically in the successive steps of a cycle, which has been extensively investigated in the last few years. For these studies, four main approaches have been followed: (a) the analysis of ribosomal distribution in bacterial lysates, (b) the investigation of polypeptide synthesis initiation *in vitro,* (c) the measurement of subunit exchange between ribosomes during protein synthesis *in vivo* and *in vitro,* and (d) the kinetics of labeling of the ribosomal particles from RNA or protein precursors, using pulse-chase experiments.

The proportions of the different ribosomal species found in bacterial lysates

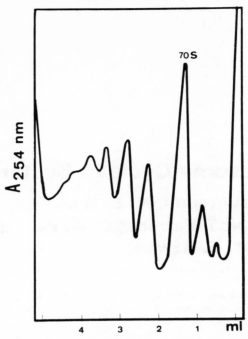

Fig. 1. *Ribosomal distribution pattern of an extract from growing* E. coli. Lysates were obtained as described previously (13) from exponentially growing cells harvested by fast cooling of the cultures. Bacterial extracts were centrifuged on 15-40% linear sucrose gradients for 90 min at 50,000 rpm in a Spinco SW65 rotor, and the absorbance was recorded with an Isco ultraviolet analyzer.

depend strictly on the physiological state of the cells and vary according to the conditions employed during the preparation and analysis of the extracts.

Several investigators have reported that lysates of growing bacteria contained substantial amounts of polyribosomes and subunits but only traces or no 70S ribosomes (5). These results were interpreted to mean that 70S particles do not exist *in vivo*, but can be formed artificially by degradation of polyribosomes (5-8) or association of subunits in the presence of mRNA (9,10).

However, more careful studies carried out in many laboratories have led to different conclusions: when exponentially growing cells were rapidly cooled, immediately broken with very mild methods, and the concentration of ions was maintained as close as possible to the intracellular levels, the corresponding bacterial lysates contained about 65-75% of their ribosomes as polysomes, around 15-20% as 70S monomers, and the remaining 6-12% as subunits. Figure 1 shows a typical ribosomal profile obtained by sucrose gradient centrifugation analysis of an extract corresponding to growing *Escherichia coli* D10. This pattern did not change after the addition of aurintricarboxylic acid to the lysing medium in order to prevent the attachment of mRNA to subunits and therefore the formation of artificial initiation monosomes. Similar results were reported for several other strains of *E. coli* (11,12), *B. stearothermophilus* (13), *B. licheniformis* (14), *A. vinelandii* (15), and *B. megaterium* (16).

A large proportion of the 70S ribosomes do not bear nascent polypeptide chains, as can be shown in extracts prepared immediately after a pulse of radioactive amino acids (13,17). Other experiments have also demonstrated that these monomers are not bound to mRNA (13,18). Therefore, they are neither a product of polysomal degradation nor an initiation or termination monosome. They represent instead free 70S ribosomes which are formed after termination of each round of translation. These run-off particles accumulate with a concomitant decrease of polyribosomes in several conditions, namely, when the culture is slowly cooled, after glucose starvation, by inhibition of protein synthesis initiation, or in stationary phase cells (13).

Our results, as well as those of others, show that in addition to polysomes and subunits, bacterial lysates contain two kinds of 70S ribosomes: (a) monosomes or complexed ribosomes, fairly stable and formed by subunits, mRNA, and either fMet-tRNA or peptidyl-tRNA, and (b) free monomers or 30-50S couples, which are easily dissociated at about 1-3 mM Mg^{2+} concentration (16), in the presence of Na ions (18,19), by very mild treatment with RNase (20) or dissociation factor (11), and even by the high hydrostatic pressure generated during centrifugation at high speed (21). For these reasons, some investigators have observed only traces of 70S monomers in their extracts.

Recently, Kaempfer (22-24) has studied the exchange of the two ribosomal subparticles between the ribosomes engaged in translation and the pool of free subunits. He has concluded that on completion of polypeptide synthesis, the 30S and 50S particles are released from mRNA and join the pool of subunits. These can directly reinitiate a new round of translation, but in suboptimal conditions for protein synthesis, they reassociate to form free monomers, which would be "sidetrack" products of the ribosome cycle. According to Kaempfer's scheme, single ribosomes would not be in equilibrium with subunits; perhaps the monomers constitute a reserve of inactive ribosomes that could return to the translation process by the action of dissociation factor, when the cell needs a higher rate of protein synthesis. However, the experiments of pulse and chase carried out *in vivo* with protein or RNA precursors strongly suggested that a major part of the 70S population participates actively as an intermediate in the ribosomal cycle (3). Moreover, Spirin (25) has shown the existence of a dynamic equilibrium between free monomers and subunits. In accordance with these

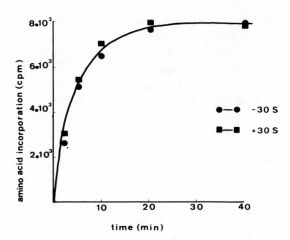

Fig. 2. Kinetics of amino acid incorporation in a cell-free system from E. coli *D10.* Reaction mixture and assay conditions were as already indicated (28).

results, we have observed that the subunit exchange of ribosomes occurs during protein synthesis as well as after its completion (26,27).

We have used a cell-free system with endogenous mRNA to study the polypeptide synthesis and the exchange between the 70S particles formed in the reaction and the radioactive subunits added to the mixture. Polyribosomes were obtained by very mild lysis of *E. coli* D10 cells harvested after rapid cooling of exponentially growing cultures. The extracts were centrifuged on a sucrose layer using conditions such that only the polysomes and a small fraction of the 70S particles reached the bottom of the tube, and the resuspended pellet was used. The S_{100} supernatant fluid was again centrifuged at high speed for a long time to eliminate the subunits; therefore, our initial reaction mixture did not contain ribosomal subparticles unless they were added.

Figure 2 shows the kinetics of polypeptide synthesis. The addition of purified 30S subunits did not change amino acid incorporation into the hot TCA-insoluble material.

The protein synthesis termination process has been measured by counting the radioactive polypeptide present in the supernatant fractions after sucrose gradient centrifugation of the samples.

Amino acid incorporation into the presumably completed polypeptides was the same either in the presence or in the absence of added 30S particles. All these controls indicated that the addition of 30S subunits to our *in vitro* system modified neither protein synthesis nor the completion and release of polypeptides. Thus we have been able to study the 30S subunit exchange between 70S ribosomes and the labeled smaller subparticles during protein synthesis. The ribosomal profiles were obtained after sucrose gradient centrifugation of samples taken at different times during protein synthesis carried out in the presence of ^{32}P-labeled 30S subunits (Fig. 3). When translation proceeds, the polyribosomes gradually disappear with a concomitant increase of the monomer. The radioactivity which sediments together with the 70S peak is a measure of the exchange.

Figure 4 shows the exchange of subunits between 70S and 30S particles during polypeptide synthesis and after its completion. In both cases, the kinetics of exchange were very similar, indicating that at any moment the 70S ribosomes can be in equilibrium with the subunit pool.

The results already described from our laboratory and several others are

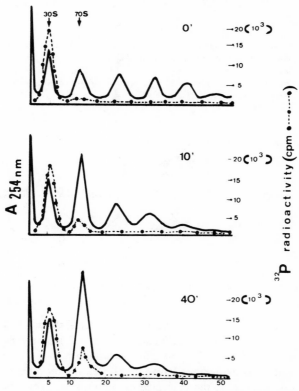

Fig. 3. Sucrose density gradient profiles after different times of polypeptide synthesis in the presence of labeled 30S subunits. Conditions were as in Fig. 2. Samples were layered on top of 5-20% (w/v) linear sucrose gradients and centrifuged for 75 min at 35,000 rpm in a SW40 rotor.

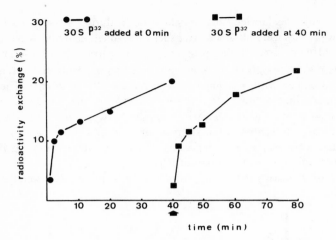

Fig. 4. Kinetics of the exchange between 70S ribosomes and
³²P-labeled 30S subunits during and after polypeptide chain termination. Experiments were carried out as in Fig. 3. The exchange
of radioactivity is expressed as percentage of the total radioactivity present in the assay.

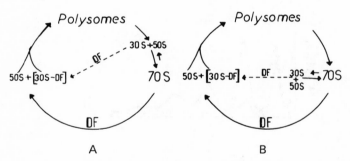

Fig. 5. Two possible models for the ribosome cycle.

compatible with both models of the ribosome cycle shown in Fig. 5. These
schemes differ only in the termination step, because it is not yet clear whether
ribosomes are released from the polysome as subunits or as 70S monomers. In
order to elucidate this matter, we have investigated the termination of polypeptide synthesis by measuring the exchange of subunits between ribosomes in the
presence of spermidine. It is well known that this polyamine, normally present
in bacteria, strongly stabilizes the 70S particles (29). On the other hand, in our
conditions spermidine did not alter amino acid incorporation or the release of
completed polypeptide chains. If the ribosomal subparticles are liberated from

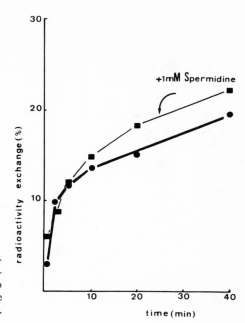

Fig. 6. Effect of spermidine on the kinetics of subunit exchange during protein synthesis. Conditions were similar to those described in Figs. 2 and 3, with the addition of spermidine where indicated.

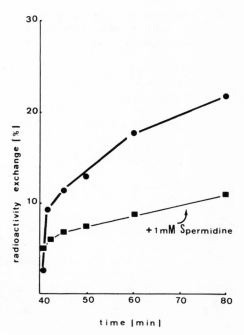

Fig. 7. Kinetics of subunit exchange after polypeptide termination in the absence or presence of spermidine. Reactions were performed as in Figs. 2 and 3. Where indicated, the spermidine was present from the beginning of the experiment; in both cases, ^{32}P 30S particles were added after 40 min of incubation.

mRNA, as shown in model A, it would be expected that spermidine would not substantially modify the exchange of subunits. On the contrary, if 70S monomers are released from polysomes on termination of translation (model B), these free ribosomes would be stabilized by spermidine with a concomitant marked decrease of the exchange.

Figure 6 demonstrates that the subunit exchange produced during protein synthesis was not affected by spermidine. On the other hand, the post-termination exchange, obtained when labeled 30S particles were added after 40 min of incubation, was clearly reduced by the presence of spermidine throughout the experiment (Fig. 7). Therefore, when the 70S particles are already formed, the polyamine can indeed stabilize them and inhibit their equilibrium with the subunits.

Table I indicates that either in the absence or in the presence of spermidine, the exchange of subunits depends on protein synthesis. When sparsomycin is added during the first incubation, the exchange is completely blocked, exclusively through the effect of this antibiotic on polypeptide elongation. This conclusion is supported by the fact that sparsomycin added during the second incubation does not inhibit the post-termination exchange of subunits.

All the results presented here, as well as the pulse-chase experiments re-

Table I. Effect of Sparsomycin on the Exchange Between 70S Particles and 30S Subunits During and After Polypeptide Synthesis[a]

First incubation	Second incubation	Exchange (%)
+ ^{32}P-30S	—	22.1
+ ^{32}P-30S + 1mM spermidine	—	22.5
+ ^{32}P-30S + 1mM spermidine + 0.1mM sparsomycin	—	7.3
+ ^{32}P-30S + 0.1mM sparsomycin	—	4.8
—	+ ^{32}P-30S	25.4
—	+ ^{32}P-30S + 0.1 mM sparsomycin	24.0
Control without incubation		3.5

[a] Labeled 30S subparticles, spermidine, and sparsomycin were added to the complete system at zero time (first incubation) or after 40 min (second incubation) as indicated. Assay conditions were as in Figs. 2 and 3. First incubation was for 40 min and the second for 20 min.

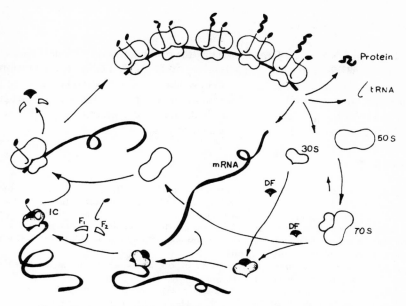

Fig. 8. Proposed model for the ribosome cycle during protein synthesis.

ported by Van Dijk-Salkinoja and Planta (3), are in agreement with model A that we have postulated for the ribosome cycle. This model is shown in detail in Fig. 8.

The initiation complex is formed by the interaction of 30S subunit, F3 or dissociation factor, mRNA, f-Met-tRNA, and initiation factors F1 and F2. The 50S subunit is then added and the monosome is formed, in this way starting the translation process. After elongation, when nascent polypeptide chains are completed, the ribosomes are released as 30S and 50S particles which can freely exchange with the pool of subunits. They readily reassociate and reach a dynamic equilibrium strongly shifted toward 70S monomers. These free ribosomes are split into their subunits through the action of dissociation factor and can then return to active protein synthesis.

It is interesting to point out that we have recently found a new factor which causes *in vitro* association of 30S and 50S subunits at a magnesium concentration close to the physiological level (30). This association factor could also participate in the ribosome cycle.

We wish to emphasize that it is necessary to be very cautious in the interpretation of the results. Most of the conclusions about the ribosome cycle are drawn from *in vitro* experiments, and these are indeed extrapolations of *in vivo* conditions.

ACKNOWLEDGMENTS

I.D.A. and N.S.G. are Career Investigators of the Consejo Nacional de Investigaciones Científicas y Técnicas (Argentina). M.G.-P. is a Fellow of the Organization of American States. C.A.P. is a Fellow of the Consejo Nacional de Investigaciones Científicas y Técnicas (Argentina) under the auspices of an exchange program with the Conselho Nacional de Pesquisas (Brasil). M.E.A. is a Fellow of the Instituto Nacional de Farmacología (Argentina).

SUMMARY

The ribosomal distribution in bacterial lysates obtained with the different methods described up to the present may not reflect the *in vivo* state. However, the utilization of several mild disrupting procedures which include ionic concentrations very similar to the physiological levels has shown that ribosomes can be found in the following forms: (a) particles engaged in protein synthesis as monosomes or polyribosomal aggregates, (b) free monomers, and (c) 30S and 50S subunits.

A cycle of dissociation and reassociation of ribosomes occurs during the successive rounds of translation in growing bacteria.

Although the initiation, elongation, and termination steps of protein synthesis have been thoroughly investigated, it is not yet clear whether ribosomes are released from the messenger as subunits or as 70S monomers.

In our laboratory, we have studied polypeptide synthesis in an *in vitro* system containing polyribosomes and S_{100} supernatant from *E. coli* D10. Labeled 30S subunits were added in several conditions and at different moments of the process. The exchange of radioactivity between 30S and 70S particles has been measured during protein synthesis as well as after its completion, in the presence or in the absence of spermidine, used to stabilize the 70S ribosomes. The results allow us to analyze in detail some aspects of the termination step. The most likely schemes of the ribosome cycle are discussed.

RESUMEN

Los diferentes métodos utilizados hasta ahora para el estudio de la distribución de ribosomas en lisados bacterianos pueden no reflejar el estado real existente *in vivo*. Sin embargo el uso de varios procedimientos menos drásticos en condiciones iónicas similares a las fisiológicas han permitido establecer que los ribosomas se encuentran en tres formas: (a) partículas que intervienen en la síntesis de proteínas ya sea como monosomas o como agregados poliribosómicos; (b) monómeros libres; y (c) subunidades 30S y 50S.

Los ribosomas participan repetidamente en un ciclo de disociación y reasociación que tiene lugar durante los sucesivos procesos de traducción de las bacterias en crecimiento.

Aunque las etapas de iniciación, elongación y terminación de la síntesis de proteínas han sido exhaustivamente investigadas, aún no se ha aclarado completamente si los ribosomas se liberan del RNA mensajero como subunidades o como monómeros 70S.

En nuestro laboratorio hemos estudiado la síntesis de polipéptidos en un sistema *in vitro* que contenía poliribosomas y sobrenadante S_{100} de *E. coli* D10. En varias condiciones y en diferentes momentos del proceso se agregó subunidades 30S marcadas. Se midió el intercambio de radioactividad entre las partículas 30S y 70S tanto durante como después de la síntesis de proteínas, y en presencia o ausencia de espermidina, que fue usada como agente estabilizante de los ribosomas 70S. Los resultados permiten analizar en detalle algunos aspectos de la etapa de terminación y postular los esquemas más probables del ciclo de ribosomas.

REFERENCES

1. Meselson, M., Nomura, M., Brenner, S., Davern, C., and Schlessinger, D., *J. Mol. Biol., 9,* 696 (1964).
2. Kaempfer, R., Meselson, M., and Raskas, H. J., *J. Mol. Biol., 31,* 277 (1968).
3. Van Dijk-Salkinoja, M. S., and Planta, R. J., *Arch. Biochem. Biophys., 141,* 477 (1970).
4. Kelley, W. S., and Schaechter, M., in Rose, A. H., and Wilkinson, J. F. (eds.), *Advances in Microbial Physiology,* Vol. II, Academic Press, New York (1968), pp. 89-142.
5. Mangiarotti, G., and Schlessinger, D., *J. Mol. Biol., 20,* 123 (1966).
6. Mangiarotti, G., and Schlessinger, D., *J. Mol. Biol., 29,* 395 (1967).
7. Schlessinger, D., Mangiarotti, G., and Apirion, D., *Proc. Natl. Acad. Sci. U.S.A., 58,* 1782 (1967).
8. Varricchio, F., *Nature, 223,* 1364 (1969).
9. Phillips, L. A., Hotham-Iglewski, B., and Franklin, R. M., *J. Mol. Biol., 40,* 279 (1969).
10. Phillips, L. A., Hotham-Iglewski, B., and Franklin, R. M., *J. Mol. Biol., 45,* 23 (1969).
11. Subramanian, A. R., Davis, B. D., and Beller, R. J., *Cold Spring Harbor Symp. Quant. Biol., 34,* 223 (1969).
12. Godson, G. N., and Sinsheimer, R. L., *Biochim. Biophys. Acta, 149,* 489 (1967).
13. Algranati, I. D., González, N. S., and Bade, E. G., *Proc. Natl. Acad. Sci. U.S.A., 62,* 574 (1969).
14. Van Dijk-Salkinoja, M. S., Stoof, T. J., and Planta, R. J., *Europ. J. Biochem., 12,* 474 (1970).
15. Oppenheim, J., Scheinbuks, J., Biava, C., and Marcus, L., *Biochim. Biophys. Acta, 161,* 386 (1968).
16. Kelley, W. S., and Schaechter, M., *J. Mol. Biol., 42,* 599 (1969).
17. Flessel, C. P., Ralph, P., and Rich, A., *Science, 158,* 658 (1967).
18. Algranati, I. D., *FEBS Letters, 10,* 153 (1970).
19. Beller, R. J., and Davis, B. D., *J. Mol. Biol., 55,* 477 (1971).
20. Uchida, T., Abe, M., Matsuo, K., and Yoneda, M., *Biochim. Biophys. Acta, 224,* 628 (1970).
21. Infante, A. A., and Baierlein, R., *Proc. Natl. Acad. Sci. U.S.A., 68,* 1780 (1971).
22. Kaempfer, R., *Proc. Natl. Acad. Sci. U.S.A., 61,* 106 (1968).
23. Kaempfer, R., *Nature, 228,* 534 (1970).
24. Kaempfer, R., *Proc. Natl. Acad. Sci. U.S.A., 68,* 2458 (1971).
25. Spirin, A. S., *FEBS Letters, 14,* 349 (1971).
26. Perazzolo, C. A., Azzam, M. E., and Algranati, I. D., submitted for publication.
27. Subramanian, A. R., and Davis, B. D., *Proc. Natl. Acad. Sci. U.S.A., 68,* 2453 (1971).
28. Azzam, M. E., Perazzolo, C. A., and Algranati, I.D., *21,* 165 (1972).
29. Hardy, S. J. S., and Turnock, G., *Nature New Biol., 229,* 17 (1971).
30. García-Patrone, M., González, N. S., and Algranati, I. D., *Proc. Natl. Acad. Sci. U.S.A., 68,* 2822 (1971).

DISCUSSION

R. P. Perry (Philadelphia, U.S.A.): One comment in relation to your last statement on eukaryotic organisms. It has been shown in several laboratories that the pool of free subunits is not in complete equilibrium with the subunits which are being released at termination, so that in an *in vivo* situation you might have preferential attachment of the recently terminated subunits and not rapid equilibrium with the free subunit pool. This is one facet which you might not pick up in *in vitro* system when things are much slower: you might not see this preferential reincorporation.

I. D. Algranati (Buenos Aires, Argentina): Yes, but it should be mentioned that in eukaryotic *in vitro* systems the exchange of subunits is slower after translation than during it. In our case, the situation is different because both exchanges occur at the same rate.

A. S. Spirin (Moscow, USSR): I would like to make a few comments. One is about hydrostatic pressure-induced dissociation. I think that it is not necessary to think in terms of hydrostatic pressure-induced dissociation because if you have equilibrium between 70S particles and subunits, and you centrifuge this equilibrium in some zonal way, that means the zone is moving into the same equilibrium; then you can lose the slower-moving subunits. You will have a smaller amount of the couples in comparison with the equilibrium mixture in static conditions. Usually, if you use long tubes there is dissociation during moving of the zone because of tailing of the smaller ribosomal subunits. Therefore, I think it is not necessary to appeal in every case to pressure-induced dissociation. My other comment concerns the discrepancy in the literature about the 70S termination form or the 50S and 30S termination form. The point is that in all the states where ribosomes are not translating they are in equilibrium with subunits. The state depends on the ionic conditions of homogenization or operation, because many factors, dissociation or initiation factor, aminoacyl-tRNA, or other proteins, may just shift the equilibrium. The selective conditions of homogenization determine which form of ribosomes (70S or their subunits) can predominate. My feeling is that this discussion is more semantic than real, that is, about the 70S form or the 50S plus the 30S form. What do you think about it?

I. D. Algranati: In our studies, we have centered our interest on two points of the ribosomal cycle. One is related to the mechanism of the whole process, because even though nontranslating ribosomes are in equilibrium with their subunits, the sequence of the reactions (and possibly their controls) is different if 70S particles are liberated on termination of translation and then they partially dissociate, or if subunits are released and subsequently reassociate to give couples. We can distinguish both situations in the presence of spermidine, which is a normal physiological component of bacterial extracts. The spermidine can stabilize the 70S ribosomes (or shift the equilibrium) in such a way as to substantially block exchange when the experiment is done with spermidine throughout the protein synthesis and labeled smaller subparticles are added afterward. However, the exchange of radioactivity between 30S and 70S during translation was exactly the same in the absence or in the presence of spermidine. The second point is related to the functional meaning of free 70S ribosomes: are they real intermediates of the cycle or do they constitute a reserve pool of ribosomes which only appear when the rate of protein synthesis decreases? Although there is not yet a conclusive answer to this question, we think that 70S monomers do participate as intermediates in the ribosomal cycle of growing bacteria.

28

Antibiotic Action in Protein Synthesis

D. Vazquez

Instituto de Biología Celular
Madrid, España

Most of the antibiotics known to inhibit protein synthesis block some of the steps taking place at the ribosome level by interacting with either the ribosomes or other components required in the reactions leading to protein synthesis. Broadly speaking, there are at least two classes of systems for protein synthesis including those of the prokaryotic type (bacteria, blue-green algae, mitochondria, chloroplasts, and possibly nuclei) and those of the eukaryotic type (cytoplasmic systems from yeast, fungi, green algae, protozoa, higher plants, and mammalian cells). Functional diffences between the prokaryotic and eukaryotic types of systems for protein synthesis are found not only in the ribosomes but also in the supernatant factors; i.e., there is ample evidence that ribosomes and supernatants can be crossed between widely different systems belonging to the same type but not between systems of different types.

Since there are at least two types of protein-synthesizing systems, the antibiotics can be classified according to their specificity into those affecting systems of (a) the prokaryotic type, (b) the eukaryotic type, and (c) both the prokaryotic and the eukaryotic types (Table I) (for reviews, see refs. 1-8). A few of these antibiotics (e.g., fusidic acid and emetine) are known to affect some of the supernatant factors, but in most cases the inhibitors interact directly with the ribosome. Different experimental approaches have determined the subunit of prokaryotic ribosomes on which inhibitors act (Table II). Although fusidic acid is known to directly affect the G supernatant factor, it is included in Table II among the inhibitors acting on the 50S subunit because it has been shown to bind to this subunit in the presence of GTP and G factor, forming the complex 50S-fusidic acid-G-GDP (9-11).

Table I. Inhibitors of Protein Synthesis

Acting on prokaryotic systems

Chloramphenicol group: Lincomycin group:

Chloramphenicol   Lincomycin
D-AMP-3   Clindamycin
D-Thiomycetin (Thiamphenicol) Celesticetin
D-Win-5094
                                      Streptomycin group:
Macrolides group:
                                      Streptomycin
Angolamycin   Neomycin
Carbomycin   Kanamycin
Erythromycin   Paromomycin
Lancamycin   Gentamycin
Leucomycin   Hygromycin B
Methymycin
Oleandomycin   Siomycin group:
Spiramycin
Neospiramycin   Siomycin
Forocidin   Thiostrepton (Bryamycin)
Tylosin   Thiopeptin
                                 Sporangiomycin
                                 Kasugamycin
Streptogramin A group:
                                 Spectinomycin
Streptogramin A (Vernamycin A)
Ostreogrycin G   Viomycin

Streptogramin B group: Multhiomycin

Streptogramin B   Berninamycin
Viridogrisein
Staphylomycin S   Micrococcin

                                 Althiomycin

Acting on prokaryotic and eukaryotic systems

Actinobolin   Polydextran sulfate

Amicetin   Polyvinyl sulfate

Aurintricarboxylic acid   Puromycin

Blasticidin S   Pactamycin

Bottromycin A_2 Sparsomycin

Table I. (Continued)

Edeine	Tetracycline group:
Fusidic acid	Chlortetracycline
Gougerotin	Doxycycline
	Oxytetracycline
Nucleocidin	Tetracycline
Chartreusin	

Acting on eukaryotic systems

Anisomycin	Pederin
Emetin	Phenomycin
Enomycin	Tenuazonic acid
Glutarimide group:	Tylophora alkaloids:
Actiphenol	Cryptopleurine
Cycloheximide	Tylocrebrine
Streptimidone	Tylophorine
Streptovitacin A	

Patterns and modes of antibiotic action on bacterial ribosomes have been elucidated considerably in recent years, but corresponding studies on inhibition of eukaryotic protein synthesis are not so well developed, primarily due to our incomplete knowledge of ribosomal structure and function in eukaryotic systems. However, it has been reported that the ribosomal subunits in eukaryotic-type ribosomes perform functions similar to their prokaryotic counterparts, namely, peptide bond formation on the larger subunit (12-14) and codon-anticodon recognition in the smaller one (12,15). It can then be assumed that a number of antibiotics, known to act on both bacterial and eukaryotic protein synthesis, do so by blocking homologous steps in the two systems. Taking this into account, and considering the reported results of antibiotic action on eukaryotic ribosomes, we can summarize (Table III) what is known about the ribosome subunits of eukoryotic cells as specific targets of inhibitor action.

Work in our laboratory has been concerned with active centers integrated in the larger ribosomal subunit of both prokaryotic and eukaryotic ribosomes. We have also studied the mechanism of action of antibiotics acting on these ribosome active centers; the results obtained will be summarized in this paper.

Table II. Inhibitors of Protein Synthesis Acting on Prokaryotic Ribosomes: Site of Action

Smaller subunit

Streptomycin group: Aurintricarboxylic acid

   Streptomycin   Polydextran sulfate
   Neomycin
   Kanamycin   Polyvinyl sulfate
   Paromomycin
   Gentamycin   Tetracycline group:
   Hygromycin B
                                  Chlortetracycline
Kasugamycin   Doxycycline
                                  Oxytetracycline
Pactamycin   Tetracycline

Spectinomycin

Edeine

Larger subunit

Chloramphenicol group: Streptogramin A group:

   Chloramphenicol   Streptogramin A
   D-AMP-3   Ostreogrycin G
   D-Thiomycetin
   D-Win-5094   Streptogramin B group:

Macrolides group: Streptogramin B
                                  Viridogrisein
   Angolamycin   Staphylomycin S
   Carbomycin
   Erythromycin   Lincomycin group:
   Lancamycin
   Leucomycin   Lincomycin
   Methymycin   Clindamycin
   Oleandomycin   Celesticetin
   Spiramycin
   Neospiramycin   Siomycin group:
   Forocidin
   Tylosin   Siomycin
                                  Thiostrepton
Actinobolin   Thiopeptin
                                  Sporangiomycin
Gougerotin   Althiomycin

Table II. (Continued)

Puromycin	Blasticidin S
Sparsomycin	Bottromycin A$_2$
Amicetin	Fusidic acid

Table III. Inhibitors of Protein Synthesis Acting on Eukaryotic Ribosomes: Site of Action

Smaller subunit

Edeine	Tetracycline group:
Aurintricarboxylic acid	Chlortetracycline
	Doxycycline
Polydextran sulfate	Oxytetracycline
	Tetracycline
Polyvinyl sulfate	
Sodium fluoride	
Pactamycin	

Larger subunit

Actinobolin	Glutarimide group:
Amicetin	Actiphenol
	Cycloheximide
Gougerotin	Streptimidone
	Streptovitacin A
Puromycin	
	Tylophora alkaloids:
Blasticidin S	
	Cryptopleurine
Fusidic acid	Tylocrebrine
	Tylophorine
Sparsomycin	
Anisomycin	Tenuazonic acid

ANTIBIOTIC INHIBITORS OF PEPTIDE BOND FORMATION

Antibiotic Action on the Peptidyl Transferase Center

The peptidyl transferase center, known to be integrated in the larger subunit of both prokaryotic and eukaryotic ribosomes (2-5,16), catalyzes the peptide bond formation step in protein synthesis. This has been clearly demonstrated in a simplified system known as the "fragment reaction," in which either formyl-methionyl- or acetyl-leucyl-oligonucleotides and puromycin act as substrates in the peptide bond formation step, replacing f-Met-tRNA (donor substrate) and aminoacyl-tRNA (acceptor substrate), respectively.

In addition to the above substrates, the "fragment reaction" requires the larger ribosome subunit, monovalent and divalent cations, and alcohol, but neither mRNA nor the smaller subunits are required. The advantage of the fragment reaction is that it must be limited to a part of the larger ribosomal subunit in the immediate vicinity of the catalytic center, since both substrates are of relatively small size. From this consideration, it can be expected that interactions which normally take place between tRNA and other parts of the ribosome are lacking in the fragment reaction. Using this system, either f-Met- or N-acetyl-aminoacyl puromycin is formed, and neither GTP nor the supernatant factors G and T nor the initiation factors are required for peptide formation. With this experimental system, it has been shown that a number of antibiotics which interact with the larger subunit block the peptidyl transfer step (Table IV). Similar results have been found by other workers, using different experimental systems (for reviews, see ref. 2-8). As would be expected, inhibitors blocking the function of the smaller subunit specifically do not affect the "fragment reaction." On the other hand, the macrolide antibiotic erythromycin does not inhibit the "fragment reaction" but blocks the inhibitory effect of chloramphenicol and lincomycin on peptide bond formation (8).

The peptidyl transfer reaction presumably takes place in several steps, among which are the binding of the peptidyl donor and acceptor substrates at the P and the A sites of the peptidyl transfer center. There is ample evidence that only the terminal moieties of tRNA interact with the center, and we have developed systems to resolve the binding steps using simple substrates containing the CpCpA oligonucleotide of tRNA. To study substrate interaction at the peptidyl transferase center, we have used assays based on the measurement of binding of CACCA-N-acetyl-Leu and UACCA-Leu to the P and A sites, respectively, of the larger ribosomal subunits in the presence of ethanol. The effects of inhibitors acting on the peptidyl transferase center have been studied in these systems, and the results obtained are presented in Table V (17-19). Inhibition of fragment binding by an antibiotic does not necessarily imply that substrate and antibiotic compete directly for binding at overlapping sites. The substrate and antibiotic

Table IV. Inhibitors of the Ribosomal Peptidyl Transferase Activity

Blocking the activity of the larger subunit of prokaryotic ribosomes	Blocking the activity of the larger subunit of both prokaryotic and eukaryotic ribosomes	Blocking the activity of the larger subunit of eukaryotic ribomes
Chloramphenicol group:	Actinobolin	Anisomycin
Chloramphenicol	Amicetin	Trichodermin
D-AMP-3	Blasticidin S	Tenuazonic acid
D-Thiomycetin	Gougerotin	
D-Win-5094	Sparsomycin	
Macrolides group:		
Angolamycin		
Carbomycin		
Spiramycin		
Streptogramin A group:		
Streptogramin A		
Ostregogrycin G		
Lincomycin group:		
Lincomycin		
Clindamycin		
Celesticetin		

Table V. Substrate Binding to the Peptidyl
Transferase Center

Inhibitors of CACCA-N-acetyl-Leu binding to the P site	Inhibitors of UACCA-Leu binding to the A site

50S ribosomal subunits

Macrolides group:

   Carbomycin
   Spiramycin

Streptogramin A group:

   Steptogramin A
   Ostreogrycin G

Lincomycin group:

   Lincomycin
   Clindamycin

Macrolides group:

   Carbomycin
   Spiramycin

Streptogramin A group:

   Streptogramin A
   Ostreogrycin G

Lincomycin group:

   Lincomycin
   Clindamycin

Chloramphenicol group:

   Chloramphenicol
   D-AMP-3
   D-Thiomycetin
   D-Win-5094

60S ribosomal subunits

Anisomycin   Anisomycin

binding sites might be spatially separated but allosterically linked. However, the above results clearly show that some antibiotics inhibit peptide bond formation by specifically blocking substrate binding to the A site of the peptidyl transferase center, whereas others block substrate binding to the P site of the peptidyl transferase center, and a number of antibiotics block binding of the donor as well as the acceptor substrate.

When the effect of sparsomycin was tested on binding of CACCA-N-acetyl-Leu to either 50S or 60S ribosomal subunits, it was found that this antibiotic induces formation of a substrate-ribosome complex which does not carry out the "fragment reaction" (19,20). Requirements for this "sparsomycin reaction" are similar to those of the "fragment reaction" except that puromycin is replaced by sparsomycin. Quantitative studies suggest that the complex formed contains ribosome, sparsomycin, and CACCA-N-acetyl-Leu in a ratio of 1-1-1 (16,20). The "sparsomycin reaction" may be similar in some respects to the "fragment reaction." In the first step, a CCA-peptidyl group binds at the P site on the larger subunit at the peptidyl transferase center. In the second step, the bound fragment either reacts with puromycin or interacts with sparsomycin to give, respectively, peptidyl-puromycin or the sparsomycin complex; both puromycin and sparsomycin act on the A site. The "sparsomycin reaction" is inhibited by all inhibitors of CACCA-N-acetyl-Leu binding (obviously by blocking the first step of the "sparsomycin reaction") but also by chloramphenicol in the case of prokaryotic ribosomes, by cycloheximide in the case of eukaryotic ribosomes, and by amicetin, gougerotin, and blasticidin S in the case of both eukaryotic and prokaryotic ribosomes (Table VI). At certain ethanol concentra-

Table VI. Sparsomycin-Induced Binding of CACCA-N-acetyl-Leu to the Larger Ribosomal Subunit

Inhibitors of the reaction by 50S ribosomal subunits	Inhibitors of the reaction by 60S ribosomal subunits
Chloramphenicol group:	Anisomycin
Chloramphenicol D-AMP-3 D-Thiomycetin D-Win-5094	Amicetin
	Blasticiden S
	Cycloheximide
Macrolides group:	Gougerotin
Carbomycin Spiramycin	
Streptogramin A group:	
Streptogramin A Ostreogrycin G	
Lincomycin group:	
Lincomycin Clindamycin	
Amicetin	
Blasticidin S	
Gougerotin	

tions, amicetin and gougerotin (and probably blasticidin S), in the absence of sparsomycin, induce formation of a substrate-ribosome complex which is apparently similar to that formed with sparsomycin. It is possible that the modes of action of amicetin, gougerotin, and blasticidin S are related to that of sparsomycin and that they compete for the same site, but that the nonreactive complexes formed in their presence are less stable. This suggests that amicetin, blasticidin S, and gougerotin act like sparsomycin at the A site of the peptidyl transferase center. Neither chloramphenicol nor cycloheximide directly affects CACCA-N-acetyl-Leu binding, and their blocking of the "sparsomycin reaction" might be due to inhibition by these antibiotics of sparsomycin binding by acting either at or near the A site of the peptidyl transferase center.

Antibiotic Binding Site at the Peptidyl Transferase Center

Chloramphenicol binds to ribosomes from bacteria (21,22), chloroplasts, and blue-green algae (23,24) at a site located on the 50S subunit (25). Chloramphenicol binding is inhibited by a number of other antibiotic inhibitors of protein synthesis, including members of the lincomycin, streptogramin A, and macrolide groups, thus suggesting that all of these compounds interact with the 50S subunit at related sites (26). Binding to the 50S subunit has been directly confirmed in the cases of lincomycin (27-29,37), members of the streptogramin A group (30-32), and the macrolides spiramycin (31,33) and erythromycin (34-37). By use of the experimental system known as the "fragment reaction," these antibiotics have been shown to act on the peptidyl transferase center of the 50S subunit. Although erythromycin does not directly inhibit the "fragment reaction," it completely blocks the effects of lincomycin and chloramphenicol in this reaction, suggesting that it also acts at or near the peptidyl transferase center (8).

Detailed studies were carried out in our laboratory on the binding of ^{14}C-chloramphenicol, ^{14}C-lincomycin, and ^{14}C-erythromycin to *Escherichia coli* ribosomes either in the presence of ethanol (conditions of the "fragment reaction") or in more physiological conditions in a buffer not containing ethanol (37). It was found in both experimental conditions that there is one binding site per ribosome for lincomycin, chloramphenicol, and erythromycin. These antibiotics act at closely related sites, but there are some differences in the properties of the three sites, such as (a) erythromycin clearly blocks chloramphenicol binding, whereas chloramphenicol only partially inhibits erythromycin binding; (b) in some cases, the ribosomal binding site for lincomycin is damaged without the chloramphenicol binding site being affected; (c) the presence of ethanol enhances the affinity of ribosomes for lincomycin and erythromycin but decreases the affinity of ribosomes for chloramphenicol; and (d) puromycin partially inhibits chloramphenicol and lincomycin binding to ribosomes but does not affect erythromycin binding (37). Differential responses were also found when the effects of a number of antibiotics acting on the 50S subunits were tested on chloramphenicol, lincomycin, erythromycin, and spiramycin binding (Table VII) (8,33,37). All the antibiotics found to compete for binding are known to act on the 50S subunit, and most of them, but not all, are inhibitors of peptide bond formation, as determined by the "fragment reaction" assay. Important exceptions are erythromycin, oleandomycin, neospiramycin, forocidin, streptogramin B, and viridogrisein, all of which inhibit binding of the antibiotics studied but have little or no effect on the fragment reaction. Among these, neospiramycin is of particular interest. It has the same structure as spiramycin but lacks one of the sugar residues. It is therefore probable that it binds at the same site as spiramycin and that it is the extra sugar residue of spiramycin which interferes with binding of donor and acceptor substrates at the peptidyl transferase center. Neospiramycin only inhibits binding of the donor substrate and to a lesser extent than spiramycin. Since lincomycin and carbomycin have a similar effect to that of spiramycin on substrate binding, it is reasonable to suppose that the binding site for lincomycin overlaps other parts of the spiramycin binding site. It is probable that the binding site for lincomycin also overlaps the binding sites for the other macrolides and that the variable effects of the macrolides on the peptidyl transferase center are due to differences in size of the molecules, as illustrated by the spiramycin-neospiramycin example (8,37).

All the results considered above support the proposition that there is one peptidyl transferase center on every 50S subunit and that lincomycin, chloramphenicol, sparsomycin, and a number of other antibiotics act on protein synthesis by binding at the center or at nearby sites. In order to investigate the relationships of these sites to the ribosome structure, we have made use of systems developed for the dissociation and reconstitution of 50S ribosomal subunits (38,39). A series of cores (α, β, γ) can be prepared from 50S subunits of E. coli ribosomes by isopycnic centrifugation in CsCl-MG^{2+} solutions. The cores contain intact 23S and 5S RNA, but lack increasing numbers of the proteins required to make up the 50S subunit. The β cores lack all of the acidic proteins and at least one of the basic proteins. The γ cores lack, in addition, approximately six more of the basic proteins. When the particles were tested for activity in different assays, it was found that the β cores possess good activity for (a) catalysis of the "fragment reaction," (b) release of formylmethionine activity, (c) chloramphenicol binding, (d) lincomycin binding, (e) erythromycin binding, and (f) the sparsomycin reaction (Table VIII and refs. 16 and 40).

In contrast, the γ cores were devoid of all these activities. The protein fractions split off in preparation of the cores were also inactive, but restoration of activity was achieved by readdition of "split" proteins to the γ cores. The proteins required for such a restoration are confined to the "split" proteins obtained in the conversion of β cores to γ cores. Although sparsomycin and

Table VII. Effects of Antibiotics on Binding to Ribosomes of Chloramphenicol, Lincomycin, Erythromycin, and Spiramycin[a]

Antibiotic	Concentration (mM)	Inhibition of binding of			
		^{14}C-chloramphenicol	^{14}C-lincomycin	^{14}C-erythromycin	^{14}C-spiramycin
Chloramphenicol	0.1	+	+	–	
	5			30%	33%
Lincomycin	0.1	+	+	–	
	10			52%	50%
Celesticetin	1	57%	+	25%	
Erythromycin	0.1	+	+	+	+
Spiramycin	0.1	+	+	+	+
Neospiramycin	0.1	+	+	+	+
Forocidin	0.1	+	+	35%	+
Carbonmycin	0.1	+	+	+	+
Oleandomycin	0.1	+	+	33%	22%
Angloamycin	0.1	37%	+	–	
Lancamycin	0.1	+		–	
Methymycin	0.1	+	46%	–	
Chalcomycin	0.1	+	+		
Streptogramin A	0.1	+	+	+	+
Streptogramin B	0.1	63	+	+	
Viridogrisein	0.1	42	+	+	+
Amicetin	1	–	–	–	
Sparsomycin	0.5	–	20	–	

Gougerotin	1		-	-	-
Puromycin	1	20	20	20	-
	5	40	40	40	-
Siomycin	0.1	-	-	-	-
Thiostrepton	0.01	-	-	-	-
Bottromycin A$_2$	0.1	-	-	-	-

[a] In this table, a plus sign indicates inhibition greater than 70% and a minus sign indicates inhibition less than 20%. The concentrations of the labeled antibiotics, whose binding was estimated, were in the range from 1 to 5 μM. E. coli ribosomes were used in the experiments on ^{14}C-chloramphenicol, ^{14}C-lincomycin, and ^{14}C-erythromycin binding, whereas B. subtilis ribosomes were used in ^{14}C-spiramycin binding. (Data are taken from refs. 8 and 33.)

Table VIII. Activities of Protein-Deficient Cores from 50S Subunits[a]

Assay				Activity		
	β Cores	γ Cores	"Split" proteins	γ+SP$_{\beta-\gamma}$	γspar+SP$_{\beta-\gamma}$	γNEM+SP$_{\beta-\gamma}$
(a) "Fragment reaction"	+	-	-	+	+	+
(b) Release of formylmethionine	+	-	-	+		
(c) Chloramphenicol binding	+	-	-	+		-
(d) Lincomycin binding	+	-	-	+	-	
(e) Erythromycin binding	+	-	-	+	+	+
(f) "Sparsomycin reaction"	+	-	-	+		
(g) G-dependent GTPase activity	+	±		+		

[a] Abbreviations: γ, γ cores; γspar, γ cores pretreated with sparsomycin; γNEM, γ cores pretreated with N-ethyl maleimide; SP$_{\beta-\gamma}$, "split" proteins released in the preparation of γ cores from β cores. (Data are taken from refs 40 and 50.)

NEM do not affect ^{14}C-lincomycin binding to ribosomes, they do prevent reconstitution of the lincomycin binding sites using γ cores and the "split" protein fraction (40).

The results of this study provide further support for the model in which lincomycin, chloramphenicol, and sparsomycin act directly on the peptidyl transferase center of 50S subunits, since all these activities are lost simultaneously on removal of about six proteins from the β cores without a major conformational change. Our reconstitution experiments are in agreement with previous reports that peptidyl transferase plays an important role in release of formylmethionine in protein chain termination (41,42). Also, these results suggest a close relationship between the erythromycin binding site and the binding site of the peptidyl transferase inhibitors tested. The study is also a step toward the correlation of the structure and function of the 50S subunit. The observation that β cores are fully active clearly eliminates the acidic proteins and certain basic proteins from being possible components of the peptidyl transferase center. The reversible loss of activity in going from β to γ cores makes further identification of the active component(s) difficult. It seems probable that the "split" proteins obtained in the conversion of β to γ cores contain the component(s) responsible for the catalysis of the peptidyl transfer and the binding of substrates and peptidyl transfer inhibitors, but that in order for this component(s) to be active it must be situated in the special environment provided by the ribonucleoprotein particle. Alternatively, it is possible (a) that the center is still intact on the γ cores but the "split" proteins are required for its active conformation, or (b) that the core and "split" protein fractions contain complementary components of the center, more than one of which is needed for activity.

We know very little about antibiotic binding sites on the 60S subunit of eukaryotic ribosomes, because we did not have appropriate radioactive labeled

Table IX. Inhibitors of 50S Subunit-Dependent GTP Hydrolysis

Inhibitors of G-dependent GTPase activity		Inhibitors of T-dependent GTPase activity acting on procaryotic systems
Acting on prokaryotic systems	Acting on prokaryotic and eukaryotic systems	
Siomycin	Fusidic acid*	Siomycin
Thiostrepton		Thiostrepton
Thiopeptin		Thiopeptin
Sporangiomycin		Sporangiomycin

* In fact fusidic acid allows hydrolysis of one GTP molecule but stabilizes the resultant complex of fusidic acid-G-GDP-ribosome, blocking subsequent rounds of uncoupled GTP hydrolysis.

compounds. Studies on peptide bond formation activity of 60S subunits, pre-treated with the required antibiotics, have clearly shown that a number of them certainly act on the 60S subunit (Table III and ref. 19). Studies on the effect of these antibiotics on functional activities of these subunits have also shown that some of the antibiotics act on the peptidyl transferase center. From the results obtained on the effects of anisomycin on the binding of the donor and acceptor substrates, it appears that anisomycin has a similar action on 60S subunits to that of either streptogramin A or spiramycin or lincomycin on 50S subunits (19). We have recently obtained ^{3}H-anisomycin by tritium exchange labeling, and the antibiotic specifically binds to the 60S subunit but not to the 40S subunit. Further studies with this antibiotic are in progress in our laboratory.

ANTIBIOTIC INHIBITORS OF G-DEPENDENT GTPase ACTIVITY

Antibiotic Action on the G site

In protein synthesis, G-dependent GTP hydrolysis is further coupled to other reactions. It is generally believed that the role of this reaction is to provide the energy required for the translocation step (for review, see ref. 43). Combined 50S and 30S subunits are more effective in complementing G than either subunit alone (44,45). However, the rate of G-dependent GTP hydrolysis with 50S subunits is 25-40% of that with 70S ribosomes, whereas the 30S subunits alone do not have a significant activity in complementing G. This implies that the primary interaction in hydrolysis of GTP takes place between G and the 50S subunit. The 50S site at which G interacts is known as the G site (45).

A number of antibiotics have been found to block the G-dependent GTPase activity (Table IX). Whereas fusidic acid is equally active on eukaryotic and prokaryotic systems, the other antibiotics are only active on ribosomes of the prokaryotic type. These groups of antibiotics differ not only in their inhibitory spectra but also in their mode of action. Fusidic acid interacts with G (46-48) and allows the hydrolysis of one GTP molecule, but then stabilizes the resultant complex of fusidic acid-G-GDP- and the ribosome or its larger subunit (9-11). On the other hand, siomycin and thiostrepton are known to act on the 50S ribosomal subunit (45,49). These two antibiotics interfere with the action of G by preventing its attachment to the 50S ribosomal subunit (45). This has been clearly demonstrated, as siomycin inhibits both (a) formation of a complex between fusidic acid, G factor, and the ribosome in the presence of either GTP or GDP and (b) G interaction with ribosomes in the absence of fusidic acid (45).

The G site and the peptidyl transferase center are on distinct parts of the 50S subunit. Siomycin does not inhibit either the fragment reaction or binding of chloramphenicol, lincomycin, and erythromycin. On the other hand, none of the known inhibitors of peptidyl transfer block the G-dependent GTPase reaction. Failure to obtain cross effects with specific inhibitors suggests that the functioning of the two sites is not interconnected through a mechanism involving allosteric changes in the 50S subunit (45).

Evidence presented above clearly shows the existence of an active center in the 50S ribosomal subunit, responsible for the G-dependent hydrolysis of GTP (45). The use of protein-deficient nucleoprotein core particles derived from the 50S ribosome subunit (38,39), is a very valuable tool for studying the minimal ribosomal structural components required for some ribosomal activities. We have studied the G-dependent GTP hydrolysis in 50S-derived cores and reconstituted particles, and have found that most of the activity is lost in the β- to γ-core step (Table VII) (50). However, there is a residual G-dependent GTPase activity in the γ cores which is insensitive to thiostrepton. It has recently been reported that two specific proteins of the 50S subunit known as L7 and L12 are implicated in G-dependent GTPase activity (51). Recent analyses of our "split" protein fractions, carried out in collaboration with Drs. H. G. Wittmann and K. Nierhaus, have shown that neither L7 nor L12 is present in the "split" protein fraction released in the preparation of β cores, whereas protein L7 (but not L12) is present in the SPβ-γ fraction. These results suggest that the residual GTPase activity of the γ cores is due to the L12 protein remaining integrated in the ribonucleoprotein structure.

Antibiotic Binding at the G Site

Recent studies have shown that ^{3}H-hydrofusidic acid forms a complex with G factor, GTP, and 70S ribosomes (11). GTP and 70S ribosomes can be replaced by GDP and 50S subunits, respectively, but the antibiotic binds very little to either G factor, GTP, or ribosomes separately. These observations confirm the complex observed in the presence of the nonradioactive antibiotic using radioactive GTP or GDP (9,10).

There is conclusive evidence for binding of thiostrepton (49) and siomycin (45) to the 50S subunit. When ribosomal subunits were pretreated with siomycin and the unbound molecules separated by centrifugation, no binding of the antibiotic to the 30S subunits was detected. The treated 50S subunits were inactive in the G-dependent GTP hydrolysis, clearly showing that the antibiotic interacts with the 50S subunit, presumably at the G site (45).

ANTIBIOTIC ACTION ON THE T SITE

It is well known that the elongation factor T (T_s plus T_u) stimulates aminoacyl-tRNA binding to bacterial ribosomes. Coupled to this binding, there is a T-dependent hydrolysis of GTP. This T-dependent GTP hydrolysis can be observed in the absence of the 30S subunit, like the case of the G-dependent GTPase activity. However, the T-dependent reaction can be distinguished from the G-dependent GTP hydrolysis by the insensitivity of the former to fusidic acid and its dependence on aminoacyl-tRNA (43,52).

A number of compounds active on the smaller ribosomal subunit are known to block enzymic binding of aminoacyl-tRNA to ribosomes by interfering with the codon-anticodon interaction at the level of the 30S subunit (tetracyclines, edeine, pactamycin, aurintricarboxylic acid, and polydextran sulfate). However, these compounds do not interfere directly with the function of T, and, as expected, they do not block the T-dependent GTPase coupled to aminoacyl-tRNA binding.

On the other hand, a number of antibiotics, by binding to the 50S ribosomal subunit, inhibit aminoacyl-tRNA binding to the ribosome; these include streptogramin A, sparsomycin, thiostrepton, and siomycin (53). Sparsomycin and streptogramin A are known to have a strong inhibitory effect on the binding of the CCA-aminoacyl end of aminoacyl-tRNA to the A site of the peptidyl transferase center (for reviews, see refs. 2,8). Therefore, it is likely that the inhibitory effect of sparsomycin and streptogramin A on aminoacyl-tRNA binding is not due to a direct effect on the T site. In support of this assumption is the finding that these antibiotics do not inhibit the T-dependent GTP hydrolysis coupled to aminoacyl-tRNA binding. On the other hand, siomycin and thiostrepton do not affect the peptidyl transferase center but do block the T-dependent binding of aminoacyl-tRNA to the ribosomal A site, using as mRNA either R17-RNA or poly U (53). Siomycin and thiostrepton also inhibit GTP hydrolysis associated with T-dependent binding of Phe-tRNA, suggesting that these antibiotics prevent interaction between the GTP-Tu-aminoacyl-tRNA and the ribosome by interacting with the A site of the 50S subunit (54) (Table IX). Similarly, as indicated above, siomycin and thiostrepton, by interacting with the 50S ribosomal subunit, prevent binding of factor G and by doing so inhibit G-dependent GTPase. All the experimental evidence so far suggests that a single-site interaction of siomycin and thiostrepton on the 50S ribosomal subunit is responsible for their effects on both the binding of the GTP-Tu-aminoacyl-tRNA and that of factor G to the ribosome (54).

ACKNOWLEDGMENTS

This work was supported by grants from the United States National Institutes of Health (AI 08598) and Division Farmaceutica Lepetit and Lilly Indiana of Spain. The experimental work described as performed in our laboratory was carried out in collaboration with Drs. R. E. Monro, J. Modolell, J. P. G. Ballesta, A. Jimenez, M. L. Celma, R. Fernandez-Muñoz, E. Battaner, B. Cabrer, V. Montejo, L. Carrasco, and M. Barbacid.

SUMMARY

Most of the antibiotics known to block protein synthesis act at the ribosome level. Since, broadly speaking, there are at least two classes of ribosomes (corresponding to prokaryotic and eukaryotic types of cells or organelles), antibiotics acting on protein synthesis can be classified according to their specificity toward the ribosomes in those affecting (a) prokaryotic systems, (b) eukaryotic systems, and (c) both prokaryotic and eukaryotic systems. This classification shows that although there are important differences between prokaryotic and eukaryotic ribosomes, both types must have a number of common structural features as there are a number of inhibitors acting on both types of ribosomes. In many cases, we also know the ribosome subunit and functions which are the targets of antibiotics, and these are briefly described.

We are particularly interested in studying the activities of the larger ribosome subunit (either from 70S- or 80S-type ribosomes) and the specific action of a number of compounds blocking these activities. We have found, and it is widely accepted, that specific centers responsible for the peptidyl transferase and G-dependent GTPase activities are integrated in the larger ribosomal subunits. We have also found a number of antibiotics inhibiting this peptidyl transferase center in either (a) bacterial ribosomes or (b) eukaryotic ribosomes or (c) both types of ribosomes. Our studies with a number of radioactive antibiotics have shown that, at saturation, one molecule of antibiotic binds per ribosome. Our evidence also suggests that certain members of these groups specifically compete with the terminus of the CCA-peptidyl donor substrate for binding at the P site on the peptidyl transferase center, whereas other compounds interfere with substrate binding at the A site.

Studies carried out recently in our laboratory have demonstrated that two antibiotics (siomycin and thiostrepton) block the G-dependent GTPase center of the 50S ribosome subunit by interfering with binding of the G supernatant factor with this center. Siomycin and thiostrepton also block T-dependent binding of aminoacyl-tRNA; all the results obtained so far suggest that both inhibitory effects of siomycin and thiostrepton are a consequence of a single interaction of the antibiotics with the 50S subunit. Our antibiotic studies have clearly shown in 50S subunits that peptidyl transferase and G-dependent GTPase centers in the subunit are separated and independent.

Analyses of protein-deficient cores from 50S subunits also indicate a close relationship between the peptidyl transferase center and the sites for binding of antibiotics known to act on this center (chloramphenicol, lincomycin, and clindamycin). These studies have shown different structural components and requirements for activities of the G-dependent GTPase and peptidyl transferase centers. On the other hand, activities for peptide bond formation and releasing formyl-methionine, both of which appear to implicate the peptidyl transferase center, have similar structural requirements.

RESUMEN

La mayoría de los antibióticos que bloquean la síntesis de proteínas actúan a nivel ribosomal. Puesto que, hablando en términos generales, hay por lo menos dos clases de ribosomas (que corresponden a los tipos de células u organoides procariotes y eucariotes), los antibióticos que actúan sobre la síntesis de proteínas pueden clasificarse según su especificidad hacia los ribosomas, en aquellos que actúan sobre (a) sistemas de tipo procariote, (b) sistemas eucariotes y (c) ambos sistemas. Esta división demuestra que aunque hay importantes diferencias entre ribosomas procarióticos y eucarióticos, ambos tipos deben tener un cierto número de rasgos estructurales comunes, ya que hay diversos inhibidores que actúan sobre los dos tipos de ribosomas. En muchos casos se conoce la subunidad y función del ribosoma que son afectadas por el antibiótico y éstas serán brevemente descriptas.

Estamos particularmente interesados en estudiar las actividades de la subunidad ribosómica mayor (ya sea de los ribosomas 70S u 80S, y la acción específica de determinados compuestos que bloquean estas actividades. Hemos encontrado, y ello es aceptado generalmente, que los centros específicos responsables de las actividades de peptidil transferasa y GTPasa G-dependiente están integrados en la subunidad mayor del ribosoma. También hemos encontrado algunos antibióticos que inhiben el centro de la peptidil transferasa, ya sea en (a) ribosomas bacterianos, o (b) ribosomas eucariotes, o (c) ambos tipos de ribosomas. Nuestros estudios con antibióticos radioactivos han demostrado que en la saturación, se une una molécula de antibiótico por ribosoma. Nuestros resultados también sugieren que ciertos miembros de estos grupos compiten específicamente con el grupo terminal CCA-peptidil del sustrato dador para la unión en el sitio P del centro de la peptidil transferasa, en tanto que otros compuestos interfieren con la unión del sustrato en el sitio A.

Estudios llevados a cabo recientemente en nuestro laboratorio han demostrado que dos antibióticos, siomicina y thiostreptona, bloquean el centro GTPasa G-dependiente en la subunidad 50S del ribosoma al interferir con la unión del factor sobrenadante G con este centro. La siomicina y la thiostreptona también bloquean la unión T-dependiente del aminoacil-tRNA; todos los resultados obtenidos hasta ahora sugieren que ambos efectos inhibitorios de siomicina y thiostreptona son consecuencia de una única interacción del antibiótico con la subunidad 50S. Nuestros estudios con antibióticos han demostrado claramente que en las subunidades 50S los centros de peptidil transferasa y de GTPasa G-dependiente se hallan separados e independientes.

Los análisis de "corazones" ribosómicos ("cores") deficientes en proteínas, de subunidades 50S, también indican una relación estrecha entre el centro de peptidil transferasa y los sitios para la unión de los antibióticos que se conoce que actúan en este centro (cloramfenicol, lincomicina y clindamicina). Estos estudios también han demostrado componentes estructurales y requerimientos diferentes para las actividades de los centros de peptidil transferasa y GTPasa G-dependiente. Por otra parte las actividades para la formación de la unión peptídica y para la liberación de la formyl-metionina, ambas de las cuales parecen implicar al centro peptidil transferasa, tienen requerimientos estructurales semejantes.

REFERENCES

1. Vazquez, D., and Monro, R. E. *Biochim. Biophys. Acta, 142,* 155 (1967).
2. Vazquez, D., and Monro, R. E., *Abhandlungen der Deutschen Akademie der Wissenchaften zu Berlin, Klasse für Medizin, No. 1,* (1968), pp. 569-580.
3. Vazquez, D., and Monro, R. E. *Agrochimica, 12,* 489 (1968).
4. Vazquez, D., Staehelin, T., Celma, M. L., Battaner, E., Fernandez-Muñoz, R., and Monro, R. E., *Inhibitors, Tools in Cell Research,* Bücher, T., and Sies, H., (eds.), Springer-Verlag, Berlin-Heidelberg-New York, (1969), pp. 100-123.
5. Vazquez, D., Staehelin, T., Celma, M. L., Battaner, E., Fernandez-Muñoz, R., and Monro, R. E., *FEBS Symposium, 21,* 109 (1970).
6. Weisblum, B., and Davies, J., *Bacteriol. Rev., 32,* 493 (1969).
7. Pestka, S., *Ann. Rev. Microbiol., 25,* 487 (1971).
8. Monro, R. E., Fernandez-Muñoz, R., Celma, M. L., and Vazquez, D., in Mitsuhashi, S. (ed.), *Drug Action and Drug Resistance in Bacteria,* University of Tokyo Press, Tokyo (1971), pp. 303-333.
9. Bodley, J. W., and Lin, L., *Nature, 227,* 60 (1970).

10. Bodley, J. W., Lin, L., and Highland, J. H., *Biochem. Biophys. Res. Commun., 41,* 1406 (1970).
11. Okura, A., Kinoshita, T., and Tanaka, N., *Biochem. Biophys. Res. Commun., 41,* 1545 (1970).
12. Vazquez, D., Battaner, E., Neth, R., Heller, G., and Monro, R. E., *Cold Spring Harbor Symp. Quant. Biol., 34,* 369 (1969).
13. Falvey, A. K., and Staehelin, T., *J. Mol. Biol., 53,* 1 (1970).
14. Silverstein, E., *Biochem. Biophys. Res. Commun., 36,* 671 (1969).
15. Leader, D. P., Wool, I. G., and Castles, J. J., *Proc. Natl. Acad. Sci. U.S.A., 67,* 523 (1970).
16. Monro, R. E., Staehelin, T., Celma, M. L., and Vazquez, D., *Cold Spring Harbor Symp. Quant. Biol., 34,* 357 (1969).
17. Celma, M. L., Monro, R. E., and Vazquez, D., *FEBS Letters, 6,* 273 (1970).
18. Celma, M. L., Monro, R. E., and Vazquez, D., *FEBS Letters, 13,* 247 (1971).
19. Battaner, E., and Vazquez, D., *Biochim. Biophys. Acta, 254,* 316 (1971).
20. Monro, R. E., Celma, M. L., and Vazquez, D., *Nature, 222,* 356 (1969).
21. Vazquez, D., *Biochem. Biophys. Res. Commun., 12,* 409 (1963).
22. Vazquez, D., *Nature, 203,* 257 (1964).
23. Anderson, L. A., and Smillie, R. M., *Biochem. Biophys. Res. Commun., 23,* 535 (1966).
24. Rodriguez-Lopez, M., and Vazquez, D., *Life Sci., 7,* 327 (1968).
25. Vazquez, D., *Biochem. Biophys. Res. Commun., 15,* 464 (1964).
26. Vazquez, D., *Biochim. Biophys. Acta, 114,* 277 (1966).
27. Chang, F. N., Sih, C. J., and Weisblum, B., *Proc. Natl. Acad. Sci. U.S.A., 55,* 431 (1966).
28. Chang, F. N., and Weisblum, B., *Biochemistry, 6,* 836 (1967).
29. Rodriguez-Lopez, M., Celma, M. L., Fernandez-Muñoz, R., and Vazquez, D., in *Atti VII Simposio Internationale di Agrochimica su la Sintesi Biologica delle Proteine* (1968), pp. 63-68.
30. Ennis, H. L., *Mol. Pharmacol., 2,* 444 (1966).
31. Vazquez, D., *Life Sci., 6,* 381 (1967).
32. Ennis, H. L., *Biochemistry, 10,* 1265 (1971).
33. Vazquez, D., *Life Sci., 6,* 845 (1967).
34. Oleinick, N. L., and Corcoran, J. W., *J. Biol. Chem., 244,* 727 (1969).
35. Mao, J. C. H., and Putterman, M., *J. Mol. Biol., 44,* 347 (1969).
36. Teraoka, H., *J. Mol. Biol., 48,* 511 (1970).
37. Fernandez-Muñoz, R., Monro, R. E., Torres-Pinedo, R., and Vazquez, D., *Europ. J. Biochem., 23,* 185 (1971).
38. Maglott, D. R., and Staehelin, T., *Methods Enzymol., 20,* 408 (1971).
39. Staehelin, T., Maglott, D., and Monro, R. E., *Cold Spring Harbor Symp. Quant. Biol., 34, 39 (1969).*
40. Ballesta, J. P. G., Montejo, V., and Vazquez, D., *FEBS Letters, 19,* 75 (1971).
41. Vogel, Z., Zamir, A., and Elson, D., *Biochemistry, 8,* 5161 (1969).
42. Tompkins, R. K., Scolnick, E. M., and Caskey, C. T., *Proc. Natl. Acad. Sci. U.S.A., 65,* 702 (1970).
43. Lucas-Lenard, J., and Lipmann, F., *Ann. Rev. Biochem., 40,* 409 (1971).
44. Nishizuka, Y., and Lipmann, F., *Arch. Biochem. Biophys., 116,* 344 (1966).
45. Modolell, J., Vazquez, D., and Monro, R. E., *Nature New Biol., 230,* 109 (1971).
46. Kuwano, M., and Schlessinger, D., *Proc. Natl. Acad. Sci. U.S.A., 66,* 146 (1970).
47. Kinoshita, T., Kawano, G., and Tanaka, N., *Biochem. Biophys. Res. Commun., 33,* 769 (1968).

48. Tocchini-Valentini, G. P., Felicetti, L., and Rinaldi, G. M., *Cold Spring Harbor Symp. Quant. Biol., 34,* 463 (1969).
49. Weisblum, B., and Demohn, V., *J. Bacteriol., 101,* 1073 (1970).
50. Ballesta, J. P. G., Montejo, V., and Vazquez, D., *FEBS Letters, 19,* 79 (1971).
51. Kischa, K., Möller, W., and Stöffler, G., *Nature New Biol., 233,* 62 (1971).
52. Gordon, J., *J. Biol. Chem., 244,* 5680 (1969).
53. Modolell, J., Cabrer, B., Parmeggiani, A., and Vazquez, D., *Proc. Natl. Acad. Sci. U.S.A., 68,* 1796 (1971).
54. Cabrer, B., Vazquez, D., and Modolell, J., *Proc. Natl. Acad. Sci. U.S.A. 69,* 733 (1972).

29

Mechanisms of Mammalian Protein Synthesis

Kivie Moldave

California College of Medicine
University of California, Irvine
Irvine, California, U.S.A.

Most of the information on protein synthesis in mammalian cells has concerned the elongation of nascent polypeptide chains on ribosomes. This process represents the mechanism for translating the internal codons in mRNA which are expressed as amino acids, beyond the one which specifies initiation. Information that may relate to the initiation or termination of protein synthesis in eukaryotes is now becoming available (1-18), but these processes are not as well understood as they are in bacterial cells (19,20).

In mammalian systems, the transfer of amino acids from tRNA to ribosome-bound polypeptides requires aminoacyl-tRNAs, ribosomes, two soluble protein factors (aminoacyl transferase I, TI; and aminoacyl transferase II, TII), GTP, a sulfhydryl compound, and ammonium and magnesium ions. The tRNAs are charged with radioactive amino acids in the presence of ATP and aminoacyl-tRNA synthetases (21,22). Ribosomes containing endogenous peptidyl-tRNA and mRNA, but free of soluble protein factors, are prepared from microsomes by extraction with deoxycholate and purified with 0.5 M NH$_4$Cl (23). The endogenous peptidyl-tRNA (as well as mRNA) can be removed from these ribosomes, which then require an exogenous source of template mRNA for protein synthesis (24). Other ribonucleoprotein preparations that have been used in these experiments consist of subunits (40S and 60S particles) prepared from stripped rat liver ribosomes (25,26).

The two transfer factors obtained from the soluble portion of rat liver homogenates can be resolved by chromatography on Sephadex G200 (27) or on hydroxyapatite by a batch fractionation procedure (28). TI can be purified further and resolved completely from contaminating traces of TII by chromatography of the TI-containing hydroxyapatite batch eluate on DEAE-Sephadex or cellulose phosphate columns. Purification of TII can be accomplished by chromatographing the TII-containing hydroxapatite batch eluate on cellulose phosphate and DEAE-Sephadex columns, followed by electrofocusing in a pH-gradient apparatus (29). Both TI and TII are necessary for the polymerization of tRNA-bound amino acids into a peptide-bound form.

GTP is the only nucleotide required for the aminoacyl transfer reaction, from tRNA to protein. Other naturally occurring nucleotides do not replace GTP. The products of the reaction are GDP and inorganic phosphate. Evidence indicates that at least two intermediate steps in polypeptide chain elongation, which involve ribosome-bound intermediates, result in the hydrolysis of the nucleotide (30). Two other steps have been recognized which involve the transfer factors and require a guanine nucleotide specifically but which do not result in a hydrolytic cleavage of the molecule (30) since the β-γ methylene analogue of GTP (5'-guanylyl methylene diphosphonate, GDPCP) is active. Whether these latter two steps reflect allosteric or conformational effects of GTP on the transfer factors remains to be determined. The requirement for a sulfhydryl compound (reduced glutathione, mercaptoethanol, or dithiothreitol) is related to the activation of TII (31); a sulfhydryl requirement in peptide chain elongation, other than for the activation of TII, has not been detected.

Polypeptide chain elongation is the translation of internal codons by ribonucleoprotein particles carrying a peptidyl-tRNA, an N-acylaminoacyl-tRNA, or an aminoacyl-tRNA. Amino acids from aminoacyl-tRNA are added one at a time, through a cyclic series of reactions, resulting in the elongation of the polypeptide chain from the N-terminal residue toward the C-terminal amino acid residue. Figure 1 is a schematic representation of the individual steps which must be considered as each amino acid is added to the nascent peptide chain. One of the transfer factors (designated as transferase I in Fig. 1) catalyzes the interaction of aminoacyl-tRNAs with 80S ribosomes, placing the incoming aminoacyl-tRNA at the A site of the ribosome. This interpretation is based on the observation that in the presence of TI and GTP or GDPCP, radioactive aminoacyl-tRNA is bound to ribosomes stripped of endogenous peptidyl-tRNA. It is recovered with ribosomes isolated from the reaction mixture by gradient centrifugation or filtration on Millipore membranes (32). This binding reaction is a fairly intricate one (33-35) which appears to involve the formation of a complex between TI and the aminoacyl-tRNA (reaction 1) in the presence of guanine nucleotide, followed by the integration of the factor-substrate complex with the ribosome (reaction 2):

$$\text{Aminoacyl-tRNA} + \text{TI} \xrightarrow{\text{GTP}} [\text{aminoacyl-tRNA} \cdot \text{TI}] \tag{1}$$

$$[\text{Aminocyl-tRNA} \cdot \text{TI}] + \text{ribosomes} \xrightarrow{\text{GTP}} \text{ribosomes} [\text{aminoacyl-tRNA} \cdot \text{TI}] \tag{2}$$

The binding of aminoacyl-tRNA to ribosomes requires TI and GTP or GDPCP, and binding of TI factor to ribosomes requires aminoacyl-tRNA and GTP or GDPCP (32,34). Evidence for a series of reactions between the binding factor, aminoacyl tRNAs, and GTP prior to the reaction with ribosomes has also been obtained with bacterial preparations (19,20).

If peptidyl-tRNA is present at the P site of the ribosome (as shown in Fig. 1), the binding reaction with GTP is followed by the formation of a peptide bond between the carbonyl group in the peptidyl-tRNA ester and the amino group in the aminoacyl-tRNA. Peptide bond formation is catalyzed by a ribosome-associated activity, peptidyl transferase, and does not require any soluble transfer factors or GTP (30,36-44). However, when the β-γ methylene analogue of GTP is used in the binding reaction, aminoacyl-tRNA is integrated with the ribosome, but it is not incorporated into a peptide-bound form (30). These data suggest the participation of an intermediate step between the initial binding of aminoacyl-tRNAs to ribosomes and their reaction with peptidyl-tRNA to form a new peptide bond; both steps require a guanine nucleotide, but the former does not involve hydrolysis of GTP while the latter step requires it.

Figure 2 shows the peptidyl transfer reaction schematically. The reaction on the left side of the figure leads to the formation of a new peptidyl-tRNA, one

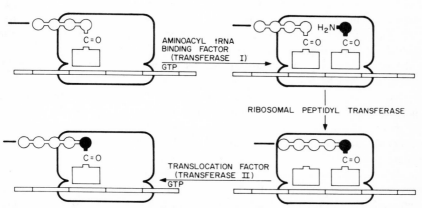

Fig. 1. Intermediate steps in peptide chain elongation. The small circles represent individual amino acids bound to tRNA (squares), within the ribosome composed of two attached subunits. The mRNA with its component codons is represented by the bar attached to the small subunit, at the lower part of the ribosome. Similar symbols are used in the other figures.

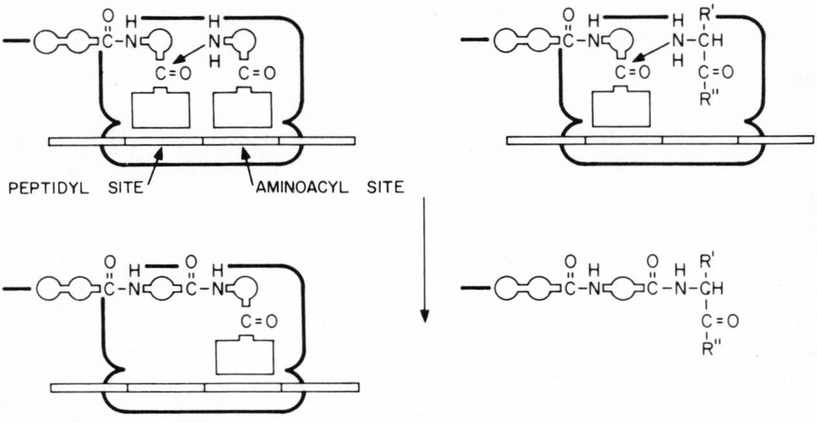

Fig. 2. Peptidyl transferase with aminoacyl-tRNA and puromycin.

amino acid longer, as the result of a nucleophilic attack of the amino nitrogen in aminoacyl-tRNA on the carbonyl carbon in the peptidyl-tRNA ester. The right side of the figure shows the analogous reaction when the antibiotic puromycin (represented by the compound with R' and R'' at the A or aminoacyl site of the ribosome) is used at low concentrations; under the appropriate conditions, puromycin reacts with peptidyl-tRNA at the P or peptidyl site only (30). Thus a convenient assay for peptidyl transferase consists of determining the amount of acid-soluble radioactive puromycin which is converted to the hot ($90°$) acid-insoluble form, as peptidyl puromycin is synthesized by the ribosomal activity.

If the peptidyl transferase reaction is carried out with aminoacyl-tRNA, the newly formed peptidyl-tRNA arises at the A site. It is translocated to the P site in the presence of the other transfer factor (designated transferase II in Fig. 1), making the A site available for the interaction of the next codon with the appropriate aminoacyl-tRNA (44). Translocation has also been studied using labeled puromycin, since at low concentrations it reacts with peptidyl-tRNA at the P site. Two types of ribosomes are obtained from rat liver using the procedures designed in this laboratory. As shown in Fig. 3, some ribosomes contain peptidyl-tRNA at the P site and others contain peptidyl-tRNA at the A site. When a preparation of control ribosomes is treated with puromycin, only those with endogenous peptidyl-tRNA at the P site react (also shown by the open circles in the inset in this figure) to yield radioactive peptidyl puromycin; approximately 10-20% of the ribosomes isolated from rat liver react in this manner. However, after preincubation with translocation factor TII and GTP, ribosomes with peptidyl-tRNA at the A site are translocated, the peptidyl-tRNA is transferred to the P site, and the ribosomes now react with puromycin (closed circles in inset). The number of ribosomes which react with puromycin or with aminoacyl-tRNA after treatment with TII and GTP is many times greater than the number of control ribosomes (30,44). An additional role of GTP has been detected in the TII-dependent reaction. TII binds to ribosomes in the presence of GTP or GDPCP (43,45-47), prior to the translocation step itself, which requires GTP specifically and results in hydrolysis of the nucleotide. If the sulfhydryl group(s) on TII is not reduced with mercaptan, the translocation factor does not bind to ribosomes (43). These steps are summarized in reactions (3) and (4):

$$\text{TII + ribosomes-(peptidyl-tRNA}_a) \xrightarrow[\text{R-SH}]{\text{GDPCP}} [\text{TII} \cdot \text{ribosomes-(peptidyl-tRNA}_a)] \tag{3}$$

$$[\text{TII} \cdot \text{ribosomes-(peptidyl-tRNA}_a)] \xrightarrow{\text{GTP}} \text{TII + ribosomes-(peptidyl-tRNA}_p) + \text{GDP} + \text{P}_i \tag{4}$$

Just as translocation of peptidyl-tRNA from the A to the P site increases the reactivity with puromycin, the addition of aminoacyl-tRNA to ribosomes (Fig. 4) and peptidyl transfer result in a decrease in the number of ribosomes with peptidyl-tRNA at the P site and consequently in the reactivity toward puromycin. The open circles in the inset of Fig. 4 represent peptidyl puromycin formed with translocated ribosomes which were incubated with aminoacyl-tRNA under

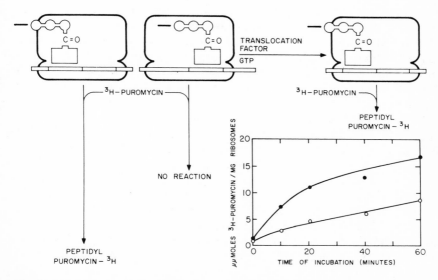

Fig. 3. Translocation. ○, Puromycin reaction before translocation; ●, puromycin reaction after incubation with TII and GTP.

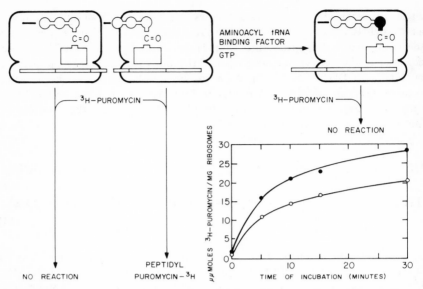

Fig. 4. Aminoacyl-tRNA binding and peptidyl transferase. ○, Puromycin reaction after an incubation in the presence of aminoacyl-tRNA; ●, puromycin reaction after an incubation in the absence of aminoacyl-tRNA.

nonenzymatic (20 mM Mg^{2+}) binding conditions; the closed circles refer to the reaction with ribosomes treated with puromycin directly after translocation.

The code-specific interaction between various tRNA derivatives and template codons requires ribonucleoprotein particles and results in the binding of the tRNA to the particle. Although this interaction involves weak bonds, it results in the firm integration of tRNA with the particle; the bound tRNA can be recovered with the particle isolated from the reaction mixture. Binding can be carried out nonenzymatically in the presence of relatively high concentrations of magnesium ions, and in many cases enzymatically in the presence of protein factors at low magnesium ion concentrations (Table I). When the reactions are carried out in low magnesium ion-containing solutions, binding is completely dependent on GTP and TI, consistent with participation as an intermediate step in peptide chain elongation on 80S ribosomes. It was considered of interest, however, to examine codon-specific tRNA-ribonucleoprotein interactions, other than those which occur during chain elongation, for a number of reasons: (a) the established role of N-formylmethionyl-tRNA and the participation of ribosomal subunits in peptide chain initiation with prokaryotic ribosomes (19,20); (b) the requirement for initiation factors, distinct from peptide chain elongation factors, for the interaction of mRNA with the small ribosomal subunit, then with fMet-tRNA, and finally with the large ribosomal subunit to form the prokaryotic initiation complex [see reviews by Lengyel and Söll (19) and by Lucas-Lenard and Lipmann (10); these reactions are presented schematically in Fig. 5] ; (c) the requirement for initiation factors for incorporation of N-acetylphenylalanine at the N-terminal position of polyphenylalanine, with *Escherichia coli* preparations, at low magnesium ion concentrations (48-50); (d) the requirement for "initiation" factors obtained from "washes" of mammalian ribosomes, in addition to those required for chain elongation, for the synthesis of some proteins (1,6,12); (e) the apparent existence of a ribosome cycle in mammalian cells, in which subunits participate in one of the stages in protein synthesis (2,4,5); (f) the implication of specific tRNAs (7-10,11,15) or N-acylaminoacyl-tRNAs (51-53) in chain initiation with mammalian ribosomes; (g) the fact that TI, the binding factor for peptide chain elongation on 80S ribosomes, does not recognize these specific eukaryotic tRNAs, e.g., Met-tRNA$_f$ in contrast to Met-tRNA$_m$ (54-57); (h) the binding of aminoacyl-tRNAs and N-acylaminoacyl-tRNAs to 40S subunits in the presence of protein factor(s) distinct from TI which catalyzes binding of aminoacyl-tRNAs to 80S ribosomes (14,16,17). These data suggest that the decoding of the first codon to be translated in an mRNA cistron is

Table I. Binding of Various tRNAs to Ribosomes[a]

Substrate	Deletions	Ribosome-bound radioactivity	
		Enzymatic (cpm)	Nonenzymatic (cpm)
Aminoacyl-tRNA	None	1300	850
	GTP	180	800
	TI	210	810
Phenylalanyl-tRNA	None	6500	5800
	GTP	560	5600
	TI	140	5400
N-acetylphenylalanyl-tRNA	None	30	3300
	GTP	20	3000
	TI	15	3500

[a] Binding of the tRNA derivatives to 80S ribosomes was carried out as described for aminoacyl-tRNA (32), phenylalanyl-tRNA (24), and N-acetylphenylalanyl-tRNA (24,49). The radioactive substrates were incubated with ribosomes, TI partially purified on hydroxyapatite, and GTP, in buffered salts solution containing 6 mM MgCl$_2$ (enzymatic) or 20 mM MgCl$_2$ (nonenzymatic). When aminoacyl-tRNA was used, the ribosomes were stripped of endogenous peptidyl-tRNA. When phenylalanyl-tRNA or N-acetylphenylalanyl-tRNA was used, the ribosomes were stripped of both peptidyl-tRNA and mRNA, and the incubations also contained poly U. Analyses were carried out by filtration through Millipore membranes (32).

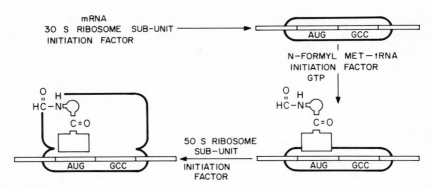

Fig. 5. Peptide chain initiation in prokaryotic cells. Three distinct initiation factors are involved, at various factor-dependent steps.

carried out by a ribonucleoprotein particle (subunit) which does not carry an endogenous aminoacyl, N acylaminoacyl, or peptidyl moiety. The translation of all subsequent codons is then carried out by a ribonucleoprotein particle (ribosome) carrying an aminoacyl- N-acylaminoacyl-, or peptidyl-tRNA. Therefore, the reactions between aminoacyl-tRNAs, N-acylaminoacyl-tRNAs, ribosomes, and ribosomal subunits were investigated.

The effect of the binding factor which catalyzes aminoacyl-tRNA binding in peptide chain elongation (TI) on the binding of phenylalanyl-tRNA with various ribonucleoprotein particles is shown in Table II. The TI preparation, purified by chromatography on cellulose phosphate after elution from hydroxyapatite, is very active with 40S plus 60S particles, as it is with 80S ribosomes. The effect

Table II. Effect of Purified TI on the Binding of Phenylalanyl-tRNA to Various Ribosomal Particles[a]

Ribosomal particles	Incubation additions	Particle-bound radioactivity (cpm)
40S	None	150
40S	TI	300
40S + 60S	None	150
40S + 60S	• TI	5300

[a] Radioactive phenylalanyl-tRNA was incubated with 40S subunits or 40S plus 60S particles in buffered salts-dithiothreitol solution (6 mM MgCl$_2$), in the presence of GTP and poly U. Some incubations, where noted, received TI partially purified by chromatography on hydroxyapatite.

on 40S particles is small and varies considerably from preparation to preparation; some TI fractions, although fully active with 80S ribosomes or 40S plus 60S particles, are completely inactive with 40S subunits.

The effect of purified TI on the binding of N-acetylphenylalanyl-tRNA to various ribosomal particles was also investigated (Table III). In contrast to the very extensive binding of phenylalanyl-tRNA to 80S ribosomes (40S plus 60S particles) catalyzed by TI, binding of either substrate to 40S subunits, or of N-acetylphenylalanyl-tRNA, is not usually observed. Occasionally, some TI preparations appear to stimulate binding of both phenylalanyl-tRNA and N-acetylphenylalanyl-tRNA to 40S subunits, suggesting that some TI preparations are contaminated with additional activities related to 40S subunits. This possibility was investigated by carrying out the binding reactions with a crude supernatant fraction from the soluble portion of rat liver homogenates, "pH 5 supernatant," the starting material for the preparation of TI and TII (Table IV). As seen in this table, "pH 5 supernatant" markedly stimulates the binding of N-acetylphenylalanyl-tRNA to 40S subunits. Highly purified TI, which is active in polyphenylalanine synthesis in the presence of TII, does not stimulate this binding; indeed, it appears to inhibit it. Although not shown here, "pH 5 supernatant" fraction also stimulates the binding of phenylalanyl-tRNA to the 40S subunits, but is inactive when either substrate is incubated with 60S subunits alone.

The results obtained with "pH 5 supernatant" and purified TI suggest the presence of an activity (or activities), distinct from TI, which brings about these additional interactions between 40S subunits and tRNA derivatives. Additional

Table III. Effect of Purified TI on the Binding
of Phenylalanyl-tRNA and N-Acetylphenylalanyl-tRNA
to Various Ribosomal Particles[a]

Ribosomal particles	Substrate	Particle-bound radioactivity (cpm)
40S	Phe-tRNA	250
40S	N-acetyl-Phe-tRNA	200
40S + 60S	Phe-tRNA	4300
40S + 60S	N-acetyl-Phe-tRNA	300

[a] Radioactive phenylalanyl-tRNA (Phe-tRNA) or N-acetylphenylalanyl-tRNA (N-acetyl-Phe-tRNA) was incubated with 40S subunits or 40S plus 60S particles in buffered salts-dithiothreitol solutions (6 mM MgCl$_2$), in the presence of GTP, poly U, and TI purified chromatographically on hydroxyapatite and DEAE-Sephadex (0.4 M KCl eluate).

Table IV. Effect of Soluble Proteins
on the Binding of N-Acetylphenylalanyl-tRNA
to 40S Ribosomal Subunits[a]

Incubation additions	Particle-bound radioactivity (cpm)
None	1000
TI	600
"pH 5 supernatant"	3800

[a] Radioactive N-acetylphenylalanyl-tRNA was incubated with 40S subunits and GTP in buffered salts-dithiothreitol solution (6 mM MgCl$_2$). Where noted, purified TI protein or "pH 5 supernatant" fraction (27,28) was added.

Table V. Effect of DEAE-Sephadex Eluate on the Binding
of N-Acetylphenylalanyl-tRNA to various Ribosomal Particles[a]

Ribosomal particles	Incubation additions	Particle-bound radioactivity (cpm)
40S	None	550
40S	0.25 M eluate	2300
40S + 60S	None	200
40S + 60S	0.25 M eluate	400

[a] Radioactive N-acetylphenylalanyl-tRNA was incubated with 40S subunits or 40S plus 60S particles in buffered salts-dithiothreitol solution (6 mM MgCl$_2$), in the presence of GTP and poly U. Some incubations, where noted, received supernatant protein obtained by chromatography on hydroxyapatite and recovered from DEAE-Sephadex in the 0.20-0.25 M KCl eluate.

support for this suggestion is based on the observations that the activity which carries out binding to 40S subunits is sensitive to sulfhydryl compounds, while TI is not, and that the heat stability of the activity which binds tRNAs to 40S subunits differs from that which binds aminoacyl-tRNAs to 80S ribosomes. More definitive evidence is obtained by chromatographing the TI-containing eluate from hydroxyapatite columns (48) on DEAE-Sephadex. The activity which catalyzes binding of tRNA derivatives to 40S subunits is eluted from the DEAE at KCl concentrations of approximately 0.25 M(see Table V), while the activity which catalyzes binding of aminoacyl-tRNA to 80S ribosomes (TI) is eluted at about 0.4 M KCl. The two binding activities are thus resolved from each other. The new binding activity has been tentatively designated as TX.

The template specificity of the new binding factor which catalyzes the interaction with 40S particles, eluted at 0.25 M KCl from DEAE, was examined with a number of polynucleotides. In the presence of polyuridylic acid or MS2 phage RNA, TX catalyzes the binding of N-acetylphenylalanyl-tRNA to 40S subunits. Binding does not occur when polyadenylic acid or ApUpG is used as template; however, binding of E. coli fMet-tRNA to rat liver 40S subunits is observed in the presence of TX and ApUpG or MS2 RNA. Whether the preparation responsible for the binding of aminoacyl-tRNA and N-acylamino-acyl-tRNA to 40S subunits represents one or several activities is not conclusively established.

The presence of 60S subunits in the TX-catalyzed reaction results in the complete inhibition of the binding of N-acetylphenylalanyl-tRNA to 40S subunits (Table VI), probably due to the reaction between 40S and 60S particles to form 80S ribosomes. However, if binding of N-acetylphenylalanyl-tRNA to 40S subunits is allowed to occur in the presence of TX, prior to the addition of 60S subunits, 40-50% of the N-acetylphenylalanyl-tRNA can be recovered with the particles isolated from the reaction mixture.

The data summarized above indicate the existence of at least two different types of binding activities which carry out specific interactions between tRNAs

Table VI. Effect of 60S Subunits on the Binding of
N-Acetylphenylalanyl-tRNA to Ribonucleoprotein Particles[a]

Incubation additions		Particle-bound radioactivity (%)
First incubation	Second incubation	
TX	None	100
TX, 60S	None	0
TX	60S	45

[a] The first incubation contained radioactive N-acetylphenylalanyl-tRNA, GTP, 40S subunits, and TX obtained by chromatography on DEAE-Sephadex in buffered salts-dithiothreitol solution (6 mM $MgCl_2$). One incubation also received 60S subunits at the beginning; another one received 60S subunits after 15 min and incubation was continued for 10 min (second incubation). One-hundred percent activity, in the control incubation in the absence of 60S subunits, represented about 1200 cpm, corrected for binding in the absence of TX.

and ribonucleoprotein particles. One factor (TI) is required for the binding of aminoacyl-tRNA to 80S ribosomes only; the available evidence indicates that TI is the aminoacyl-tRNA-binding factor for polypeptide chain elongation which places the aminoacyl-tRNA at the A site of the ribosome. The other binding activity catalyzes the interaction of aminoacyl-tRNA and N-acylaminoacyl-tRNA with 40S subunits, but is not appreciably active with 80S ribosomes. Some of the characteristics of this novel binding reaction, the properties of the new binding factor, the template specificity, the role of the small ribosomal subunit, and the effect of the large one are similar to those exhibited by prokaryotic systems. This might suggest that the reaction could play a role in peptide chain initiation in eukaryotic systems, but this interpretation remains to be established.

ACKNOWLEDGMENTS

These studies were supported in part by research grants from the American Cancer Society (P-177) and the U.S. Public Health Service (AM-01397, AM-11032; and AM-15156). THe author expresses his appreciation to Drs. E. Gasior, F. Ibuki, R. A. Schroer, J. Siler, L. Skogerson, and D. Young for their contributions and participation in the experiments described herein.

SUMMARY

Polypeptide chain elongation on mammalian ribosomes requires aminoacyl-tRNAs, two soluble protein factors, GTP, sulfhydryl compound, and various cations. One of the transfer factors, aminoacyl transferase I (TI), catalyzes the interaction between aminoacyl-tRNAs and 80S ribosomes, placing the aminoacyl-tRNA at the A site of the ribosomes; this binding reaction is a complex one involving several intermediary steps. A ribosome-associated activity, peptidyl transferase, then catalyzes the reaction between the peptidyl-tRNA on the P site and the newly bound aminoacyl-tRNA, resulting in the formation of a peptide bond; the peptidyl moiety, bound in an ester linkage to tRNA, is transferred to the amino group of the aminoacyl-tRNA, in a reaction which does not require soluble protein factors or GTP. The newly formed peptidyl-tRNA at the A position is translocated to the P site in the presence of aminoacyl transferase II (TII) and GTP. This complex reaction, involving at least one intermediary step, places the next codon to be translated at the unoccupied A site, ready to participate in another cycle of reactions leading to peptide chain extension. Recent studies in a number of laboratories have revealed data that may relate to the initiation of protein synthesis in mammalian systems. In this laboratory, studies on a model chain initiation system based on information from prokaryotic cells have led to an investigation of the interactions of aminoacyl-tRNAs, N-acylaminoacyl-tRNAs, and ribosomal subunits from rat liver. TI, which catalyzes the binding of aminoacyl-tRNA to 80S ribosomes and to 40S plus 60S particles, is inactive with 40S subunits and with N-acylaminoacyl-tRNAs. An activity is present in the crude soluble fraction of rat liver homogenates which stimulates binding of phenylalanyl-tRNA and N-acetylphenylalanyl-tRNA to 40S subunits but which is inactive with 80S ribosomes. The new binding activity, which is specific for 40S subunits, can be resolved from TI on DEAE-Sephadex. The binding reaction is strongly inhibited by

60S subunits; however, if 60S subunits are added to the incubation after the binding reaction has been allowed to occur with 40S subunits, a considerable amount of the substrate remains associated with the particles.

RESUMEN

La elongación de la cadena polipeptídica sobre ribosomas de mamíferos requiere aminoacil-tRNAs, dos factores proteicos solubles, GTP, compuestos con grupos sulfhidrilos y varios cationes. Uno de los factores de transferencia, la aminoacil transferasa I (TI), cataliza la interacción entre los aminoacil-tRNAs y los ribosomas 80S, colocando el aminoacil-tRNA en el sitio A del ribosoma; esta reacción de unión es compleja y comprende varias etapas intermedias. Una actividad ligada al ribosoma, la de la peptidil transferasa, cataliza entonces la reacción entre el peptidil-tRNA en el sitio P y el aminoacil-tRNA recientemente unido, lo que conduce a la formación de un enlace peptídico; la porción peptidilo, unida por medio de un enlace éster al tRNA, es transferida al grupo amino del aminoacil-tRNA en una reacción que no requiere factores proteicos solubles ni GTP. El peptidil-tRNA recientemente formado en la posición A es translocado al sitio P en presencia de la aminoacil transferasa II (TII) y GTP. Esta reacción compleja, que incluye por lo menos una etapa intermedia, coloca al próximo codón a traducir en el sitio A que se halla desocupado, listo para participar en otro ciclo de reacciones que conducen a la extensión de la cadena peptídica.

Estudios en este laboratorio de un modelo para la iniciación de la cadena, basado en información obtenida en células eucarióticas, nos ha llevado a investigar las interacciones entre los aminoacil-tRNAs, N-acilaminoacil tRNAs y las subunidades ribosomales del hígado de rata. TI, la cual cataliza la unión del aminoacil-tRNA a los ribosomas 80S y a las partículas 40S y 60S, es inactivo con subunidades 40S y con N-acilaminoacil tRNAs. Alguna actividad se encuentra en la fracción cruda y soluble del homogenizado del hígado de rata, la cual estimula la unión de fenilalanil tRNA y N-acetilfenilalanil t-RNA a las subunidades 40S, pero es inactiva con las subunidades 80S. Esta nueva actividad de unión, la cual es específica para las subunidades 40S, puede resolverse de la de TI en DEAE-Sephadex. La reacción de unión es altamente inhibida por la subunidades 60S; sin embargo, si las subunidades 60S son agregadas a la incubación después que la reacción de unión con las subunidades 40S ha ocurrido, una cantidad considerable de substrato se queda asociado a estas partículas.

REFERENCES

1. Miller, R. L., and Schweet, R., *Arch. Biochem. Biophys., 125,* 632 (1968).
2. Kaempfer, R., and Meselson, M., *Cold Spring Harbor Symp. Quant. Biol., 34,* 209 (1969).
3. Moldave, K., Galasinski, W., Rao, P., and Siler, J., *Cold Spring Harbor Symp. Quant. Biol. 34,* 347 (1969).
4. Adamson, S. D., Howard, G. A., and Herbert, E., *Cold Spring Harbor Symp. Quant. Biol. 34,* 547 (1969).
5. Baglioni, C., Vesco, C., and Jacobs-Lorean, M., *Cold Spring Harbor Symp. Quant. Biol., 34,* 555 (1969).
6. Heywood, S. M., *Nature, 225,* 696 (1970).
7. Smith, A. E., and Marcker, K. A., *Nature, 226,* 607 (1970).
8. Jackson, R., and Hunter, T., *Nature, 227,* 672 (1970).
9. Wigle, D. T., and Dixon, G. H., *Nature, 227,* 676 (1970).
10. Houseman, T., Jacobs-Lorean, M., RajBhandary, U. L., and Lodish, H. A., *Nature, 227,* 913 (1970).

11. Bhaduri, S., Chatterjee, N. J., Bose, K. K., and Gupta, N. K., *Biochem. Biophys. Res. Commun., 40,* 402 (1970).
12. Shafritz, D. A., and Anderson, W. F., *J. Biol. Chem. 245,* 5553 (1970).
13. Goldstein, J., Beaudet, A., and Caskey, C. T., *Proc. Natl. Acad. Sci. U.S.A., 67,* 99 (1970).
14. Leader, B. P., Wool, I. G., and Castles, J. C., *Proc. Natl. Acad. Sci. U.S.A., 67,* 523 (1970).
15. Marcus, A., Weeks, T. P., Leis, J. P., and Keller, E. P., *Proc. Natl. Acad. Sci. U.S.A., 67,* 1681 (1970).
16. Moldave, K., and Gasior, E., *Fed. Proc., 30,* 1289 (1971).
17. Heywood, S. M., and Thompson, W. C., *Biochem. Biophys. Res. Commun., 43,* 470 (1971).
18. Beaudet, A. L., and Caskey, C. T., *Proc. Natl. Acad. Sci. U.S.A., 68,* 619 (1971).
19. Lengyel, P., and Söll, D., *Bacteriol. Rev., 33,* 264 (1969).
20. Lucas-Lenard, J., and Lipmann, F., *Ann. Rev. Biochem., 40,* 409 (1971).
21. Moldave, K., in Colowick, S. P., and Kaplan, N. O. (eds.), Vol. 6, *Methods in Enzymology,* Academic Press, New York (1963), pp. 757-761.
22. Yamane, T., and Sueoka, N., *Proc. Natl. Acad. Sci. U.S.A., 50,* 1093 (1963).
23. Skogerson, L., and Moldave, K., *Biochem. Biophys. Res. Commun., 27,* 568 (1967).
24. Siler, J., and Moldave, K., *Biochim. Biophys. Acta, 195,* 123 (1969).
25. Martin T. E., and Wool, I. G., *Proc. Natl. Acad. Sci. U.S.A., 60,* 569 (1968).
26. Rao, P., and Moldave, K., *J. Mol. Biol., 46,* 447 (1969).
27. Gasior, E., and Moldave, K., *J. Biol. Chem., 240,* 3346 (1965).
28. Schneir, M., and Moldave, K., *Biochim. Biophys. Acta, 166,* 58 (1968).
29. Galasinski, W., and Moldave, K., *J. Biol. Chem., 244,* 6527 (1969).
30. Skogerson, L., and Moldave, K., *Arch. Biochem. Biophys., 125,* 497 (1968).
31. Sutter, R. P., and Moldave, K., *J. Biol. Chem., 241,* 1698 (1966).
32. Ibuki, F., and Moldave, K., *J. Biol. Chem., 243,* 791 (1968).
33. Ibuki, F., Gasior, E., and Moldave, K., *J. Biol. Chem., 241,* 2188 (1966).
34. Ibuki, F., and Moldave, K., *J. Biol. Chem., 243,* 44 (1968).
35. Rao, P., and Moldave, K., *Biochem. Biophys. Res. Commun., 28,* 909 (1967).
36. Traut, R. R., and Monro R. E., *J. Mol. Biol., 10,* 63 (1964).
37. Leder, P., and Bursztyn, H., *Biochem. Biophys. Res. Commun., 25,* 233 (1966).
38. Bretscher, N. S., and Marcker, K. A., *Nature, 211,* 380 (1966).
39. Monro, R. E., *J. Mol. Biol., 26,* 147 (1967).
40. Monro, R. E., and Marcker, K. A., *J. Mol. Biol., 25,* 347 (1967).
41. Gottesman, M. E., *J. Biol. Chem., 242,* 5564 (1967).
42. Pestka, S. *J. Biol. Chem., 243,* 2810 (1968).
43. Skogerson, L., and Moldave, K., *J. Biol. Chem., 243,* 5354 (1968).
44. Skogerson, L., and Moldave, K., *J. Biol. Chem., 243,* 5361 (1968).
45. Parmeggiani, A., and Gottschalk, E. M., *Biochem. Biophys. Res. Commun., 35,* 861 (1969).
46. Brot, N., Spears, C., and Weissbach, H., *Biochem. Biophys. Res. Commun., 34,* 843 (1969).
47. Kuriki, Y., Inoue, N., and Kaziro, Y., *Biochim. Biophys. Acta, 224,* 487 (1970).
48. Lucas-Lenard, J., and Lipmann, F., *Proc. Natl. Acad. Sci. U.S.A., 57,* 1050 (1967).
49. Nakamoto, T., and Hamel, E., *Proc. Natl. Acad. Sci. U.S.A., 59,* 238 (1968).
50. Klem, E. B., and Nakamoto, T., *Proc. Natl. Acad. Sci. U.S.A., 61,* 1349 (1968).
51. Arnstein, H. R. V., and Rahminoff, H., *Nature, 219,* 942 (1968).
52. Laycock, D. G., and Hunt, J. A., *Nature, 221,* 1118 (1969).

53. Liew, C. C., Haslett, G. W., and Allfrey, V. G., *Nature, 226,* 414 (1970).
54. Kerwan, S., Shear, C., and Weissbach, H., *Biochem. Biophys. Res. Commun., 41,* 78 (1970).
55. Tarrago, A., Monasterio, O., and Allende, J. E., *Biochem. Biophys. Res. Commun., 41,* 765 (1970).
56. Shafritz, D. A., and Anderson, W. F., *Nature, 227,* 918 (1970).
57. Gosh, K., Grishko, A., and Gosh, H. P., *Biochem. Biophys. Res. Commun., 42,* 462 (1971).
58. Moldave, K., Galasinski, W., and Rao, P., in Moldave, K., and Grossman, L. (eds.), *Methods in Enzymology, Nucleic Acids,* Vol. 20, Academic Press, New York (1971), pp. 337-348.
59. Siler, J., and Moldave, K., *Biochim. Biophys. Acta, 195,* 130 (1969).

DISCUSSION

H. N. Torres (Buenos Aires, Argentina): In the elongation step, you have two factors, TI and TII, and these factors require GTP. Which is the limiting step in this elongation reaction, the reaction that requires TI factor or the reaction that requires TII factor? And another question: the first reaction, the reaction that requires TI factor, has been formed in the absence of TI factor and the presence of a high amount of magnesium. Is it possible to carry out the second reaction by addition of TII factor and GTP?

K. Moldave (Irvine, U.S.A.): No, binding of aminoacyl-tRNA is not catalyzed by TII and GTP; the binding reactions that I described are quite similar, I think, to the ones that were described by Dr. Spirin. We also visualize that the ribosome, let us say it has a growing peptide chain on the P site, has an open A site; this latter site can be filled either nonenzymatically with high magnesium or enzymatically with TI. But in the reaction with TI, we find that there is an intermediate step which I did not mention in my talk, and I am glad that you have brought it up. This intermediate step, which we came across a number of years ago, occurs in mammalian and bacterial systems. In the reaction, TI brings aminoacyl-tRNA to the ribosome and puts it on the "proper" site. It is a codon-specific reaction, but it cannot react in the peptidyl transferase reaction, possibly because it is not in the right position or configuration. We found that we can isolate this step by incubating in the presence of GMP-PCP because a guanine nucleotide is required for this binding reaction, but GTP hydrolysis is not required and does not occur. GTP hydrolysis occurs in the next step, and I have intentionally drawn the initially bound aminoacyl-tRNA out of line, not just to show that I am a bad artist, but because I do not want to align the two tRNAs, the peptidyl-tRNA and the aminoacyl-tRNA, in such a position that they would react. If you now allow these two tRNAs to align properly, they can react in the peptidyl transferase reaction. Peptidyl transferase does not require GTP, and the initial binding reaction I just mentioned does not require GTP hydrolysis; but between these two steps, you have to add GTP for alignment, and it is at this intermediate step that GTP hydrolysis takes place. So there is this intermediate step which occurs on the ribosome, after binding, and we feel that it is at this point that the hydrolysis of GTP takes place. Nonenzymatically, the aminoacyl-tRNA goes to the A site in the presence of high magnesium, and it is placed in a position or configuration which will react in the peptidyl transferase reaction, so it skips the intermediate step. We feel that the "alignment" or "accommodation" relates to a ribosomal event that is catalyzed by GTP and requires hydrolysis of the nucleotide; we picture a very similar thing occurring in translocation of peptidyl-tRNA from one site to the other. The sequence I just described shows two steps involving GTP hydrolysis. However, I think I should add a word of caution. The fact that one does observe two distinct GTP steps at which hydrolysis occurs need not mean that two GTPs are hydrolyzed per amino acid added during protein synthesis, as I suggested several years ago. I do not think that it is necessarily a strict prerequisite; I do not think it need be an obligatory requirement. Dr. Lipmann has suggested that these two GTP-dependent events are coupled and that one GTP molecule may well catalyze both, concomitantly. I think this question has to remain open for the present. With regard to your first question as to which is the limiting step in the elongation reactions, our data would suggest that the rate-limiting step is translocation.

H. N. Torres: I do not understand the first reaction carried out in the presence of high magnesium concentration and in the absence of TI factor. Is it possible that there is some kind of exchange reaction between aminoacyl-tRNA and peptidyl-tRNA? For example, if one of the amino acids contained in the peptidyl-tRNA bound to the ribosome is labeled and the aminoacyl-tRNA is cold, is there some exchange reaction? If there is, the formation of radioactive aminoacyl-tRNA in this condition is nonenzymatic.

K. Moldave: I do not really know if I can answer that question specifically. We do not feel that there is an interaction as you suggest with anything on the P site of the ribosome. We do not observe exchange of that type. Labeled aminoacyl-tRNA in high magnesium ion concentrations binds to the ribosome, reacts in the peptidyl transferase reactions, and becomes incorporated into a peptide-bound form; but in the absence of TII, it is quantitatively recovered in the *C*-terminal position of the nascent peptide. Our experiments without peptidyl-tRNA on the P site seem to show that there is a little bit of a difference in the stability of the complex containing aminoacyl-tRNA on the A site as compared to the P site, but I do not think that I can really say very much about this particular kind of interaction. We can say that in high magnesium, we can certainly put aminoacyl-tRNA in a position that makes a peptide bond, and that this is a codon-specific reaction; thus it goes through or skips the intermediate reaction. Beyond that, we have not observed more nor do we know more about the particular sequence that is catalyzed by high magnesium.

30

The Effect of Sodium Fluoride, Edeine, and Cycloheximide on Peptide Synthesis with Reticulocyte Ribosomes

Boyd Hardesty, Tom Obrig, James Irvin, and William Culp

Clayton Foundation Biochemical Institute
The University of Texas
Department of Chemistry
Austin, Texas, U.S.A.

Our purpose in studying antibiotics and other inhibitors of protein synthesis has been to use these compounds to elucidate and characterize reaction mechanisms. The followng discussion is limited to three compounds, sodium fluoride, edeine, and cycloheximide, that have related but dissimilar effects on peptide initiation. Portions of the material presented were published previously (1,2,5).

METHODS

Antibiotics

The source of the antibiotics has been reported elsewhere (1,2).

Preparation of Biological Materials and Assay Systems

Techniques for the preparation of aminoacyl-tRNA, ribosomes, and the transfer enzymes are presented in a single reference source (3,4).

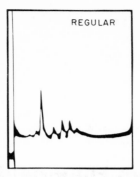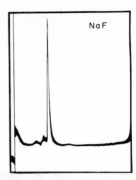

Fig. 1. Schlieren profiles of regular and NaF ribosomes
Ribosomes at 4.0 mg/ml in a solution containing 10 mM
Tris-HCl (pH 7.5), 1.0 mM KCl, and 0.10 mM MgCl$_2$ were
centrifuged at 20° and 40,000 rpm in a Beckman model E
analytical centrifuge.

Incorporation of free amino acids into globin peptides was measured in the
complete reaction mixture as previously described (5). The reaction mixture
contains, in a total volume of 1.4 ml, 50 μmoles of Tris-HCL (pH 7.5), 100 μmoles
of KCl, 5 μmoles of MgCl$_2$, 20 μmoles of GSH, 0.05 μmole of each of 20
common L-amino acids excluding cystine and the radioactive amino acid, 0.1
μmole of ^{14}C-L-leucine (2-10 mc/mmole) or ^{14}C-L-valine (4-40 mc/mmole), 1
μmole of ATP, 0.25 μmole of GTP, 10 μmoles of creatine phosphate, 0.05 mg of
creatine phosphokinase, 1 mg of protein from the 40-70% ammonium sulfate
enzyme fraction, 0.15 mg of reticulocyte tRNA, and 4 mg of unwashed ribosomes from cells that have or have not been previously incubated with NaF. The
former are termed "NaF ribosomes," while the latter are "regular ribosomes."
Incubations were at 37° unless otherwise indicated. Incorporation of radioactivity into peptides was measured as hot trichloroacetic acid-insoluble material.

RESULTS

Sodium Fluoride

Marks *et al.* (6) observed a decrease in polysomes and an increase in 78S
ribosomes isolated from intact reticulocytes following incubation of these cells
with NaF. Polysomes and globin synthesis could be re-established in these cells if
they were transferred to an incubation mixture that did not contain NaF.
Typical results for this effect of NaF on intact reticulocytes are depicted in Fig.
1. Conversion of polysomes to monomeric ribosomes is associated with a
concomitant loss of nascent peptide chains from the ribosomes (5). *In vitro*

studies indicate that most of the nascent peptides attached to polysomes are completed and released from the ribosomes as the a and β chains of rabbit globin. NaF has little or no detectable effect on these reactions by which peptides are completed and released in the cell-free system. Data of these types have been interpreted to indicate that NaF inhibits peptide synthesis by blocking one or more reactions involved in the initiation of peptides on the ribosomes. This interpretation is supported by the amino-terminal data presented in Table I.

For these experiments, preparations of either "regular ribosomes" that bear nascent peptides attached to polysomes or "NaF ribosomes" isolated from reticulocytes that had been incubated with NaF were used *in vitro* to synthesize peptides containing ^{14}C-valine. Amino-terminal ^{14}C-valine was determined by the fluorodinitrobenzene method and is expressed as a percent of the total ^{14}C-valine in these peptides. Valine is the animo-terminal amino acid of both a and β chains of rabbit hemoglobin. The peptides are synthesized from their amino-terminal to their carboxyl-terminal ends; thus the proportions of chains that contain ^{14}C-valine in the amino-terminal position provide an index of peptides that were initiated during the *in vitro* incubation.

Peptides formed with regular ribosomes in the *in vitro* system had 5.7%

Table I. Percentage of N-Terminal Valine Incorporated
with NaF Ribosomes and Regular Ribosomes Inhibited
by NaF or Cycloheximide[a]

Source of peptides	*In vitro* inhibitor	Percentage N-terminal valine	Percentage N-terminal methionine
Randomly labeled hemoglobin	—	8.2	2
Regular ribosomes	None	5.7	2
NaF ribosomes	None	8.3	—
Regular ribosomes	NaF	0.9	—
Regular ribosomes	Cycloheximide	0.2	3

[a] A complete reaction mixture as described in *Methods* was incubated for 60 min in the presence of ^{14}C-L-valine (4mc/μmole) or ^{14}C-L-methionine (20 c/mole) at 40 μc/mole, or ^{14}C-L-methionine (200 c/mole) was used when inhibitors were employed. The percent N-terminal valine or methionine was measured as described previously (5). Globin randomly labeled with valine or methionine in whole cells was used as a standard.

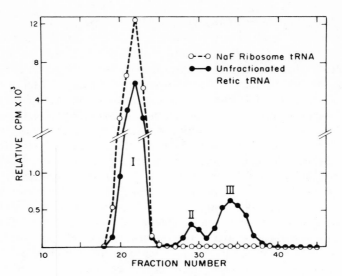

Fig. 2. Chromatography of tRNA from NaF ribosomes. Ribosomes
were prepared from rabbit reticulocytes incubated with NaF and
then washed by sedimenting them through a 5-20% linear sucrose
gradient containing 10 mM Tris-HCl (pH 7.5), 35 mM KCl, and 1.0
mM MgCl$_2$. The isolated ribosomes were resuspended, and soluble
RNA was extracted with phenol as previously described (17). Bulk
reticulocyte tRNA was prepared by phenol extraction of intact
reticulocytes. The tRNA preparations were subjected to pH 9.2 to
hydrolyze aminoacyl-tRNA. Transfer RNA, 0.25 mg, was acylated
in a 1.0 ml reaction mixture containing 20 mM tris-HCl (pH 7.5), 8
mM KCl, 6 mM MgCl$_2$, 10 mM GSH, 10^{-5} M methionine, and 0.5
mg protein from a 40-70% ammonium sulfate fraction prepared
from a postribosomal reticulocyte lysate. Transfer RNA isolated
from NaF ribosomes was acylated with ^{3}H-methionine, 186
mc/mmole. Acylation of bulk reticulocyte tRNA was carried out
using ^{14}C-methionine, 233 mc/mmole. Details of the procedures
used are reported elsewhere (10). The methionyl-tRNAs were isolated, pooled, and run on a reversed phase column (RPC-2) as
described by Weiss and Kelmers (9).

amino-terminal valine. This value is to be compared with 8.2% amino-terminal
valine for hemoglobin that was randomly labeled with ^{14}C-valine during a
relatively long incubation of intact cells. The difference between these values
reflects completion of nascent peptides and *de novo* initiation with regular
ribosomes in the *in vitro* system. In contrast to these results with regular
ribosomes, peptides formed *in vitro* with NaF ribosomes have values expected
for randomly labeled globin. We have interpreted these results to indicate that
^{14}C-valine is incorporated into the amino-terminal position of nearly all peptides

formed with NaF ribosomes (5). Furthermore, the addition of either NaF or cycloheximide to the *in vitro* reaction mixture blocks incorporation of amino-terminal valine with regular ribosomes. At these concentrations, the inhibitors reduce *in vitro* synthesis with NaF ribosomes to levels which make it impractical to determine amino-terminal incorporation of ^{14}C-valine.

The data presented in Fig. 2 indicate that NaF ribosomes carry $tRNA_f^{Met}$, the tRNA species involved in peptide initiation in eukaryotes (7,8). For these experiments, tRNA was extracted from washed NaF ribosomes. The tRNA was charged with ^{3}H-methionine and then mixed with ^{14}C-Met-tRNA formed with tRNA extracted from intact reticulocytes. The mixture of Met-tRNAs was chromatographed on a reversed phase column (9), and the distribution of the radioactive carbon and tritium was determined. Nearly all of the Met-tRNA formed with tRNA from NaF ribosomes is eluted in a single peak, even though two additional peaks of Met-tRNA are observed with tRNA isolated from intact cells. In contrast, three Met-tRNA peaks were observed with tRNA isolated from regular ribosomes. The Met-tRNA from the NaF ribosomes can be formylated with bacterial enzymes and appears to be $tRNA_f^{Met}$ (10). This species, $tRNA_f^{Met}$, accounts for about half of the total amino acid acceptor capacity observed with tRNA extracted from NaF ribosomes.

Considered together, we interpret these data to indicate that NaF blocks a reaction of peptide initiation after $tRNA_f^{Met}$ is bound to ribosomes. The sensitive reaction must precede incorporation of valine into the amino-terminal position of the completed chains.

Edeine

Edeine is a broad-spectrum antibiotic that is a mixture of two closely related basic peptides (11). Kurylo-Borowska and her colleagues have shown it to inhibit DNA synthesis *in vivo* in *Escherichia coli* with little or no inhibitory effect on the synthesis of RNA or protein (12). They observed that edeine was a potent inhibitor of poly U-directed binding of Phe-tRNA or polyphenylalanine synthesis with *E. coli* ribosomes, but that it had much less inhibitory effect on peptide synthesis directed by f2 phage RNA or endogenous mRNA. Inhibition of poly U-directed synthesis could be overcome by formation of a poly U-Phe-tRNA-ribosome complex (13).

We have observed that edeine blocks initiation of either polyphenylalanine or globin peptides in the *in vitro* reticulocyte systems at a molar ratio of about one edeine per ribosome (1). Resistance to edeine inhibition of polyphenylalanine synthesis can be established by preliminary incubation of poly U, uncharged tRNA, and ribosomes to form an initiation complex of these components. Resistance to inhibition is not established if the tRNA is treated with periodate to oxidize the hydroxyl group of the 3'-terminal ribose. These results

Table II. Effect of Ribosome Complex Formation on
Subsequent Edeine Inhibition of Polyphenylalanine Synthesis[a]

Components in the preliminary incubation	Polyphenylalanine polymerized (pmoles)		Inhibition (%)
	No. edeine	0.2 μM edeine	
Ribosomes	28	2	93
Ribosomes, poly U	30	9	70
Ribosomes, tRNA	27	2	93
Ribosomes, poly U, tRNA	32	32	0
Ribosomes, poly U, IO_4-treated tRNA	27	9	67

[a] A preliminary incubation was carried out at 37° for 5 min in a total
volume of 0.25 ml in a solution of the following composition: 0.02 M
tris-HCl (pH 7.5), 8 mM MgCl$_2$, 70 mM KCl, and 5 mM dithiothreitol.
The following were added to the incubation mixture where indicated:
0.25 mg deoxycholate-washed ribosomes from cells incubated with
NaF, 100 μg poly U, 50 μg deacylated tRNA, and 70 pmoles Phe-tRNA
(100 μg tRNA acylated with ^{14}C-L-phenylalanine, 40 mc/mmole).
Periodate treatment of tRNA is described elsewhere (14). The reaction
mixture was cooled to 0°, and then edeine plus additional salts and the
complementary components required for polyphenylalanine synthesis
were added. Polyphenylalanine was formed during a final incubation at
37° for 5 min.

are presented in Table II. Earlier work demonstrated a high dependence on the
formation of a complex of ribosomes, poly U, and deacylated (uncharged)
tRNA^{Phe} for initiation of polyphenylalanine peptides on reticulocyte ribosomes
at moderate concentrations of Mg^{2+} (14). Other experiments have shown that
edeine is a potent inhibitor of deacylated tRNA^{Phe} binding during the preincubation in which the initiation complex is formed (1).

The effect of edeine appears to be primarily on the smaller or 40S ribosomal
subunit, as shown by the data presented in Table III. Binding of either labeled
ApUpG or Met-tRNA in the presence or absence of the other compound was
measured in these experiments. Considered together with the low molar ratio of
edeine to ribosomes that causes inhibition of peptide synthesis, these data
suggest that the primary site for edeine is located on the small ribosomal
subunit. This hypothesis is supported by the results for inhibition of globin

synthesis with NaF ribosomes presented below. It is not clear whether the primary effect of edeine is on binding of mRNA or tRNA. Edeine may affect functional binding of both tRNA and mRNA to 40S subunits. *In vivo*, these may be mutually dependent phenomena of the type observed for binding of ApUpG or Met-tRNA in Table III.

As described above, NaF appears to block a reaction of peptide initiation in intact reticulocytes with the concomitant accumulation of an initiation complex that contains tRNA$_f^{Met}$ and presumably mRNA. Synthesis *in vitro* with NaF ribosomes occurs with peptides that are initiated from two starting points: those that are initiated *de novo*, and peptides that are formed on ribosomes involved in the initiation complex accumulated in the presence of NaF. As shown in Fig. 3A, leucine incorporation *in vitro* with these ribosomes is nearly abolished by NaF. However, edeine blocks only about half of the synthesis that can take place during a 15 min incubation. These results are in sharp contrast to those observed with ribosomes that have been dissociated into subunits with 0.5 M KCl. Synthesis with these ribosomes is completely blocked by edeine (1). The tRNA$_f^{Met}$ is removed from NaF ribosomes by treatment with 0.5 M KCl. For comparison, the corresponding data with regular ribosomes that retain nascent peptides attached to polysomes are given in Fig. 3B. With regular ribosomes,

Table III. Effect of Edeine on Binding of ApUpg and
Met-tRNA to 40S Ribosomal Subunits[a]

	Edeine	Additions		
		Met-tRNA	ApUpG	ApUpG and Met-tRNA
		(pmoles)		
[3]H-ApUpG bound	−	−	30.3	86.5
	+	−	37.6	32.0
[35]S-Met-tRNA bound	−	0.26	−	4.0
	+	0.24	−	1.6

[a] Details of the procedures used are reported elsewhere (1). The 0.20 ml reaction mixture contained 0.01 M Tris-HCL (pH 7.5), 70 mM KCl, 30 mM MgCl$_2$, 1 mM 2-mercaptoethanol, 1 μM edeine where indicated, 1 A_{260} unit of 40S subunits, 0.2 A_{260} unit of unlabeled ApUpG or 0.02 A_{260} unit of ^{3}H-ApUpG (5.9 × 10[5] cpm per A_{260} unit), and 29 pmoles of unlabeled or ^{35}S-Met-labeled (1790 mc/mmole) Met-tRNA. ^{3}H-ApUpG binding was carried out at 24° for 15 min, while ^{35}S-Met-tRNA binding was performed at 37° for 15 min. Data presented represent material bound to Millipore filters.

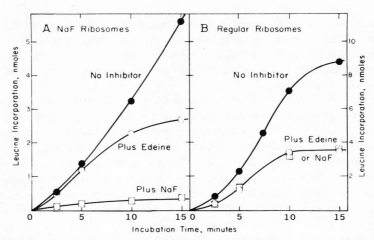

Fig. 3. Effect of edeine and NaF on incorporation of free leucine into globin. A description of the experimental procedure and the incubation mixture containing 0.1 μmole of ^{14}C-L-leucine (2 mc/mmole) is presented in *Methods.* Edeine (1 μM) or NaF (10 mM) was added first to the mixture.

NaF and edeine cause very similar levels of inhibition. We interpret these results to indicate that synthesis from the initiation complex accumulated in the presence of NaF in intact cells is inhibited by NaF but not by edeine. This suggests that the edeine-sensitive step precedes the reaction inhibited by NaF.

Cycloheximide

Cycloheximide (actidione) is a glutarimide antibiotic that inhibits the transfer of amino acids from aminoacyl-tRNA to protein in systems that utilize ribosomes of the 80S type. The time courses for *in vitro* peptide synthesis on regular or NaF ribosomes are shown in Fig. 4. Cycloheximide slows but does not completely block extension of nascent chains that remain attached to regular ribosomes during isolation. Inhibition of the initial rate of synthesis in this *in vitro* system is about 85%. An inhibition in excess of 99% is observed for protein synthesis in intact reticulocytes (5). The rate of amino acid incorporation per ribosome is 50-100 times higher in intact cells than in this *in vitro* system.

There is a striking difference in the effect of cycloheximde on *in vitro* synthesis with NaF ribosomes from that observed in regular ribosomes. Although uninhibited synthesis is nearly the same with the two types of ribosomes, cycloheximide reduces the rate of synthesis with NaF ribosomes to about one tenth the corresponding inhibited rate observed with regular ribosomes. This difference appears to reflect a differential effect of cycloheximide on synthesis from the initiation complex formed in the presence of NaF and extension of nascent peptides on regular ribosomes.

The proportion of valine incorporated into the amino-terminal position of peptides formed in the cell-free system with regular ribosomes is given in Table I. Amino-terminal valine is reduced from 5.7% to 0.2% by cycloheximide. It is important to note that these values were for peptides formed during 60 min of incubation. These data also appear to indicate differential inhibition of peptide initiation. They preclude the possibility that low values for amino-terminal valine observed for valine incorporated with regular ribosomes in the presence of cycloheximide are due to amino-terminal methionine. In other experiments, we have studied the effect of cycloheximide on incorporation of N-formylmethionine from yeast Met-tRNA$_f^{Met}$ formylated with bacterial enzymes and on incorporation of N-acetylmethionine formed with reticulocyte Met-tRNA$_f^{Met}$. The results indicate a greater degree of inhibition of amino-terminal methionine incorporation than of leucine and appear to reflect differential inhibition of peptide initiation.

Cycloheximide appears to slow peptide extension by inhibiting TII-dependent translocation of aminoacyl-tRNA or peptidyl-tRNA from the acceptor to the donor ribosomal sites. This conclusion is supported by the data of Fig. 5. The rationale for this experiment is based on the observation that Phe-tRNA nonenzymatically bound to reticulocyte ribosomes will not react with puromycin to form phenylalanyl puromycin until the system is incubated with TII and

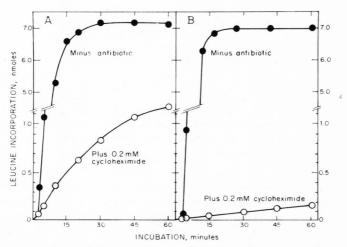

Fig. 4. Effect of cycloheximide on incorporation of free leucine into globin. The reaction mixture contained components as described in *Methods.* (A) regular ribosomes; (B) NaF ribosomes.

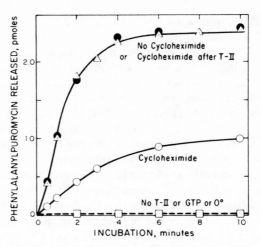

Fig. 5. The effect of cycloheximide on TII-dependent translocation and the peptidyl transferase reaction. Ribosomes carrying 16 pmoles of nonenzymatically bound ^{14}C-phenylalanyl-tRNA per milligram were prepared as previously described (2). Four-tenths milligram of these ribosomes was incubated for the indicated times in 0.25 ml containing 60 mM Tris-HCl (pH 7.5), 7 mM MgCl$_2$, 120 mM KCl, 5 mM dithiothreitol, 0.4 mM GTP, and 4 μg TII protein. Cycloheximide (1 mM) was added to the reaction mixture either before or after this incubation. After incubation, the reaction mixtures were diluted to a final volume of 0.5 ml by adding salts and puromycin (0.1 mM). Following an additional incubation at 0° for 20 min, phenylalanyl puromycin was determined as described previously (16). △, No antibiotic added; ○, cycloheximide added in TII incubation; ●, cycloheximide added in puromycin incubation; □, TII incubation performed in absence of either TII enzyme or GTP, or by incubation of the complete mixture at 0°.

GTP (14). This has been interpreted to indicate that the Phe-tRNA is bound into the acceptor site, then translocated to the donor site by a reaction requiring hydrolysis of GTP by TII. When Phe-tRNA is in the donor site, it may react with puromycin by the peptidyl transferase reaction without the further involvement of TII. The peptidyl transferase reaction can occur at 0° (15). In the experiments presented in Fig. 5, Phe-tRNA was nonenzymatically bound to the ribosomes, then the ribosomes were removed from the reaction mixture by centrifugation. The ribosomes were resuspended in a reaction mixture containing TII and GTP plus cycloheximide where indicated, then incubated at 37°. The reaction mixtures were chilled, cycloheximide was added as noted, then puromycin was added to all reaction vessels. Incubation was continued at 0° for 20 min. Phenylalanyl puromycin formed during this incubation was determined by an ethyl acetate extraction procedure (16).

The data of Fig. 6 indicate that cycloheximide inhibition of TII-dependent translocation is not caused by inhibition of ribosome-dependent hydrolysis of GTP by this enzyme. Preparations of TII used in these experiments contain no detectable GTPase activity in the absence of ribosomes and are estimated to contain about 50% TII protein (4). Cycloheximide causes about a 10% inhibition of the rate of GTP hydrolysis at concentrations that cause over 90% inhibition of the rate of peptide synthesis. Extensive experiments have failed to show any detectable effect of either glutathione or dithiothreitol on inhibition of TII GTPase activity by cycloheximide in this system.

CONCLUSIONS

We conclude that the accumulation of $tRNA_f^{Met}$ on NaF ribosomes is due to inhibition of a reaction of peptide initiation by NaF. More than 98% of this tRNA appears to be present on these ribosomes in the deacylated or uncharged form (10). The significance of deacylated $tRNA_f^{Met}$ for peptide initiation on these ribosomes is unclear. They support efficient *in vitro* peptide synthesis, relative to synthesis observed with regular ribosomes that bear nascent peptides.

Fig. 6. Effect of cycloheximide, fusidic acid, and cephalosporin P_1 on TII-dependent GTP hydrolysis. Assay procedures are described in detail elsewhere (18). The reaction mixture contained, in a volume of 0.5 ml, 0.02 M Tris-HCl (pH 7.5), 6 mM MgCl$_2$, 70 mM KCl, 5 mM dithiothreitol, 0.50 mg ribosomes from cells incubated with NaF and washed with deoxycholate and 0.5 M KCl, 4 µg purified TII enzyme free of detectable nonspecific GTPase activity, and 4 µM γ-^{32}P-GTP (about 150 cpm/pmole). ^{32}P$_i$ liberated was determined by the procedure of Conway and Lipmann (19) with minor modification (18). Where indicated, reaction mixtures contained 1 mM cycloheximide, 0.4 mM fusidic acid, or 0.4 mM cephalosporin P_1.

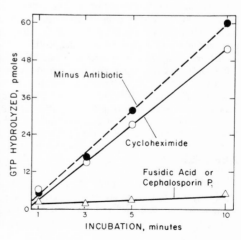

This synthesis is relatively insensitive to edeine and appears to take place on ribosomes that bear tRNA$_f^{Met}$ and mRNA as the initiation complex accumulated in the presence of NaF.

In vitro synthesis on NaF ribosomes is relatively sensitive to both NaF and cycloheximide. The studies on peptide elongation indicate that cycloheximide inhibits TII-dependent translocation of peptidyl-tRNA into the donor ribosomal site involving the 60S ribosomal subunit. Grollman and his coworkers have shown cycloheximide resistance in yeast to be a property of this subunit (20). It should be noted that this "translocation" is measured by a change in the reactive state of peptidyl-tRNA; physical movement of the tRNA on the ribosome may not be involved. The effect of cycloheximide on initiation in the *in vitro* system may reflect inhibition of "translocation" of tRNA into the donor reactive state. It is not clear whether this differential inhibition of initiation relative to elongation is due to a direct effect on the reactions involved or to an indirect effect related to a loss of initiation activity during the course of the *in vitro* incubation.

ACKNOWLEDGMENTS

The authors are grateful to Merle Batty and Mildred Hardesty for their excellent technical assistance and to Margaret Cooper for her help in preparing the typescript. This work was supported in part by Grants HD 03803 from the National Institutes of Health and GB-30902 from the National Science Foundation.

SUMMARY

Sodium fluoride inhibits peptide initiation in rabbit reticulocytes with little or no direct effect on peptide completion. It causes an accumulation of tRNA$_f^{Met}$ on ribosomes isolated from inhibited cells. These NaF ribosomes support *in vitro* synthesis during which valine is incorporated into the amino-terminal position of globin peptides. This synthesis is relatively insensitive to inhibition by edeine, a small basic peptide inhibitor that also blocks peptide initiation with little or no effect on peptide completion. Edeine appears to block binding of mRNA or tRNA$_f^{Met}$ to 40S ribosomal subunits at a point that precedes the NaF-sensitive reaction of peptide initiation. Cycloheximide slows peptide elongation by inhibiting TII-dependent translocation of peptidyl-tRNA from the acceptor to the donor ribosomal site or reactive state. Synthesis on NaF ribosomes is more sensitive to cycloheximide inhibition than synthesis on regular ribosomes.

RESUMEN

El fluoruro de sodio inhibe la iniciación de péptidos en reticulocitos de conejo, pero tiene muy poco o ningún efecto en la terminación de los mismos. Este inhibidor ocasiona una acumulación de tRNA$_f^{Met}$ en ribosomas aislados de células inhibidas. Estos ribosomas FNa, permiten la síntesis *in vitro,* durante la cual valina es incorporada en la posición amino-terminal en péptidos de globina. Esta síntesis es relativamente insensible a la inhibición por edeína, un inhibidor pequeño y alcalino el cual también bloquea la iniciación de péptidos pero no tiene ningún efecto en la terminación de los mismos. La edeína parece bloquear la unión del mRNA o tRNA$_f^{Met}$ a la subunidad ribosomal 40S en un punto que precede a la reacción sensitiva a FNa durante la elongación del péptido. La cicloheximida, la cual es dependiente de TII y del sitio aceptador, retarda la elongación del péptido mediante la inhibición de la translocación del peptidil-tRNA al sitio ribosomal o sitio activo. La síntesis de ribosomas FNa es más sensitiva a la inhibición por cicloheximida que la síntesis con ribosomas normales.

REFERENCES

1. Obrig, T., Irvin, J., Culp, W., and Hardesty, B., *Europ. J. Biochem., 21,* 31 (1971).
2. Obrig, T., Culp, W., McKeehan, W., and Hardesty, B., *J. Biol. Chem., 246,* 174 (1971).
3. Hardesty, B., McKeehan, W., and Culp, W., in Grossman, L., and Moldave, K. (eds.), *Methods in Enzymology,* Vol. 20, Academic Press, New York (1971), p. 316.
4. Hardesty, B., and McKeehan, W., in Grossman, L., and Moldave, K. (eds.), *Methods in Enzymology,* Vol. 20, Academic Press, New York (1971), p. 330.
5. Lin, S., Mosteller, R., and Hardesty, B., *J. Mol. Biol., 21,* 51 (1966).
6. Marks, P., Burka, E., Rifkind, R., and Danon, D., *Cold Spring Harbor Symp. Quant. Biol., 28,* 223 (1963).
7. Takeishi, K., and Ukita, T., *J. Biol. Chem., 243,* 5761 (1968).
8. Smith, A., and Marcker, K., *Nature, 226,* 607 (1970).
9. Weiss, J., and Kelmers, A., *Biochemistry, 6,* 2507 (1967).
10. Culp, W., Morrisey, J., and Hardesty, B., *Biochem. Biophys. Res. Commun., 40,* 777 (1970).
11. Borowski, E., Chmara, H., and Jareczek-Marawska, E., *Biochim. Biophys. Acta, 130,* 560 (1966).
12. Hierowski, M., and Kurylo-Borowska, Z., *Biochim. Biophys. Acta, 95,* 578 (1965).
13. Kurylo-Borowska, A., and Hierowski, M., *Biochim. Biophys. Acta, 95,* 590 (1965).
14. Culp, W., McKeehan, W., and Hardesty, B., *Proc. Natl. Acad. Sci. U.S.A., 63,* 1431 (1969).
15. Monro, R. E., *J. Mol. Biol., 26,* 147 (1967).
16. Leder, P., and Bursztyn, H., *Biochem. Biophys. Res. Commun., 25,* 233 (1966).
17. Mosteller, R., Culp, W., and Hardesty, B., *J. Biol. Chem., 243,* 6343 (1968).
18. McKeehan, W., and Hardesty, B., *J. Biol. Chem., 244,* 4330 (1969).
19. Conway, T., and Lipmann, F., *Proc. Natl. Acad. Sci. U.S.A., 52,* 1462 (1964).
20. Rao, S., and Grollman, A., *Biochem. Biophys. Res. Commun., 29,* 696 (1967).

DISCUSSION

G. D. Novelli (Oak Ridge, U.S.A.): Did you say that when you isolated the ribosomes from the cells incubated with sodium fluoride, the acceptor activity of the tRNA on the ribosome was 50% methionine?

B. Hardesty (Austin, U.S.A.): Roughly 50% of the total acceptor capacity was for methionine. The other 50% was divided more or less equally among all other amino acids.

G. D. Novelli: Were these aminoacylated, or were they vacant?

B. Hardesty: As we have isolated it, the tRNA$_f^{Met}$ from these sodium fluoride ribosomes is almost exclusively in the deacylated form. However, there are technical difficulties that must be considered in the interpretation of this result. I hesitate to take the time to expound on this point.

G. D. Novelli: In the reversed phase diagram you showed, were the tRNAs preaminoacylated with methionine or were they aminoacylated later?

B. Hardesty: They were preaminoacylated.

G. Favelukes (La Plata, Argentina): I have more than a question, it is really a comment. If I may be allowed to do so, I would like to offer the following for the problem Dr. Novelli has in mind. In a very recent experiment here, my student Enzo Bard has found the following: He has prepared a lysate from reticulocytes and incubated it according to Lamfrom and Knopf. This incubation is in the presence of ^{14}C-valine and ^{3}H-methionine for a short time, 10 min at 25°. Under these conditions, the polysomes are completely preserved and the system is still completely functional. What he has found is that the profiles of ^{14}C and ^{3}H distributions in the gradient differ. ^{14}C counts coincide with the polysomal distribution and are almost absent in the 80S and subunit peaks. The ^{3}H distribution parallels that of ^{14}C in the polysomes. Also, the 80S ribosomes are devoid of ^{3}H. However, there is a small, but very distinct peak of ^{3}H-methionine in the 40S region. There is little or no ^{14}C-valine in this region. We take this to indicate that at least some of the subunits in the 40S peak are bound to a mRNA and that these may carry initiator Met-tRNA$_f^{Met}$. Now, when this same experiment is done, but in the presence of sodium fluoride which is added before methionine, in 10 min all the polysomes disappear, we have a very large peak of 80S ribosomes, and we find very few ^{14}C-valine counts distributed along the gradient. Instead, ^{3}H-methionine is present as a small peak on the 40S region, so that under these conditions we believe that the 40S subunits are still able to bind to mRNA, which is essentially what Dr. Hardesty has said, but that they bind methionyl-tRNA. What I think this indicates, or at least suggests, is that, besides the presence of deacylated tRNA$_f^{Met}$ in these complexes, there is methionyl-tRNA in the initiator complexes and that this can be seen directly. We have a third experiment in which we used aurintricarboxylic acid. Although this was only one experiment, it suggests that the amount of methionyl-tRNA on the 40S subunits has decreased a lot.

B. Hardesty: I want to make it very clear that the tRNA$_f^{Met}$ that we have studied, in sharp contrast to the results that Dr. Favelukes has just described, is accumulated on the 80S or, rather, on the shoulder of the 80S ribosomes. This may be a very important distinction. The results Dr. Favelukes has described are what we have been looking for. Perhaps this involves the answer to why we get accumulation on the 80S, as was not anticipated. This may be related to deacylation on the 40S subunits, which we now believe is enzymatic.

P. Lengyel (New Haven, U.S.A.): What is the sucrose gradient pattern after edeine treatment?

B. Hardesty: That is a difficult question. I failed to mention that edeine apparently is not permeable to intact cells, which grossly compromises its utility for these types of studies. In our cell-free system, which is not a lysate system, it appears to cause some acceleration of polysome breakdown to 80S.

A. S. Spirin (Moscow, USSR): Did you really show the existence of 1½-somes?

B. Hardesty: No, McCarty has dealt extensively with this. We have not pursued this. The only thing that I could offer on this point is that it seems clear that we get an accumulation of the tRNA$_f^{Met}$ on the heavy shoulder of the 80S peak. As you correctly imply, this observation might reflect any of a number of phenomena. It might, and I emphasize the uncertainty, be related to 1½-somes.

G. Favelukes: When you dialyze a lysate against low magnesium, you may observe certain changes in the distribution of the ribosomes. My student Celina Martone finds that when a regular lysate (which has a well-defined profile of polysomes) is dialyzed against, for example, 0.5 mM Mg^{2+} and salts, there will be shifts in the ribosomal distribution. The individual polysome peaks become somewhat shorter, and there appear shoulders and bands in intermediate regions which suggest intermediate components. Besides, we find that there is an increase in the 60S peak, but *not* in the 40S peak. We do not know what this really means. We can interpret it in at least two different ways. One is that initiation complexes in any of these polysomes may undergo partial dissociation in low magnesium by releasing the 60S subunit but not the 40S, which remains bound to the mRNA. The other interpretation is suggested by the fact that preincubation with cycloheximide abolishes this effect. It could mean that what we are really looking at is a change in the properties of the polysomes, or rather of the individual ribosomal subunits in the polysomes, which all tend to be with their chains in the A site. Therefore, as has been suggested before, they would have a more compact conformation. These ribosomes would tend not to give the rather open structures which then may be observed as the intermediate peaks. Really, I cannot make a choice between these interpretations at this moment.

A. S. Spirin: Complicated sedimentation profiles, especially in sucrose gradients, may be a consequence just of equilibrium between associating and disassociating forms. Because of this, some components—especially intermediate components—may not be new components in reality but just a reflection of existence of the equilibrium.

G. Favelukes: As far as this is concerned, we were worried about the possibility that what we were looking at was an artifact due to the high-speed gradients that we were using. Once we ran a low-speed gradient, and we saw exactly the same thing. Maybe it can tell us something about the speed with which this process takes place. You are reflecting on an equilibrium, and we see this kind of thing in 1 hr or in 14 hr.

R. P. Perry (Philadelphia, U.S.A.): Dr. Hardesty, is there any evidence for or against the proposition that the initial translocation from the first initiator site might require different factors than the elongation translocation?

B. Hardesty: There is a great deal of evidence both for and against. You are asking now specifically about the initiation factors?

R. P. Perry: What is the first translocation from the initiator—the first initiator site over to the P site—does it require a different translocation factor than the ones that are involved in the subsequent elongation?

B. Hardesty: This certainly appears to be the case in *E. coli.* I am sure that you know that Dr. French Anderson has some data that indicate that this is very likely the case in the reticulocyte system. I would rather not comment on his observations in terms of our own data.

R. P. Perry: You said you had a differential type of inhibition with cycloheximide when you measured *N*-acetylmethionine incorporation *vs.* the elongation of the peptides. I wonder whether you supported the idea that there was a different setup.

B. Hardesty: The way we would like to interpret this effect on chain initiation is that cycloheximide is, in fact, a slightly better inhibitor of one or more of the early translocation steps into what is functionally the donor site than it is an inhibitor of subsequent steps. The reason this might occur is not clear. It might reflect differences in the strength of the interaction between cycloheximide and ribosomes during initiation and ribosomes that bear longer nascent peptides. We believe that cycloheximide does exactly the same thing in either initiation or extension by blocking translocation or conversion of aminoacyl-tRNA into the donor site, or reactive state, as we prefer to call it.

R. P. Perry: Could I make just one more comment in regard to the runoff particles. We have been studying the runoff of ribosomes that occurs when cells are incubated at elevated temperatures. One gets a particle somewhere around 98S or 110S. We found that this runoff particle consists of the monosomes which do not contain the message, but that the monosomes from the total polysome complex, which carry the message, band as an 80S monosome. It seems that the noncoded monosomes tend to dimerize while the ones that carry the message do not.

31

Intermediate Stages in the Ribosomal Cycle of Reticulocytes

G. Favelukes, D. Sorgentini, E. Bard, and C. Martone de Borrajo

Departamento de Bioquímica
Facultad de Ciencias Exactas
Universidad Nacional de La Plata
La Plata, Argentina

The mechanisms of initiation and termination of the synthesis of protein chains have been the subject of many studies in recent years, both in mammalian and in bacterial systems (for review, see ref. 1). Those studies emphasize the utilization of ribosomal subunits in the process of chain initiation and polyribosome formation either as derived subunits in the presence of defined initiation factors (2-6) or as native ribosomal subparticles pre-existent as such in the cytoplasm (7-10).

On the other hand, free inactive ribosomes are normally found in the cell together with the polysomes and subparticles, and several lines of evidence suggest that they do have a potential role in protein synthesis. In whole cells cultured in widely different conditions, large reversible shifts can be observed (11-16) in the distribution of particles among polysomes and free ribosomes at the expense of each other, which demonstrates their metabolic convertibility (13,14). Other experiments, done with bacteria (17-19) and with yeast (20), have shown protein synthesis-dependent hybridization of the component sub-units in free ribosomes. Moreover, in cell-free systems which are deficient in initiation, free inactive ribosomes arise and accumulate as a result of termination and release of completed protein chains, accompanied by the orderly disassembly of the polysomes (21-23).

All this suggests that, in the cyclic functioning of the polysomes already proposed by Rich (21), free ribosomes which may arise as a by-product of chain termination may also participate again in protein synthesis, and this would result from their dissociation into precursor subunits (24) for the build-up of initiation complexes in the polysomes.

In this paper, we review results obtained in this laboratory showing that (a) the reticulocyte subparticles are able to form polysomes and (b) free ribosomes incubated with a ribosomal extract which promotes chain initiation (25) and polysome assembly (26) dissociate into native-like subparticles. The dissociation reaction, which can be separated from initiation, resembles the ribosome dissociation step in bacteria described by Subramanian et al. (27) and by Bade et al. (28), but exhibits a rather specific requirement for ATP.

POLYSOME FORMATION IN RETICULOCYTE CELL-FREE SYSTEMS

The role of ribosomal subparticles in the formation of active initiation complexes in eukaryotes is indicated by several types of evidence, such as the stimulatory action of subparticles for initiation in reticulocyte cell-free systems (7), their preferential metabolic equilibration with polysomes in nucleated cells (9,31-35), and the ability of native 40S subparticles to associate with mRNA (10,36).

Additional evidence has been obtained in our laboratory in studies made with rabbit reticulocyte native subparticles. Early experiments done by Zylber (37) showed that ^{32}P-labeled subparticles, isolated and purified, were incorporated into the polysomes when they were added to a reticulocyte cell-free system made up of polysomes and supernatant enzymes; this incorporation was temperature and energy dependent. In those conditions, the addition of subparticles also stimulated amino acid incorporation into protein severalfold, in accordance with previous results of Bishop (7). In Table I, a similar experiment is described, in which [32]P-40S or [32]P-60S native subparticles were incubated with polysomes and unfractionated lysate supernatant, under protein synthesis conditions. After 10 min at 25°, there was a transfer of 16% of [32]P-40S material and 18% of [32]P-60S material to 80S and heavier ribosomal aggregates. Similar results have been obtained recently by Hoerz and McCarty (38). In another type of experiment pointing to this role of the subparticles (E. B. and R. F. de Schuttenberg, unpublished results), a crude ribosomal fraction exhausted of capacity for protein synthesis (composed of 40S, 60S, and 80S particles) was briefly incubated with fresh supernatant in a cell-free system for hemoglobin synthesis made up according to Lamfrom and Knopf (39). The results showed not only a good amino acid incorporating activity (which in these conditions

Table I. Attachment of Native Ribosomal Subparticles to Polysomes During Protein Synthesis[a]

	Increment of ^{32}P (% of total)		
	40S	60S	80S and heavier
^{32}P-40S subparticles	–	4.0	16.6
^{32}P-60S subparticles	–	–	18.7

[a] Native ^{32}P ribosomal subparticles labeled *in vivo* were
isolated by fractionating the crude whole ^{32}P ribosomal
fraction in a preparative sucrose gradient, in a medium
with 2 mM MgAc$_2$, 70 mM KCl, 2 mM Tris-HCl (pH 7.5),
and 3 mM MEO (solution 1). Purified ^{32}P-40S (1819
cpm) or ^{32}P-60S (1738 cpm) subparticles were incubated
for 10 min at 25°, either alone in solution 2 [2 mM
MgAc$_2$, 70 mM KCl, 26 mM Tris-HCl (pH 7.5), 15 mM
MEO] or in solution 2 with the addition of cold polysomes, particle-free lysate supernatant, 0.2 mM Mg-GTP,
1 mM Mg-ATP, and 0.025 mM hemin. The mixtures were
analyzed in 15-50% linear surcose gradients in solution 1,
run at 40,000 rpm for 135 min. After monitoring $A_{254 nm}$
40 fractions were collected and filtered through nitrocellulose membranes, and the retained ribosomes were
counted in a gas-flow counter. ^{32}P radioactivity transferred to 80S and heavier regions, expressed as percent of
total radioactivity in the gradient, was calculated from the
difference of ^{32}P plots of pairs of gradients as shown in
Fig. 1.

essentially reflects initiation of globin chains) but also a considerable build-up of
polysomes at short incubation times, at the expense of the subparticles, while
the free ribosomes remained practically constant. This suggests that it was the
subparticles (and not the 80S ribosomes) that formed the polysomes.

The participation of 80S free ribosomes in polysome build-up is known to
occur in whole reticulocytes during the recovery from inhibition of protein
synthesis caused by sodium fluoride (13) or by depletion of iron (11). The
question of whether this participation of 80S ribosomes also takes place in a
cell-free system was explored by adding purified ^{32}P-80S free ribosomes to a
complete cell-free system made up with polysomes and lysate supernatant (Fig.
1A, B). After incubating for 10 min at 25°, the conversion of ^{32}P-80S particles
into polysomes, or into subparticles, was not significant, as evidenced by the
difference between curves B and A (shown in the differential plot B-A). This is
to be compared with the results obtained with ^{32}P subparticles, mentioned
before, and suggests that the 80S free ribosomes *per se* are unable to act as
initiators of protein synthesis.

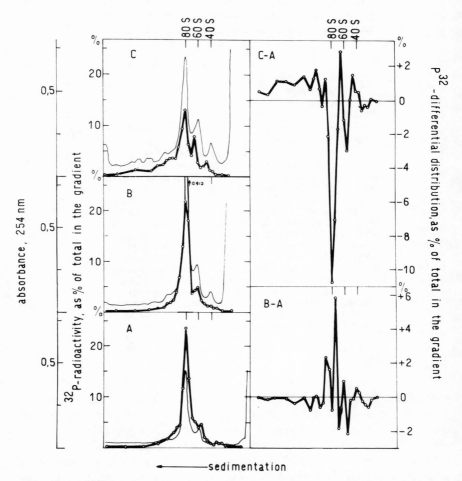

Fig. 1. *Attachment of native* ^{32} *P-80S free ribosomes to polysomes during cell-free protein synthesis: the effect of the ribosomal extract.* The experiment was performed as described in Table I. ^{32} P-80S ribosomes (1296 cpm), isolated and purified, were incubated for 10 min at 25°, and the ribosomal distribution was analyzed as before. (A) In solution 2 without additions (control); (B) as A, with the addition of cold polysomes, supernatant, energy, and other components listed in Table I; (C) as B, plus 4 μl of crude RE (adjusted to final K$^+$ concentration as in A and B). Crude RE was the 150,000 × g supernatant of a suspension of 37 mg/ml crude whole ribosomes in 1 M KCl, extracted for 15 min at 0°. ———, Absorbance, 254 nm; ○, ^{32} P radioactivity of the fractions, expressed as percent total cpm in the gradients. (B−A and (C−A) Differential plots showing the shifts in ^{32} P distribution.

Table II. Separation of Ribosomal Dissociation Effect
and Stimulation of Protein Synthesis by RE

Additions	Dissociation effect[a] (vs. 80S + energy)		Cell-free protein synthesis[b]	
	RE:Rb	Dissociation (%)	RE:Rb	^{14}C-valine incorporation (pmoles/mg Rb)
Crude RE	3.4:1	2.0	5:1	185
D-RE	2.8:1	13.7	4.2:1	3
G25-RE	3.4:1	25.6	4:1	4

[a] Derived 80S ribosomes were incubated and analyzed as described in Fig. 2. The results are expressed as percent decrease of the area under the 80S peak, measured by planimetry, compared with the 80S ribosomes plus energy.
[b] The complete cell-free system, containing derived 80S ribosomes (0.5 mg), AS supernatant enzymes, and other components, was incubated 60 min at 37°. Incorporation of ^{14}C-valine without additions was 3 pmoles/mg Rb.

Miller and Schweet (25) and Cohen (26) have shown that in the presence of a high KCl ribosomal wash, 80S ribosomes acquire the ability to initiate chains and build polysomes. We prepared a crude extract of whole ribosomes in 1 M KCl (RE*), which, as expected, greatly stimulated amino acid incorporating activity of exhausted 80S ribosomes (Table II). When RE was added to the incubation mixture C, in the experiment described in Fig. 1, a considerable amount of ^{32}P ribosomal material (about 20%) was transferred from the 80S peak to the polysome region (Fig. 1, C-A). This is predictable, in accord with Cohen's observations on the formation of polysomes promoted by RE (26). However, in addition to this, significant amounts of ^{32}P-40S and ^{32}P-60S subparticles were formed (2.5% and 2.8% of total radioactivity, respectively) which behaved as stable native-like subparticles. This provides a clue as to the mechanism of polysome formation at the expense of 80S ribosomes: in the presence of RE, free ribosomes would dissociate into native subparticles, which, as shown before, are able by themselves to initiate the synthesis of peptide chains and build polysomes.

* Abbreviations: RE, ribosomal extract; G25-RE, ribosomal extract treated with Sephadex G25; D-RE, dialyzed ribosomal extract; MEO, mercaptoethanol; Mg-GTP or Mg-ATP, an equimolar mixture of magnesium acetate and GTP or ATP; RE:Rb, proportion of RE added to a unit amount of 80S ribosomes, expressed as the corresponding amount of crude whole ribosomes (Rb) originally extracted; MgAc$_2$, magnesium acetate.

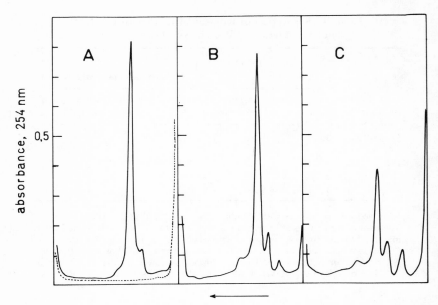

Fig. 2. *Dissociation of 80S ribosomes.* Derived 80S ribosomes (100 μg) were incubated for 10 min at 25° in 62.5 μl 2 mM MgAc$_2$, 70 mM KCl, 26 mM Tris-HCl (pH 7.5), 0.2 mM Mg-GTP, 1 mM Mg-ATP, and 16 mM MEO. (A) Without additions, (B) with crude *RE* (97 μg protein, RE:Rb ratio 1.66:1), (C) with G25-RE (423 μg protein, 7.2:1 ratio). The mixtures were analyzed as described in Table I in sucrose gradients run at 40,000 rpm for 165 min. Derived 80S ribosomes were prepared by exhaustive incubation of polysomes in a complete cell-free system and isolated in a preparative sucrose gradient. Crude RE was desalted (G25-RE) by passing through a short column of Sephadex G25 equilibrated with 100 mM KCl, 2 mM Tris-HCl (pH 7.5), and 3 mM MEO. The broken line tracing in A represents the profile of crude RE alone.

DISSOCIATION OF 80S FREE RIBOSOMES

If the dissociation of 80S ribosomes into subparticles is a part of the overall process of protein synthesis in the cell, we can predict some expected properties of the dissociation step: (a) it should be able to occur in a medium adequate for protein synthesis (that is, in the presence of Mg^{2+} and K$^+$ (free) ions in concentrations that are adequate for that process, as well as nucleoside triphosphates and a source of energy); (b) it should require a specific stimulation factor, and it should be irreversible by itself (because in the conditions mentioned before, free ribosomes as well as native subparticles are stable by themselves and do not tend to dissociate or reassociate spontaneously); (c) it should precede the initiation of protein synthesis (which requires subparticles) and should be separable from this later step.

We have studied the dissociation of free ribosomes into subparticles directly, by incubating them with RE (Fig. 2). 80S ribosomes held for 10 min at 25° in a medium adequate for globin synthesis and chain initiation (25), with 2 mM (free) Mg^{2+} ions, 70 mM K^+ ions, and energy (Mg-ATP and Mg-GTP), show very little dissociation (Fig. 2A). Coincidently, mixtures of 40S and 60S native subparticles do not tend to associate in that medium (unpublished experiments). Instead, when crude RE (gradient B) or Sephadex-treated, RE (gradient C) is present in the incubation, a substantial proportion of the 80S particles are converted to 40S and 60S subparticles (the larger dissociation observed in C compared with B was due to an increase in the ratio of RE:Rb and to the use of Sephadex-treated instead of crude RE—see below).

This dissociation fulfills conditions (a) and (b): the medium is apt for protein synthesis, the reaction requires the presence of RE (80S ribosomes do not spontaneously dissociate by themselves), and it is not reversible (the degree of dissociation is variable, which means that it does not reflect a simple dissociation-association equilibrium dependent only on the relative concentrations of the particles). Experiments described in Table II indicate that condition (c) also holds: D-RE and G25-RE, which have lost the capacity of crude RE to stimulate protein synthesis and chain initiation (60 times the basal protein synthesis by the 80S ribosomes), are quite active in ribosome dissociation. This shows that the dissociating activity is resistant to dialysis and that the two activities are separable and distinct. The basis for the loss of initiation-promoting activity is not known; it leads to an apparent enhancement of the dissociating activity. We believe that this reflects the true dissociating capacity of RE. The low dissociations obtained with crude extracts, which have been observed consistently, would be due to a reutilization of the released subparticles, which in the presence of the crude extract would make ribosomal aggregates (monosomes and polysomes), thus being masked by the 80S free ribosomes.

The extent of dissociation is dependent on the amount of RE added (Table III). We express this as a ratio (RE:Rb) between the amounts of crude ribosomes extracted and of 80S ribosomes in the assay: we have tested input ratios as high as 11.4:1. The dissociation can be quite extensive, but large amounts of RE are definitely inhibitory. In Fig. 3, the effect of a dialyzed RE added in 5.7:1 ratio is shown. This resulted in 56% of the initial 80S ribosomes being dissociated into subparticles.

We shall discuss briefly some salient features of this reaction: (a) The dissociating activity of RE is lost by heating at 55° for 10 min, suggesting that the factor is protein-like.

(b) The temperature dependence of the reaction (optimal at 37°, very slow at low temperatures, and with a sharp decrease at 45°) is behavior typical of biochemical reactions mediated by proteins (in this case, the factor or the substrate ribosomes might be inactivated at 45°).

**Table III. Dependency of
Dissociation on the Levels of RE[a]**

D-RE added (RE:Rb)	Percent dissociation (vs. 80S + energy)
2.8:1	13.7
5.7:1	40
11.4:1	16

[a] The experiment was performed as described in Table II. D-RE had been dialyzed against 100 mM KCl, 2 mM Tris-HCl (pH 7.5), and 3 mM MEO.

(c) The time course of the dissociation, which at $25°$ or $37°$ is essentially completed, suggests that the dissociation factor(s) is being used up, instead of acting catalytically. This is also supported by the dependency on the input ratio RE:Rb, which suggests a stoichiometric action and by the gross accord between the amount of dissociated subparticles and the quantity of these in the extracted original ribosomal preparation.

(d) The dissociation is equally effective with ribosomes obtained in three different ways—(i) native 80S free ribosomes isolated from a lysate of normal cells, (ii) polysome-derived 80S ribosomes isolated after incubation of the polysomes in a cell-free system until exhaustion, and (iii) 80S ribosomes from fluoride-treated, polysome-depleted cells. These three types of preparations contain populations of ribosomes that may differ, e.g., in the state of phosphorylation of some ribosomal proteins (40,41) or in the tendency to form polysomes and participate in protein synthesis (40). However, these possible differences were not reflected in their dissociability in the presence of ATP.

(e) Dissociation is markedly enhanced in the presence of Mg-ATP. Table IV shows that, while the RE (either crude or dialysed) has a small but significant dissociating activity of its own, addition of a mixture of 1 mM Mg-ATP and 0.2 mM Mg-GTP increases dissociation two- or even fourfold. It should be noted also that the nucleotides by themselves are able to induce some dissociation. These three effects, of RE, or of nucleotides alone, or of both together, have been repeatedly observed. The enhancing effect of nucleotides is not due to a decrease in free Mg^{2+} concentration through its chelation by the nucleotides, because these are added as Mg compounds. Other experiments have shown that the effect of the nucleoside triphosphates can be ascribed solely to Mg-ATP, as GTP has no synergistic or additive effect. In Table V, the effect of each of the four nucleoside triphosphates is shown. At equal concentrations of each, added as 1 mM Mg salts, only ATP shows a definite stimulation. GTP in particular is inactive; there is slight stimulation by UTP, but this is not considered as significant. Other experiments (not shown) indicate that under the same conditions ADP and AMP are not active in the dissociation. Further, although in this dissociation system optimal levels of ATP usually lie between 1 and 2 mM, when an ATP-generating system is added (creatine phosphate and creatine kinase) there is a maximal effect on dissociation of ATP levels as low as 0.2 mM. This suggests that the true levels of ATP required for dissociation are not high, but the supply is critical either because of the very active ATPases in reticulocyte lysates (41) or because the products of ATP degradation are inhibitory.

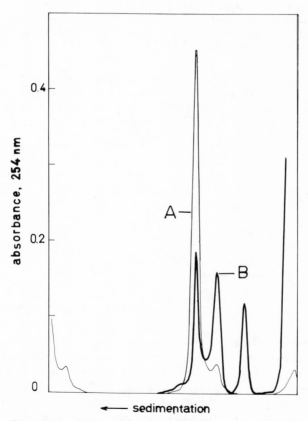

Fig. 3. Dissociation of derived 80S ribosomes by dialyzed RE. The experiment was performed as in Fig. 2. (A) 80S ribosomes incubated with energy alone; (B) same as A, with the addition of D-RE (RE:Rb ration 5.7:1)

Table IV. Effect of Energy on Dissociation[a]

	Percent dissociation (vs. 80S)
1. 80S + crude RE	12.0
2. As 1, + 0.2 mM Mg-GTP + 1 mM Mg-ATP	23.5
3. 80S + D-RE	14.5
4. As 3, + 0.2 mM Mg-GTP + 1 mM Mg-ATP	56.5
5. 80S + 0.2 mM Mg-GTP + 1 mM Mg-ATP	14.2

[a] Incubations were performed as in Fig. 2, and results are expressed as in Table II. RE:Rb ratios were 3.4:1 for crude RE and 5.7:1 for D-RE.

Table V. Effect of Nucleoside Triphosphates on RE-Dependent Ribosome Dissociation[a]

	Percent dissociation (vs. 80S)
1. 80S + G25-RE	23
2. As 1, + 1 mM ATP	3i
3. As 1, + 1 mM GTP	21
4. As 1, + 1 mM CTP	21
5. As 1, + 1 mM UTP	26

[a] Experiments were performed as in Table II. RE:Rb ratio was 6.4:1.

(f) The following inhibitors of protein synthesis, in concentrations that severely inhibit initiation or elongation, have no effect on dissociation (Table VI): cycloheximide, fusidic acid, puromycin, sparsomycin, and sodium fluoride. Thus interaction of the dissociation factor (and ATP) with the 80S ribosomes does not involve, at least directly, those areas of the active center of the ribosome that are engaged in the task of binding aminoacyl-tRNA, or translocating it, or catalyzing formation of the peptide bond. It is interesting to note that NaF does not inhibit (or stimulate) dissociation. It had been observed that in animal cells treated with fluoride, there occurs a substantial decrease in the

Table VI. Effects of Inhibitors of Protein Synthesis[a]

	Percent dissociation (vs. 80S)
1. 80S + G25-RE	20
2. As 1, + 10^{-3} M cycloheximide	20
3. As 1, + 10^{-4} M sparsomycin	21
4. As 1, + 10^{-3} M puromycin	23
5. As 1, + 10^{-4} M fusidic acid	24
6. As 1, + 0.02 M sodium fluoride	21

[a] Experiments were performed as in Table II. Re:Rb ratio was 6.2:1.

amount of subparticles (15,24). On the grounds that in the presence of fluoride the cell supply of ATP is greatly decreased (13), Colombo et al. (24) have suggested that ribosome dissociation is ATP dependent. Our results strongly support this contention.

CONCLUSIONS

The experiments reported here support the generally accepted view that the native ribosomal subparticles are direct precursors of active ribosomal complexes in mammalian systems. The specific requirements for initiation are met in crude systems made up of polysomes, fresh supernatant, and the isolated purified subparticles. 80S free ribosomes, which in reconstituted systems devoid of subparticles are unable to build up polysomes, can do so when they dissociate into native subparticles. Dissociation requires a factor present in the high salt ribosomal wash, and it takes place in an ionic medium adequate for protein synthesis and in which both the free ribosomes and the native subparticles are stable by themselves. The existence of a dissociation factor in reticulocytes has been recently mentioned by Davis (42). Pètre (43) has described, in yeast, a ribosome dissociation factor extracted from a ribosomal preparation enriched with native subparticles. The properties of the yeast dissociation reaction are similar to those of the reticulocyte system described here.

The requirement for dissociation in the build-up of active ribosomal complexes suggests that the dissociation factor functions as one of the initiation factors. In *Escherichia coli*, the dissociation factor of Subramanian and Davis (44) has been shown to be identical with pure initiation factor F3 of Sabol *et al.* (44). In animal cells, three initiation factors have been isolated from high salt ribosomal washes or reticulocytes (45) and of chicken embryonic muscle (46); these factors are required for the initiation of the synthesis of globin and myosin, respectively. It remains to be established whether any of these factors are related to the dissociation factor of RE.

Dissociation of 80S ribosomes promoted by the sole addition of dialyzed RE is stimulated markedly in the presence of Mg-ATP, but not by other nucleoside triphosphates. This effect is not caused by Mg sequestration. The inability of GTP to replace ATP in this stimulation should be noted. GTP had been found to stimulate dissociation of bacterial ribosomes by preparations of dissociating factors (47,29). Recent results show that with pure *E. coli* dissociation factor, GTP is not required for the reaction (30). That the requirement of ATP in the reticulocyte system is not absolute suggests a heterogeneity of the reaction, in which part of the ribosomes (or perhaps the dissociation factor) are able to dissociate in the absence of ATP, while in the presence of ATP extra ribosomes or factor can be converted to a reactive form.

An ATP requirement for "activation" of a quiescent population of ribosomes and initiation of protein synthesis in nongerminated wheat embryos was shown years ago by Marcus (48,49). The parallelism between these reports and the ATP stimulation of ribosome dissociation in reticulocytes suggests that in wheat embryos one effect of ATP could be on the dissociation of 80S ribosomes into subparticles, thus readying the protein-synthesizing machinery for initiation of translation required during germination.

The function of ATP in the dissociation reaction in the reticulocyte system is not known. The phosphorylation of ribosomal proteins has been reported in reticulocytes (40,41), in rat liver (50), and in adrenal cortex (52). In the latter two systems, but not in reticulocytes, phosphorylation is dependent on cyclic AMP. In reticulocytes, Kabat (40) has reported that the different types of ribosomal particles characteristically carry specific phosphorylated proteins. In particular, one phosphorylated protein, S_u, is found only in the 40S ribosomal subparticle (40). It could well be that the dissociation of a ribosome implies the attachment of this S_u protein to the newly formed subparticle, together with its phosphorylation by ATP.

The question of the metabolic role of the free ribosomes and their relation to the polysomal cycle has been debated by many authors (*cf.* the discussion on bacterial systems by Algranati *et al.*, Chapter 27 of this volume). While it is accepted that the free ribosomes may become engaged in protein synthesis, it is recognized in animal cells that the free ribosomes in the cytoplasm (or at least the bulk of them) are not actively participating in the polysomal cycle, and certainly not at the rate of one particle per round of protein synthesis in the polysomes (31-35,52). Similar conclusions have been reached in a reticulocyte cell-free system (53). The possibility that a small fraction of the free ribosomes are obligatory participants in the polysomal cycle has been discussed by Baglioni *et al.* (9). This would introduce a functional heterogeneity of the whole population of free ribosomes, which has not been detected with the usual methods of gradient analysis. The functional diversity of 80S ribosomes could be simply due to the conformation of the polysomes together with the topographical distribution of ribosomes in the cytoplasm, favoring the participation of only a fraction of them (9). Selective modification of some components of ribosomes would be another possible way of modulating their functional capacity. Recent findings of Kabat (40) on the selective phosphorylation of ribosomal particles show that, on recovery of reticulocytes from fluoride inhibition, the nonphosphorylated, newly accumulated ribosomes are selectively used to form polysomes, while the normally existing, phosphorylated ribosomes are excluded from this utilization. Our results do not clarify whether free ribosomes and the dissociation step are obligatory components of the polysome cycle in reticulocytes or only side-products convertible to a storage form which can be salvaged for reutilization. These results do provide, however, a pathway for the participation of free 80S ribosomes in the process leading to protein synthesis.

ACKNOWLEDGMENTS

This research was supported by grants from the Consejo Nacional de Investigaciones Científicas y Técnicas, the Comisión de Investigaciones Científicas de la Provincia de Buenos Aires, and the Comisión de Investigaciones Científicas de la Universidad Nacional de La Plata. C. M. de B. is a Fellow of the Consejo Nacional de Investigaciones Científicas y Técnicas, Argentina. Results reported here will be published in detailed form elsewhere.

SUMMARY

In mammalian cells, native 40S and 60S ribosomal subparticles are generally accepted to be the immediate precursors of mRNA-ribosome initiation complexes. On the other hand, free 80S ribosomes can participate in protein synthesis in the cell and contribute to the build-up of polyribosomes. Also, the 80S ribosomes appear as by-products of the release of terminated chains in cell-free systems. This suggests that in the cyclic operation of the polysomal machinery, there must exist a step in which free 80S ribosomes dissociate into subparticles.

This contention, which has also been demonstrated in bacteria, is supported by experiments with the reticulocyte cell-free system: (a) ribosomal subparticles are incorporated into polysomes during protein synthesis; (b) free 80S ribosomes do not enter the polysomes under similar conditions; (c) addition of a high salt extract of the whole ribosomal fraction stimulates incorporation of 80S ribosomal material into polysomes; (d) the ribosomal extract (RE) can induce dissociation of 80S ribosomes into subparticles. This dissociation activity takes place in a physiological milieu, is independent of the initiation-promoting activity of RE, is heat labile, and requires time and temperature. ATP, but not other nucleotides, markedly stimulates the dissociation. The reaction is not inhibited by common antibiotic inhibitors nor by NaF. The significance of this reaction and the requirement for ATP are discussed in relation to the role of free ribosomes and the activation of ribosomes in dormant and other systems.

RESUMEN

Es generalmente aceptado que en las células de maníferos las subpartículas ribosómicas de 40S y 60S, nativas, son los precursores inmediatos de los complejos de iniciación mRNA-ribosoma. Por otra parte, en la célula los ribosomas 80S libres pueden participar de la síntesis proteica y contribuir a la formación de polirribosomas. Además de ello, aparecen como productos colaterales de la liberación de proteínas terminadas, en sistemas acelulares. Esto sugiere que, en relación con el funcionamiento cíclico de la maquinaria polisómica, debe existir un paso en el que los ribosomas 80S libres se disocien a subpartículas.

Esta proposición, que ha sido ya demostrada en bacterias, está apoyada por experimentos con el sistema acelular de reticulocitos: (a) Las subpartículas ribosómicas se incorporan a polisomas durante la síntesis de proteínas. (b) Los ribosomas 80S libres no se incorporan a polisomas por sí mismos, en esas condiciones. (c) El agregado de un extracto en sales concentradas, de la fracción ribosómica total, estimula la incorporación de material ribosómico 80S a polisomas. (d) El extracto ribosómico (RE) puede inducir la disociación de ribosomas 80S en subpartículas: esta actividad de disociación tiene lugar en un medio fisiológico, es independiente de la actividad de RE que estimula la iniciación, es termolábil, y requiere tiempo y temperatura. La disociación es marcadamente estimulada por el ATP, pero no por otros nucleótidos. La reacción no es inhibida por inhibidores antibióticos comunes, ni por el FNa. La significación de esta reacción, y su requerimiento de ATP, son discutidos en relación con el papel de los ribosomas libres, y la activación de los ribosomas en sistemas "dormidos," y otros.

REFERENCES

1. Lucas-Lenard, J., and Lipmann, F., *Ann. Rev. Biochem., 40,* 409 (1971).
2. Nomura, M., and Lowry, C. V., *Proc. Natl. Acad. Sci. U.S.A., 58,* 946 (1967).
3. Nomura, M., Lowry, C., and Guthrie, C., *Proc. Natl. Acad. Sci. U.S.A., 58,* 1487 (1967).
4. Hille, M. B., Miller, M. J., Iwasaki, K., and Wahba, A. J., *Proc. Natl. Acad. Sci. U.S.A., 58,* 1652 (1967).
5. Ghosh, H. P., and Khorana, H. G., *Proc. Natl. Acad. Sci. U.S.A., 58,* 2455 (1967).
6. Shafritz, D. A., Laycock, D. G., Crystal, R. G., and Anderson, W. F., *Proc. Natl. Acad. Sci. U.S.A., 68,* 2246 (1971).
7. Bishop, J. O., *Biochim. Biophys. Acta, 119,* 130 (1966).
8. Eisenstadt, J. M., and Brawerman, G., *Proc. Natl. Acad. Sci. U.S.A., 58,* 1560 (1967).
9. Baglioni, C., Vesco, C., and Jacobs-Lorena, M., *Cold Spring Harbor Symp. Quant. Biol., 34,* 555 (1969).
10. Heywood, S. M., *Nature, 225,* 696 (1970).
11. Waxman, H. S., and Rabinovitz, M., *Biochim. Biophys. Acta, 129,* 369 (1966).
12. Hori, M., Fisher, J., and Rabinovitz, M., *Science, 155,* 83 (1967).
13. Marks, P. A., Burka, E. R., Conconi, F. M., Perl, W., and Rifkind, R. A., *Proc. Natl. Acad. Sci. U.S.A., 53,* 1437 (1965).
14. Hogan, B. L. M., and Korner, A., *Biochim. Biophys. Acta, 169,* 129 (1968).
15. Hogan, B. L. M., *Biochim. Biophys. Acta, 182,* 264 (1969).

16. Godchaux, W., Adamson, S. D., and Herbert, E., *J. Mol. Biol., 27,* 57 (1967).
17. Kaempfer, R., Meselson, M., and Raskas, M., *J. Mol. Biol., 31,* 277 (1968).
18. Kaempfer, R., *Proc. Natl. Acad. Sci. U.S.A., 61,* 106 (1968).
19. Kaempfer, R., *Nature, 228,* 534 (1970).
20. Kaempfer, R., *Nature, 222,* 950 (1969).
21. Rich, A., Warner, J. R., and Goodman, H. M., *Cold Spring Harbor Symp. Quant. Biol., 28,* 269 (1963).
22. Hardesty, B., Miller, R., and Schweet, R., *Proc. Natl. Acad. Sci. U.S.A., 50,* 924 (1963).
23. Noll, H., Staehelin, T., and Wettstein, F. O., *Nature, 198,* 632 (1963).
24. Colombo, B., Vesco, C., and Baglioni, C., *Proc. Natl. Acad. Sci. U.S.A., 61,* 651 (1968).
25. Miller, R. L., and Schweet, R., *Arch. Biochem. Biophys., 125,* 632 (1968).
26. Cohen, B. B., *Biochem. J., 110,* 231 (1968).
27. Subramanian, A. R., Ron, E. Z., and Davis, B. D., *Proc. Natl. Acad. Sci. U.S.A., 61,* 761 (1968).
28. Bade, E. G., González, N. S., and Algranati, I. D., *Proc. Natl. Acad. Sci. U.S.A., 64,* 654 (1969).
29. González, N. S., Bade, E. G., and Algranati, I. D., *FEBS Letters, 4,* 331 (1969).
30. Subramanian, A. R., and Davis, B. D., *Nature, 228,* 1273 (1970).
31. Girard, M., Latham, H., Penman, S., and Darnell, J. E., *J. Mol. Biol., 11,* 187 (1965).
32. Joklik, W. K., and Becker, Y., *J. Mol. Biol., 13,* 496 (1965).
33. Perry, R. P., and Kelley, D. E., *J. Mol. Biol., 16,* 255 (1966).
34. Hogan, B. L. M., and Korner, A., *Biochim. Biophys. Acta, 169,* 139 (1968).
35. Kabat, D., and Rich, A., *Biochemistry, 8,* 3742 (1969).
36. Lebleu, B., Marbaix, G., Wérenne, J., Burny, A., and Huez, G., *Biochem. Biophys. Res. Commun., 40,* 731 (1970).
37. Zylber, E., Doctor's thesis, Universidad Nacional de La Plata, Argentina (1967).
38. Hoerz, W., and McCarty, K. S., *Biochim. Biophys. Acta, 228,* 526 (1971).
39. Lamfrom, H., and Knopf, P. M., *J. Mol. Biol., 9,* 558 (1964).
40. Kabat, D., *Biochemistry, 9,* 4160 (1970).
41. Kabat, D., *Biochemistry, 10,* 197 (1971).
42. Davis, B. D., *Nature, 231,* 153 (1971).
43. Pètre, J., *Europ. J. Biochem., 14,* 399 (1970).
44. Sabol, S., Sillero, M. A. G., Iwasaki, K., and Ochoa, S., *Nature, 228,* 1269 (1970).
45. Prichard, P. M., Gilbert, J. M., Shafritz, D. A., and Anderson, W. F., *Nature, 226,* 511 (1970).
46. Heywood, S. M., *Proc. Natl. Acad. Sci. U.S.A., 67,* 1782 (1970).
47. Subramanian, A. R., Davis, B. D., and Beller, R. J., *Cold Spring Harbor Symp. Quant. Biol., 34,* 223 (1969).
48. Marcus, A., and Feeley, J., *Proc. Natl. Acad. Sci. U.S.A., 56,* 1770 (1966).
49. Marcus, A., *J. Biol. Chem., 245,* 962 (1970).
50. Loeb, J. E., and Blat, C., *FEBS Letters, 10,* 105 (1970).
51. Walton, G. M., Gill, G. N., Abrass, I. B., and Garren, L. D., *Proc. Natl. Acad. Sci. U.S.A., 68,* 880 (1971).
52. Vesco, C., and Colombo, B., *J. Mol. Biol., 47,* 335 (1970).
53. Adamson, S. D., Howard, G. A., and Herbert, E., *Cold Spring Harbor Symp. Quant. Biol., 34,* 547 (1969).

DISCUSSION

H. N. Torres (Buenos Aires, Argentina): What was the effect of sodium fluoride when the dissociation was carried out in the presence of Mg-ATP?

G. Favelukes (La Plata, Argentina): The results I showed with sodium fluoride were done in the presence of Mg-ATP, so sodium fluoride does not inhibit the action of Mg-ATP, either. We even see an increase in the dissociation, which I attribute to the fact that in those conditions any residual chain initiation that is left is completely inhibited, so that we see the subparticles just as they are being made, and they are not utilized for ribosome construction again.

H. N. Torres: Have you carried out experiments in which the ribosomal particles were preincubated in the presence of Mg-ATP and then the dissociating factor was added, and also the reverse experiment, preincubation of the dissociation factor with Mg-ATP and then incubation with tne ribosomal particles?

G. Favelukes: No, we did not do that. We have some indirect indications that preincubation of the ribosomes will not lead to an increase of the dissociation effect, because we have been using ribosomes which are derived ribosomes, that is, ribosomes which have been isolated after runoff in a cell-free system in which there is 1 mM Mg-ATP; these derived ribosomes dissociated equally well in the treatment with dissociating factor.

G. D. Novelli (Oak Ridge, U.S.A.): Did you check to see if your derived particles in the presence of ATP still have methionyl-tRNA?

G. Favelukes: No, I did not do that.

K. Moldave (Irvine, U.S.A.): Do you know if the activity that stimulates protein synthesis is the same as the activity that dissociates, by heating, inactivation, or chromatography?

G. Favelukes: No, but we have indirect evidence that the two activities are different. The stimulatory activity for protein synthesis is very labile, while the dissociating activity is rather stable.

K. Moldave: And are the subunits active, for example, in globin or polyphenylalanine synthesis, when they are reisolated?

G. Favelukes: We do not have a direct experiment on that.

H. N. Torres: Do you have any cyclic AMP effect?

G. Favelukes: We did not test that because I think our system is very crude at this stage. We should probably do some purification.

H. N. Torres: Your extract is an ideal system to study the cyclic AMP effect.

G. Favelukes: There are some indications (at least according to Kabat) that phosphorylation of the different components of the ribosomal cycle would not be influenced by cyclic AMP. In the presence of sodium fluoride, which tends to change cyclic AMP availability, he does not see such effects reflected on the phosphorylation of the monomers and the subunits.

H. R. Mahler (Bloomington, U.S.A.): Exploring this a little further, although your system is quite crude, have you explored the nature of this dissociating factor any further, is it protein or nucleic acid, is it heat labile or heat stable?

G. Favelukes: It is heat labile. It will be inactivated by incubating for 10 min at 55°.

R. Soeiro (New York, U.S.A.): In some of your sucrose gradients, it appears as though some material went to the top of the gradient. Is there anything specific that is eluted from these particles during this dissociation?

G. Favelukes: I do not know.

I. D. Algranati (Buenos Aires, Argentina): You mentioned that after dialysis the dissociation activity increased. During this dialysis, do you have a precipitate?

G. Favelukes: Yes, we do have a slight precipitate, and a precipitate results just by mere dilution of the extract.

NOTE ADDED IN PROOF

After presentation of this paper, two publications have appeared on the presence and activity of a mammalian ribosome dissociation factor, in rat liver [Lawford, G. R., Kaiser, J., and Hey, W. C., *Can. J. Biochem., 49,* 1301 (1971)], and in rabbit reticulocytes [Lubsen, N. H., and Davis, B. D., *Proc. Natl. Acad. Sci. U.S.A. 69,* 353 (1972)]. The characteristics of the dissociation reaction promoted by purified preparations in both systems are similar to those observed by us; studies on ATP effects were not mentioned in those reports.

32

Studies on the Binding
of Aminoacyl-tRNA
to Wheat Ribosomes

Jorge E. Allende, Adela Tarragó,
Octavio Monasterio, Marta Gatica,
José M. Ojeda, and María Matamala

Departamento de Biologla
Facultad de Ciencias
and
Departamento de Bioqulmica y Química
Facultad de Medicina
Universidad de Chile
Santiago, Chile

The correct positioning of specific aminoacyl-tRNAs on the ribosome-mRNA complex is a key reaction in protein synthesis (translation). Although the intimate mechanism of the reaction is still mysterious, much information has been obtained about the components and products of aminoacyl-tRNA binding to ribosomes in bacterial systems (1). We know much less about how this process occurs in eukaryotic cells.

During the past few years, we have been interested in looking at the mechanism of protein synthesis in a wheat embryo system, and in this communication we shall relate some of our findings that deal with the binding of aminoacyl-tRNA to wheat ribosomes.

MATERIALS AND METHODS

Wheat embryo ribosomes, partially purified T_1 elongation factor from wheat embryos, tRNA, and radioactive aminoacyl-tRNA were prepared as described previously (2).

Radioactive amino acids and nucleotides were purchased from New England Nuclear Corporation.

Binding of Aminoacyl-tRNA to Wheat Ribosomes

The incubation mixture contained 50 mM Tris-HCl (pH 7.5), 7.5 mM or 20 mM $MgCl_2$ for the enzymatic and nonenzymatic binding, respectively, 120 mM NH_4Cl, 5 mM GTP, and 2.5 A_{260} units of wheat ribosomes expressed as RNA; 0.8 A_{260} units of poly U was added when the binding of phenylalanyl- or N-acetylphenylalanyl-tRNA was assayed and 0.18 A_{260} of AUG when the binding of methionyl-tRNA was measured. When crude preparations of T_1 enzyme were used, the reaction mixture contained 10^{-4} M sparsomycin to prevent polymerization of phenylalanine. The incubation was carried out for 20 min and was stopped by addition of saline buffer as described by Nirenberg and Leder (3).

Detection of Ternary Complex T_1-GTP-Aminoacyl-tRNA on Nitrocellulose Filters

Reaction mixtures contained 10 mM Tris-HCl (pH 7.5), 50 mM NH_4Cl, 10 mM $MgCl_2$, 1 mM dithiothreitol, 3 μM ^{3}H-GTP, wheat T_1 factor, and aminoacyl-tRNA. After 5 min incubation at $0°$, the reaction was stopped by addition of 3 ml of a buffer containing the same salt concentrations as the incubation mixture. The solution was filtered immediately in a refrigerated filter and washed three times with 5 ml of the same buffer. The filters were counted in a liquid scintillation counter.

Isolation of Ternary Complex T_1-GTP-Aminoacyl-tRNA by Gel Filtration on Sephadex G100

The complex was formed by incubating 1 ml containing 50 mM sodium cacodylate buffer (pH 7.0), 10 mM $MgCl_2$, 150 mM NH_4Cl, 1 mM dithiothreitol, 150 μM GTP, between 40 and 100 pmoles of aminoacyl-tRNA, and enough enzyme to bind 150 pmoles of GTP, during 10 min at $0°$. After the incubation, the mixture was passed through a Sephadex G100 column (1.45 by 55 cm), equilibrated, and eluted with 50 mM sodium cacodylate (pH 7.0), 1 mM $MgCl_2$, 150 mM NH_4Cl, 1 mM mercaptoethanol, and 75 μM GTP. Aliquots of 1 ml were precipitated with cold 5% trichloroacetic acid, filtered on nitrocellulose membranes, and counted in a scintillation system.

Fractionation of Both Species of Wheat Methionyl-tRNA on Benzoylated DEAE-Cellulose Columns

A column of benzoylated DEAE-cellulose (Schwarz Bioresearch) of 1.5 by 35 cm was equilibrated with a buffer containing 10 mM sodium acetate (pH 5.2), 10 mM MgCl$_2$, 0.5 mM 2-mercaptoethanol, and 0.4 M NaCl. The radioactive methionyl-tRNA was eluted with a linear gradient of salt from 0.4 to 1.0 M NaCl in the same buffer (400 ml in each chamber) (4).

Preparation of Ribosomal Subunits

Approximately 90 A_{260} units of washed ribosomes from wheat embryos

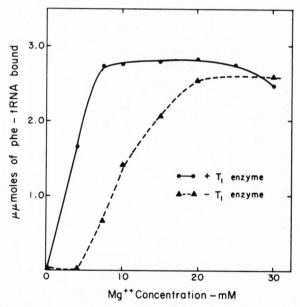

Fig. 1. The effect of magnesium ion concentration on the binding of phenylalanyl-tRNA to wheat ribosomes. The binding of approximately 10 pmoles of ^{14}C-phenylalanyl-tRNA to 2.3 A_{260} units of wheat ribosomes was measured under the conditions described in *Materials and Methods* for enzymatic and nonenzymatic binding. Approximately 10 μg of T$_1$ enzyme was added to each enzymatic assay.

was incubated in a buffer containing 0.01 M MgCl$_2$, 0.01 M Tris-HCl (pH 7.5), 0.005 M mercaptoethanol, and 0.5 M NH$_4$Cl at 37° for 10 min. This solution was then layered on a 25 ml 5-20% linear sucrose gradient in the same buffer as above. The gradients were centrifuged at 0° and 20,000 rpm for 12 hr in a SW25 rotor. Fractions were collected, and the ribosomal subunits were detected by the absorbance at 260 nm. Ribosomal particles from *Escherichia coli* were used as standards to determine the approximate sedimentation coefficient of the subunits. The fractions containing the 40S and 60S subunits were pooled, diluted in the same buffer, and pelleted by centrifugation at 105,000 × g for 8 hr.

RESULTS

It has been previously reported (2) that wheat embryo extracts contain a protein factor which binds GTP specifically and which is required for polypeptide synthesis. This factor has been partially purified by (NH$_4$)$_2$SO$_4$ precipitation, DEAE-cellulose chromatography, and more recently by phosphocellulose

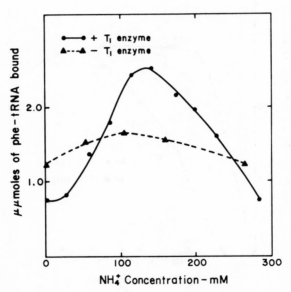

Fig. 2. The effect of ammonium ion concentration on the binding of ^{14}*C-phenylalanyl-tRNA to wheat ribosomes.* Enzymatic and nonenzymatic binding of ^{14}C-phenylalanyl-tRNA was assayed at the indicated NH$^+$ concentrations with other conditions as described in *Materials and Methods.* Approximately 10 μg of T$_1$ enzyme was used in these assays.

column chromatography. The factor, elongation factor T_1 (EF T_1), promotes the binding of aminoacyl-tRNA to wheat ribosomes (Fig. 1). It is evident that EF T_1 stimulates phenylalanyl-tRNA binding to wheat ribosomes in the presence of poly U only at low Mg^{2+} concentrations (3-10 mM). At higher Mg^{2+} concentrations (higher than 20 mM), there is equivalent aminoacyl-tRNA binding in the presence and absence of EF T_1. Figure 2 shows the effect of NH_4^+ concentrations on enzymatic Phe-tRNA binding at 7.5 mM Mg^{2+} and on the nonenzymatic reaction at 20 mM. It is apparent that enzymatic binding requires the presence of NH_4^+, reaching an optimum reaction at 120 mM concentration of the monovalent cation, while nonenzymatic binding is not appreciably affected by the presence of NH_4^+.

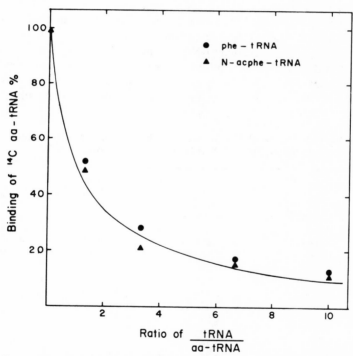

Fig. 3. *The effect of deacylated tRNA on the nonenzymatic binding of phenylalanyl-tRNA and N-acetylphenylalanyl-tRNA to wheat ribosomes.* The assay was performed as described in *Materials and Methods* for nonenzymatic binding. The 100% values of ^{14}C-phenylalanyl-tRNA and ^{14}C-acetylphenylalanyl-tRNA in the absence of added tRNA were 3.23 and 2.80 pmoles of each, respectively. The ratio of the deacylated to charged tRNA was calculated on the basis of 260 nm absorbance. All assays contained 1.2 and 1.3 A_{260} units of phenylalanyl-tRNA and N-acetylphenylalanyl-tRNA, respectively.

Nonenzymatic binding is nonspecific, since N-acetylphenylalanyl-tRNA binds to ribosomes under similar conditions and deacylated-tRNA also binds to ribosomes in the presence of mRNA. This is illustrated by the results shown in Fig. 3. In these experiments, the binding of radioactive Phe-tRNA and N-acetyl-Phe-tRNA to wheat ribosomes in the presence of poly U was assayed in the presence of different ratios of deacylated tRNA. If one assumes that the deacylated Phe-tRNA binds to the ribosomes with an efficiency similar to that of the acylated Phe-tRNA, one can draw the theoretical dilution curve that different amounts of the tRNA would have on the binding of aminoacyl-tRNA to a limiting amount of ribosomes. It is clear that the experimental points obtained in these experiments fit very well the theoretical curve, represented by the solid line in Fig. 3.

A different result is obtained when the enzymatic binding of aminoacyl-tRNA is studied. In Table I, one can see the inhibitory effect of the addition of a fourfold amount of deacylated tRNA on the binding of Phe-tRNA to wheat ribosomes at different concentrations of Mg^{2+}. It is clear that in the absence of enzyme, the inhibition obtained is close to the expected 80%. In the presence of T_1 and a low Mg^{2+} concentration, however, there is practically no inhibition. As

Table I. Effect of tRNA on Enzymatic and Nonenzymatic Binding of Phenylalanyl-tRNA at Different Mg^{2+} Concentrations[a]

Mg^{2+} (mM)	T_1 enzyme and GTP	Picomoles of phenylalanyl-tRNA bound		
		tRNA absent	tRNA present	Percent inhibition
4	–	0.00	0.00	–
7.5	–	0.68	0.11	84
10	–	1.42	0.36	75
15	–	2.07	0.59	73
20	–	2.55	0.60	76
4	+	1.60	1.49	7
7.5	+	2.76	1.93	30
10	+	2.77	1.69	39
15	+	2.81	1.32	53
20	+	2.83	1.10	61

[a] The enzymatic and nonenzymatic conditions for the assay of phenylalanyl-tRNA binding to wheat ribosomes were as described in *Materials and Methods* except for the magnesium ion concentrations. In all reactions, 9 pmoles of ^{14}C-phenylalanyl-tRNA (0.5 A_{260} units) and 2.2 A_{260} units of washed ribosomes were used. Where indicated, 2 A_{260} units of deacylated tRNA and T_1 enzyme (12 μg) were added to the enzymatic binding assays.

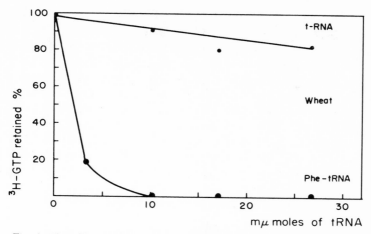

Fig. 4. The effect of aminoacyl-tRNA and deacylated tRNA on the retention of ^{3}*H-GTP on nitrocellulose membranes in the presence of* T_1. The assay for ^{3}H-GTP retention is as described in detail in *Materials and Methods*. The amounts of Phe-tRNA and tRNA were calculated from A_{260} measurements.

the Mg^{2+} increases and the reaction loses its enzymatic character, the inhibitory effect rises and approaches the theoretical value. Direct experiments have also shown that there is no enzymatic binding of N-acetylphenylalanyl-tRNA.

The basis for the specificity of the enzymatic reaction lies in the capacity of the enzyme to discriminate in the formation of the ternary complex T_1-GTP-aminoacyl-tRNA. As shown previously (2), the specificity in the formation of this complex can be assayed conveniently by the nitrocellulose membrane retention method, since the ternary complex goes through the filter while the T_1-GTP complex is retained. Figure 4 shows that aminoacyl-tRNA does interact with the T_1-GTP complex while deacylated tRNA does not.

In addition, it is possible to isolate the ternary complex by gel filtration on Sephadex G75 and G100 (Fig. 5). In columns using these gels, free aminoacyl-tRNA is retained and is clearly separated from the T_1 factor assayed by its GTP binding capacity (A). When aminoacyl-tRNA is incubated with T_1 in the presence of GTP, a considerable fraction of the aminoacyl-tRNA forms a complex and emerges from the column considerably earlier than the free aminoacyl-tRNA (B,D). It can be seen that the formation of this complex depends on the presence of GTP and that N-acetylphenylalanyl-tRNA is unable to form the ternary complex.

Figure 6 shows the results obtained when fractions obtained from a Sephadex G100 column, run as described in Fig. 5B, were incubated with ribosomes

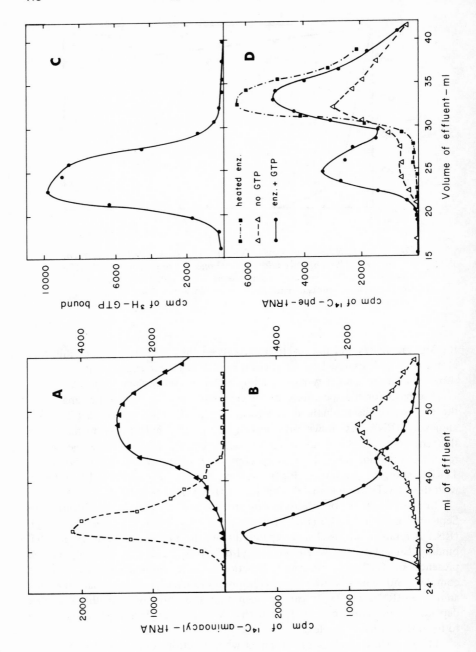

and poly U in the presence of 5 mM Mg^{2+}. It can be seen that phenylalanyl-tRNA present in the ternary complex fractions binds efficiently to the ribosomes but that the free Phe-tRNA fractions bind only very slightly. This last result was expected, since we already had observed that there was no nonenzymatic binding at the Mg^{2+} concentration used.

Since it has been shown by Ono et al. (5) that E. coli methionyl-tRNA$_f$ did not form a ternary complex with the bacterial elongation factor T_u, it was of some interest to determine whether both major methionyl-tRNA species from wheat could form the ternary complex with T_1 and GTP.

Figure 7 shows that methionyl-tRNA$_2$ does form the ternary complex with T_1 and GTP, but methionyl-tRNA$_1$ does not appear to form this complex. This finding supports the evidence obtained by Leis and Keller (6) that wheat Met-tRNA$_1$ has initiator properties.

Richter and Lipman (7), however, published work that demonstrated that Met-tRNA$_f$ of yeast did interact with GTP and T_1 factor from that organism. These authors, however, used a different method to detect formation of the ternary complex. The apparent discrepancy between their findings and ours, however, was resolved in a collaborative effort (8). In this work, it was determined that the initiator methionyl-tRNA from both wheat and yeast does interact with the homologous T_1 factor and GTP and this interaction can be detected by rapid methods such as the nitrocellulose retention method (Fig. 8). However, the interaction of the initiator Met-tRNA species differs from that observed with all other aminoacyl-tRNAs in that the complex formed is too

---

Fig. 5. Formation of the ternary complex, wheat binding factor-GTP-phenylalanyl-tRNA. The elution profiles of A and B were obtained using a Sephadex G75 column of 1.5 by 55 cm. The graph in A represents the calibration runs obtained by passing separately 1.5 mg of the wheat protein (40-80% ammonium sulfate) and 20,000 cpm of ^{14}C-Phe-tRNA in the column equilibrated and eluted with 50 mM cacodylate buffer (pH 7.1), 120 mM NH$_4$Cl, 5mM MgCl$_2$, and 1 mM glutathione. Fractions of 1.5 ml were collected, and the enzyme was assayed (□) by measuring the capacity of 200 μl aliquots to retain ^{3}H-GTP on nitrocellulose filters. The position of the ^{14}C--Phe-tRNA was determined by precipitating 50 μl aliquots with cold 5% TCA, filtering, and counting the radioactivity of the filters (▲). In graph B are included the elutions of 20,000 cpm of ^{14}C-Phe-tRNA (●) and 10,000 cpm of N-acetyl-Phe-tRNA (△), both of specific activity 100 μc/μmole, when passed through the column after the incubation with 1.5 mg of the enzyme to form the ternary complex as detailed in Materials and Methods. The elution buffer was the same as given in A except that it contained 0.15 μM GTP. Graphs in C and D were obtained using a Sephadex G75 column of 1.5 by 26 cm. C is the calibration of the GTP binding protein, and D is the elution of 120,000 cpm of ^{14}C-Phe-tRNA previously incubated with the complex system (●); incubated in the absence of GTP and eluted from the column with a buffer that also lacks GTP (△), and incubated with an enzyme that had been exposed to 50° for 10 min (■).

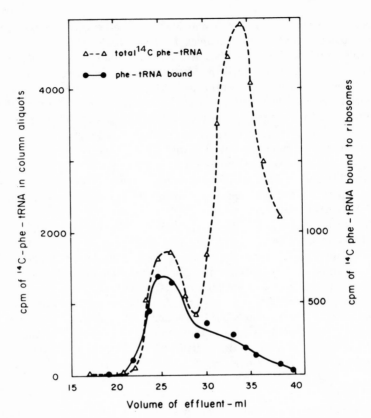

Fig. 6. Binding of ¹⁴C-phenylalanyl-tRNA from the ternary complex to wheat ribosomes. The procedure for the formation and isolation of the ternary complex was as described in Fig. 2. Aliquots of 400 μl of the fractions tested were incubated with 2 A_{260} units of wheat ribosomes and 40 μg of polyuridylic acid in the column eluting buffer in a final column of 500 μl. The incubation was 15 min at 20°, the reaction was stopped by addition of 5 ml of the same buffer at 0°, and the mixture was passed through nitrocellulose membranes (0.45 μ pore). The radioactivity retained on the membranes was counted in a scintillation counter (70% efficiency for ¹⁴C).

labile to be isolated by the Sephadex G100 method. The complex also seems to be abortive, since the binding of the initiator methionyl-tRNA to ribosomes is not enhanced by T_1 and GTP.

The previous studies induced us to look into the mechanism of binding of the initiator methionyl-tRNA to wheat ribosomes. Contrary to what has been described by other authors for bacterial systems and some eukaryotic systems (1), the proteins obtained by washing the ribosomes with high salt (0.5-1.0 M NH_4Cl) do not stimulate the binding of initiator methionyl-tRNA to wheat ribosomes in the presence of GTP and the coding triplet ApUpG. However, it was discovered that ribosomes washed with 0.5 M NH_4Cl bound preferentially the initiator species of methionyl-tRNA at low Mg^{2+} (9). Figure 9 shows that this preferential binding occurs with *E. coli* as well as wheat ribosomes. In

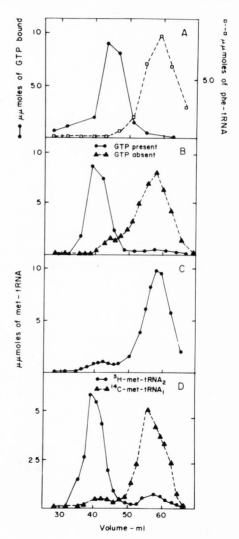

Fig. 7. Formation of ternary complex by the two major species of methionyl-tRNA from wheat. The general method was as described in Fig. 5C,D. In all experiments, 250 µg of wheat T_1 enzyme was used. (A) The elution columns of the wheat T_1 enzyme measured by the capacity of aliquots (100 µl) to retain ^3H-GTP on nitrocellulose filters and of ^{14}C-Phe-tRNA run separately on the same column. (B) The elution of wheat ^{14}C-Met-tRNA$_2$ (100 pmoles) incubated with wheat T_1 enzyme and GTP. Also shown in this figure is a control experiment in which GTP was left out of the incubation and of the elution buffer. (C) The elution of wheat ^{14}C-Met-tRNA$_1$ (90 pmoles) incubated and eluted with the complete system. (D) The elution of an incubation to form ternary complex in which 50 pmoles of ^{14}C-Met-tRNA$_1$ and 50 pmoles of ^3H-Met-tRNA$_2$ were added together. Aliquots were precipitated, filtered, and counted in a scintillation system that discriminated between the ^3H and ^{14}C radioactivity (4).

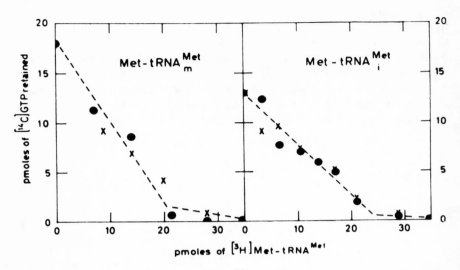

Fig. 8. Interaction of both wheat Met-tRNA ^{Met} species with T_1 and GTP as measured by the nitrocellulose retention method. All tubes contained (in 200 μl) approximately 20 μg of wheat T_1 factor and 3 μM ^{14}C-GTP(374 c/mol), 10 mM tris-HCl (pH 7.5), 10 mM MgCl$_2$, and 50 mM NH$_4$Cl. After incubation for 5 min at 0° C. ^{3}H-Met-tRNA (specific activity of ^{3}H-methionine, 3470 c/mol) was added where indicated and the incubation was continued for 5 min at 0°. The reaction was stopped by the addition of 5 ml of cold buffer (containing the same concentrations of Tris-HCl, MgCl$_2$, and NH$_4$Cl as above), and the mixture was passed immediately through a cool, wet nitrocellulose filter. The filter was washed three times with 5 ml of the same cold buffer and dried, and the ^{14}C was counted in a scintillation counter. The points • and × constitute averages of duplicates of two separate experiments (8).

this regard, it is interesting to note that the same preparation of *E. coli* ribosomes also bound preferentially *E. coli* Met-tRNA$_f$ in the presence of ApUpG, but required the addition of initiation factors to bind fMet-tRNA$_f$. Figure 10 shows that the separated 40S ribosomal subparticles from wheat have the capacity to bind preferentially the initiator species of wheat methionyl-tRNA. The 60S subparticles do not bind aminoacyl-tRNA.

CONCLUSIONS

The results presented in this report indicate that the binding of aminoacyl-tRNA to wheat ribosomes has properties very similar to those described for bacterial systems.

The occurrence of nonenzymatic binding of aminoacyl-tRNA and tRNA to wheat ribosomes at high magnesium ion concentrations demonstrates that, as pointed out by Dr. Spirin in Chapter 26 of this volume, the ribosomal particles

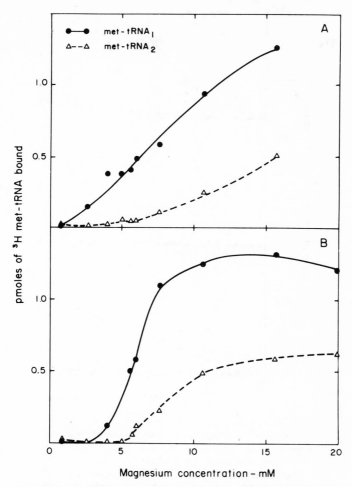

Fig. 9. The binding of wheat Met-tRNA species to wheat and E. coli *ribosomes at different magnesium ion concentrations.* The binding reaction was carried out by the procedure of Nirenberg and Leder (3). Incubation was for 15 min at 25° in a 50 μl mixture. In A, 2 A_{260} units of washed ribosomes from wheat and, in B, 2 A_{260} units of washed E. coli ribosomes were employed. Both experiments contained 0.18 A_{260} units of ApUpG and, where indicated, 3 pmoles of ^{3}H-Met-tRNA^{Met}. The tRNA-^{Met} was 1% acylated, and the tRNA-^{Met} was 3.4% acylated.

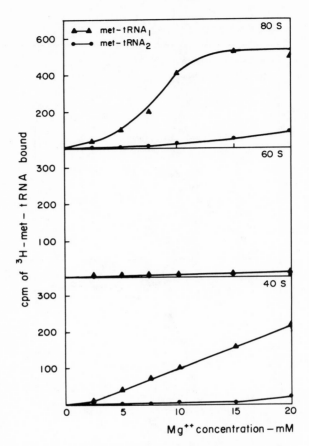

Fig. 10. *The binding of both methionyl-tRNA species to wheat ribosomal subparticles.* The ribosomal subparticles were prepared as described in *Materials and Methods.* The amount of subparticles used, where indicated, is expressed as units of absorbance at 260 nm: 0.26 of 40S, 0.33 of 60S, and 1.6 of 80S. In all experiments, 2.25 pmoles of ^{3}H-Met-tRNA^{Met} and 3.2 pmoles of ^{3}H-Met-tRNA^{Met} were used.

possess inherent structural features that favor an interaction with transfer RNA with specificity for correct codon recognition. At the physiological Mg^{2+} concentrations, however, the entry to the correct ribosomal site is limited to aminoacyl-tRNA that has previously complexed with elongation factor T_1 and GTP. Although the exact function of T_1, or its bacterial counterpart EF T_u is not known, it is clear from our results that in wheat this factor lends specificity to ribosomal binding. The importance of this specificity is clear from the fact that the imperfect and labile complex formed by T_1 with the initiator methionyl-tRNA prevents this aminoacyl-tRNA from transferring its methionine moiety into internal positions of the polypeptide chain.

It is interesting to note that several investigators have been unable to isolate an active ternary complex T_1-GTP-aminoacyl-tRNA using the factor from mammalian systems. It would seem that the complex in those cases is more unstable.

We have examined the possibility that complexing of aminoacyl-tRNA to wheat T_1 or *E. coli* T_u and GTP might serve as a purification procedure for the specific aminoacyl-tRNA, since it produces a shift in the elution of the bound aminoacyl-tRNA on gel filtration. The method, therefore, would depend on the specificity of T_1, which would only recognize the aminoacylated species of tRNA leaving the unacylated tRNA to elute in their normal positions. Preliminary tests with several aminoacyl-tRNAs show that the method does yield a ten- to fifteenfold purification in a single pass through a Sephadex G100 column. This work, however, has purely academic interest, since there are now many good methods for tRNA purification.

One of the most interesting differences between the known features of the elongation process in eukaryotes and prokaryotes is the existence of an extra factor, elongation factor T_s, which was first described in bacteria by Lucas-Lenard in Dr. Lipmann's laboratory (10). The main function of this factor is apparently to permit the regeneration of free T_u from the product of the binding reaction, T_u-GDP, by decreasing the affinity of T_u for the nucleoside diphosphate (11). We are presently studying the possibility that such a factor may exist in wheat embryo extracts.

The preferential binding of the initiator methionyl-tRNA species to the 40S subunit of wheat ribosomes is of some interest, since it may be related to a special entry site for the initiator aminoacyl-tRNA. Although our ribosomes were washed with $0.5\ M$ NH_4Cl, we cannot rule out the possibility that the preferential binding observed was mediated through initiation factors remaining on our particles. We did not find any stimulatory effects by the ribosomal wash in the binding of the initiator methionyl-tRNA. In light of the results presented here by Drs. Moldave and Heredia, however, we will certainly look for this activity in the supernatant fraction. Indeed, Dr. Marcus (12) has found initiation factors in the supernatant fraction of wheat extracts.

ACKNOWLEDGMENTS

This work was supported by a grant from CONICYT, Chile, and CIC, Universidad de Chile. A. T. and O. M. are Graduate Fellows of CONICYT, Chile.

SUMMARY

Aminoacyl-tRNA can bind to wheat embryo ribosomes either enzymatically or nonenzymatically. Nonenzymatic binding of aminoacyl-tRNA requires high concentrations of Mg^{2+} (10-30 mM) and is not affected by the presence of NH_4^+. Enzymatic binding occurs at more physiological concentrations of Mg^{2+} (3-7 mM) and is greatly enhanced by the addition of NH_4^+. Enzymatic binding is specific for aminoacyl-tRNA, while nonenzymatic binding occurs at a similar efficiency with deacylated tRNA and N-acetyl-phenylalanyl-tRNA. The enzymatic binding is catalyzed by wheat elongation factor T_1, isolated and partially purified using its capacity to retain radioactive GTP on nitrocellulose membranes as an assay. This enzymatic factor interacts specifically with aminoacyl-tRNA and GTP to form a ternary complex T_1-GTP-aminoacyl-tRNA; this complex is not retained on nitrocellulose filters. The ternary complex can be isolated by gel filtration and can be shown to be active by its capacity to transfer its aminoacyl-tRNA moiety to the ribosome-mRNA complex. The initiator methionyl-tRNA species from wheat differs from the other major methionyl-tRNA species and from all other aminoacyl-tRNAs from this source in that it forms a very labile ternary complex with T_1 and GTP. The initiator methionyl-tRNA species also has the property of binding to ribosomes at low Mg^{2+} concentrations in the absence of added factors. This preferential binding of the initiator species can be obtained with the isolated 40S ribosomal subparticles.

RESUMEN

El aminoacil-tRNA se une a los ribosomas provenientes del embrión de trigo, enzimáticamente no enzimáticamente. La unión no enzimática del aminoacil-tRNA requiere altas concentraciones de Mg^+ (10-30 mM) y no es afectada por la presencia de NH_4^+. La unión enzimática ocurre a concentraciones fisiológicas de Mg^+ (3-7 mM) y es altamente aumentada cuando se agrega NH_4^+. La unión enzimática es específica para el aminoacil-tRNA, mientras que la unión no enzimática ocurre con igual eficiencia con tRNA no acilado y con N-acetil-fenilalanil RNA. La unión enzimática es catalizada por el factor de elongación T_1 obtenido del trigo, y el cual se obtiene parcialmente purificado por su capacidad de retener GTP radioactivo al filtrarlo a través de membranas de nitrocelulosa. Este factor enzimático reacciona específicamente con aminoacil-tRNA y GTP para formar el complejo ternario, T_1-GTP-aminoacil-tRNA. Este complejo no se adhiere a los filtros de nitrocelulosa. El complejo ternario puede ser aislado utilizando filtración gel y puede demostrarse que es activo por su habilidad de tranferir su aminoacil-tRNA al complejo ribosoma-mRNA. La especie del iniciador metionil-tRNA del trigo difiere de las otras especies de metionil-tRNA y de los otros aminoacil-tRNA del trigo en que forma un complejo muy inestable con T_1 y GTP. El iniciador metionil-tRNA tiene además la propiedad de unirse a ribosomas, a concentraciones bajas de Mg^+ y en la ausencia de los factores solubles. Esta unión preferencial del iniciador se obtiene con las subunidades ribosomales 40S.

REFERENCES

1. Lucas-Lenard, J., and Lipmann, F., *Ann. Rev. Biochem., 40,* 409 (1971).
2. Jerez, C., Sandoval, A., Allende, J. E., Henes, C., and Ofengand, J., *Biochemistry, 8,* 3006 (1969).
3. Nirenberg, M. W., and Leder, P., *Science, 145,* 1399 (1964).
4. Tarragó, A., Monasterio, O., and Allende, J. E., *Biochem. Biophys. Res. Commun., 41,* 765 (1970).

5. Ono, Y., Skoultchi, A., Klein, A., and Lengyel, P., *Nature, 220,* 1304 (1968).
6. Leis, J. P., and Keller, E. B., *Biochem. Biophys. Res. Commun., 40,* 416 (1970).
7. Richter, D., and Lipmann, F., *Nature, 227,* 1212 (1970).
8. Richter, D., Lipmann, F., Tarragó, A., and Allende, J. E., *Proc. Natl. Acad. Sci. U.S.A., 68,* 1805 (1971).
9. Monasterio, O., Tarragó, A., and Allende, J. E., *J. Biol. Chem., 246,* 1539 (1971).
10. Lucas-Lenard, J., and Lipmann, F., *Proc. Natl. Acad. Sci. U.S.A., 55,* 1562 (1966).
11. Miller, D. L., and Weissbach, H., *Biochem. Biophys. Res. Commun., 38,* 1016 (1970).
12. Marcus, A., Weeks, D. P., Leis, J. P., and Keller, E. B., *Proc. Natl. Acad. Sci. U.S.A., 67,* 1681 (1970).

DISCUSSION

H. N. Torres (Buenos Aires, Argentina): What is the stoichiometry for the reaction in the formation of the complex; what is the proportion of T_1 factor, GTP, and aminoacyl-tRNA?

J. E. Allende (Santiago, Chile): We cannot say, because our T_1 factor is still not completely pure and there are problems in the determination of its molecular weight. We can say, however, that in the nitrocellulose membrane assay 1 pmole of aminoacyl-tRNA titrates 1 pmole of ^{3}H-GTP to form the ternary complex.

B. Hardesty (Austin, U.S.A.): Is the T_1 GTPase activity stimulated by the initiator Met-$tRNA_1$ on the ribosome? Have you tested that?

J. E. Allende: I am sorry, we have not done the experiment. I think that it is an interesting experiment that you are suggesting, since the initiator Met-tRNA from wheat does form a ternary complex with T_1 and GTP but cannot bind in a stable form to the ribosome. A lack of GTPase activity might point to the nature of the deficiency that makes this an abortive complex.

R. P. Perry (Philadelphia, U.S.A.): I just want to comment on the experiments done by Dr. Abraham Marcus in my Institute using the same type of system that you have. He uses ribosomal subunits from wheat embryos, but instead of using poly U he uses TMV RNA as his message. In this case, I believe that the binding required specific factors, isolated from the supernatant. This was binding to the 40S subunit.

J. E. Allende: Yes, Dr. Marcus has performed very interesting experiments using TMV RNA, which has the advantage of being a natural messenger. I don't think, however, that I have seen his experiments with ribosomal subunits published.

H. Mahler (Bloomington, U.S.A.): Have you tried to carry out reactions in the formation of this complex with the third methionyl-tRNA which is present in eukaryotic cells, namely, mitochondrial fMet-tRNA?

J. E. Allende: We have not. This Met-tRNA, mitochondrial Met-$tRNA_f$, was found in wheat, however, by Dr. Betty Keller and her coworkers. I do not think she has done the experiment of finding the interaction with T_1, but I believe Dietmar Richter in Dr. Lipmann's laboratory has been studying the fact that there is a different set of elongation factors in the organelles of yeast. I think that it would be interesting to do it, to determine whether there is specificity.

H. Mahler: This mitochondrial Met-$tRNA_f$ can be formylated by an enzyme present in the organelle?

J. E. Allende: That's right.

D. Novelli (Oak Ridge, U.S.A.): I would like to take exception to your statement that separation on Sephadex of the tRNA is simply academic. We have encountered some situations where it is necessary to aminoacylate and then derivatize a group of tRNAs and isolate them first over BD-cellulose and subsequently by reversed phase chromatography. Unfortunately, to my surprise, some of the derivatized ones are much more labile than the aminoacylated ones, and we have to keep going through consecutive rounds of this. In these instances I think yours would be an excellent method of separating a class of tRNAs, then subsequently subfractionating it.

J. E. Allende: A student in my laboratory, Oscar Reyes, who is here in the audience, has worked on this in his undergraduate thesis, and he has a lot of information about this purification method. It does work and it really does not require a lot of enzyme. A few grams of *E. coli* can yield, after one day's work, enough T factor to complex many picomoles of aminoacyl-tRNA.

K. L. Manchester (Kingston, Jamaica): Could I just make two general comments. I want to congratulate Dr. Allende on a very trivial point, and that is that the scale of many of his slides was in micromoles or picomoles rather than in counts per minute. I do not want to sound self-righteous on this, because I am sure my own work will be criticized the same way, but the use of only numbers of counts gives us no indication of how many micromoles of a particular compound will bind into equivalent micromoles of the other material. There certainly are published papers on the binding studies which, if you follow the authors' footnotes, suggest that the authors were unaware of what ratio of materials they were actually getting in the complex. The second point is again a rather trivial one, which is not meant to be any criticism of anyone's work, but when we do studies like the effect of ammonium chloride at different magnesium concentrations, most people are well aware of complex formation between magnesium and ATP and to a lesser degree between phosphoenolpyruvate and creatine phosphate and so on, but in the chemistry literature today there are data for the complexing value of even chloride with magnesium. Therefore, when one gets a curve which goes up and then comes down, the down portion could well be, if one is low in magnesium, due to the high concentration of chloride. Of course, there are other explanations as well on that.

J. E. Allende: I agree completely.

33

Polymerization Factors in Yeast

C. F. Heredia, A. Toraño, M. S. Ayuso, A. Sandoval, and C. San José

Instituto de Enzimología
Centro de Investigaciones Biológicas
Censejo Superior de Investigaciones Científicas
Madrid, España

It is now apparent that elongation of the peptide chain on the ribosomes requires the participation of several protein factors (elongation factors) which have been isolated from the soluble fraction of the cell. Three elongation factors have been obtained from bacteria (1,2) and designated as T_u, T_s, and G. Factor T (T_u plus T_s) is involved in the binding of the aminoacyl-tRNA to the ribosome-mRNA complex in a GTP-dependent reaction (2-4). This binding reaction is preceded by the formation of a ternary complex between factor T, GTP, and aminoacyl-t-RNA (5-8). Once the aminoacyl-tRNA has been bound to the ribosome, a peptide bond is formed between the carboxyl group of the carboxy-terminal amino acid of the peptidyl-tRNA (bound to the donor site of the ribosome) and the amino group of the newly bound amino acid. This reaction is catalyzed by peptidyl transferase, a protein located in the large ribosomal subunit (9). Elongation factor G then catalyzes the translocation of the nascent peptide chain from the acceptor to the donor site of the ribosome (10). A simultaneous release of the tRNA from the donor site occurs together with the movement of the ribosome along the mRNA (5). In this way, the acceptor site is ready to bind a new aminoacyl-tRNA molecule, and a new elongation cycle starts.

Elongation factors functionally similar to those from bacteria have also been obtained from eukaryotes. Yeast possess two protein-synthesizing systems: a bacterial-like system derived from the mitochondria (11,12) and another from the cytoplasm with characteristics similar to those from mammalian cells (13). Peptide chain mitochondrial (12,14) and cytoplasmic (15,16) elongation factors have been isolated from yeast cells. This communication deals with the isolation and partial purification of yeast cytoplasmic elongation factors and their role in the peptide chain elongation cycle. Evidence is also presented which suggests the existence of a protein factor, different from the elongation factors, which promotes a GTP-dependent binding of N-acetylphenylalanyl-tRNA to yeast ribosomes.

METHODS AND MATERIALS

A yeast hybrid *Saccharomyces fragilis* X *Saccharomyces dobzhanskii* was used in these experiments. Conditions of growth, composition of the growth medium, and preparation of crude extracts have been previously described (17). Preparation and purification of yeast ribosomes were as described elsewhere (18).

Partially purified soluble protein preparations were obtained by treating the $105,000 \times g$ supernatant with alumina Cγ as previously described (16). After centrifugation, the gel was washed with 0.1 M phosphate buffer (pH 6.5). The soluble proteins adsorbed on the gel were then eluted with 0.5 M phosphate buffer (pH 6.5). The eluate was dialyzed overnight against a standard buffer (18). This fraction is referred to as "soluble protein fraction."

Binding of Aminoacyl-tRNA

The reaction mixtures (0.1 ml) for the binding of ^{14}C-phenylalanyl-tRNA or N-acetyl-^{14}C-phenylalanyl-tRNA to the ribosomes contained the following components: 50 mM Tris-acetate (pH 6.5), 100 mM ammonium acetate, 50 μg poly U, 1 mM GTP, 10 mM magnesium acetate, 2 A_{260} units of purified ribosomes, aminoacyl-tRNA, soluble proteins, and other components as indicated in each case. After incubation at 30° for 20 min, the mixtures were diluted with 3 ml of a cold buffer containing 50 mM Tris-acetate (pH 6.5), 100 mM ammonium acetate, and 10 mM magnesium acetate and filtered through Millipores (19). After washing of the filters three times with 3 ml of the above mentioned buffer, they were dried and the radioactivity was estimated in a liquid scintillation spectrometer.

Materials

Uniformly labeled L-^{14}C-phenylalanine and ^{3}H-GTP were obtained from the Radiochemical Centre (England). The GTP and yeast ribonucleic acid were from Sigma Chemical Company. Puromycin was from Nutritional Biochemicals.

5'-Guanylyl-βγ-methylene diphosphonate (GMP-PCP) was from Miles Chemical Company. Polyuridylic acid (poly U) was from Boehringer.

Soluble ribonucleic acid (tRNA) was charged with ^{14}C-phenylalanine as previously described (18). Acetylation of phenylalanyl-tRNA was performed by the method described (18).

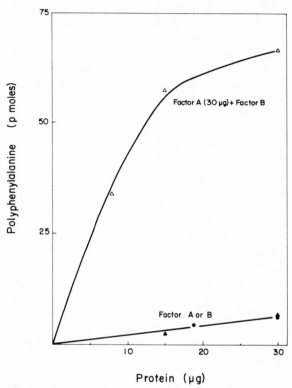

Fig. 1. *Complementarity of yeast elongation factors for the polymerization of phenylalanine.* Reaction mixtures (0.4 ml) contained 50 mM ammonium maleate buffer (pH 6.5) (about 90 mM ammonium), 1 mM spermidine, 0.05 mM mercapto-ethanol, 50 µg poly U, 13 mM magnesium acetate, 1.25 mM GTP, 1 A_{260} unit purified ribosomes, 70 µg ^{14}C-phenyla-lanyl-tRNA (containing 80 pmoles ^{14}C-phenylalanine), and elongation factors as indicated. Incubations were at 20° for 30 min. Phenylalanine polymerization was followed as previously described (18).

RESULTS

Dissociation of the Yeast Amino Acid Transfer System into Complementary Protein Fractions

Yeast ribosomes can be obtained free of soluble proteins by washing them with solutions of high ionic strength. After washing with a buffer containing 0.5 M ammonium chloride, the ribosomes are completely dependent on the soluble protein fraction for the polymerization of amino acids from aminoacyl-tRNA (18). Dissociation of this soluble protein into two complementary factors (elongation factors) has been achieved by different procedures (15,20). One of these procedures takes advantage of the different affinity of the yeast elongation factors toward gels of alumina $C\gamma$ under controlled conditions of pH and ionic strength (16). At pH 6.5 and low salt concentrations, both factors are adsorbed on the gel, and they can be eluted with 0.5 M phosphate buffer (pH 6.5). As the salt concentration is increased in the 105,000 $\times$ g supernatant, fractions enriched in one of the two elongation factors are obtained. At 0.2 M phosphate, only one of the factors (factor B) is adsorbed on the gel, while the other factor (factor A) remains in the supernatant. Factor B can be eluted from the gel by treatment with 0.5 M phosphate buffer (pH 6.5). The preparations of factor A obtained by this procedure usually contain some factor B. The factor B contaminating these preparations can be eliminated by heat treatment. After 2 min at 55°, factor B is completely inactivated, while factor A remains fully active. An alternative procedure to obtain preparations of factor A practically free of contamination with factor B is to adsorb both factors on alumina $C\gamma$ at low ionic strength, elute them with 0.5 M phosphate buffer (pH 6.5), and heat the eluates at 55° for 2 min. The complementarity of the two soluble protein fractions in the poly U-dependent polymerization of phenylalanine from phenylalanyl-tRNA is shown in Fig. 1. A great increase in the activity was observed with the combination of the two fractions over the sum of the activities shown by each of these two fractions tested separately.

Involvement of One of the Yeast Elongation Factors in the Binding of the Aminoacyl-tRNA to the Ribosomes

The binding of the aminoacyl-tRNA to the ribosome-mRNA complex can be considered as the first step in the peptide chain elongation cycle. This binding reaction has been shown to occur in all the systems so far studied under two different experimental conditions, depending on the magnesium concentration in the medium. Schweet and his group, working with the reticulocyte system, were the first to demonstrate the participation of one of the soluble elongation factors (TF_1) in the binding of phenylalanyl-tRNA to the ribosome-poly U complex in a reaction which required GTP (21). At high magnesium concentrations, the binding reaction was independent of the presence of these two components. The results presented in Table I indicate that one of the yeast elongation factors (factor A) and GTP are both involved in the binding of phenylalanyl-tRNA to purified yeast ribosomes at low magnesium concentrations. GTP cannot be replaced by its analogue GMP-PCP, which acts as an inhibitor of the binding reaction. This enzymatic type of binding reaction has characteristics different from those of the nonenzymatic one which occurs at high magnesium concentrations. While the former has a requirement for ammo nium or potassium ions and is not inhibited by deacylated tRNA, the latter does not require monovalent cations and is inhibited by deacylated tRNA. The inhibition by deacylated tRNA is counteracted by the presence of both factor A and GTP in the reaction mixtures (18). The presence of spermidine (1 mM) lowers the magnesium requirement for the enzymatic binding of aminoacyl-tRNA to concentrations below 5 mM. The phenylalanyl-tRNA bound to the ribosomes in response to elongation factor A and GTP is unreactive with puromycin, which suggests that it is bound to the A site of the ribosome.

The formation of a ternary complex between elongation factor T, GTP, and aminoacyl-tRNA has been shown to be a step prior to the binding of aminoacyl-tRNA to bacterial ribosomes. Our results (Fig. 2) and those reported by Richter (20) show that in yeast, as in other systems, the aminoacyl-tRNA binding factor forms a complex with radioactive GTP which is retained on nitrocellulose filters. When phenylalanyl-tRNA is added to the incubation mixtures, the radioactivity retained in the filters decreases in response to increasing amounts of the

Table I. Requirements for the Enzymatic Binding of
Phenylalanyl-tRNA to Yeast Ribosomes[a]

Experiment No.	Conditions	Phenylalanyl-tRNA bound (pmoles)
1.	Complete mixture	7
	Factor A and GTP	1
	Factor A	3.5
	GTP	2
	Factor A, heated 2 min at 70°	3
2.	Complete	11
	GTP omitted	1.5
	GTP replaced by GMP-PCP	0.7
	Complete + GMP-PCP	3.8

[a] Taken from Ayuso and Heredia (18).

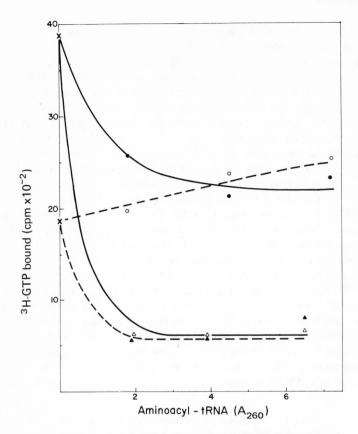

Fig. 2. *Effect of phenylalanyl-tRNA and* N-*acetylphenylalanyl-tRNA on the formation of the complex between* ^{3}*H-GTP and the yeast-soluble factors.* Reaction mixtures (0.1 ml) containing 50 mM Tris-acetate (pH 6.5), 100 mM ammonium chloride, 10 mM magnesium acetate, 2.5 μM ^{3}H-GTP (specific activity 1 mc/μmol), soluble protein fraction (about 150 μg protein), and aminoacyl-tRNA as indicated were incubated at 0° for 20 min. After incubation, the mixtures were diluted with 3 ml of a cold buffer containing 50 mM Tris-acetate (pH 6.5), 100 mM ammonium chloride, and 10 mM magnesium acetate, filtered through Millipore filters, and washed five times with 3 ml of the above buffer; the radioactivity retained in the filters was counted in a liquid scintillation spectrometer. When indicated, the soluble protein fraction was preincubated for 20 min at 20° with 20 mM N-ethylmaleimide. Solid lines, untreated soluble preparations; dashed lines, N-ethylmaleimide-treated preparations; ○, ●, N-acetylphenylalanyl-tRNA; △, ▲, phenylalanyl-tRNA; x, without aminoacyl-tRNA.

aminoacyl-tRNA present. In accordance with current views, this is due to the formation of a ternary complex between aminoacyl-tRNA binding factor, GTP, and phenylalanyl-tRNA which passes through the filter. When N-acetylphenyl-alanyl-tRNA is substituted for the phenylalanyl-tRNA, the amount of ^{3}H-GTP retained in the filters is only partially affected by the presence of this compound. This effect of the N-acetylphenylalanyl-tRNA disappears when the soluble protein fraction has been preincubated with N-ethylmaleimide. As shown below, this treatment inactivates the capacity of the soluble fraction to bind N-acetylphenylalanyl-tRNA to the ribosomes, leaving unimpaired its phenylala-nyl-tRNA binding activity due to the presence of the elongation factor A. After treatment of the soluble fraction with N-ethylmaleimide, the amount of ^{3}H-GTP retained in the filter is lower than in control experiments and is only sensitive to phenylalanyl-tRNA. Neither N-acetylphenylalanyl-tRNA (Fig. 2) nor deacylated tRNA has any effect. This seems to indicate that blocking the NH_2 group of the amino acid moiety renders the resulting compound unable to be recognized by the elongation factor A responsible for the binding of the aminoacyl-tRNA.

Factors Involved in the Binding of N-acetylphenylalanyl-tRNA to Yeast Ribosomes

Crude yeast ribosomes bind N-acetylphenylalanyl-tRNA at low magnesium concentrations in a GTP-dependent reaction. The capacity of the crude ribosomes to carry out this binding reaction is lost after they are washed with solutions containing 0.5 M ammonium chloride. However, these washed ribosomes retain their ability to bind N-acetylphenylalanyl-tRNA at high magnesium concentrations in the absence of GTP (18). Addition of the ammonium chloride

Table II. Requirements for the Enzymatic Binding of
N-acetylphenylanyl-tRNA to Yeast Ribosomes[a]

Conditions	N-acetylphenylalanyl-tRNA bound (pmoles)
Complete system	4.5
Soluble protein fraction	0.6
GTP	0.5
Ammonium ion	1.2
GTP replaced by GMP-PCP (1 mM)	0.5

[a] Conditions for the binding reaction were as indicated in *Methods and Materials,* using 25 pmoles of N-acetylphenylalanyl-tRNA and 50 μg of the soluble protein fraction.

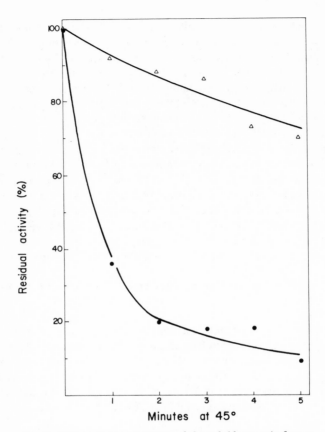

Fig. 3. Differential inactivation of the soluble protein factors.
Aliquots of the soluble protein fraction (0.2 ml) in 0.5 *M*
phosphate buffer (*p*H 6.5) were maintained at 45° for the
times indicated. After cooling in an ice bath, the binding of
N-acetylphenylalanyl-tRNA (●) or the polymerization of
phenylalanine from phenylalanyl-tRNA (△) was followed in a
final volume of 0.4 ml as described in *Methods and Materials*
and in the caption of Fig. 1.

wash fluid to these purified ribosomes does not result in a stimulation of the
binding of *N*-acetylphenylalanyl-tRNA at low magnesium concentrations, even
in the presence of GTP. However, a considerable amount of *N*-acetylphenyl-
alanyl-tRNA is bound to purified yeast ribosomes at 10 m*M* magnesium in
response to a soluble protein fraction in a GTP-dependent reaction (Table II).
This protein factor apparently has characteristics different from those of the
elongation factors. As shown in Fig. 3 the factor implicated in the binding of

N-acetylphenylalanyl-tRNA to purified yeast ribosomes is lost after heating for 2 min at $45°$, while the activities of the elongation factors remain unaltered, as shown by their ability to polymerize phenylalanine. The factor responsible for the binding of N-acetylphenylalanyl-tRNA is sensitive to sulfhydryl reagents. The activity is practically lost after incubation for 5 min at $30°$ with 20 mM N-ethylmaleimide, while this treatment does not affect the capacity of elongation factor A to promote the GTP-dependent binding of phenylalanyl-tRNA to purified yeast ribosomes (Table III). Dithioerythritol (50 mM) protects the factor against inactivation by N-ethylmaleimide. Finally, as shown in Table III, neither of the two isolated elongation factors is able to catalyze the GTP-dependent binding of N-acetylphenylalanyl-tRNA to yeast ribosomes. Taken together, these data strongly suggest the existence of a new factor present in the soluble fraction of the cell, responsible for the binding of N-acetylphenylalanyl-tRNA to purified yeast ribosomes.

As in the case of phenylalanyl-tRNA, the factor-dependent binding of N-acetylphenylalanyl-tRNA to purified yeast ribosomes requires GTP and a monovalent cation (NH_4^+). GTP cannot be replaced by its structural analogue GMP-PCP, which acts as an inhibitor of the binding reaction.

Table III. Factor-Dependent Binding of Aminoacyl-tRNA to Purified Yeast Ribosomes and Effect of N-Ethylmaleimide (NEM)[a]

		Aminoacyl-tRNA bound	
Experiment No.	Additions	N-acetyl-Phe-tRNA (pmoles)	Phe-tRNA (pmoles)
1	None	0.3	0.4
	Soluble protein fraction	2.3	—
	NEM-treated soluble protein fraction	0.3	4.3
2	Elongation factor A	—	3.1
	NEM-treated factor A	—	2.7
3	None	0.5	0.4
	Soluble protein fraction	2.5	—
	Elongation factor A	0.4	2.5
	Elongation factor B	0.4	—

[a] Conditions for the binding of aminoacyl-tRNA were those described in *Methods and Materials,* using N-acetylphenylalanyl-tRNA, 15 pmoles, or phenylalanyl-tRNA, 35 pmoles (experiments 1 and 2) or 20 pmoles (experiment 3). Approximately 50 μg of protein of each of the protein fractions was used. When indicated, protein fractions were preincubated with N-ethylmaleimide (20 mM) at $30°$ for 5 min.

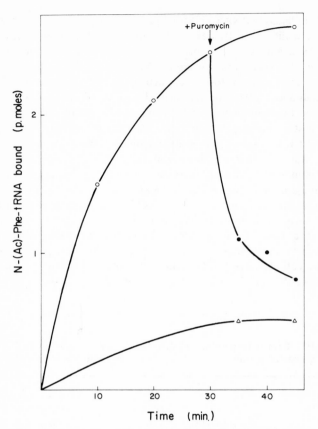

Fig. 4. *Reactivity with puromycin of the* N-*acetylpheny-lalanyl-tRNA enzymatically bound to the ribosomes.* The binding of *N*-acetylphenylalanyl-tRNA (13 pmoles) to the ribosomes was followed as described in *Methods and Materials* with (○) or without (△) soluble protein fraction (50 μg). At 30 min, puromycin was added (●) in a volume of 75 μl to give a final concentration of 4 m*M*. A control with 75 μl of water was run in parallel. Radioactivity retained in the filters was estimated as described in *Methods and Materials*.

Reactivity of the *N*-acetylphenylalanyl-tRNA Enzymatically Bound to the Ribosomes

N-acetylphenylalanyl-tRNA enzymatically bound to purified yeast ribosomes is reactive with puromycin (Fig. 4), which implies that it is bound to the donor or peptidyl site of the ribosomes. Since our crude soluble protein

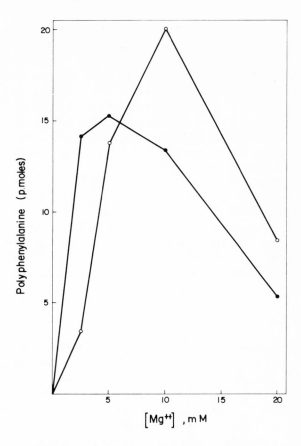

Fig. 5. *Magnesium requirements for the polymerization of phenylalanine by ribosomes bearing enzymatically bound* N-*acetylphenylalanyl-tRNA.* Purified ribosomes (1.8 A_{260} units) were preincubated at 30° for 5 min with (●) or without (○) N-acetylphenylalanyl-tRNA (10 pmoles) in a reaction mixture (0.1 ml) containing 100 mM tris-HCl (pH 6.5), 50 mM ammonium chloride, 50 μg poly U, 1 mM GTP, 10 mM magnesium acetate, and 55 μg of soluble protein fraction. After incubation, the reaction mixtures were supplemented with ^{14}C-phenylalanyl-tRNA (35 pmoles), 100 μg of soluble protein fraction, and GTP, ammonium, and Tris-HCl (pH 6.5) to give the final concentrations shown, in a final volume of 0.4 ml. Magnesium was added when necessary to adjust for the concentrations shown in the figure. After incubation for 2 min at 30°, the amounts of polyphenylalanine were estimated as described (18).

preparations also contain the activity responsible for the process of translocation, we do not yet know if N-acetylphenylalanyl-tRNA enters directly at the
donor site of the ribosome or if its location at this site involves translocation. A
lack of translocation is suggested by the fact that fusidic acid, a compound
known to inhibit translocase (22,23), does not affect the enzymatic binding of
N-acetylphenylalanyl-tRNA, under conditions in which polyphenylalanine
synthesis is completely inhibited. Contrary to the result with enzymatically
bound N-acetylphenylalanyl-tRNA, when this compound is bound at high magnesium concentrations in the absence of soluble protein fraction and GTP, it
does not react with puromycin.

Enzymatic binding of N-acetylphenylalanyl-tRNA to ribosomes leads to a
marked lowering of the magnesium ion requirement for the polymerization of
phenylalanine from phenylalanyl-tRNA. As can be seen from the results presented in Fig. 5, after binding of N-acetylphenylalanyl-tRNA to ribosomes
optimal polymerization of phenylalanine is attained at magnesium concentrations (2.5 mM) at which the rate of polymerization is very low when normal
ribosomes are used. Part of the N-acetylphenylalanine enzymatically bound is
incorporated into the nascent polyphenylalanine chain.

DISCUSSION

The results presented above and those reported by other workers indicate
that in the soluble fraction of yeast extracts there exist three different protein
factors implicated in the process of polypeptide synthesis. Two of these protein
factors (A and B) have been isolated and partially purified. Their functional
characteristics are equivalent to those of elongation factors T and G from
bacterial systems. Factor A promotes a GTP-dependent binding of the aminoacyl-tRNA to the ribosomes. Factor B is probably involved in the process of
translocation. The yeast aminoacyl-tRNA binding factor forms a complex with
GTP and aminoacyl-tRNA prior to the binding of the aminoacyl-tRNA to the
ribosomes.

A third activity has been detected in the soluble fraction of yeast extracts
which catalyzes the binding of N-acetylphenylalanyl-tRNA to yeast ribosomes.
Although we have not yet been successful in separating this factor from the
elongation factors, there are several properties by which they can be differentiated: (a) the factor is much more susceptible to heat inactivation than the
elongation factors; (b) it is inactivated by treatment with N-ethylmaleimide,
which does not affect the elongation factor A responsible for the binding of
phenylalanyl-tRNA to the ribosomes; (c) neither of the elongation factors is able
to catalyze binding of N-acetylphenylalanyl-tRNA to yeast ribosomes; (d) elongation factor A can discriminate against N-acetylphenylalanyl-tRNA for the
formation of a ternary complex with aminoacyl-tRNA and GTP.

Binding of *N*-acetylphenylalanyl-tRNA to yeast ribosomes, in response to this protein factor, leads to a shift in the magnesium requirements for the polymerization of phenylalanine from phenylalanyl-tRNA to concentrations at which the rate of polymerization is very low with normal ribosomes. The *N*-acetylphenylalanyl-tRNA bound is reactive with puromycin and is incorporated into the nascent polyphenylalanine chain. Although we do not know yet the nature of its function, this factor has characteristics similar to those found for a soluble factor present in rat liver (24) and *Artemia salina* (25) which seems to be implicated in peptide chain initiation.

ACKNOWLEDGMENTS

Part of this work was supported by a grant from the United States Public Health Service (TW 00303). The authors are indebted to Miss Carmen Moratilla for very able technical assistance and to Miss Clotilde Estévez for the typing of the manuscript. A. T. is a fellow of the Ministerio de Educación y Ciencia; C. S. is the recipient of a fellowship from the Fundación Juan March; A. S. is on leave of absence from the Departamento de Bioquímica, Facultad de Medicina, Universidad de Chile.

SUMMARY

Two soluble protein factors functionally equivalent to the elongation factors T and G from bacteria have been isolated from the cytoplasmic fraction of yeast extracts. One of these factors is involved in the binding of aminoacyl-tRNA to purified yeast ribosomes. The other factor is probably implicated in translocation. The aminoacyl-tRNA binding factor forms a ternary complex with GTP and phenylalanyl-tRNA but not with *N*-acetylphenylalanyl-tRNA or deacylated tRNA.

A third activity has been detected in the soluble fraction of yeast extracts which catalyzes a GTP-dependent binding of *N*-acetylphenylalanyl-tRNA to purified yeast ribosomes. This factor can be distinguished from the aminoacyl-tRNA binding factor by its greater sensitivity to heat and its inactivation by sulfhydryl reagents. The *N*-acetylphenylalanyl-tRNA bound in response to this factor is reactive with puromycin and is incorporated as the amino-terminal residue in the nascent polyphenylalanine chain.

RESUMEN

Se han aislado en levadura dos factores proteicos solubles funcionalmente equivalentes a los factores de crecimiento de la cadena peptídica T y G aislados en bacterias. Uno de estos factores está implicado en la fijación de aminoacil-tRNA a ribosomas de levadura. El otro factor interviene verosímilmente en el proceso de translocación. El factor responsable de la fijación del aminoacil-tRNA forma un complejo con GTP y fenilalanil-tRNA pero no con *N*-acetil-fenilalanil-tRNA o tRNA deacilado.

Se ha detectado una tercera actividad en la fracción proteica soluble de extractos de levadura que cataliza la fijación dependiente de GTP, de *N*-acetilfenilalanil-tRNA a ribosomas purificados. Este factor puede distinguirse del factor fijador de aminoacil-tRNA por su mayor sensibilidad al calor y por su inactivación por reactivos de grupos sulfhidrilos. El N-acetilfenilalanil-tRNA fijado a los ribosomas con el concurso de este factor, reacciona con puromicina y se incorpora como aminoácido terminal a la cadena de polifenilalanina.

REFERENCES

1. Lucas-Lenard, J., and Lipmann, F., *Proc. Natl. Acad. Sci. U.S.A., 55,* 1562 (1966).
2. Skoultchi, A., Ono, Y., Moon, H. M., and Lengyel, P., *Proc. Natl. Acad. Sci. U.S.A., 60,* 675 (1968).
3. Ravel, J. M., *Proc. Natl. Acad. Sci. U.S.A., 57,* 1811 (1967).
4. Haenni, A.-L., and Lucas-Lenard, J., *Proc. Natl. Acad. Sci. U.S.A., 61,* 1363 (1968).
5. Lucas-Lenard, J., and Haenni, A.-L., *Proc. Natl. Acad. Sci. U.S.A., 59,* 554 (1968).
6. Gordon, J., *Proc. Natl. Acad. Sci. U.S.A., 59,* 179 (1968).
7. Ravel, J. M., Shorey, R. L., and Shive, W., *Biochem. Biophys. Res. Commun., 29,* 68 (1967).
8. Skoultchi, A., Ono, Y., Waterson, J., and Lengyel, P., *Cold Spring Harbor Symp. Quant. Biol., 34,* 437 (1969).
9. Monro, R. E., *J. Mol. Biol., 26,* 147 (1967).
10. Lipmann, F., *Science, 164,* 1024 (1969).
11. Scragg, A. H., Morimoto, H., Villa, V., Nekhorocheff, J., and Halvorson, H. O., *Science, 171,* 908 (1971).
12. Richter, D., and Lipmann, F., *Biochemistry, 9,* 5065 (1970).
13. Bretthauer, R. K., Marcus, L., Chaloupka, J., Halvorson, H. O., and Bock, R. M., *Biochemistry, 2,* 1079 (1963).
14. Scragg, A. H., *FEBS Letters, 17,* 111 (1971).
15. Klink, F., and Richter, D., *Biochim. Biophys. Acta, 114,* 431 (1966).
16. Ayuso, M. S., and Heredia, C. F., *Biochim. Biophys. Acta, 145,* 199 (1967).
17. Heredia, C. F., and Halvorson, H. O., *Biochemistry, 5,* 946 (1966).
18. Ayuso, M. S., and Heredia, C. F., *Europ. J. Biochem., 7,* 111 (1968).
19. Nirenberg, M., and Leder, P., *Science, 145,* 1399 (1964).
20. Richter, D., *Biochem. Biophys. Res. Commun., 38,* 864 (1970).
21. Arlinghaus, A. G., Shaeffer, J., and Schweet, R. S., *Proc. Natl. Acad. Sci. U.S.A., 51,* 1291 (1964).
22. Tanaka, N., Kinoshita, T., and Nasukawa, M., *Biochem. Biophys. Res. Commun., 30,* 278 (1968).
23. Malkin, M., and Lipmann, F., *Science, 164,* 71 (1969).
24. Leader, D. P., Wool, I. G., and Castles, J. J., *Proc. Natl. Acad. Sci. U.S.A., 67,* 523 (1970).
25. Zasloff, M., and Ochoa, S., personal communication.

DISCUSSION

K. Moldave (Irvine, U.S.A.): Do you know whether the N-acetyl-Phe-tRNA is bound initially to the small subunit? Are there small subunits in your ribosome preparations?

C. F. Heredia (Madrid, Spain): No, we have run some sucrose gradients to see whether there are subunits other than the 80S, and we found only a peak of 80S ribosomes.

K. Moldave: I might tell you about an experience in our laboratory with a reaction which has these characteristics also and it may bear on it. We find that we do get a small stimulation by soluble proteins, not as good as yours, when we work with the 80S ribosomes. We can get binding to 80S ribosomes with other factors, either N-acetyl-Phe-tRNA or Phe-tRNA. When we work with the intact ribosomes or the reconstituted ribosomes, we always require GTP. When we work with a small subunit, the GTP requirement is lost, and our tentative interpretation is that there is perhaps a conformational change in the interaction of the two subunits in which GTP is required to allow for binding to the upper sites on the 80S.

C. F. Heredia: This is one possibility. We are trying to get ribosomal subunits, but it is quite hard and we only get the subunits in an inactive form. With the active subunits, we plan to study the binding of this N-acetyl-Phe-tRNA.

34

Modifications of Polysome-Associated RNA After Poliovirus Infection

G. Contreras, T. Cárdenas, Carmen Grado, S. Yudelevich, and D. F. Summers

Unidad de Virología
Departamento de Microbiología y Parasitología
Facultad de Medicina y Facultad de Ciencias
Universidad de Chile
Santiago, Chile
and

D. F. Summers
Department of Cell Biology
Albert Einstein College of Medicine
New York, New York, U.S.A.

It is reasonable to assume that viral infection triggers a number of host cell responses; some produced by oncogenic viruses are already well documented (1). It would be surprising that, among viruses lytic for eukaryotic cells, replication would be solely a cytoplasmic event. Since there are data suggesting the existence of signals that reach the cell nucleus after poliovirus infection (2,3), we decided to look for alterations of polysome-associated RNA as one of the early HeLa cell responses to the viral stimulus. This paper will describe the alterations detected and a preliminary characterization of the RNA molecules involved.

MATERIALS AND METHODS

Suspension cultures of S3 HeLa cells grown in Eagle's medium and a plaque-purified strain of type-1 poliovirus were used throughout the studies. Cell growth, harvesting, infection, and labeling procedures have been described (4). In every experiment, actinomycin D (0.04 μg/ml) was added to the cell culture, 15 min prior to infection (5). The cells (4 $\times$ 10^6/ml) were infected with different multiplicities (ranging from 30 to 300 PFU/cell) as indicated in each experiment, in a serum-free medium. The uninfected cells received an equal volume of CsCl solution corresponding in density to that of the virus band. Bovine serum (5%) was added 5 min later, in order to minimize cell physiological variations, and the time of the serum addition was taken as zero experimental time. ^{3}H-5-uridine (20 c/mmole) was obtained from Bioschwarz; the same amount of isotope was added to both cultures at the selected time postinfection (p.i.). The pulse was stopped upon emptying the cultures into centrifuge tubes containing crushed frozen Earle's solution. As previously described (6), cells were fractionated by Dounce homogenization after a 5 min period swelling in hypotonic buffer, termed "RSB" (reticulocyte standard buffer: 0.01 M NaCl, 0.015 M MgCl$_2$, 0.01 M Tris, pH 7.4). The homogenate was centrifuged at 1500 rpm for 5 min at 0°. The supernatant was made to 0.5% in deoxycholate, termed "cytoplasmic extract," and was layered on a 7-47% w/v linear sucrose gradient (dissolved in RSB the previous day and autoclaved), prepared in the cold room. After sedimenting, the optical density (OD) at 260 nm was recorded in a Gilford instrument, and the desired number of fractions was collected on an ice-water bath. Radioassay of samples was performed as previously described (4).

Selected polysome gradient fractions were pooled, made to 0.5% in sodium dodecyl sulfate (SDS), ethanol precipitated, kept at $-20°$ for several hours, and centrifuged. The RNA pellet was dissolved in about 2 ml of an isotonic SDS buffer, termed "NETS" (0.15 M NaCl, 0.001 M EDTA, 0.01 M Tris, pH 7.2, and 0.2% SDS), and aliquots were layered on fifteen 15-30% w/v sucrose gradients in NETS. Other aliquots were again ethanol precipitated, centrifuged, and dissolved in 0.01 M PO$_4$ buffer, pH 7.0. Once dissolved, ^{14}C-labeled RNA from *Escherichia coli* was added; the samples were made to 10% in formaldehyde and to 0.5% in SDS, heated to 65° in a water bath for 15 min, and rapidly chilled with crushed ice. Aliquots of formaldehyde-treated RNA were layered on 5-20% w/v sucrose gradients in 3% formaldehyde-0.1 M PO$_4$ buffer. Other samples of this RNA were layered on 20 cm long gels prepared with 2.4% polyacrylamide plus 0.5% agarose (7). The electrophoresis was carried out at 10 ma per gel during 12 hr, using Bromophenol Blue as marker. The gels were crushed and counted as described by Maizel (8).

RESULTS

The cytoplasmic extract of HeLa cells incorporates ^{3}H-5-uridine into RNA in the region of RNA molecules smaller than 5S (3) when analyzed in a 15-30%

sucrose gradient after a radioactive pulse of 10-20 min. Similar results are obtained in the presence of 0.04 μg/ml of actinomycin D. Therefore, the experiments to be reported here were done in the presence of this antibiotic, in order to minimize radioisotope uptake by ribosomal RNA (5). With this procedure, a low radioactive background is obtained, allowing an analysis of the polysome region as shown in Fig. 1. The OD of the large polysomes is seen as a broad peak (fractions 9-13), followed by smaller decreasing peaks, assumed to be polysomes from about ten to two ribosomal units. Within the first hour of infection, we have not detected any differences regarding OD among the infected and uninfected cells. The radioactive profile follows the OD pattern, except for some clear distinct peaks which are observed in the infected cells' polysomes, in fractions 6-13 and 15-21. Thereafter, the radioactive counts level off in relation to ribosomes and subunits, increasing again in the lighter gradient

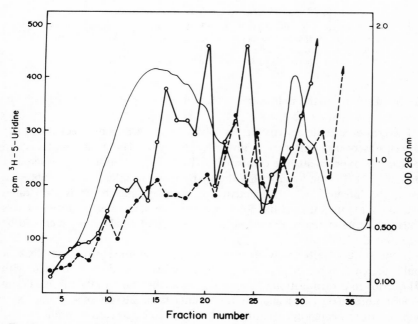

Fig. 1. *Analysis of the polysome region.* The cytoplasmic extracts, obtained from 40 million uninfected cells and from an equal number of infected cells that had been exposed to 100 μc of ³H-5-Uridine from 15 to 30 min after poliovirus infection (30 PFU/cell) were layered on a 7-47% w/v sucrose gradient, in RSB, and sedimented in a Spinco SW27 rotor at 23.5 K for 180 min at 4°. ————, the OD of both experimental series is the same; •, cpm of the extract from uninfected cells; ○, cpm of the extract from infected cells. Fraction 1 is the bottom of the gradient tube.

Table I. Specific Activity of the Polysomes Labeled with
[3]H-5-Uridine Given as Pulses Within 11-35 min Post-Infection[a]

| | Mean specific activity[b] | | Specific activity ratio: $\frac{infected}{uninfected}$ |
Gradient area	Uninfected	Infected	
Polysomes (fractions 9-24)	7.007	10.161	1.45± 0.11
Ribosomes and subunits (fractions 25-30)	3.936	4.303	1.09
Gradient top (fractions above 31)	21.253	23.218	1.09
Total	34.380	41.003	1.19± 0.08

[a] The experiments were done as described in Fig. 1. The isotope pulses were given at the following times p.i. (min): 11-21, 12-24, 15-30, 18-30, 20-30, and 20-35 min.
[b] Mean specific activities of six experimental series.

zone (gradient top); the radioactivity of both series is practically the same in these other gradient areas.

The greater specific activity of the polysomes derived from infected cultures has been observed consistently in several experiments. The mean specific activities from six experiments are compared in Table I. ^{3}H-5-uridine was given as a short pulse, 10-15 min long, within the first 35 min of infection. It can be seen that in the infected cells, radioactivity of the polysome region is 1.45 times greater ($\pm$ 0.11) than that of the polysomes from uninfected cells; moreover, it is in this polysome region where the slight difference of total counts seems to be concentrated.

If the tracer is effectively incorporated into polysome-associated RNA, it should decrease substantially when the cytoplasmic extract is treated with EDTA prior to centrifugation (5). Figure 2 shows the effect of 0.01 M EDTA on the OD profile (Fig. 2A) and on the counts (Fig. 2B) of such gradients as compared to untreated cytoplasmic extract from infected cells. A similar reduction of both OD and cpm of the polysome area has been observed when cytoplasmic extracts from uninfected cells are treated with 0.01 M EDTA.

The greater radioactivity observed in the polysomes prepared from infected cells implies a faster polysome turnover. Since 10^{-2} M cycloheximide seems to prevent polysome turnover through inhibition of polysome breakdown (9), it should have a marked effect on those polysomes which are turning over faster. The effect of 2 $\times$ 10^{-2} M cycloheximide added during the last 3 min of the

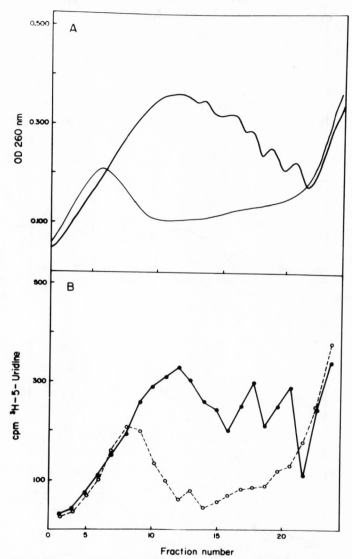

Fig. 2. Effect of 0.01 M *EDTA on OD profile and radioactive counts.*
The cytoplasmic extract from 40 million HeLa cells, infected with 100
PFU/cell and exposed to 100 μc of ³H-5-uridine from 11 to 21 min p.i.,
was divided in halves before layering on the sucrose gradient. One half
was made to 0.01 *M* EDTA and left at room temperature for 15 min;
the remaining half received the same amount of RSB and was treated
likewise. Both the sucrose gradient and sedimentation conditions are
the same as described in Fig. 1. OD profiles in Fig. 2A: heavy line,
nontreated; light line, EDTA treated. Cpm in Fig. 2B: ●, nontreated; ○,
EDTA treated.

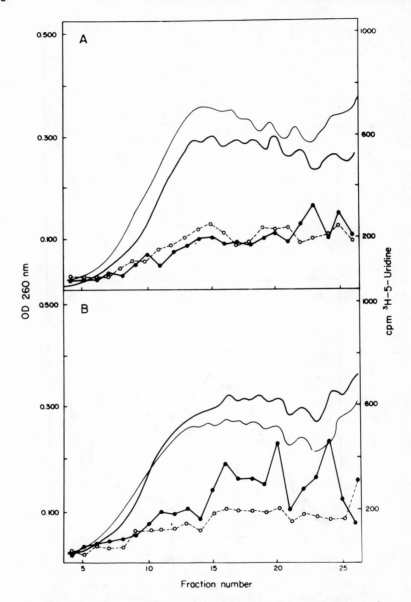

Fig. 3. Effect of 2 × 10⁻²M cycloheximide during last 3 min of isotope pulse.
HeLa cells (40 × 10⁶) were exposed to ³H-5-uridine from 18 to 30 min after
infection with 300 PFU/cell. Three minutes before completion of the pulse
(i.e., 27 min p.i.), the cultures were quickly divided in halves, and one was
treated with 2 × 10⁻²M cycloheximide. The cytoplasmic extracts were

isotope pulse is shown in Fig. 3. The brief exposure to the drug results in the increase of polysome OD, with a concomitant decrease of polysome specific activity in uninfected cells; the effect of cycloheximide on the infected cell polysomes is more pronounced. The specific activities of fractions 9-25 are the following: uninfected-untreated, 1185; uninfected plus cycloheximide, 1053; infected-untreated, 1463; infected plus cycloheximide, 1085.

Another observation lending support to the hypothesis that uridine is incorporated into messenger-like RNA, associated with polysomal and not with ribosomal RNA, comes from experiments using labeled amino acids as precursors. Similar results to those presented in Fig. 1 are obtained using radioactive phenylalanine, trytophan, and lysine.

The phenomenon we have been describing seems to be restricted to a certain period within the first hour of infection, since the radioactive peaks described are not observed if the isotope pulses are given either before the first 15 min of infection or after 40 min p.i. These results are shown in Table II, in which the gradient counts have been grouped in three areas as described in Table I; for the purpose of comparison, the ratios presented in Table I are also included. The gradient top (1.27 ratio), observed with pulses given between 40 and 60 min p.i.,

Table II. Specific Activity Ratios[a] from
Polysome Gradients Obtained After ^{3}H-5-
Uridine Pulses Given Within 1 hr of Infection

Gradient area	Isotope pulses (min p.i.)		
	0-15	10-30[b]	40-60
Polysomes	0.93	1.45	1.10
Ribosomes and subunits	0.87	1.09	1.02
Gradient top	1.07	1.09	1.27
Total	1.04	1.19	1.22

[a] Infected/uninfected cell specific activities ratios.
[b] Ratios already given in Table I.

layered on a sucrose gradient and sedimented as stated in Fig. 1. Figure 3A uninfected culture: heavy line, nontreated OD; •, nontreated cpm; light line, plus cycloheximide OD; o, plus cycloheximide cpm. Figure 3B infected culture: heavy line, nontreated OD; •, nontreated cpm; light line, plus cycloheximide OD; o, plus cycloheximide cpm.

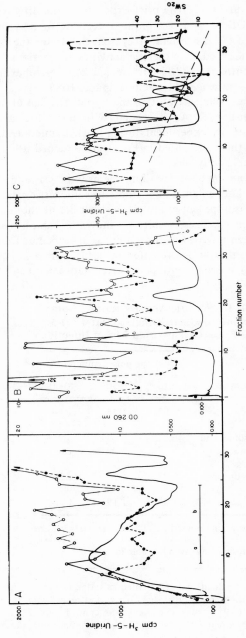

Fig. 4. Characterization of polysome-associated RNA. The cytoplasmic extracts from 80 million uninfected and an equal number of infected HeLa cells (300 PFU/cell) were sedimented each in two sucrose gradients as stated in Fig. 1. The OD profiles and the radioactive counts were recorded as usual from one of the gradients. With this information, the remaining two fraction sets were pooled as indicated in Fig. 4A, made 0.5% in SDS followed by ethanol precipitation. The RNA was then layered on 15-30% w/v sucrose gradients in NETS and sedimented in a Spinco SW27 rotor at 16.5 K for 16 hr at 20°. Heavy line, OD profiles, ●, uninfected cpm; ○, infected cpm.

could be an indication that lighter molecules are being liberated from the polysome after completing its cycle in protein synthesis.

In order to characterize the polysome-associated RNA, two polysome regions (a and b), as indicated in Fig. 4A, were pooled and treated with SDS followed by ethanol precipitation. The extracted RNA was dissolved in buffer and layered on a 15-30% w/v sucrose gradient; 28S and 18S ribosomal RNAs

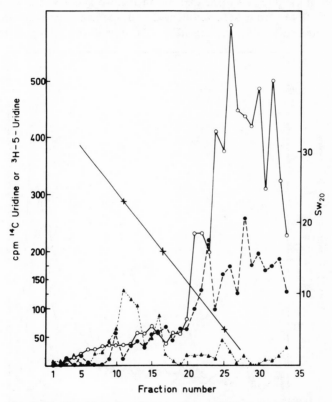

Fig. 5. Profile obtained on heat treatment. RNA was extracted, as indicated in Fig. 4, from a pool of large and small polysomes. HeLa cells had been infected with 300 PFU/cell and exposed to ^{3}H-5-uridine from 15 to 30 min p.i. The polysome-associated RNA was made 10% in formaldehyde-0.01 M PO_4 buffer and 0.5% SDS; it was heated to 65° for 15 min, together with ribosomal and *E. coli* ^{14}C-labeled 5S RNA. After heat treatment, RNA was layered on a 5-20% w/v sucrose gradient in 3% formaldehyde-0.1 M PO_4 buffer and sedimented in a SW27 Spinco rotor at 25 K for 14 hr at 20°. •, Uninfected cell RNA; ○, infected cell RNA; ▲, *E. coli* ^{14}C-labeled RNA.

provide a useful OD marker. The radioactive profiles show that (a) there are more counts in the RNA derived from both large (Fig. 4B) and small (Fig. 4C) polysomes from infected cells; (b) there are areas, fractions 19-23 and 29-35 in Fig. 4B plus fractions 9-16 in Fig. 4C, in which the radioactive profiles from both uninfected and infected cells coincide; (c) the latter observation lends further interest to those radioactive peaks which are seen only in the RNA from infected cell polysomes, i.e., fractions 3-8 in Fig. 4B and 5-9 plus 24-29 in Fig. 4C; and (d) RNAs from both uninfected and infected cells show differences when associated either with the large (Fig. 4B) or small (Fig. 4C) polysomes.

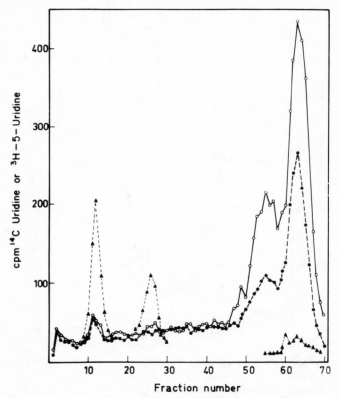

Fig. 6. *Profile obtained in polyacrylamide plus agarose.* Another sample of the polysome-associated RNA, formaldehyde treated, was layered on a 20 cm long gel made with 2.4% polyacrylamide plus 0.5% agarose. The electrophoresis of each gel was made at 10 ma for 12 hr, using Bromophenol Blue as an indicator of migration. The gel fractions were collected through a gel crusher, precipitated with TCA, and counted. ●, Uninfected cell RNA; ○, infected cell RNA; ▲, *E. coli* [14] C-labeled RNA.

Before attempting to measure the size of the RNA molecules sedimenting under the conditions shown in Fig. 4, it is necessary to carry out a heat treatment in the presence of formaldehyde, in order to dissociate possible molecular aggregates and/or internal hydrogen bonds. The profile obtained is shown in Fig. 5. Since under these conditions OD markers are no longer sharp and precise, *E. coli* ^{14}C-labeled ribosomal RNA and 5S RNA were used as markers. It can be seen that most of the large molecules seen in Fig. 4B and 4C have now disappeared, although some from the infected RNA remain (fractions 5-9 and 13-15). However, now the main difference between both series is seen around 10S, 7S to 8S, and smaller RNA molecules. A very similar pattern is obtained if formaldehyde-treated RNA samples are analyzed in 2.4% polyacrylamide gels plus 0.5% agarose, as shown in Fig. 6.

CONCLUSIONS

The synthesis of some cellular macromolecules is inhibited shortly after poliovirus infection; 45S rRNA precursor is particularly sensitive. Although this is a well-documented observation (2), its mechanism remains obscure. It has been postulated that the input viral material is responsible for this inhibition (2). Another alternative would be that this inhibition is mediated through the action of cellular proteins which are synthesized in response to the cellular imbalance created by the viral stimulus. This imbalance of cellular activity could explain the observation that the inhibition of 45S rRNA seems to be preceded by a short period of increased synthesis (3). The alternative of cellular imbalance would agree with a recent trend envisioning virus-host cell relationships as more complex and subtle than they were previously thought to be, and would encourage a search for early cellular responses to the viral stimulus. The best candidate to study is mRNA turnover in poliovirus-infected cells, which could be involved in the synthesis of "early inhibitory proteins."

Our results suggest the existence of cellular mRNA which shows a faster turnover for a clearly restricted period of 15-20 min within the first 30 min p.i. The possibility that other cellular RNA is being detected in our experiments is remote. Besides, all these experiments have been performed in the presence of a low concentration of actinomycin D, thus minimizing incorporation of the tracer into cellular rRNA (5). Moreover, the cell batches used were derived from PPLO-free stocks and were checked for this microorganism, since its contamination could blur our results. The remaining alternative is that we are witnessing a very early viral RNA replication, which, according to available information (2,10), would be 15-30 min ahead of the translation of newly synthesized viral RNA.

The preliminary characterization of polysome-associated RNA suggests molecules of at least two sizes, some rather large RNA messengers on the order of

30S and a few small ones of the order of 8S. It is worth noting that histones are synthesized on small polysomes (11), and preliminary isolations of the nuclear proteins of this system show a highly different pattern in the infected cells (12). However, at this stage, it would be speculative to try to ascertain which are the proteins being synthesized.

The alternative, i.e., that the small RNA molecules are breakdown products resulting from the procedure used, does not agree with the following evidence: (a) there are small polysomes, thus bound by small mRNA, which show high specific activity; (b) there is no detectable breakdown of the *E. coli* ribosomal RNA used as marker. Obviously, if we had a large cellular mRNA, we would have used it as marker; our next choice would have been poliovirus RNA.

Hybridization experiments in progress will try to determine whether cellular or viral genetic material is coding for this RNA. While testing for DNA-RNA hybrids, competition experiments with cellular rRNA are in line. These hybridization experiments, together with a thorough characterization of the polysome-associated RNA, will be essential in the elucidation of the early changes of poliovirus-infected human aneuploidic cells.

ACKNOWLEDGMENTS

A substantial part of this work was performed by one of the authors, G. C., at Albert Einstein College of Medicine as a Senior Research Fellow, John Simon Guggenheim Memorial Fund, 90 Park Avenue, New York. Part of this work was supported by grant No. 145 from Comisión Nacional de Investigación Científica y Tecnológica, Santiago, Chile. We thank Miss Marie Lancia (in New York) and Miss Carmen Cortez (in Santiago) for the excellent technical support they provided in maintaining the HeLa cell cultures. We wish to thank Drs. Jacob V. Maizel and Jonathan R. Warner for their advice and stimulating discussions.

SUMMARY

The cytoplasmic extracts of uninfected and infected cells were analyzed in sucrose gradients after short pulses with ^{3}H-5-uridine given at different times, within the first hour of poliovirus one-step growth cycle in HeLa (S3) cells. The specific activity of some polysome regions (3-5 and 7-10 ribosomal units) has been consistently greater in the polysomes obtained from infected cells if the pulse is given within 10-35 min postinfection; the same pattern is observed with labeled amino acid pulses. The radioactivity is considerably reduced if the cytoplasmic extract is treated with 0.01 M EDTA before layering on the 7-47% sucrose gradient. The addition of $2 \times 10^{-2}M$ cycloheximide during the last 3 min of the pulse results in a marked decrease of polysome specific radioactivity; the effect is more pronounced in the infected material. The RNA isolated from selected polysome regions shows distinct peaks of greater specific activity in 8S and 30S RNA molecules in the infected cells. Similar sedimentation values are obtained after heat treatment in the presence o. formaldehyde, as determined by sucrose gradients and polyacrylamide gels.

RESUMEN

Los extractos citoplasmáticos de células infectadas y no infectadas han sido analizados en gradientes de sacarosa, después de pulsos cortos con ^{3}H-5-uridina suministrados en diferentes tiempos, durante la primera hora de un ciclo de multiplicación del virus de polio en células HeLa (S_3). La actividad específica de algunas regiones de polisomas (de 3 a 5 y de 7 a 10) ha sido consistentemente mayor en los polisomas obtenidos de células infectadas, si el pulso es dado entre 10 a 35 minutos después de la infección; un patrón similar se observa con pulsos de aminoácidos radioactivos. La radioactividad se reduce considerablemente si el extracto citoplasmático es tratado con 0.01 M EDTA antes de depositarlo sobre el gradiente de 7-47% de sacarosa. Si se agrega cicloheximida durante los últimos 3 minutos del pulso, se observa una reducción marcada en la actividad específica de los polisomas; el efecto es más acentuado en material infectado. El RNA de regiones seleccionadas de polisomas, muestra claras máximas de mayor actividad específica en moléculas de RNA 8S y 30S de células infectadas. Valores similares de sedimentación son obtenidos después de tratamiento con calor, en presencia de formaldehido según se determina en gradientes de sacarosa y gels de poliacrilamida.

REFERENCES

1. Dulbecco, R., *Science, 166,* 962 (1969).
2. Darnell, J. E., Girard, M., Baltimore, D., Summers, D. F., and Maizel, J. V., in Colter, J. S., and Parenchych, W. (eds.), *The Molecular Biology of Viruses,* Academic Press, New York, (1967), p. 375.
3. Contreras, G., Summers, D. F., Maizel, J. V., and Ehrenfeld, E., "Hela Cell Nucleolar RNA Synthesis After Poliovirus Infection," to be published.
4. Penman, S., Becker, Y., and Darnell, J. E., *J. Mol. Biol., 8,* 541 (1954).
5. Penman, S., Vesco, C., and Penman, M., *J. Mol. Biol., 34,* 49 (1968).
6. Penman, S., Scherrer, K., Becker, Y., and Darnell, J. E., *Proc. Natl. Acad. Sci. U.S.A., 49,* 654 (1963).
7. Dingman, C. W., and Peacock, A. C., *Biochemistry, 7,* 659 (1968).
8. Maizel, J. V., *Science, 151,* 988 (1966).
9. Godchaux, W., III, Adamson, S. D., and Herbert, E., *J. Mol. Biol., 27,* 57 (1967).
10. Baltimore, D., Girard, M., and Darnell, J. E., *Virology, 29,* 179 (1966).
11. Robbins, E., and Borun, T. W., *Proc. Natl. Acad. Sci. U.S.A., 57,* 409 (1967).
12. Contreras, G., and Pederson, T., unpublished results.

DISCUSSION

R. T. Schimke (Stanford, U.S.A.): I have a suggestion that might help you in supporting your idea that you have messengers made, which are relatively small in size and presumably cannot be the polio coat protein messenger, which I understand should be fairly large. I was wondering whether in these cells after infection you are in fact making preferentially several small proteins that are not being made in the normal cells. I think you might be able to do this by a combination of ^{3}H and ^{14}C amino acids and then display them on SDS gels and ask whether in the infected state you have more small proteins synthesized.

G. Contreras (Santiago, Chile): Part of this work has been done already by Summers and collaborators; it was done in the presence of 3 mM guanidine, which inhibits markedly the synthesis of cellular proteins. When they looked for the proteins being made within the virus cycle, they were able to characterize four which are viral capsid proteins and perhaps six which are nonviral capsid proteins, which are not clearly well defined up to now. Maybe these are the small molecules that you are suggesting.

35

On the Relationship Between Transcription, Translation, and Ribosomal RNA Synthesis During Microsomal Hydroxylase Induction

Friedrich J. Wiebel, Edward J. Matthews, and Harry V. Gelboin

Chemistry Branch
National Cancer Institute
National Institutes of Health
Bethesda, Maryland, U.S.A.

The microsomal enzyme complex, aryl hydrocarbon hydroxylase (AHH*), belongs to the group of mixed-function oxygenases (1) which catalyze the metabolism of numerous xenobiotics such as drugs, pesticides, and carcinogens (2). The enzyme system is found in most mammalian tissues and in a variety of cells in culture (3,4).

Addition of polycyclic hydrocarbons to the culture medium of monolayer cells causes a manyfold increase in AHH activity. Enzyme activity rises rapidly after a 30-60 min lag period and reaches a plateau level after 12-24 hr, depending on inducer concentration and cell type (5). During the continuous presence of

---

* Abbreviations: BA, benz(a)anthracene; BP, benzo(a)pyrene; Act D, actinomycin D; rRNA, ribosomal RNA; mRNA, messenger RNA; TCA, trichloroacetic acid; AHH, aryl hydrocarbon hydroxylase.

inducer, AHH activity remains at an elevated level. After maximum induction, removal of inducer either by metabolic conversion or by replacement with control medium causes a decrease in enzyme activity with a half-life of 3-6 hr (4).

We previously reported that the increase in enzyme activity initially requires RNA synthesis and continuously requires protein synthesis (4,5). The present studies are primarily concerned with the following aspects of AHH induction: (a) the synthesis, transport, and phenotypic expression of the RNA species which is required for induction; (b) the relationship of induction-related RNA synthesis to ribosomal RNA (rRNA) synthesis and transport; and (c) the role of the inducer in translation and enzyme degradation.

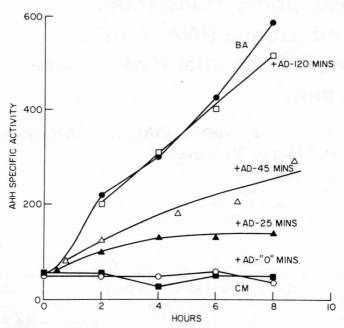

Fig. 1. Requirement of RNA synthesis for the induction of aryl hydrocarbon hydroxylase in hamster embryo cell cultures. Actinomycin D (AD) (1 μg/ml medium) was added simultaneously with, or at various times after, the inducer benz(a)anthracene (BA) (3 μg/ml medium). The base line represents AHH activity in cultures incubated in medium free of BA or AD (CM). The preparation of monolayer cultures from hamster embryos and the assay of AHH activity were carried out as described previously (6). Specific activity of AHH is expressed as μμmoles of alkali-extractable product formed per milligram protein per 30 min.

RESULTS

Requirement of RNA and Protein Synthesis for Induction

We have previously found that the inhibitors of protein synthesis, cyclohexi-mide and puromycin, completely prevent AHH induction when applied simul-taneously with inducer, or halt any further increase in enzyme activity during the course of induction (4,5). This suggests that the induction depends on the continuous synthesis of protein. This protein might either constitute part of the enzyme complex or be a short-lived protein functioning as an enzyme activator.

Figure 1 shows that AHH induction also requires the synthesis of RNA. However, this requirement is transient. After RNA synthesis is permitted during a short period in the presence of inducer, the inhibitor actinomycin D (Act D) is no longer effective in preventing an increase in enzyme activity. During a 2 hr exposure to inducer, sufficient induction-specific RNA accumulates to sustain maximum induction for a subsequent 6 hr (Fig. 1).

Previous observations (5) and the data shown in Table I and Fig. 7B indicate

Table I. Effect of Various Inhibitors of RNA Synthesis on the Induction of AHH

Inhibitory agent	(% of control)[a]	
	Exposure to inhibitor concomitant with BA	Exposure to inhibitor after BA + CY[b] treatment
Act D (1 μg/ml)	<1	103 ± 10
UV irradiation 1050 erg/mm^2	34 ± 2	111 ± 10
21000 erg/mm^2	9 ± 2	63 ± 4
Ethidium bromide (1 μg/ml)	87 ± 4	—

[a] Effect of the inhibitors is expressed as percent of control, i.e., of the amount of induction observed in cells that were exposed to BA only. AHH specific activity (see Fig. 1) increased from 8 to a level of 40 during the 3 hr exposure to BA.

[b] Cultures of the mouse thymus-spleen cell line, JLSV$_5$, were exposed to benz(a)anthracene (BA) (3 μg/ml) and cycloheximide (CY) (10 μg/ml) for 2 hr. The inhibitory agents were applied immediately after removal of the cycloheximide from the culture medium, and AHH induction was determined 3 hr later.

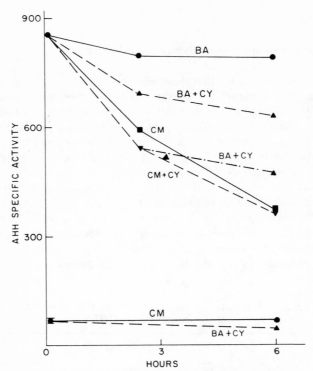

Fig. 2. The decay of aryl hydrocarbon hydroxylase activity in hamster embryo cell cultures and the stabilization by benz-
(a) *anthracene.* Secondary cultures were exposed to benz*(a)* anthracene (3 µg/ml medium) for 16 hr. The medium was replaced by conditioned medium from cell cultures of the same age without any additions (CM) or with cycloheximide (CM + CY), benz(*a*)anthracene (BA), or benz(*a*)anthracene and cycloheximide (BA + CY). The two bottom lines show the AHH activity in previously untreated cultures incubated with control medium or medium containing benz(*a*)anthra-cene and cycloheximide (BA + CY). Cycloheximide was used at a final concentration of 10 µg/ml medium. Cultures were washed three times with the appropriate medium prior to the change of medium. Other conditions were as described in Fig. 1.

that the induction-specific RNA is synthesized during a cycloheximide block of protein synthesis. The transient requirement for RNA synthesis is further dem-onstrated by the effects of UV irradiation, which is known to impair DNA template activity by thymine-dimer formation (7). When cultures are UV-irradiated immediately before the addition of inducer, enzyme induction is largely inhibited (Table I). However, irradiation of the cells 2 hr after their simultaneous exposure to inducer and to an inhibitor of protein synthesis does not appreciably affect the increase in enzyme activity when the protein synthesis block is released. Ethidium bromide, which specifically inhibits the formation of mitochondrial RNA (8), has no apparent effect on AHH induction (Table I).

These data suggest that AHH induction involves the activation of specific genes whose transcription results in the synthesis and accumulation of an induction-specific RNA. The transcription and the translation of this RNA appear to be independent processes, since each can occur in the other's absence (Fig. 7B, refs. 4,5).

Post-transcriptional Regulation of AHH

Enzyme activity decreases rapidly when inducer is removed from preinduced cultures (Fig. 2). The rate of decay is virtually the same in the presence or absence of cycloheximide. This indicates that induction-specific protein synthesis ceases immediately on removal of the inducer. As shown in Fig. 1, induction-specific RNA accumulates in sufficient amounts and has a sufficiently long half-life to direct protein synthesis for several hours. This is supported by the observation that in fully induced cultures (22 hr) inhibition of RNA synthesis does not result in a decrease in enzyme activity for at least 3 hr. The cessation of specific protein synthesis while the induction-related RNA is still present indicates that the inducer is a requirement for translational function.

Figure 2 also shows that in the presence of inducer enzyme activity decays at a slower rate than in the absence of inducer. To exclude a possible stimulatory effect of the polycyclic hydrocarbon on protein synthesis, cycloheximide (10 μg/ml) was used to block protein synthesis by more than 95%. The two bottom lines in Fig. 2 demonstrate that under these conditions benz(a)anthracene (BA) does not cause an increase in enzyme activity.

It is unlikely that the difference in enzyme level in the presence and absence of the polycyclic hydrocarbon is due to an activation of the enzyme system, since addition of BA during the decay of enzyme activity does not cause an absolute increase in the enzyme level but only lowers its rate of disappearance (Fig. 2). Thus the findings suggest that BA stabilizes the enzyme system and protects it against degradation.

Effect of Low Concentration of Act D on Induction of AHH

In the following experiments, we used low concentrations of Act D that inhibit preferentially the synthesis of rRNA (9). When Act D (0.1 μg/ml) is present 90 min before and during a 3.5 hr exposure to the inducer, AHH activity

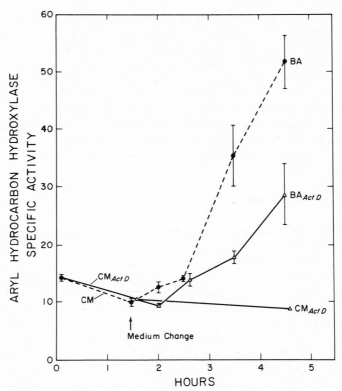

Fig. 3. *Effect of a low concentration of actinomycin D on the induction of aryl hydrocarbon hydroxylase in JLSV_s cells.* Cells were exposed to growth medium containing 0.1 μg/ml Act D (CM $_{Act\ D}$) or to fresh medium without any additions (CM) for 90 min. The medium of Act D treated cultures was then replaced by medium containing the inducer, benz(*a*)anthracene (2 μg/ml), and 0.1 μg/ml Act D (BA$_{Act\ D}$) or by medium containing Act D without the inducer (CM$_{Act\ D}$). The medium of control cultures was changed to inducer-containing medium (BA). At various times after treatment, AHH specific activity (see Fig. 1) was determined in two to four cultures. The graph indicates mean and range of observed values.

increases at a rate that is approximately half that observed with inducer only (Fig. 3). The period of exposure to Act D prior to the addition of inducer can be extended up to 180 min without any significant reduction in the degree of induction.

As shown in Fig. 4, induction of enzyme activity decreases linearly as the Act D concentrations are increased and is reduced by 75% with 0.12 μg/ml of

Act D. AHH induction is entirely prevented by Act D concentrations above 0.25 μg/ml.

Effect of Act D on RNA Synthesis

Parallel to the examination of AHH activity, we determined the effect of low concentrations of Act D on RNA synthesis and the appearance of the newly synthesized RNA in the cytoplasm. After a 90 min period of pretreatment with Act D, ^{3}H-uridine was added simultaneously with the inducer and allowed to be

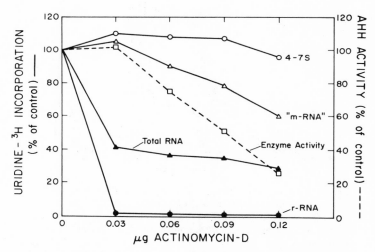

Fig. 4. Correlation of aryl hydrocarbon hydroxylase induction and ^{3}H-uridine incorporation into cytoplasmic RNA: effect of low concentrations of actinomycin D. Cultures were exposed to growth medium containing Act D at various concentrations (0.03-0.12 μg/ml) or growth medium free of Act D for 90 min. Then BA was added in 0.5 ml of medium to give a final 0.5 μg/ml simultaneously with 250 μc of ^{3}H-uridine, and cultures were incubated for another 180 min. At the end of this period, AHH activity and ^{3}H-uridine incorporation were measured. For fractionation of cells and separation of cytoplasmic RNA samples on gel electrophoresis, see Fig. 5. "Total RNA" represents trichloroacetic acid precipitable material in the cytoplasmic fraction. The amount of radioactivity in ribosomal RNA (rRNA), low molecular weight RNA (4S-7S), and heterodisperse RNA ("mRNA") was determined from electropherograms (Fig. 5). The amount of "mRNA" was derived by subtraction of counts comprising the peaks of rRNA and 4S-7S RNA from the total counts in the electrophoretic fractions. AHH activity and radioactivity in RNA fractions from Act D treated cultures are expressed as percent of control, i.e., of corresponding activities in cultures not exposed to Act D.

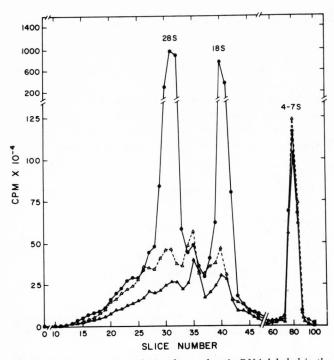

Fig. 5. Electrophoretic analysis of cytoplasmic RNA labeled in the presence of low concentrations of actinomycin D. Experimental conditions were as described in the text and in Fig. 2. △, 0.06 μg/ml Act D; ▲, 0.12 μg/ml Act D; •, control (no Act D). The profile of cytoplasmic RNA after treatment with 0.03 μg/ml and 0.09 μg/ml follows closely the one after 0.06 μg/ml or is intermediate to those of 0.06 and 0.12 μg/ml, respectively. Cells were fractionated as described by Penman *et al.* (10), and RNA was isolated by phenol extraction. RNA samples were analyzed on composite gels (2% acrylamide, 0.5% agarose) that were run for 90 min at 200 v at a temperature of 12.5° (11). Details of the experimental procedures are described elsewhere (12). Values represent counts per minute per slice. Note the changes in scale on ordinate and abscissa.

incorporated for 3 hr. Electrophoretic analysis of the cytoplasmic RNA (Fig. 5) demonstrates the almost complete absence of labeled rRNA species (28S and 18S) in the cytoplasm of Act D treated cells. A small peak of radioactivity in the 24S region appeared to be increased in the presence of Act D. The nature of this peak was not resolved.

Figure 4 summarizes the data on the effect of Act D on the synthesis of cytoplasmic RNA. ³H-uridine incorporation into total cytoplasmic RNA is inhibited about 60% by Act D concentrations from 0.03 to 0.12 μg/ml. Much of this inhibition is accounted for by a more than 90% suppression in the appearance of rRNA.

RNA species in the 4S-7S region seem virtually unaffected. In contrast, radioactivity in cytoplasmic heterodisperse RNA ("mRNA") declines gradually with Act D concentrations above 0.03 μg/ml. Thus the labeling of this RNA fraction correlates best with the inhibition of AHH induction by Act D.

The high sensitivity of rRNA synthesis to Act D can also be seen in the profile of labeled nuclear RNA (Fig. 6): radioactivity in the ribosomal precursor region is largely suppressed, the 32S peak disappears entirely, and in the 45S

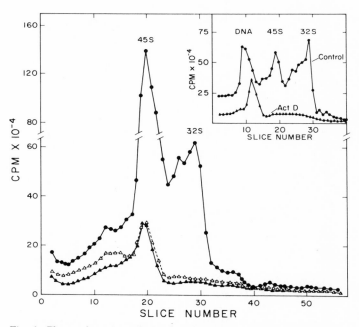

Fig. 6. *Electrophoretic analysis of nuclear RNA labeled in the presence of low concentrations of actinomycin D.* Experimental conditions were as described in the text and in Fig. 2. $\triangle$, 0.06 μg/ml Act D; $\blacktriangle$, 0.12 μg/ml Act D; $\bullet$, control (no Act D). The profiles of nuclear RNA after treatment with 0.03 and 0.09 μg/ml Act D are very similar to those shown. For cell fractionation, isolation of RNA, and electrophoretic conditions, see caption of Fig. 5. Note the change of scale on the ordinate. The inset shows separation of nuclear RNA from control cultures and cultures treated with 0.12 μg/ml Act D on acrylamide gels that were run for 6 hr at 50 v at a temperature of 12.5°. Values represent counts per minute per slice.

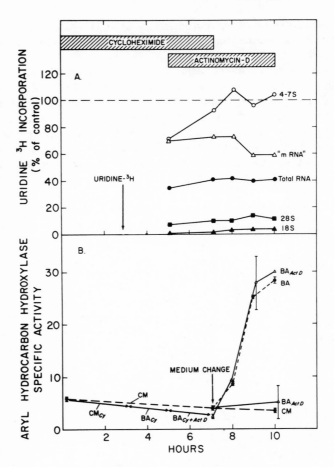

Fig. 7. *Induction of aryl hydrocarbon hydroxylase and appearance of newly labeled RNA in the cytoplasm: effect of inhibition of protein synthesis by cycloheximide.* The experimental conditions are described in the text. The time periods during which the cultures were exposed to 10 μg/ml cycloheximide and/or 1 μg/ml Act D are shown schematically at the top of the figure. (A) Appearance of labeled RNA in the cytoplasm was determined at various times after addition of ^{3}H-uridine (50 μc/medium). RNA samples were analyzed on polyacrylamide gels (see Fig. 5). The amounts of radioactivity in cytoplasmic, acid-precipitable RNA (total RNA), low molecular weight RNA (4S-7S), ribosomal RNA (18S and 28S), and heterogeneous RNA ("mRNA") were evaluated as described in Figs. 4 and 5. Radioactivity in RNA fractions from cycloheximide-treated cultures is given as percentage of the radioactivity in corresponding frac-

region only a small peak persists which remains unchanged with all Act D concentrations used. In contrast, the rapidly labeled heterogeneous RNA seen in gel slices 1-20 is much less affected by low Act D concentrations.

With different electrophoretic conditions (see inset to Fig. 6 and caption), the Act D "resistant" labeled material no longer migrates in the 45S region but appears in the region where DNA bands. Since it is susceptible to ribonuclease treatment, possibly it represents a fraction of heterodisperse RNA that is more closely associated with DNA and is not separated by our extraction procedure.

Thus the data presented in Figs. 4 and 6 demonstrate that maximum induction of AHH occurs in the near absence of newly formed rRNA in the nucleus or the cytoplasm.

Cycloheximide as Inhibitor of rRNA Synthesis: Correlation with AHH Induction

A number of investigators have shown that inhibition of protein synthesis inhibits the synthesis and maturation of rRNA (13,14). In order to suppress the synthesis and hence the availability of rRNA in the nucleus at the onset of induction, we exposed cell cultures to cycloheximide (10 μg/ml) for a period of 3 hr before the addition of inducer. ^{3}H-uridine was added simultaneously with the inducer, and RNA synthesis was allowed to occur for 2 hr in the presence of cycloheximide (Fig. 7). From this point on, RNA synthesis was blocked continuously for periods of 2-5 hr by a high dose of Act D (1 μg/ml). During the first 2 hr, both Act D and cycloheximide were present. Cycloheximide was then removed from the medium to release the block to protein synthesis.

As shown in Fig. 7, cycloheximide inhibits the synthesis of total cytoplasmic RNA and its transport by about 60%. The appearance of 28S and 18S rRNAs is suppressed by 90% and 98%, respectively, at the time of the onset of AHH induction. During the following hours, the absolute amount of labeled cytoplasmic rRNA species shows virtually no increase, even though the block of protein synthesis is removed and rRNA transport could take place. In contrast to rRNA appearance of "mRNA" in the cytoplasm is inhibited by only 30%. The apparent increase in cytoplasmic low molecular weight RNA (4S-7S) might be due to continuing export of these species from the nucleus, but might also be due to an accumulation of breakdown products caused by the Act D treatment (15). Figure 7B clearly demonstrates that induction occurs although rRNA synthesis and transport are largely suppressed during the entire induction period.

---

tions from control cultures 2 hr after addition of the label. (B) For time intervals indicated, cultures were exposed to growth medium (CM) or BA-containing medium, 3 μg/ml (BA), to some of which cycloheximide, 10 μg/ml (CY), and/or Act D, 1 μg/ml (Act D), were added.

Thus the results are essentially consistent with the data obtained by use of low concentrations of Act D; i.e., the treatment with both inhibitors specifically prevents the formation of cytoplasmic rRNA but permits the synthesis and expression of the induction-specific RNA.

CONCLUSIONS

The results indicate that AHH induction depends on the continuous synthesis of protein but requires RNA synthesis only during an initial 2 hr period. The nature of this induction-specific RNA is not known. Although some changes were observed in the RNA profile during enzyme induction *in vivo*, analysis by sedimentation and by gel electrophoresis of RNA species formed during induction in hamster embryo cells in culture revealed no significant difference before and after exposure to inducer (16). Several conclusions concerning the induction-specific RNA may be drawn from the present studies: (a) The essentially complete absence of newly formed rRNA in nucleus or cytoplasm during enzyme induction indicates that rRNA does not specify the synthesis of induction-related proteins. (b) Since Act D concentrations that inhibit induction do not affect the synthesis of low molecular weight RNA (7S), it is unlikely that these species contain the induction-specific RNA. (c) The correlation of inhibition of AHH induction with the inhibition of appearance of newly formed heterogeneous RNA in the cytoplasm suggests that the induction-specific RNA is contained in this fraction, which is usually associated with messenger RNA. (d) The studies with ethidium bromide indicate that mitochondrial RNA does not have a major role in AHH induction.

A number of investigators have postulated (17-21) that mRNA transfer across the nuclear membrane depends on concomitant transfer of rRNA. Thus mRNA was thought to be transferred from the nucleus to the cytoplasm in association with the smaller ribosomal subunit (17-19). Ribosomal RNA and ribosome formation have also been implicated in the regulation of growth and development of mammalian cells by partially controlling mRNA transport and expression (20). Furthermore, a functional nucleolus, site of rRNA synthesis (22), appeared to be required for the transfer of genetic information from the nucleus to the cytoplasm (23).

Our present results show that a selective inhibition of rRNA synthesis does not prevent the newly formed "informational" RNA from reaching the cytoplasmic site of protein synthesis, where it acts to increase the formation of the induction-specific protein(s).

It is possible that a pre-existing pool of unlabeled nuclear RNA is involved in a step of mRNA transfer, but this appears unlikely in view of our results that show prolonged inhibition of rRNA synthesis preceding the transfer of the informational RNA. Under normal growth conditions, labeled 28S and 18S RNA appear in the cytoplasm of $JLSV_5$ cells 45 min and 30 min, respectively, after addition of ^{3}H-uridine (unpublished observations). Other studies (9,24) indicate that Act D does not cause an extended preservation of an rRNA pool in the nucleus.

The independence of the appearance of heterodisperse RNA in the cytoplasm from rRNA synthesis and transfer, seen in the present studies, has been observed by others (25,26). It is presumed in these studies that the transferred, heterodisperse RNA represents mRNA. Our studies indicate that this informational RNA species, reaching the cytoplasm in the absence of concomitant rRNA transfer, is phenotypically expressed as increased enzyme activity.

In the other studies reported here, we have shown that the inducer is required for the translational process. The inducer also stabilizes the induced enzyme and thereby decreases its rate of degradation.

ACKNOWLEDGMENTS

We thank Dr. C. W. Dingman for suggesting the procedure that produced the results shown in Fig. 6 (inset), and J. L. Leutz and D. Ray for excellent technical assistance.

SUMMARY

The mammalian microsomal enzyme system, aryl hydrocarbon hydroxylase, is highly inducible in cell culture. After the addition of inducer, there is a 35 min lag period, after which the enzyme level increases a hundredfold during a 16 hr period. The rise in enzyme activity is prevented by actinomycin D only when the latter is added within 1-2 hr after the inducer. After this period, the further 6 hr rise in enzyme activity is insensitive to actinomycin D. Thus RNA synthesis is required only during the initial induction period. The cells can pass from actinomycin D sensitivity to insensitivity in the presence of cycloheximide. Thus the induction-specific RNA may be synthesized in the absence of protein synthesis. We conclude that transcription and translation of the induction-specific RNA are independent processes. The results of differentially inhibiting RNA synthesis with low concentrations of actinomycin D, high doses of cycloheximide, or ethidium bromide suggest that the induction-specific RNA is not ribosomal RNA, not low molecular weight RNA, and not mitochondrial RNA, but rather is present in the cytoplasmic heterodisperse RNA presumed to contain messenger RNA. The synthesis of the induction-specific RNA is dissociable from the synthesis and transfer of ribosomal RNA, since a low concentration of actinomycin D that completely prevents the latter does not inhibit enzyme induction.

Other results presented indicate that the translation process requires the presence of inducer, since removal of inducer from the medium terminates the translation of accumulated messenger RNA. The inducer has also been found to stabilize partially the induced enzyme.

RESUMEN

El sistema enzimático aril hidrocarburo hidroxilasa de microsomas de maníferos, es altamente inducible en cultivos de células. Después del agregado del inductor hay un período de latencia de 35 minutos después del cual el nivel de enzima aumenta 100 veces en un período de 16 horas. El aumento de la actividad enzimática es impedido por actinomicina D, sólo si esta última es agregada 1-2 horas después del inductor. Después de este período el aumento posterior en la actividad enzimática es insensible a actinomicina D. Por lo tanto, la síntesis de RNA se requiere solamente durante el período inicial de inducción. Las células pueden pasar de un estado de sensibilidad a insensibilidad a actinomicina D en presencia de cicloheximida. Por lo tanto, el RNA específico para la inducción puede ser sintetizado en ausencia de síntesis de proteínas.

Los resultados de la inhibición diferencial de la síntesis de RNA con concentraciones bajas de actinomicina D, dosis altas de cicloheximida o bromuro de etidio, surieren que el RNA específico para la inducción no es RNA ribosomal, o RNA de peso molecular bajo, ni tampoco RNA mitocondrial, pero que más bien se encuentra presente en el RNA hetero géneo citoplásmico el cual se cree contiene RNA mensajero. La síntesis del RNA específico para la inducción puede separarse de la síntesis y el transporte del RNA ribosomal ya que bajas concentraciones de actinomicina D inhiben completamente esta última pero no la inducción de la enzima.

Los otros resultados presentados indican que el proceso de traducción requiere la presencia del inductor, ya que si el inductor se remueve del medio, esto resulta en la terminación de la traducción del RNA mensajero acumulado. El inductor parece estabilizar la encima inducida.

REFERENCES

1. Mason, H. S., *Advan. Enzymol., 19,* 79 (1957).
2. Conney, A. H., *Pharmacol. Rev., 19,* 317 (1967).
3. Nebert, D. W., and Gelboin, H. V., *Arch. Biochem. Biophys., 134,* 76 (1969).
4. Nebert, D. W., and Gelboin, H. V., *J. Biol. Chem., 243,* 6250 (1969).
5. Nebert, D. W., and Gelboin, H. V., *J. Biol. Chem., 245,* 160 (1970).
6. Nebert, D. W., and Gelboin, H. V., *J. Biol. Chem., 243,* 6242 (1968).
7. Wacker, A., Dellweg, H., and Weinblum, D., *Naturwissenschaften, 47,* 477 (1960).
8. Zylber, E., Vesco, C., and Penman, S., *J. Mol. Biol., 44,* 195 (1969).
9. Perry, R. P., *Proc. Natl. Acad. Sci. U.S.A., 48,* 2179 (1962).
10. Penman, S., Greenberg, H., and Willems, M., in Habel, K., and Salzman, P. (eds.), *Fundamental Techniques in Virology,* Academic Press, New York (1969), p. 49.
11. Peacock, A. C., and Dingman, C. W., *Biochemistry, 7,* 668 (1968).
12. Wiebel, F. J., Matthews, E. J., and Gelboin, H. V., *J. Biol. Chem., 247,* 4711 (1972).
13. Ennis, H. L., *Mol. Pharmacol., 2,* 543 (1966).
14. Willems, M., Penman, M., and Penman, S., *J. Cell Biol., 41,* 177 (1969).
15. Steward, G. A., and Farber, E., *J. Biol. Chem., 243,* 4479 (1968).
16. Younger, L. R., Salomon, R., Wilson, R. W., Peacock, A. C., and Gelboin, H. V., *Mol. Pharmacol., 8,* 452 (1972).
17. Joklik, W. K., and Becker, Y., *J. Mol. Biol., 13,* 511 (1965).
18. Henshaw, E. C., Revel, M., and Hiatt, H. H., *J. Mol. Biol., 14,* 241 (1965).
19. McConkey, E. H., and Hopkins, J. W., *J. Mol. Biol., 14,* 257 (1965).
20. Tata, J. R., *Nature, 219,* 331 (1968).
21. Harris, H., *Nucleus and Cytoplasm,* 2nd ed., Clarendon Press, Oxford (1970).
22. Perry, R. P., *Progr. Nucleic Acid Res. Mol. Biol., 6,* 219 (1967).
23. Sidebottom, E., and Harris, H., *J. Cell Sci., 5,* 351 (1969).
24. Penman, S., *J. Mol. Biol., 17,* 117 (1966).
25. Spohr, G., Granboulan, N., Morel, G., and Scherrer, K., *Europ. J. Biochem., 17,* 296 (1970).
26. Woodcock, D. M., and Mansbridge, J. N., *Biochim. Biophys. Acta, 240,* 218 (1971).

36

Ribosomes in Reticulocyte Maturation

Estela Sánchez de Jiménez, Ruth Roman, and Blas Lotina

Departamento de Bioquímica
Facultad de Química
Universidad Nacional Autónoma de México
México, D. F., México

During the last stage of red cell differentiation, the ribosomal content of red cells undergoes accelerated breakdown (1-3). The sedimentation velocity coefficients of chicken red cell ribosomes have been reported to change from 82S in immature red cells to 62S in fully differentiated cells (4). This phenomenon has been suggested to be due to alterations of ribosome structure occurring during the last step of red cell differentiation (4).

To further study this phenomenon, the accessibility of both types of ribosomes to pancreatic and homologous chicken red cell RNases was explored, and a physicochemical study of their ribosomal RNAs (rRNAs) was also undertaken. For this purpose, red cells from 13-day-old chick embryos and from adult chickens were used as sources of 82S and 62S ribosomes, respectively.

METHODS

Red Cell Composition

The red cell composition of 13-day-old embryo blood is reported to be as follows: 6.6% erythrocytes of primitive type, 0.5% erythroblasts, and 92.5% proerythrocytes (5).

Ribosome Preparation

Mature red cells (erythrocytes) or embryonic red cells were used as sources of RNA. The erythrocytes were obtained from Leghorn adult chickens and the embryonic cells from lots of 20-25 13-day-old embryos of the same race. The red cells from either source were washed three times with 5 vol of an isotonic salt solution in order to lower white cell contamination to less than 1:10,000 (6). Finally, the cells were suspended in 5 vol of T-Mg-K-salt (0.01 M Tris, pH 7.2, 0.01 M MgCl$_2$, 0.015 M KCl, in a 0.45% NaCl solution), treated with saponin, and centrifuged at 33,000 $\times$ g for 20 min to eliminate nuclei and membranes; the supernatant was centrifuged again at 105,000 $\times$ g for 2½ hr to sediment the ribosomal fraction.

RNA Extraction

The ribosome pellet was washed with T-Mg (0.01 M Tris, pH 7.2, 0.001 M MgCl$_2$) and homogenized in 3 vol of T-Mg. The homogenate was treated with 3 vol of T-SDS (0.01 M Tris, pH 7.2, 1% SDS, 0.01 M sucrose) at 37° for 5 min, fast cooled, and extracted with phenol, according to Kurland's procedure (7).

Sucrose Gradient Sedimentation

Ribosomes

Linear gradients (10-28% sucrose in 0.01 M Tris buffer, pH 7.2, 0.01 M KCl/NaCl, 15/1, and 0.001 M Mg^{2+} were prepared at 4° in SW Ti56 centrifuge tubes. Three to 5 OD$_{260}$ units of ribosomes, suspended in 0.2 ml of the incubation medium, was layered on top of the gradients and centrifuged at 35,000 rpm for 85 min at 2°.

Ribosomal Subunits and RNA

Linear gradients (10-33% sucrose in 0.025 M Tris, pH 7.6, 0.01 M KCl) were prepared in SW25 tubes; 0.5 ml of a ribosomal sample was layered on top of gradients and centrifuged at 21,000 rpm for 12 hr at 2°.

Linear sucrose gradients (5-20% in 0.01 M Tris, pH 7.2, 0.01 M NaCl) were prepared at 4° in SW25 centrifuge tubes. Twenty to 25 OD$_{260}$ units of RNA was dissolved in 1 ml of 0.01 M Tris buffer, pH 7.2, placed in the upper part of each gradient, and centrifuged at 24,000 rpm for 14 hr at 2°.

The gradients were fractionated using an LKB fraction collector connected to a UV-sensitive cell (254 nm) with an automatic register; 0.2 ml samples were collected for ribosomes and 0.7 ml samples for RNA.

Disc Electrophoresis in Polyacrylamide-Agarose Gel

The method followed for the separation of RNA by electrophoresis was basically that described by Loening (8), modified by Peacock and Dingman (9).

Acrylamide (Eastman) (recrystallized in chloroform), agarose (Bio-Rad), TEMED (N,N,N'-tetramethylethyldiamine) (Eastman), and ammonium persulfate (Fisher) were used for the gel preparation. One to 1.5 OD_{260} units of RNA in 50 μl of 0.04 M Tris-acetate buffer, pH 7.8, was placed on a gel and electrophoresed in the same buffer for 70 min (current from an LKB power source type 3290B, 45 ma; voltage, 100v). Gels were then stained for 30 min with 0.1% Toluidine-0 Blue in 7% acetic acid. The excess dye was eliminated by washing with 7% acetic acid.

RNase Digestion of Ribosomes

Ribosomes from embryonic or from mature red cells in 0.2 ml of 0.01 M acetate buffer, pH 5.5, at a fixed ionic strength given by Na^+, K^+, and Mg^{2+} were incubated with either pancreatic RNase or RNase purified from chicken red cells (10) for 1½ hr at room temperature. The reaction was stopped by lowering the temperature to $0°$. The reaction mixture was then analyzed on sucrose gradients.

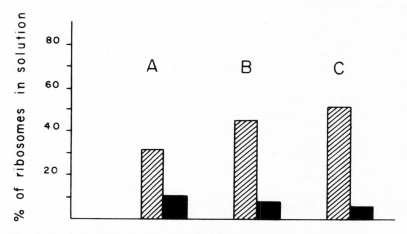

Fig. 1. Incubation of ribosomes in K^+ or Na^+ solutions. Samples (0.2 ml) containing 5-10 OD_{260} units of embryonic or adult chicken erythrocyte ribosomes were incubated for 85 min at room temperature in the following solutions: (A) 0.16 M sodium acetate (pH 5.5), 0.001 M Mg^{2+}; (B) 0.16 M potassium acetate (pH 5.5), 0.001 M Mg^{2+}; (C) 0.08 M potassium chloride, 0.08 M tris-HCl (pH 7.2), 0.001 M Mg^{2+}. The percent of UV-absorbing material moving as a peak in a 10-28% sucrose gradient sedimentation experiment (see *Methods*) is plotted. Hatched bar, adult red cell ribosomes; solid bar, embryonic red cell ribosomes.

RESULTS

The stability of the 82S and 62S ribosomes at different ionic strengths was explored in order to establish the best conditions for RNase degradation.

Figure 1 shows the results obtained when ribosomes from either mature or embryonic cells were incubated at two different ionic strengths given by either K^+ or Na^+ ions. The amount of unprecipitated ribosomes was equated with the amount of UV-absorbing material moving as a uniform peak after sucrose gradient centrifugation of the incubation mixture. As can be seen, 82S ribosomes were readily precipitated by Na^+ and even more so by K^+ alone, while 62S ribosomes showed greater stability for either ion. This effect was more pronounced when the pH of the solution was increased (Fig. 1).

In addition, the effect of different K^+/Na^+ ratios, at fixed ionic strength, was tested for both ribosomal types. Under these experimental conditions, increasing the K^+/Na^+ ratio in the medium increased the amount of either embryonic or mature ribosomes retained in suspension (Table I). It should be pointed out that for a ratio of 15 (0.15 M K^+ and 0.01 M Na^+), a higher percentage of ribosomes remained in solution than when either ion alone was placed in the medium at the same total ionic strength.

Pancreatic RNase and homologous RNase were tested with the two types of ribosomes. Approximately equivalent activities of the enzymes were used at the optimal ionic strength for ribosomal stability, and the diminution of the monosome peak with different enzyme concentrations was followed by sucrose gradient sedimentation. Figure 2 summarizes the results obtained. The 82S ribosomes were fully degraded by pancreatic RNase at all the enzyme concentra-

Table I. Effect of K^+/Na^+ Ratio on Ribosomal Stability[a]

K^+/Na (molar concentration)	Percent of ribosomes remaining in solution	
	Adult	Embryo
0.08/0.08	25.0[b]	33.8
0.14/0.02	–	85.0
0.15/0.01	70.1	95.0

[a] Ribosomes from either adult red cells for 13-day-old embryonic red cells were incubated for 60 min at room temperature in a medium containing 0.01 M acetate buffer (pH 5.5), 0.001 M $MgCl_2$, and the stated Na^+ or K^+ concentration. After incubation, ribosomes were centrifuged in a 10-28% sucrose gradient. The percentage of ribosomes remaining in solution was calculated from the size of the monosome peak.
[b] pH 5.0.

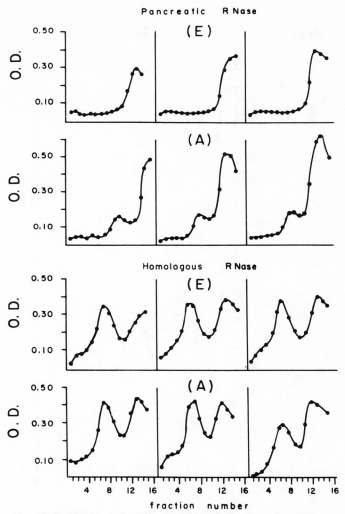

Fig. 2. Incubation of ribosomes in pancreatic or homologous RNase. Samples (0.1 ml) containing 3-5 OD $_{260}$ units of embryonic or adult ribosomes were incubated with different concentrations of pancreatic or homologous RNase in a system containing 0.001 M $MgCl^2$, 0.01 M sodium acetate (pH 5.5), 0.15 M KCl (final volume 0.2 ml) for 1½ hr at room temperature. After enzymatic digestion, the ribosomes were layered on a 10-28% sucrose gradient in 0.01 M Tris-HCl (pH 7.2), 0.01 M KCl, 0.001 M $MgCl^2$ and centrifuged at 35,000 rpm in a Spinco L centrifuge, SW Ti56 rotor, for 85 min. (A) Adult ribosomes; (E) embryonic ribosomes. From left to right, 50, 150, and 450 μg of pancreatic RNase or equivalent activity of homologous RNase.

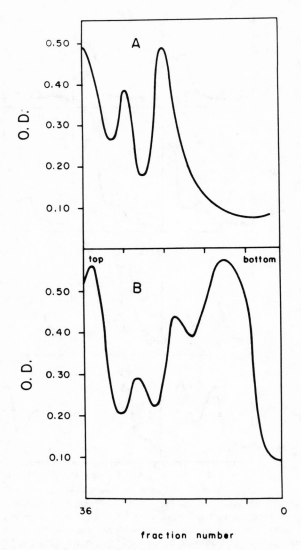

Fig. 3. Ribosomal subunit distribution. Distribution in
a 10-33% sucrose gradient of (A) embryonic or (B) adult
ribosomes after being incubated at room temperature
for 20 min in 0.025 M Tris buffer (pH 7.6), 0.01 M KCl,
and 0.050 M EDTA (see *Methods*).

tions assayed. The 62S ribosomes were also fully degraded; however, in these gradients a peak, sedimenting faster than monosomes, remained which was not further altered by increase in enzyme concentration. When homologous RNase was used for the same type of experiment, the monosomes remained as a peak sedimenting at normal speed, regardless of enzyme concentration. It should be noted, however, that the peak of adult ribosomes was partially diminished at the highest enzyme concentration.

In order to look more closely at the differences between these subcellular particles, ribosomes were allowed to stand in an incubation medium with EDTA, and the incubation mixture was then analyzed by sucrose gradient centrifuga-

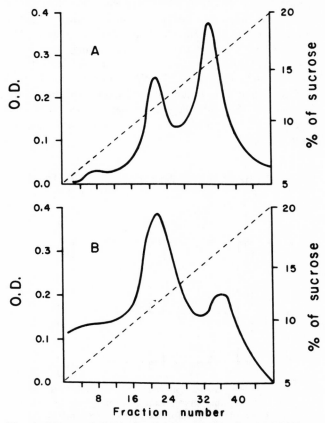

Fig. 4. Ribosomal RNA distribution. Distribution in 5-20% sucrose gradient. Centrifugation was carried out in a SW25 rotor for 12 hr at 24,000 rpm in a Spinco L centrifuge. (A) RNA from embryonic red cells; (B) RNA from adult red cells.

tion. The results of these experiments are plotted in Fig. 3. The 82S ribosomes were fully dissociated into two subunits, 60S and 40S, with a mass ratio value close to 2. On the other hand, EDTA-treated 62S ribosomes showed three peaks, two of them moving at the same velocities as the 60S and 40S particles of the embryonic cell ribosomes. The third peak, faster sedimenting, contained the majority of the UV-absorbing material and seemed to correspond to the original undissociated monosome peak (Fig. 3).

RNA was extracted from either erythrocyte or embryonic ribosomes (see *Methods*) and analyzed by sucrose gradient centrifugation. Figure 4 shows the UV absorbance profile obtained in both cases. A great difference of the ribosomal RNA distribution in the two cell types is observed. The ribosomal RNA of embryonic cells was resolved into two peaks corresponding to the 28S and 18S RNA. Calculating from the area beneath the curves gives an average value of 2.36 ± 0.13 for 28S/18S (nine determinations). This value is in accordance with reported ratios of these RNA molecules based on molecular weights of subunits (11). On the other hand, the ribosomal RNA from mature cells, although it was also distributed in two similar peaks, showed a very different profile: a small peak in the position of 28S and a large asymmetric peak corresponding to 18S. The average ratio of 28S/18S in these preparations was 0.61 ± 0.14 (four determinations).

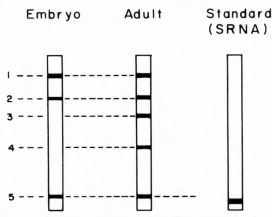

Fig. 5. *Polyacrylamide gel electrophoresis of ribosomal RNA*. The diagram represents the electrophoretic distribution of the adult and embrynic red cell ribosomal RNA; 40-60 μg of RNA was applied to each gel. One tube with *E. coli* sRNA was run as a standard in each experiment. The origin is at the top of the figure. Band Nos.: (1) 28S RNA, (2) 18S RNA, (3) 14.9S RNA, (4) 12.3S RNA, (5) 4S-5S RNA.

To analyze this phenomenon more closely, RNA from both types of ribosomes was submitted to electrophoresis in polyacrylamide-agarose gels. The banding patterns obtained are represented in Fig. 5. As is indicated in this diagram, the RNA from embryonic ribosomes showed 28S, 18S, and 4S-5S RNA bands (first, second, and fifth bands in the diagram). On the other hand, the pattern for the RNA of mature ribosomes showed bands representing 28S, 18S, and 4S-5S, and also two more bands not present in embryonic cell ribosomes (third and fourth bands in the diagram).

Assuming values of 28S and 18S for the two main ribosomal RNAs and using 4S *Escherichia coli* RNA as standard, a statistical analysis of these results was carried out. The two heavier RNA bands from mature cells gave S values of 28.3 $\pm$ 1.0 and 18.6 $\pm$ 1.5, figures not significantly different from the ones obtained for ribosomal RNA from embryonic cells: $p > 0.5$ (Table II). The S values for the two new RNA bands were calculated to be 14.9 $\pm$ 0.9 and 12.3 $\pm$ 0.8. These values correspond to molecular weights of 0.43×10^6 and 0.28×10^6 daltons, respectively (12).

CONCLUSIONS

There are several studies of ribosome structure indicating that the single-stranded regions of the ribosomal RNA are folded in the interior of the particles (13,14). That this might also be the case in chicken red cell ribosomes is supported by 82S ribosome resistance to degradation by homologous RNase, which is specific for single-stranded RNA (10) (Fig. 2).

Table II. Electrophoretic Mobility of
Ribosomal RNA from Adult and Embryonic
Red Cells[a]

Band No.	Adult red cells		Embryonic red cells	
	N	S	N	S
1	33	28.3 ± 1.0	24	28.0 ± 1.0
2	31	18.6 ± 1.5	28	18.0 ± 0.8
3	11	14.9 ± 0.9	–	–
4	21	12.3 ± 0.8	–	–
5	28	4.4 ± 0.3	28	4.4 ± 0.5

[a] The S represents the average sedimentation coefficient calculated from electrophoretic experiments in polyacrylamide gels. The number to the right represents the standard deviation. N is the number of determinations carried out. The band number corresponds to the one marked in Fig. 5.

The tertiary structure of these ribosomes seems to be profoundly altered at the last step of red cell differentiation. This change might consist of unfolding of the ribosomes, since mature particles showed a lower sedimentation coefficient (4), different ionic requirements for ribosomal stability (Fig. 1), and increased accessibility to homologous RNase degradation (Fig. 2). Furthermore, the presence of two new RNA species in the 62S ribosomes (Fig. 5) indicates that a degradative process is taking place in the "unfolded" ribosomes at specific sites along the RNA molecule, possibly determined by the ribosomal sites exposed by the unfolding of the particle.

It is also important to point out that the 62S ribosomes, when exposed to pancreatic RNase, are not completely degraded. That is, a "core" remains which is insensitive to further digestion. This phenomenon is not observed with 82S ribosomes under the same experimental conditions (Fig. 2). This fact, as well as the lack of dissociation of most 62S ribosomes into subunits during EDTA treatment, seems to indicate that there is another factor(s), beside the unfolding of the ribosomes, responsible for this phenomenon. This factor might be related to the phosphorylation-dephosphorylation process of the ribosomal proteins (15,16), which seems to play an important role in draining ribosomes from the *in vivo* ribosomal cycle (16,17).

On the other hand, some of the characteristics of 62S ribosomes indicate heterogeneity of the ribosomal population, namely, (a) partial dissociation of these ribosomes in the presence of EDTA (Fig. 3), (b) precipitation of approximately half of the 62S ribosomes when suspended in medium with either Na^+ or K^+ ions alone (Fig. 1), and (c) the simultaneous presence in the RNA extract of undegraded 28S and 18S ribosomal RNA as well as the degraded fractions, 14.9S and 12.3S RNA (Fig. 5).

The data reported above might suggest that the ribosomal cycle in the differentiating red cell is being altered as ribosomes which are unable to dissociate into subunits accumulate in the cell. Under these conditions, the lowering of the Mg^{2+} concentration known to take place during red cell maturation (18) might cause unfolding of these undissociated ribosomes, yielding ribosomal particles with increased sensitivity to RNase degradation. This sequence of events might determine the accelerated disappearance of the ribosomes and, consequently, the lack of protein synthesis in fully differentiated red cells (3,19).

SUMMARY

Ribosomes from red cells of 13-day-old chick embryos (82S) and from adult chickens (62S) were isolated. Their stabilities under different ionic environments as well as their sensitivities to ribonuclease were studied by further analysis of the particles in sucrose gradient sedimentation experiments. The results obtained in this study indicated marked structural differences between the two types of ribosomes. The 62S and 82S ribosomes differ in (a) the ion requirements for ribosome stability, (b) the dissociation behavior in the presence of EDTA, and (c) the amount of ribonuclease required for enzymatic degradation. The ribosomal RNA patterns of both cell types were also analyzed. The results indicated a dramatic change in the 28S/18S RNA ratio in mature red cell ribosomes as compared to embryonic cells, in addition to the presence of two smaller RNA molecules. The implications of these findings in the ribosomal cycle of differentiating red cells are discussed.

RESUMEN

Los ribosomas de los glóbulos rojos de embriones de pelle de 13 dias (82S) y de pollos adultos (62S) fueron aislados. Sus estabilidades en diferentes ambientes iónicos y sus sensitividades a la ribonucleasa fueron estudiadas mediante el análisis de estas partículas en experimentos de sedimentación en gradientes de sacarosa. Los resultados obtenidos en este estudio indican que existen diferencias estructurales marcadas entre las dos clases de ribosomas. Los ribosomas 62S y los 82S difieren en lo siguiente: (a) el requisito iónico necesario para la estabilidad del ribosoma, (b) el patrón de disociación en presencia de EDTA, y (c) la cantidad de ribonucleasa necesaria para la degradación enzimática.

Los patrones del RNA ribosomal de ambas células fueron también analizados. Los resultados indican un cambio drástico en la relación 28S/18S del RNA en los ribosomas de los glóbulos rojos madures al compararse con las células embriónicas, además de la presencia de dos moleculas pequeñas de RNA. Las implicaciones de estos hechos con respecto al ciclo ribosomal durante la diferenciación de los glóbulos rojos son discutidas.

REFERENCES

1. Glowacki, E. R., and Millette, R. L. *J. Mol. Biol., 11,* 116 (1965).
2. Farkas, W. R., and Marks, P. A., *J. Biol. Chem., 243,* 6464 (1968).
3. Marbaix, G., Burny, A., Huez, G., Lebleu, B., and Temmerman, J., *Europ. J. Biochem., 13,* 322 (1970).
4. Sánchez de Jiménez, E., Webb, F. H., and Bock, R. M., *Arch. Biochem. Biophys., 125,* 452 (1968).
5. Romanoff, A. L., *The Avian Embryo; Structural and Functional Development,* Macmillan, New York (1960).
6. Sánchez de Jiménez, E., Torres, J., Valles, V. E., Solis, *Biochem. J., 97,* 887 (1965).
7. Kurland, C. G., *J. Mol. Biol., 2,* 83 (1960).
8. Loening, U. E., *J. Mol. Biol., 38,* 355 (1968).
9. Peacock, A. C., and Dingman, C. W., *Biochemistry, 7,* 668 (1968).
10. Sánchez de Jiménez, E., de León, Ma. P., and Román, R., *Europ. J. Biochem.,* submitted for publication.
11. Hunt, J. A., *Nature, 226,* 950 (1970).
12. Spirin, A. S., *Progr. Nucleic Acid Res., 1,* 1 (1963).
13. Spencer, M. E., and Walker, I. O., *Europ. J. Biochem., 19,* 451 (1971).
14. Cox, R. A., *Biochem. J., 114,* 753 (1969).
15. Kabat, D., and Rich, A., *Biochemistry, 8,* 3742 (1969).
16. Kabat, D., *Biochemistry, 10,* 2 (1971).
17. Kabat, D., and Rich, A., *Biochemistry, 8,* 9 (1969).
18. Rowley, P. T., and Morris, J. A., *J. Biol. Chem., 242,* 1533 (1967).
19. Barclay, N., Master's thesis, University of Wisconsin, Madison (1965).

DISCUSSION

R. Soeiro (New York, U.S.A.): Have you been able to analyze ribosomes in the adult that remain in solution after you precipitate with high salt concentrations? Are there differences in terms of the RNA or proteins?

E. Sánchez de Jiménez (Mexico City, Mexico): No, we have not yet. We are analyzing the protein pattern that these ribosomes show, and we are isolating the different adult ribosomes to see whether they are different in protein content.

R. Soeiro: Did you have two populations?

E. Sánchez de Jiménez: Yes.

Unidentified speaker: Have you noticed, in your gel electrophoresis, the presence of messenger RNA, hemoglobin messenger RNA, in either type of polysomes?

E. Sánchez de Jiménez: No, the amount of messenger RNA that is present in relation to the ribosomal RNA is very low, and therefore it is not possible to see the messenger RNA in this type of electrophoresis. We need to add much more total RNA as we extract it from the polysomes, and then there is RNA precipitation on the upper part of the polyacrylamide gel.

R. P. Perry (Philadelphia, U.S.A.): Do you know whether something like this exists in any other species besides the chicken?

E. Sánchez de Jiménez: No, I am not aware of the existence of these types of ribosomes in other cells.

R. P. Perry: Would the same comparison, let's say in the rabbit or in the mouse, show this difference? Has anyone done this?

E. Sánchez de Jiménez: I do not know of any report, or any group which has done this; this work was done in chicken because it is rather easy to obtain cells at early stages of maturation. The anemic mammals have, in circulation, only erythrocytes and reticulocytes, and it is difficult to obtain higher than 60% reticulocyte cells in the bloodstream. So it will be very difficult to carry out work of this type with mammalian red cells.

R. T. Schimke (Stanford, U.S.A.): I would like to comment on what seems to be a remarkably different way in which ribosomes are metabolized in something like liver as opposed to red cells. It appears, from your work, that ribosomes are not being synthesized continuously, that perhaps they have a life span of some type. Certainly this is quite different in rat liver, for example, and, I presume, chicken liver, where the half-life of ribosomal RNA and ribosomal proteins is probably on the order of 2-3 days with exponential decay type kinetics. I wonder if you could comment on what you think the differences are in the mechanisms of the breakdown of the ribosomes in these two instances.

E. Sánchez de Jiménez: The life span of the ribosomes in reticulocytes has been measured, and the decrease and even cessation of ribosomal RNA synthesis do not explain the accelerated disappearance of ribosomes that is observed at the last stage of red cell differentiation. On the other hand, we should point out that in chicken red cells there is still ribosomal RNA synthesis in reticulocytes, as well as within red cells. However, there is not the same pattern of ribosomal turnover in different species of animals. So I think it would be very difficult, at the present stage of knowledge on this matter, to extrapolate our results to other tissues that have a completely different metabolism.

K. Moldave (Irvine, U.S.A.): Does the protein-synthesizing activity decrease in these ribosomes as they get converted to a 62S material?

E. Sánchez de Jiménez: We have measured the pulse incorporation of labeled amino acids in red cells. The ribosomes from red cells at different stages of differentiation up to reticulocyte show a great deal of amino acid incorporation in the area of polysomes, but at the erythrocyte stage they no longer incorporate amino acids. We have not tried *in vitro* protein-synthesizing systems.

37

Hormonal Mechanisms in Regulation of Gene Expression

Francis T. Kenney, Kai-Lin Lee, and Kenneth L. Barker

Carcinogenesis Program
Biology Division
Oak Ridge National Laboratory
Oak Ridge, Tennessee, U.S.A.

Research on the question of how genes are regulated in mammalian cells has accelerated rapidly in the last decade, with much attention being paid to systems in which gene expression is regulated by hormones. Virtually all the hormones have been implicated in this facet of regulation, including those acting via cyclic AMP as intracellular mediator; indeed, there is now firm evidence that cyclic AMP acts to regulate synthesis of specific enzymes in mammalian cells (1,2) as well as in bacteria (3,4). Our recent work, however, has involved hormones which appear to act independently of cyclic AMP, at least in the experimental system we employ. We shall review here some of our recent observations on the mechanisms involved in the stimulation of synthesis of a specific enzyme by the steroid hormone, hydrocortisone, as well as by the polypeptide hormone, insulin. As might be anticipated by the difference in structure of these hormones, we conclude that their mechanisms of enzyme induction are quite different, the steroid acting via a transcriptional mechanism and insulin clearly acting at some post-transcriptional stage of enzyme synthesis. Details of experimental approaches not fully described here can be found in our earlier publications on this work (4-7).

These experiments were carried out with cultured cells of the H35 or Reuber

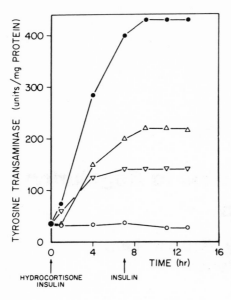

Fig. 1. *Effect of hydrocortisone plus insulin on tyrosine transaminase levels in H35 cells.* Additions were ○, none; ▽, insulin (1 milli-unit/ml at zero time and again at 7 hr); △, hydrocortisone (10^{-6} *M*) at zero time; ●, hydrocortisone plus insulin. [From Reel *et al.* (5).]

hepatoma, a chemically induced rat tumor (8) originally cultured by Pitot, *et al.* (9) and kindly made available to us by that group. These cells grow only while in contact with glass or plastic surfaces and when the culture media are supplemented with serum. Our procedure is to remove the serum from the cells 24 hr before the experiments are begun, so that the cells are not growing but remain viable and can be restored to growth phase by readdition of serum. The cells are aneuploid and have a generation time of 48 hr but retain the capacity of the normal liver to respond to hydrocortisone and insulin (but not glucagon) with a rapid and marked increase in the inducible enzyme tyrosine transaminase.

Figure 1 depicts the time course of change in tyrosine transaminase levels of these cells after treatment with hydrocortisone, insulin, or a combination of the two hormones. The insulin-induced change is quickly detectable, but the steroid has little effect for the first hour. A new steady state is reached 8-9 hr after induction is begun with either inducer; this is consistent with analyses of induction kinetics showing that the time required to reach an induced steady state depends only on the rate of degradation of the induced protein (10). From these considerations, we can infer that the half-life of induced tyrosine transaminase in cells treated with either hydrocortisone or insulin is about 2 hr. Combining the two hormonal inducers yields an additive or somewhat greater than additive response. This effect, together with the difference in kinetics of response noted above, suggests that the mechanisms involved in induction by the two hormones are not the same.

It is imperative to ensure that we are dealing with a single enzyme and not multiple proteins with the capacity to catalyze transamination between tyrosine and α-ketoglutarate. The double diffusion analysis depicted in Fig. 2 provides such verification: a single precipitin line demonstrating immunological identity is formed with enzyme from control, insulin-induced, or hydrocortisone-induced cells. Since the antiserum employed here was prepared against transaminase purified from rat liver, it is also apparent that the enzyme from cultured H35 cells is identical to that from the liver. These two points can also be made with immunological titration analyses (Fig. 3). The common equivalence point found on titration with enzyme from induced and noninduced cells establishes identity and makes the important distinction that the level of antigenically reactive enzyme parallels enzyme levels determined by activity measurements. Thus it can be stated with assurance that induction by either hydrocortisone or insulin results in more of the same enzyme present in untreated cells.

In considering how these hormones might act to increase cellular levels of tyrosine transaminase, we utilized the model depicted in Fig. 4. This is the

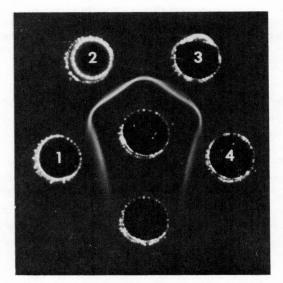

Fig. 2. Double diffusion analyses of tyrosine transaminase preparations. The center well contained antibody against purified transaminase from rat liver. Well 2 contained the purified enzyme used as antigen. Wells 1, 3, and 4 contained partially purified enzyme from H35 cells: well 1, after insulin treatment; well 3, after hydrocortisone treatment; well 4, no hormone treatment.

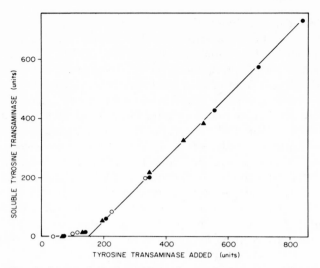

Fig. 3. Immunological titration of transaminase preparations.
Crude enzyme preparations (105,000 × *g* soluble fractions) from
hydrocortisone-treated (●), insulin-treated (▲), or control (○)
H35 cells were titrated against antitransaminase serum sufficient
to precipitate 160 units of transaminase from a fresh rat liver
soluble fraction. [From Reel *et al.* (5).]

model originally elaborated by Jacob and Monod (11), but with important
modifications that reflect the significance of degradative processes in mammalian
regulation. As shown by several investigators, messenger RNAs in mammalian
cells have a finite stability and may be stable for hours or even for days (12).
This is quite different from the situation in microbial cells, where most messenger RNAs examined have been found to be degraded within a few minutes, and
it demands that consideration be made of the lifetime of the transaminase
messenger in our measurements. Also, enzyme proteins are stable in exponentially growing bacterial cells but undergo continuous turnover in mammalian cells.
These turnover rates vary markedly for different enzymes (for review, see ref.

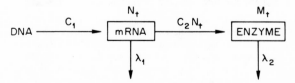

*Fig. 4. Model of cellular processes determining enzyme
level.* [From Lee *et al.* (6).]

13), and hence we must consider the rate of turnover of tyrosine transaminase in H35 cells in order to interpret the kinetics of induction.

We have established that M_t, the amount of enzyme, is increased by treatment with either hydrocortisone or insulin. It is apparent from Fig. 4 that this could be effected in several ways. The cellular mRNA content, designated N_t, could be increased either by an increase in transcription rate, C_1, or by a decrease in degradative rate, λ_1; an increase in N_t would increase the rate of enzyme synthesis, which is here assumed to be first order with respect to mRNA content. The enzyme level could be increased without change in the mRNA component either by an increase in translation rate, C_2, or by a decrease in enzyme degradative rate, λ_2.

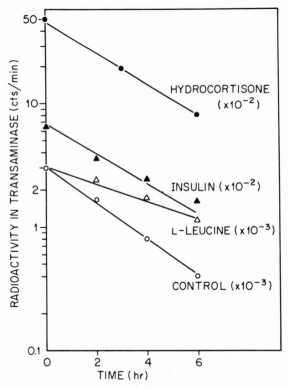

Fig. 5., Tyrosine transaminase degradation. Enzyme was prelabeled by exposure of cells for 2 hr to ^{14}C-leucine before measurements began. Unlabeled medium was substituted at zero time, and at intervals thereafter enzyme radioactivity was determined as described in the text and in ref. 14. Measurements were made after the attainment of the steady-state enzyme level in each case.

With current techniques, we cannot make direct measurements of the parameters C_1, N_t, or C_2. We can, however, by isotopic-immunochemical methods, measure the degradative rates λ_1 and λ_2.

For analysis of the rate of enzyme degradation, λ_2, we employ a "chase" measurement wherein the enzyme is prelabeled by exposure of the cells to isotopic amino acids. When measurements begin, the isotopic amino acid is replaced by its unlabeled counterpart, and the rate of loss of radioactivity is monitored as the labeled enzyme is degraded and replaced by unlabeled enzyme. In Fig. 5 are presented the results of measurements of this type with control cells, cells induced by insulin or by hydrocortisone, and cells in which the transaminase level was increased by high levels of L-leucine. In each case, the measurements are made under steady-state conditions; i.e., although the absolute enzyme level varies appreciably according to how the cells are treated, it remains constant for each treatment type. Cells are treated with isotopic amino acids for 2 hr, then placed on fresh, unlabeled medium at zero time. At this time, and at 2 hr intervals thereafter, cells from similarly treated flasks are collected and pooled, then lysed and subjected to a fast purification procedure that permits 1 hundredfold purification of tyrosine transaminase with little loss, as well as removal of most of the labeled proteins which tend to coprecipitate with antibody-transaminase complexes. Each extract is then supplemented with partially purified, unlabeled transaminase as carrier, and the enzyme is precipitated by addition of a slight excess of antitransaminase serum. A small correction is neceesary for coprecipitated, nontransaminase proteins; this is done by repeating the carrier-antibody addition to the extract (now devoid of labeled transaminase) and subtracting radioactivity of this precipitate from that of the first precipitate. These methods have been described in detail elsewhere (14). Radioactivity measurements obtained in this fashion yield linear regression lines on semilogarithmic plots (Fig. 5), as expected for a random, first-order degradative process. The data of Fig. 5 indicate that tyrosine transaminase is degraded with a half-life of about 2 hr in control cells; in cells elevated to an induced steady state by either hydrocortisone or insulin, this rate is unchanged. This rate of degradation is consistent with that inferred from analysis of the kinetics of induction (Fig. 1). It can be concluded that increased transaminase levels brought about by either hydrocortisone or insulin cannot be due to hormonal alteration of λ_2, the rate of enzyme degradation.

In contrast to the hormonal effectors, high levels of L-leucine do slow the rate of transaminase degradation and thereby contribute to the increased enzyme level brought about by this amino acid (15).

Degradation of transaminase mRNA can be measured if we accept the assumption that treatment of cells with actinomycin to prevent mRNA synthesis does not alter the rate of its degradation. In these experiments, cells are treated with actinomycin (0.2 μg/ml), and, at intervals thereafter, "pulse" labeling is used to assess the rate of enzyme synthesis. This is done by exposing cells to isotopic amino acids for a time (usually 15 min) which is sufficiently brief to prevent enzyme degradation from significantly affecting the extent of incorporation of labeled amino acid into the enzyme. Data obtained in this fashion also yield linear regression lines on semilogarithmic plots (Fig. 6), but it is important to note that on these curves each point represents a rate measurement. The rate of enzyme synthesis drops in first-order fashion after actinomycin treatment, a result consistent with random degradation of an RNA required for transaminase synthesis, which we assume is the transaminase messenger. The transaminase mRNA is degraded with a half-life essentially identical to that of the enzyme, i.e., about 2 hr, and this rate is not changed in cells wherein transaminase has been induced by treatment with hydrocortisone or insulin or by high levels of the amino acid, L-leucine. We conclude that induction by either of the hormones (or by leucine) does not involve change in λ_1, the rate of degradation of transaminase mRNA.

The measured values of the degradative rates λ_1 and λ_2 enabled us to devise a mathematical model of the processes represented in Fig. 4 (16). Values could be assigned to synthetic rates C_1 and C_2 such that when coupled with the rates

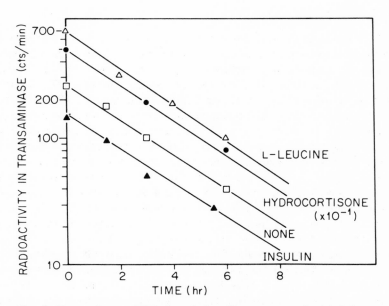

Fig. 6. *Transaminase mRNA degradation.* Enzyme was pulse labeled at zero time and at 2 hr intervals thereafter by exposure to ^{14}C-leucine for 15 min. Actinomycin (0.2 μg/ml) was added at zero time. Measurements were made after attainment of the steady-state enzyme level in each case.

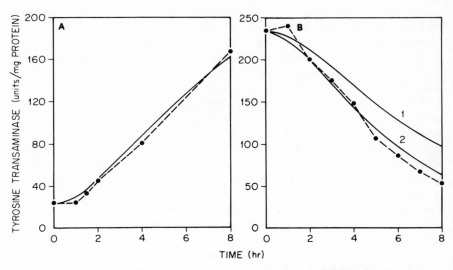

Fig. 7. Kinetics of enzyme change following hydrocortisone addition (A) and withdrawal (B). Points and broken lines are experimental data; solid lines are theoretical curves derived as described in ref. 16. [From Lee *et al.* (6).]

of mRNA and enzyme degradation the system remains in the steady state; i.e., M_t remains at a constant, low level representing the basal or uninduced condition. It is then possible to perturb the system (e.g., by increasing the rate C_1 by a factor of 10) and to ask what kinetic pattern of change in M_t, the amount of enzyme, is effected by this change in rate of transcription. Figure 7 presents the results of such theoretical measurements (solid lines) for an increased rate of transcription at zero time (Fig. 7A) and for the reverse situation wherein the elevated transcription rate is returned to the basal value at zero time (Fig. 7B). In the latter case, two theoretical curves were developed, one with the measured values of λ_1 and λ_2 (indicated as 1 in Fig. 7B) and another representing the "best fit," arrived at by increasing the degradative rates by 30% and by allowing the transcription rate to drop below the original basal value. The broken lines and points of Fig. 7 are measured values for the change in transaminase level after addition of hydrocortisone at zero time (Fig. 7A) and after withdrawal of hydrocortisone from cells that had reached an induced steady state by treatment with the steroid (Fig. 7B). It can be seen that the model predicts the pronounced lag that we observe in the hydrocortisone-mediated induction, due to the necessity of increasing N_t before enzyme synthesis and accumulation begin in earnest. The model also predicts the roughly linear increase toward the induced steady state (after the lag period) that we observe in the course of induction by the steroid hormone. Of particular importance is the prediction by the model of a slow return to the basal steady state after the transcriptional stimulus is reduced; this is observed experimentally when hydrocortisone is removed after the cells have reached an induced steady state. This kinetic pattern reflects the increased mRNA content brought about by stimulation of transcription; the mRNA disappears from the system with a half-life of about 2 hr.

The theoretical curves of Fig. 8 represent predicted kinetics of the system when the rate of translation, C_2, is elevated at zero time (Fig. 8A) and when this rate is returned to the basal rate after attainment of the induced steady state resulting from a translational induction (Fig. 8B). The points and broken lines are experimental values obtained after addition and subsequent withdrawal of the protein hormone, insulin. Here the model predicts an immediate increase in M_t followed by an exponential approach to the induced steady state; this pattern is observed after insulin treatment. After withdrawal of a translational stimulus, the model predicts an immediate first-order type of decay toward the basal state. This is what we observe after removal of insulin, but once again the absolute values observed fit better with somewhat faster degradative rates than those we determined experimentally. It is apparent that in the translational type of induction no intermediate with detectable stability is formed by inducer treatment; the data obtained with insulin as inducer are consistent with an induction mechanism of this kind.

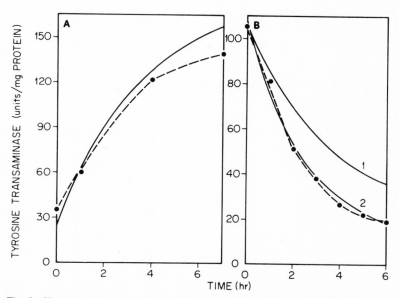

Fig. 8. Kinetics of enzyme change following insulin addition (A) and withdrawal (B). [From Lee et al. (6).]

It can be seen that with both hormonal inducers the enzyme level returns to the basal state at a rate somewhat faster than that predicted from mathematical formulations (16) derived with the measured values of the degradative rates λ_1 and λ_2. This suggests that our measured values of the half-lives of the mRNA and/or the enzyme are somewhat higher than the actual rates, or that these degradative processes are accelerated slightly after inducer removal. We prefer the former explanation, because if a consistent small error is present in measurement of these rates it would be expected to be in this direction. In measuring both λ_1 and λ_2, we follow continuously lower amounts of transaminase radioactivity, often approaching the background level; under these conditions, any contamination of transaminase-antibody precipitates with nontransaminase radioactivity will decrease the slope of the regression lines from which half-lives are estimated. For a more perfect fit of theoretical curves with the data, it was also necessary to assume that when the stimulated rates of both transcription (Fig. 7B) and translation (Fig. 8B) were reduced, they dropped transiently to a value somewhat below the usual basal rates of these processes. Whether this correction (made only to determine the conditions necessary for "best fit") is in accord with reality is unknown; our measurements are not sufficiently precise to detect a difference of this magnitude.

Inhibitor data are equally consistent with the conclusions derived from

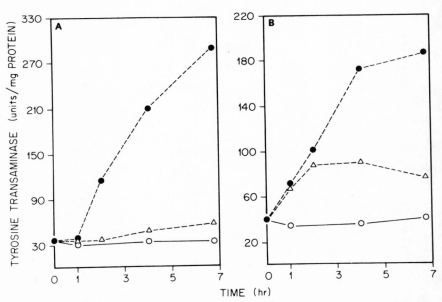

Fig. 9. Effect of actinomycin on inductions by hydrocortisone (A) and insulin (B). Actinomycin was added at 0.2 μg/ml. [From Lee et al. (6).]

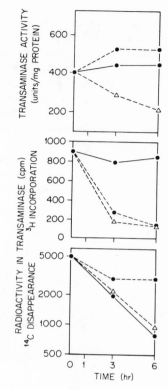

Fig. 10. Effects of high and low concentrations of actino-mycin on transaminase synthesis and degradation in H35 cells. Cells were preinduced with hydrocortisone to the induced steady state before measurements began. At zero time, actinomycin was added at 0.2 μg/ml (△－－－△), 5 μg/ml (●－－－●), or none (●——●). Top panel, enzyme levels; middle panel, pulse-labeling (^{3}H-leucine) measurements of rate of mRNA degradation; lower panel, chase (^{14}C-leucine) measurements of rate of enzyme degradation. [From Lee *et al.* (6).]

these kinetic analyses, i.e., that the steroid hormone induces via a transcriptional effect while insulin acts by increasing the rate of translation. In Fig. 9 are presented comparative data of the effects of actinomycin on induction by the two hormones. The steroid-mediated induction is almost completely blocked by actinomycin; there is no phase of this response which is insensitive to this inhibitor of RNA synthesis. In contrast, induction by insulin is insensitive to actinomycin for almost 2 hr and is not completely blocked until after 5 hr, in accord with the conclusion that this hormone acts on existing mRNA, which, however, disappears from the cells with a half-life of about 2 hr after RNA synthesis is stopped.

It is of interest that the degradative rates for tyrosine transaminase and its mRNA are essentially identical (*cf.* Figs. 5 and 6). A similar result was found in analyses of turnover of δ-aminolevulinate synthetase and its mRNA in rat liver (17), indicating that this is not an isolated phenomenon and suggesting that there may be a mechanistic basis for it. Among the possibilities is a coupling of the two degradative processes. Although such a mechanism cannot yet be excluded, the data of Fig. 10 indicate that coupling, if it occurs, is not required. In this experiment, we employed a double-labeling technique wherein "chase" analyses of enzyme degradation amd "pulse" analyses of mRNA degradation (after actinomycin treatment) are made in the same experiment. Here the effects of low (0.2 μg/ml) and high (5 μg/ml) levels of actinomycin were compared. It can be seen that at both inhibitor levels enzyme synthesis slows rapidly, presumably reflecting degradation of transaminase mRNA (middle panel). Degradation of the enzyme (lower panel) occurs at the usual rate in cells treated with low amounts of actinomycin, but slows and then virtually stops at the high

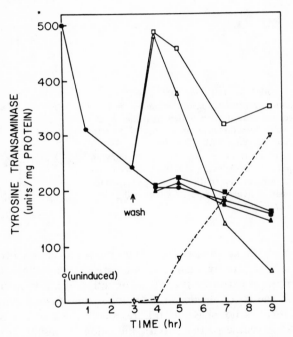

Fig. 11. Effect of cycloheximide on turnover of tyrosine transaminase in H35 cells and restoration of enzyme synthesis and degradation after removal of the inhibitor. Cells were preinduced with hydrocortisone to the induced steady state; then cycloheximide (5 μg/ml) was added. •, No further treatment. Other groups of cells were washed thoroughly 3 hr later, and the following additions were then made: △, none; □, hydrocortisone; ▲, cycloheximide; ■, hydrocortisone plus cycloheximide. The broken line indicates post-wash inducibility, i.e., the difference between those with no additions and those receiving only hydrocortisone. [From Barker et al. (7).]

inhibitor level. Degradation of the mRNA proceeds despite inhibition of enzyme degradation, and hence the two processes are not coupled in an obligatory fashion. The block in enzyme degradation brought about by high actinomycin levels can be seen to effect an increase in the enzyme level (top panel). This "superinduction" is clearly not due to accelerated enzyme synthesis resulting from interference with a translational repression mechanism (18).

Although we cannot detect evidence for coupling of enzyme and mRNA degradations, there are indications that mRNA turnover is coupled in a necessary fashion to translation. Peterkofsky and Tomkins (19) have shown that mRNA accumulates in hepatoma cells when translation is blocked by cycloheximide. This is shown in a different fashion in Fig. 11, where the cells were preinduced with hydrocortisone, then treated with cycloheximide. The transaminase level drops as expected for about 2 hr, but after this time degradation is slowed appreciably by the inhibitor. If after 3 hr of cycloheximide treatment the inhibitor is removed, the original enzyme level is restored very quickly due to synthesis on mRNA remaining in the cells. If degradation of mRNA had occurred at the usual rate during the period when translation was blocked, we would expect that less than 50% would remain intact after 3 hr. That the original enzyme level is restored indicates that the mRNA level present when cycloheximide was added is maintained essentially constant during the period of translational inhibition. Thus it would appear that the mRNA is not degraded when its translation is inhibited.

ACKNOWLEDGMENTS

This research was supported jointly by the National Cancer Institute and the U.S. Atomic Energy Commission under contract with Union Carbide Corporation. K. L. B. is a Research Career Development Awardee, National Institutes of Health. Present address: Department of Biochemistry, University of Nebraska, Omaha, Nebraska 68105, U.S.A.

SUMMARY

The mechanisms by which hydrocortisone, a steroid hormone, and insulin, a protein hormone, effect the induction of tyrosine transaminase in cultured rat hepatoma cells were analyzed kinetically. Direct measurements of the intracellular stability of this enzyme and its mRNA were made by immunochemical-isotopic analyses. Both components were degraded with half-lives of about 2 hr, and these rates were not affected by the hormonal inducers. Experimentally derived induction and de-induction curves were compared with those developed from a mathematical model of induction processes. Changes in enzyme levels brought about by hydrocortisone addition to and withdrawal from the medium were similar to those predicted by the model for an inducer acting on transcriptional processes to increase the cellular content of transaminase mRNA. Enzyme changes brought about by insulin were similar to those predicted for a translational inducer acting to increase enzyme synthesis without change in mRNA content. Effects of inhibition of RNA synthesis by actinomycin were also consistent with the conclusion that the steroid acts on transcription and insulin acts on translation. Interrelationships of cellular processes governing enzyme levels are discussed.

RESUMEN

Los mecanismos mediante los cuales la hidrocortisona, una hormona esteroide, y la insulina, una hormona polipeptídica, afectan la inducción de tirosina transaminasa en cultivos de células provenientes de hepatomas de rata fueron analizados cinéticamente. Medidas directas de la estabilidad intracelular de esta enzima y de su mRNA fueron hechas utilizando técnicas immunoquímicas-isotópicas. Ambos componentes son degradados con vidas medias de alrededor de dos horas, ye estas velocidades no son afectadas por los inductores hormonales. Las curvas de inducción y de de-inducción, obtenidas experimentalmente, se compararon con curvas obtenidas de un modelo matemático para el proceso de inducción. Cambios en el nivel de la enzima producidos cuando se agrega o se remueve la hidrocortisona del medio son similares a los cambios que predice el modelo para un inductor, el cual actúa en procesos transcripcionales aumentando el contenido celular de mRNA para la transaminasa. Cambios en el enzima causados por la insulina, son similares a los que predice el modelo para un inductor traduccional, el cual aumenta la síntesis del enzima sin cambiar el contenido de mRNA. Los efectos de la inhibición con actinomicina son consistentes con la conclusión de que el esteroide actúa al nivel de transcripción y la insulina al nivel de traducción. Las interrelaciones de los procesos celulares que controlan los niveles de la enzima son discutidos.

REFERENCES

1. Wicks, W. D., *J. Biol. Chem., 244,* 3941 (1968).
2. Wicks, W. D., Kenney, F. T., and Lee, K. L., *J. Biol. Chem., 244,* 6008 (1968).
3. Emmer, M., de Crombrugghe, B., Pastan, I., and Perlman, R., *Proc. Natl. Acad. Sci. U.S.A., 66,* 480 (1970).
4. Eron, L., Arditti, R., Zubay, G., Connaway, S., and Beckwith, J. R., *Proc. Natl. Acad. Sci. U.S.A., 68,* 215 (1971).
5. Reel, J. R., Lee, K. L., and Kenney, F. T., *J. Biol. Chem., 245,* 5800 (1970).
6. Lee, K. L., Reel, J. R., and Kenney, F. T., *J. Biol. Chem., 245,* 5806 (1970).
7. Barker, K. L., Lee, K. L., and Kenney, F. T., *Biochem. Biophys. Res. Commun., 43,* 1132 (1971).
8. Reuber, M. D., *J. Natl. Cancer Inst., 26,* 891 (1961).
9. Pitot, H. C., Peraino, C., Morse, P. A., Jr., and Potter, V. R., *Natl. Cancer Inst. Monograph,* No. 13, p. 229 (1064).
10. Berlin, C. M., and Schimke, R. T., *Mol. Pharmacol., 1,* 149 (1965).
11. Jacob, F., and Monod, J., *J. Mol. Biol., 3,* 31 (1961).
12. Wilson, S. H., and Hoagland, M. B., *Biochem. J., 103,* 556 (1967).
13. Schimke, R. T., in Munro, H. N. (ed.), *Mammalian Protein Metabolism,* Vol. IV, Academic Press, New York (1970), p. 177.
14. Lee, K. L., and Kenney, F. T., in Karolinska Symposia on Research Methods in Reproductive Endocrinology, *Acta. Endocrinol.,* Suppl. 153, p. 109 (1971).
15. Lee, K. L., and Kenney, F. T., *J. Biol. Chem., 246,* 7595 (1971).
16. Hoel, D. G., *J. Biol. Chem., 245,* 5811 (1970).

17. Tschudy, D. P., Marver, H. S., and Collins, S., *Biochem. Biophys. Res. Commun., 21,* 480 (1965).

18. Tomkins, G. M., Gelehrter, T. D., Granner, D., Martin, D. M., Jr., Samuels, H. H., and Thompson, E. G., *Science, 166,* 1474 (1969).

19. Peterkofsky, B., and Tomkins, G. M., *Proc. Natl. Acad. Sci. U.S.A., 60,* 222 (1968).

DISCUSSION

R. P. Perry (Philadelphia, U.S.A.): How did you measure the half life of the message and how did you identify the different messages for which you were measuring half lives? You mentioned that one was stable for days and another, for TKT, had a half-life of 2 hr.

F. T. Kenney (Oak Ridge, U.S.A.): For tyrosine transaminase, we measured the rate at which the enzyme is being synthesized as a function of time after blocking RNA synthesis with actinomycin. We find that the rate of synthesis decays with a half-life of 2 hr. We are inferring, of course, that synthesis of the enzyme decays because the message is disappearing. I mentioned also that we can infer from kinetic analyses that the mRNA for glutamic-alanine transaminase, a relatively stable enzyme, is also stable and appears to have a half-life of 1-3 days.

R. P. Perry: There is a case with cultured L cells in which the message for ribosomal proteins seems to have a half-life of about 2½ hr, whereas the ribosomal structural proteins themselves have almost an infinite lifetime. So this is a case where there is no relationship between the lifetime of the message and the lifetime of the protein which it makes.

F. T. Kenney: In the liver, there are six enzyme systems where we can measure directly or can make some pretty good guesses on the magnitude of degradation rates for the enzyme and its mRNA, and they seem to be the same. I did not mean to suggest that all proteins and their messengers are necessarily degraded at identical rates.

H. G. Zachau (Munich, Germany): I did not get your explanation of the superinduction by actinomycin. You made a brief comment on that; could you expand a little?

F. T. Kenney: The term "superinduction" implies that, under the condition of high actinomycin treatment, the rate of enzyme synthesis is increased. It has been argued by others that this is the case, and this result argues for a cytoplasmic repression system with which the steroid interacts. The fact is that the rate of enzyme synthesis does not increase, rather, it decreases, so I do not think the term "superinduction" is an appropriate one. Enzyme synthesis is not accelerated under these conditions, but degradation of the enzyme is blocked by high levels of actinomycin. So there is a situation where, by virtue of having preinduced the cells, you are starting with a high rate of enzyme synthesis. Now you add actinomycin, and that rate of synthesis begins to decline. However, the message has a finite life, it does not disappear immediately. So there is a period of time during which synthesis of the enzyme, although it is dropping, is still very high. Since degradation is blocked during this interval, the enzyme level increases.

R. Brentani (São Paulo, Brazil): Did you determine if the induction by insulin can be prevented by glucose?

F. T. Kenney: It cannot.

F. J. S. Lara (São Paulo, Brazil): Could you indicate why the translation of the message should cause its degradation?

F. T. Kenney: I do not know why it should, but it is well known that message degradation is associated with translation in microbial systems.

R. T. Schimke (Stanford, U.S.A.): When you measure an increased rate of synthesis of TAT with insulin as inducer, is the effect specific for TAT or do you find an accelerated rate of synthesis of other proteins?

F. T. Kenney: Insulin causes a generalized increase in protein synthesis, but a much greater increase in the rate of synthesis of this protein (TAT).

J. Allende (Santiago, Chile): Following the question that Dr. Zachau asked in relation to actinomycin, why does the rate of enzyme degradation decrease in the presence of actinomycin?

F. T. Kenney: I do not know why. Actinomycin inhibits enzyme degradation only at very high levels; it may reflect a more general toxic effect.

38

Synthesis of Mitochondrial Proteins

Karl Dawidowicz and Henry R. Mahler

Department of Chemistry
Indiana University
Bloomington, Indiana, U.S.A.

The recent discovery that the ubiquitous energy-transducing organelle of eukaryotic cells, the mitochondrion, contains its own DNA, distinct from that of the nucleus (for recent reviews, see 1-4), has generated intensive investigations in a number of related areas. They have made accessible possible answers to such fundamental questions as the nature and extent of the genetic and biogenetic autonomy of the organelle; the origin, mode of transmission, and significance of extrachromosomal, non-Mendelian hereditary determinants; and the whole chain of events that must intervene in the course of the expression of the mitochondrial genome. Central to this area is the problem of mitochondrial protein synthesis, both *in vivo* and *in vitro;* known now for some 13 years (5,6), it has been raised from its former status of relative obscurity as a laboratory curiosity to one of the fashionable fields of inquiry of contemporary biochemistry and molecular biology. Since the topic has been the subject of several recent and comprehensive reviews (7-11), I shall restrict my presentation, in the main, to our own investigations with the unicellular eukaryote *Saccharomyces cerevisiae* or baker's yeast.

   This report is in two parts. In the first, we begin by defining some remaining points of uncertainty or even controversy concerning the mechanism of protein synthesis by the mitochondrial ribosomes (mitoribosomes) of this organism; this is followed by a description of our attempts at their resolution, including the use of a somewhat different paradigm for this purpose. The second part inquires into the nature and formation of mitochondrial translational products (which in turn are also probably specified by mitochondrial transcripts) in the laying down of the mitochondrial respiratory chain.

RESULTS AND CONCLUSIONS

Translational Machinery of Yeast Mitochondria

Current State of the Art

Table I presents in a grossly abbreviated and schematic form the extent of information currently available as a result of intensive investigations in a number of laboratories during the past 5 years. Aside from certain as yet unanswered questions dealing with the protein factors for chain initiation and termination, we see that the main area of doubt resides in the properties and even the very existence of a traditional translational system, with polysomal aggregates as its core. Specifically, two questions have been raised explicitly, one technical and the other fundamental. The first concerns the sedimentation coefficient of the monomeric ribosome *active* in protein synthesis. This question is of some importance because, as has become apparent during the recent past—and is indicated in the table—the mitoribosomes of Ascomycetes, of which yeast is an example, constitute a special class of particles, quite distinct from the mitoribo-

Table I. Characteristics of Mitochondrial Protein Synthesis
(October 1971)

Parameter	Yeast	Vertebrates
Ribosomes		
Distinct[b] particle (RNA, proteins)	+	+
Active monomer, sedimentation coefficient	?[a]	55S
Presence of polysomes	?	+
Initiation		
tRNA	fMet-tRNA$_f^{Met}$	fMet-tRNA$_f^{Met}$
Distinct[b] initiation factors	±	
Elongation		
Distinct class of tRNAs	+	+
Distinct[b] elongation factors	G_{mt}, T_{mt}	
Termination		
Signal		
Distinct[b] termination factors		

[a] Isolated particles have been assigned values varying between 72 and 80S.
[b] Not identical with material found in the cytosol or active with cytoribosomes. A blank indicates that this question has not yet been investigated explicitly, a question mark that there is some controversy concerning this point.

somal particles of animals (10). So far as their RNA and protein constituents are concerned, they are also quite distinct not only from the cytoribosomes of all eukaryotic cells, including those found in their own cytoplasm, but also from those of bacteria, such as *Escherichia coli* (10,12). The latter finding is of special significance, for on the basis of earlier reports concerning their physical properties, and particularly their susceptibility to inhibitors, usually ascribed to the bacterial 30S and 50S ribosomal subunits (Table II) mitochondrial ribosomes had been commonly assigned to the "70S" class (13, 14). Isolated mitoribosomes from yeast have been variously assigned sedimentation coefficients of 72S, 74S (17), 75S (16), 76S (18), or 80S (19,20). This is an interesting discrepancy, since the last value is, of course, identical to that of yeast cytoribosomes (16-19). However, none of the investigations cited have demonstrated that the particles studied are active *in vivo,* i.e., can carry a nascent polypeptide chain; most of them also suffer from the absence of internal standards constituted by either cytoplasmic or *E. coli* ribosomes. The question has been raised explicitly by Linnane and his collaborators (9,21,22), who have proposed a unitary hypothesis of action of certain antibiotics which postulates that "the ribosome of yeast mitochondria is an integral part of the mitochondrial membrane." A logical consequence of such a postulate might well be the absence of classical polyribosome structures.

Criteria for Functional Ribosomes

Clearly, the resolution of these discrepancies requires the identification and isolation of functional mitoribosomes, free of contamination by their counterparts from other parts of the cytoplasm including its membranous elements. Although this is possible, at least in principle* (15,23,24), the steps involved may demand both the inclusion of Mg^{2+} to insure mitoribosomal integrity (14,23) and its removal by EDTA (15,24) (or the inclusion of RNase, ref. 18) to dissociate and remove the extramitochondrial contaminants, once again raising the question as to the relation of the physical properties actually observed to those characterizing the particles *in vivo.* One possible alternative, applicable even to quite crude mixtures of particles and therefore employed with those isolated from vertebrate sources such as HeLa cells (27,28), makes use of pulse label with an amino acid together with site-specific inhibitors (for a summary, see Table II, based on refs. 9,29; also refs. 30, 31) for the identification of the relevant structures. Although we too have employed this approach, specifically the couple cyclohoximide (CH) (cytoribosomes)/chloramphenicol (CAP) (mito-

---

* By virtue of the fact that the resultant particles can then be shown to be active in cell-free incorporation, in the presence of exogenous messenger and the mitochondrial elongation factors (23-26).

Table II. Antibiotic Inhibitors of Protein Synthesis

Antibiotic	Presumed mode of action	Inhibits protein synthesis by		
		Bacteria	Mitochondria	Cytoribosomes
Puromycin	Premature chain termination, polysome breakdown	+	+	+
Fusidic acid	Prevents translocation	+	−	+
Cycloheximide, emetine (glutarimides)	Blocks entry and transfer of peptidyl-tRNA on 60S subunits, slows chain propagation	−	−	+
Anisomycin	Inhibitis peptide bond formation	−	−	+
Chloramphenicol	Binds to 50S subunit,[a] blocks attachment of aa-tRNA and chain propagation	+	+	−
Erythromycin (macrolides)	Binding similar,[a] blocks binding of peptidyl-tRNA	+	+	−
Lincomycin	Binding similar,[a] blocks binding of both peptidyl- and aa-tRNA, polysome breakdown	+	+	−
Neomycin, paramomycin (aminoglycosides)	Forms abortive initiation complex with 30S subunit[a]	+	+	−
Aureomycin (tetracyclines)	Binds to 30S subunit and blocks entry of aa-tRNA[a]	+	+	−

[a] In bacteria; whether the same mode of action holds for mitochondria remains to be established. For chloramphenicol, at least, the mechanism may well be different.

ribosomes), an artificial element is introduced by this paradigm, namely, the uncoupling of what must be, in the cell, a tightly integrated interplay, not only of the two synthetic systems, but of regulatory schedules as well. We have therefore searched for an alternative not employing inhibitors and believe we have found it in the use of radioactive formate to label the nascent polypeptide chains of mitoribosomes. Our reasoning was based on the unambiguous demonstration that fMet-tRNA$_f^{Met}$ is the initiator tRNA for mitoribosomes (32-35)—as contrasted to Met-tRNA$_i^{Met}$ $_{or \; M*}$ for the cytoribosomes (36-40)—and the hope that we would make fMet the only or predominating formate-containing species by (a) using a short pulse, (b) using a purine (adenine) requiring auxotroph with exogenous adenine added, and (c) extracting and removing all RNA from samples with hot TCA (41).

The criticial experiment using sedimentation analysis in sucrose gradients for the identification of monosomes and subunits is shown in Fig. 1. The following statements summarize the observations.

(a) Incorporation of formate into molecules precipitable by hot TCA is restricted entirely to entities derived from mitochondria and in this respect is entirely analogous to the behavior of leucine incorporated in the presence of CH.

(b) In the case of mitoribosomes, there is complete coincidence of these two tracings with that for A_{260}.

(c) Incorporation of leucine and of formate into mitoribosomes is sensitive to CAP.

(d) Incorporation of leucine into cytoribosomes is insensitive to CAP. We are therefore probably justified in the inference that incorporation of formate under these conditions can be used as a highly specific means of identification for mitoribosomes active in protein synthesis *in vivo*, obviating the necessity for the use of CH (or other such inhibitors).

Comparison of Mitoribosomes with Cytoribosomes

The experiments just described also suggest that the functional mitoribosomes isolated are sufficiently homogeneous to permit a determination of their sedimentation coefficient, but they cannot tell us its precise value. For this purpose, we have carried out double-labeling experiments in which we have compared, for instance, particles labeled by long-term incorporation of uracil isolated from *E. coli*, or from yeast cytoplasm, with ones isolated from the mitochondria. One such experiment is shown in Fig. 2. If we assume the S value of the ribosome from *E. coli* to be 70S (18), then that from the cytoplasmic particle is 80S (17-19)—a good internal control—and that of the mitoribosome 75S ± 1, in complete agreement with the recent results of Grinell *et al.* on mitoribosomes active *in vitro* (17).

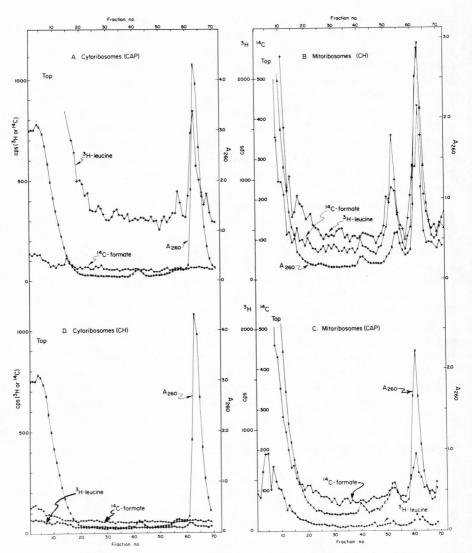

Fig. 1. Characterization of mitochondrial and cytoplasmic ribosomes and their subunits (mitoribo-somes vs. cytoribosomes). S. cerevisiae strain 4D (57,59) was grown in adenine-containing medium with 3% D,L-lactate as the carbon source and harvested by centrifugation when A_{600} reached 0.5. The cells were resuspended in one-tenth the original volume of complete medium and divided into two aliquots. To one half (for experiments B and D) was added cycloheximide (CH) to a final concentration of 100 μg/ml, to the other (for experiments A and C) chloramphenicol (CAP) to a concentration of 4 mg/ml. After a 10 min preincubation at 30°, the samples were exposed to the labeled precursors [12.5 μCi/ml of L-³H-leucine (NEN, 36 Ci/mmol) and/or 20 μCi/ml of

Mitochondrial Polysomes

Experiments such as the one shown in Fig. 2 suggest that, in addition to monomeric structures, mitoribosomes can also assume a polymeric, polysomal form and that in fact the former may simply be breakdown products—perhaps formed during isolation of the latter, fully active forms. To check this hypothesis, we have performed a number of experiments, the results of which may be summarized as follows.

(a) Polymeric, RNase-sensitive forms (differeing in sedimentation behavior from those isolated from the cytoplasm) can be identified by both continuous (steady-state) and pulse labeling with uracil, as well as by A_{260}.

(v) They carry nascent polypeptide chains, identified by labeling with both amino acids (in the presence of CH) and formate; treatment with puromycin results in a complete discharge of both labels and a dissociation of the particles to monosomes and subunits.

We conclude that mitochondrial ribosomes participate in protein synthesis—at least in part—as polyribosomes *in vivo:* the relation between fraction number and sedimentation coefficient on the one hand and number of subunits on the other is shown in Fig. 3; it obeys the relationship established for other systems (42).

---

[14]C-formate (NEN, 59 mCi/mmol)] for 5 min at 30°. Incorporation was stopped by addition of CAP to the CH-containing sample and of CH to the CAP-containing sample together with crushed ice. Cells were harvested by centrifugation at 4°C (4000 rpm for 10 min), washed twice with distilled water and once with 0.44 M sucrose-MNT buffer (10 mM MgCl$_2$, 100 mM NH$_4$Cl, 10 mM Tris, pH 7.4). Cells were broken in the same medium by mechanical disintegration in a Braun shaker at 0° in the presence of glass beads for 15 sec twice (59). Unbroken cells, nuclei, and debris were removed by repeated centrifugation at 600 × g for 20 min. For isolation of mitoribosomes (experiments B and C), the M fraction was resuspended in sucrose-MNT and centrifuged first at 600 × g for 20 min and then again at 20,000 × g for 20 min. The pellet was then washed twice with 0.65 M sorbitol containing 2 mM Tris-EDTA, pH 6.5, and once with 0.65 M sorbitol-MNT. Mitochondria were lysed by exposure to a final concentration of 2% (w/w) Triton X100 in MNT buffer, and ribonucleoprotein particles were isolated by removing membrane fragments by centrifuging at 26,000 × g for 20 min. The supernatant was then placed directly on a linear gradient of 0.3-1.4 M sucrose plus MNT and centrifuged at 26,000 rmp ($\bar{g}_{av}$ = 88,000 × g) in the SW27 rotor of a Beckman ultracentrifuge at 3°. Ordinarily, for the isolation of monomeric and polymeric ribosomes, centrifugation was for 4 or 5 hr, but for this particular experiment centrifugation was for 13 hr. At the end of the centrifugation period, 0.5 ml fractions were collected from the top by means of a ISCO fraction collector by pumping 60% sucrose into the bottom of the tube at the rate of 1 ml/min. One-tenth milliliter of each fraction was diluted and used for the determination of A_{260} and another aliquot for precipitating proteins on filter paper discs by the method of Mans and Novelli (41). This entails successive exposures to cold 10% TCA (2 hr or overnight), cold 10% TCA (twice), 5% TCA (80° for 30 min), 5% TCA (twice), ethanol-ether (3:1, twice), ether. Counting was in a Packard liquid scintillation spectrometer using a computer program with corrections for spillover and quenching as described previously (43). For cytoribosomes, the S fraction was made 0.5% in Triton X100 and incubated for 15 min at 0° and centrifuged at 26,000 × g for 20 min. The supernatant was diluted with 1 vol of MNT and subjected to sedimentation analysis as outlined above for mitoribosomes. In the display, the direction of sedimentation is from left (top) to right (bottom of tube).

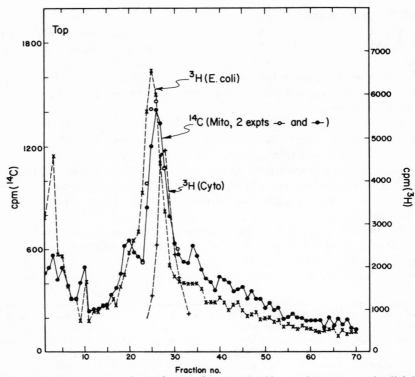

Fig. 2. Sedimentation analysis of yeast ribosomes. In this experiment, we used a diploid
strain of *S. cerevisiae* (Fleischmann) grown on 1% glucose to A_{600} = 1.6 and labeled two
aliquots with ^{14}C-uracil for 60 min [1 μCi/ml (NEN, 55 mCi/mmol) for mitoribo-
somes], and ^{3}H-uracil for 30 min [5 μCi/ml, (NEN, 40 Ci/mmol) for cytoribosomes],
respectively. The two classes of ribosomes were then isolated as described in the caption
of Fig. 1. Ribosomes from *E. coli* (auxotrophic for uracil and thymine) were isolated
from exponentially growing cells (78); the latter were labeled for 45 min at 37° with 1
μCi/ml ^{3}H-uracil as above, chilled in dry ice-ethanol, harvested by centrifugation, and
suspended in 0.4 ml of sucrose (250 g/liter) plus Tris (10 mM, pH 8.1). Lysis was by
addition of lysozyme (42.5 μg) plus EDTA (0.8 mM), followed by Brij 58 (0.1 ml of a
1% solution in 20 mM MgSO$_4$, 2 mM Tris, pH 7.4). Membranes and DNA were removed
by centrifugation at 3000 rpm for 5 min, and the lysate was subjected to gradient
analysis. For the latter, an aliquot of mitoribosomes (○) was mixed with *E. coli* lysate,
and a second (●) with cytoribosomes. Centrifugation was for 200 min at 26,000 rpm in
the SW27 rotor. Samples were precipitated with cold 10% TCA and washed repeatedly
with 5% TCA only.

Products of the Mitochondrial Translational System

Quantitative Estimates

Having once established the evidence and properties of the intramitochondrial protein-synthesizing system, the major unresolved problem is, of course, its

function in the biogenesis of the organelle and its proteins. This requires answers to three subsets of related questions: What portion of the total mitochondrial proteins originate within the organelle? Where are the proteins localized? What is their function?

Concerning the first question, most studies, in particular ones using either *Saccharomyces* or *Neurospora,* permit the inference that even when the intra-mitochondrial system is fully operative (i.e., in exponentially growing cells using a nonfermentable substrate) its contribution does not exceed 10% of the total protein of the organelle (43-48). All of these investigations, including our own, have used insensitivity to CH—and frequently also sensitivity to CAP—as the criteria, and so the resultant estimates are subject to the general criticism raised earlier concerning experiments of this type, with the additional stricture that

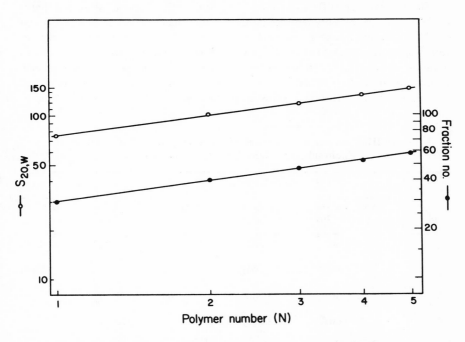

Fig. 3. Sedimentation analysis of mitoribosomes. The procedure described in the caption of Fig. 1 was followed for the isolation of mitoribosomes labeled with ^{14}C-formate. Centrifugation was for 4 hr at 26,000 rpm in the SW27 rotor. Gradient fractions were analyzed for A_{260}, material precipitable by cold TCA, and protein by the Mans and Novelli (41) procedure. The positions of the peaks (fractions 30, 40, 48, 54, and 58) coincided in all three measurements. Counts per minute per 0.1 ml aliquots for the two determinations were within ± 10% of the average and were 2550, 1250, 750, 525, and 475, respectively. The data were then converted to $s_{20, w}$ assuming 75S for the monomer. The various aggregates are shown to obey the relationship expected (42) for nascent chains on oligomeric ribosomes attached to mRNA.

here the paradigm may well lead to enchanced synthesis of one class and reduced or abolished synthesis of another, and thus render quantitative estimates meaningless.

However, when similar techniques are applied to the second essentially qualitative question, they do permit relatively strong inferences (7-9,11,43,47-51): among the four mitochondrial compartments (the outer membrane, the intermembrane space, the inner membrane including its cristae and their attachments, and the matrix), the contribution of the resident translational system is restricted to only one, the inner membrane.

Identification of Actual Components

Having established the inner membrane as the mitochondrial structure that is made up, in part, by polypeptides of local origin, the next logical step consists of the identification and isolation of these polypeptides and an assignment of their function. Here progress has been relatively slow, and the results obtained are not without ambiguity. Identification and isolation, in principle at least, of such membrane proteins can be and have been achieved by electrophoresis (or chromatography), but to be successful the procedure requires a strongly denatur-

Table III. Number and Molecular Weight (in daltons) of Product of Mitochondrial Protein Synthesis in Ascomycetes[a]

Band	Saccharomyces cerevisiae			Neurospora crassa	
	Weislogel and Butow (79)	Thomas and Williamson (80)	Yang and Criddle (81)[b]	Weiss et al. (74)	Swank et al. (82)
1	13,000	11,000	15,000	(11,000 ?)	(~13,000)
2	24,000	(15,800)	20,000	17,500	20,000
3	27,000	23,000	26,500	(21,000 ?)	
4	(34,000)	(28,000)		(25,000 ?)	
5	38,000	33,000		27,700	
6	41,000		40,000	33,500	(~33,000)
7	44,000	(48,000)			(48,000)

[a] CH-insensitive incorporation, SDS-acrylamide electrophoresis. Minor components are in parentheses, predominant species underlined.
[b] S. carlsbergensis, isolated mitochondria in vitro.

ing environment such as the presence of sodium dodecyl sulfate (SDS) (usually applied first at high temperature), and frequently urea as well. These are conditions designed to lead to the removal of prosthetic groups and to the disruption of all secondary, tertiary, and quaternary structure so as to produce monomers in a disordered conformation (52), which by their very nature preclude retention of any enzymatic or other functional activity. Results obtained recently by the application of these techniques to the mitochondria from yeast and *Neurospora* are summarized in Table III. Although apparently all investigators agree that the polypeptides synthesized within and located in the inner membrane belong to just a few molecular weight classes, there is no such agreement as to the number of such classes, their actual molecular weight, or their relative importance, even within the same organism.

Functional Tests

Clearly, an alternative approach is' required. In our laboratories, we have tried to assess the intramitochondrial contribution to inner membrane function by means of two complementary types of experiments: the use of site-specific inhibitors and of biochemical mutants. These experiments (46, 53-61), some of which go back almost 10 years and others which are still in progress, are summarized in Table IV, which also includes the results of similar studies on two components of the mitochondrial ATPase complex (F_1 and OSCF) carried out by Schatz (62) and by Tzagoloff (63). We postulate that for an inner membrane component to have its origin in the cytoplasm and be specified by a nuclear gene (a) it must be present in a cytoplasmic (ρ^-) mutant that is known to possess a completely nonfunctional mitochondrial DNA (mt-DNA) or a virtual absence of this component (designated as mt-DNA^0 in the table—both these types are known (57,64-66) and have been or are being used by us*; (b) its synthesis under derepressing or derepressed conditions must be unaffected by CAP as well as by ethidium bromide (EB) or acriflavine (AF), inhibitors which at least in this instance are known to interact with mt-DNA and block mitochondrial transcription preferentially (65-70); (c) its synthesis must be blocked by CH. Although (a) and (b) are both necessary and sufficient operational criteria, (a) is by far the more conclusive.

Conversely, a component absent in the mutant as well as blocked in synthesis by CAP, EB, and AF but not CH could be regarded as unambiguously of mitochondrial origin. Unfortunately, the first part of this last criterion is not

* The criterion may be more restrictive than needed for mitochondrial translation; so far, all ρ^- mutants studied—regardless of the extent of the aberration in their mt-DNA—lack one or more essential components required for mitochondrial protein synthesis and are therefore inactive in this regard (see ref. 9).

Table IV. Criteria for Intramitochondrial Contribution[a]

Entity or activity	Presence in ρ^- (including mt-DNA⁰)	Inhibition by Short-term exposure to		
		EB or AF	CAP	CH
Citric acid cycle enzymes (matrix)	+	−	−	+
ATPase (F$_1$)	+	−	−	+
OSCF	+	−	−	+
Majority proteins of inner membrane	+	−	−	+
NADH dehydrogenase	+	−	−	+
Succinate dehydrogenase	+	−	−	+
NADH-cytochrome c reductase*	CRM	−	−	+
Succinate-cytochrome c reductase*		−	−	+
CYTOCHROME OXIDASE	CRM	+	·+	±
Ubiquinone	+			
Nonheme iron (S)	+			
[Cu]	+			
Cytochrome b	−	±	−	+
Cytochrome c_1	−	−	−	+
Cytochrome c	+	−	−	+
CYTOCHROME aa_3	−	+	+	+

[a] EB, ethidium bromide; AF, acriflavine; CAP, chloramphenicol; CH, cycloheximide; CRM, cross-reacting material, i.e., protein showing partial immunological or enzymatic activity; OSCF, oligomycin-sensitivity conferring factor; +, strong; −, no effect; ±, effect observed depends on paradigm used; blank, not studied explicitly.
* Sensitive to antimycin A.

sufficient in this instance, since the ρ^- mutation is pleiotropic and the primary lesion is unknown. The same objection also holds for the mitochondrial inhibitors, unless attention is restricted to their immediate effects. It is quite apparent from the table that only the terminal segment of the respiratory chain, i.e., cytochrome oxidase-cytochrome aa_3, meets the criteria for requiring a mitochondrial contribution, *but,* since related protein(s) are present in the mutant (56,71) and the synthesis of cytochrome oxidase is sensitive to CH, its elaboration also requires participation of the nucleocytoplasmic system. This conclusion was also arrived at independently by Chen and Charalampous by a study of respiratory adaptation (72).

Composition and Synthesis of Cytochrome Oxidase

Our attention was therefore inexorably drawn to the synthesis of cytochrome oxidase, or its means of integration into the membrane, as a likely target for the participation of the mitochondrial system of gene expression. We set out to purify the enzyme and study its properties, particularly with respect to its polypeptide components. These studies by Shakespeare (73) have led to the conclusion that pure cytochrome oxidase of yeast (A_{280}/A_{420} = 3.25) can be isolated as a monomer (mol wt = 100,000) which is highly active enzymatically ($k \geqslant 5000$ min^{-1} mg^{-1} protein—or a specific activity of $\geqslant 200$ μmoles cytochrome oxidized $\times$ min^{-1} $\times$ mg^{-1} protein—vs. k = 1200 min^{-1} $\times$ mg for pure beef heart enzyme under identical conditions). On dissociation in the presence of SDS and mercaptoethanol at an elevated temperature, followed by electrophoresis in acrylamide gels in the presence of SDS, the enzyme can be shown to be composed of four polypeptide chains in roughly equimolar proportion (Table V). While these studies were in progress, Weiss et al. (74) and Birkmayer (75) both reported on similar studies on the cytochrome oxidase from Neurospora crassa employing different methods of purification. The preparation of Weiss et al. was examined by acrylamide gel electrophoresis in the presence of SDS (Table V) and that of Birkmayer by electrophoresis in the presence of urea and acetic acid. Although extensive and satisfactory purification was achieved on the basis of spectroscopic criteria, neither preparation showed the activity to be

Table V. Molecular Weights of Component Polypeptides in Cytochrome Oxidase (SDS-acrylamide Electrophoresis)

Band No.	Beef heart[a]	Saccharomyces cerevisiae[a]	Neurospora crassa[b]
1	9,000	7,500	8,000
2	12,000	14,000	10,000
3	17,000	23,200	13,000
4	23,000	46,000	20,000
5	55,000		30,000

[a] Shakespeare and Mahler (73)
[b] Weiss et al. (74)

expected for a pure enzyme (specific activities of 4.6 and 2.8 μmoles of cytochrome c oxidized $\times$ min^{-1} $\times$ mg^{-1} protein). This may have some bearing on what inferences are permissible from the conflicting and diametrically opposed evidence presented by the two groups concerning the function of the CH-insensitive incorporation system in the biosynthesis of proteins: Weiss *et al.* claim that cytochrome oxidase, and specifically its 20,000 dalton subunit, is contributed by the mitoribosomal system, while Birkmayer concludes that this system contributes neither to the intact enzyme nor to its subunits. Our studies on the biosynthesis of the polypeptides of yeast cytochrome oxidase are proceeding along two routes:

(a) The synthesis of immunological CRM to antibodies of pure enzyme in the presence of ethidium bromide (EB). Our preliminary results here confirm the earlier studies with a mutant (15) that in fact some (but, of course, we do not know which) component of cytochrome oxidase capable of competing with the enzyme for the binding of cytochrome c is still synthesized when mitochondrial transcription is absent.

(b) Studies on incorporation in the presence of CH, CAP, and EB.

Transcription vs. *Translation*

On the basis of our results so far—and we must emphasize that these have been restricted to a limited number of components of the inner membrane and the matrix—we have no evidence whatever for either the import of nuclear transcripts for translation by mitoribosomes (76) or its converse, the export of mitochondrial transcripts for translation by cytoribosomes (77).

ACKNOWLEDGMENTS

We are grateful to Dr. Peter Shakespeare for permitting us to report on his unpublished observations. This research was supported by Research Grant GM12228 from the National Institute of General Medical Sciences, National Institutes of Health, U.S. Department of Health, Education and Welfare. H. R. M. is a recipient of Public Health Service Research Career Award No. GM05060 from the Institute of General Medical Sciences, National Institutes of Health, U.S. Department of Health, Education and Welfare. K. D. is supported by Consejo de Desarrollo Cientifico y Humanistico, Universidad Central de Venezuela. Mrs. Joanne Cochran provided capable technical assistance in some of the experimental work.

SUMMARY

The particles responsible for protein synthesis in mitochondria of *Saccharomyces cerevisiae* are ribosomes with a sedimentation coefficient of 75S arranged in polysomal aggregates. Incorporation of labeled formate into N-termini of nascent polypeptide chains provides a specific means for their identification. The products of this synthesis are restricted to certain minority proteins of the inner mitochondrial membrane, and among the respiratory chain contribute only to the elaboration of a functional cytochrome oxidase, which also requires the participation of products of cytoplasmic protein synthesis.

RESUMEN

Las partículas responsables de la síntesis de proteínas en las mitocondrias de *Saccharomyces cerevisiae* son ribosomas con coeficientes de sedimentación de 75S arregladas en agregados polisomales. La incorporación de formato radioactivo en el N-terminal de las cadenas polipeptídicas nacientes provee una forma especifica de identificación Los productos de esta síntesis se limitan a cierto número de proteínas menores pertenecientes a le membrana mitocondrial interna, y en la cadena respiratoria, contribuyen solamente a le elaboración de un citocromo oxidasa, la cual requiere además la participación de productos de la síntesis de proteínas citoplásmicas.

REFERENCES

1. Roodyn, D. B., and Wilkie, D., *The Biogenesis of Mitochondria,* Methuen, London (1968).
2. Nass, S., *Internat. Rev. Cytol., 25,* 55 (1969).
3. Rabinowitz, M., and Swift, H., *Physiol. Rev., 50,* 376 (1970).
4. Borst, P., and Kroon, A. M., *Internat. Rev. Cytol., 26,* 107 (1969).
5. McLean, J. R., Cohn, G. L., Brandt, J. K., and Simpson, M. V., *J. Biol. Chem., 233,* 657 (1958).
6. Rendi, R., *Exptl. Cell Res., 17,* 585 (1959); see also Mager, J., *Biochim. Biophys. Acta, 38,* 150 (1968).
7. Schatz, G., in Racker, E. (ed.), *Membrane of Mitochondria and Chloroplast,* Van Nostrand and Reinhold, New York (1970), p. 251.
8. Ashwell, M., and Work, T. E., *Ann. Rev. Biochem., 39,* 251 (1970).
9. Linnane, A. W., and Haslam, J. M., *Curr. Topics Cell. Regulation, 2,* 101 (1970).
10. Borst, P., and Grivell, L. A., *FEBS Letters, 13,* 73 (1971).
11. Beattie, D., *Sub-Cell. Biochem., 1,* 1 (1971).
12. Vermia, I. M., Edelman, M., and Littauer, V. Z., *Europ. J. Biochem., 19,* 124 (1971).
13. Clark-Walker, G. D., and Linnane, A. W., *Biochem. Biophys. Res. Commun., 25,* 8 (1966).
14. Lamb, A. J., Clark-Walker, G. D., and Linnane, A. W., *Biochim. Biophys. Acta, 161,* 415 (1968).
15. Schmitt, H., *Europ. J. Biochem., 17,* 278 (1970); but see *FEBS Letters, 4,* 234, (1969).
16. Stegeman, W. J., Coper, C S., and Avers, C. J., *Biochem. Biophys. Res. Commun., 39,* 691 (1970).
17. Grinell, L. A., Reÿnders, L., and Borst, P., *Biochim. Biophys. Acta, 247,* 91 (1971).
18. Kaempfer, R., *Nature, 222,* 950 (1969).
19. Morimoto, H., and Halvorson, H. O., *Proc. Natl. Acad. Sci. U.S.A., 68,* 324 (1971).
20. Vignais, P. U., Huet, J., and Andre, J., *FEBS Letters, 3,* 177 (1969).
21. Burn, C. C., Mitchell, C. H., Lukins, H. B., and Linnane, A. W., *Proc. Natl. Acad. Sci. U.S.A., 67,* 1233 (1970).
22. Forrester, I. T., Watson, K., and Linnane, A. W., *Biochem. Biophys. Res. Commun., 43,* 409 (1971); Dixon, H., Kellerman, G. M., Mitchell, C. H., Towers, N. H., and

Linnane, A. W., *Biochem. Biophys. Res. Commun. 43,* 780 (1971).

23. Scragg, A. H., Morimoto, H., Villa, V., Nekhorocheff, J., and Halvorson, H. O., *Science, 171,* 908 (1971).
24. Richter, D., and Lipman, F., *Biochemistry, 9,* 5065 (1970).
25. Perani, A., Tiboni, O., and Ciferri, O., *J. Mol. Biol., 55,* 107 (1971); *cf.* Ciferri, O., Parisi, A., Perani, A., and Grandi, M., *J. Mol. Biol., 37,* 529 (1968).
26. Parisi, B., and Cella, R., *FEBS Letters, 14,* 209 (1971).
27. Perlman, S., and Penman, S., *Nature, 227,* 133 (1970); *Biochem. Biophys. Res. Commun., 40,* 941 (1970).
28. Brega, A., and Vesco, C., *Nature New Biol., 229,* 136 (1971).
29. Pestka, S., *Ann. Rev. Biochem., 40,* 697 (1971).
30. Grandi, M., Helms, A., and Küntzel, H., *Biochem. Biophys. Res. Commun., 44,* 864 (1971).
31. DeVries, H., Agsteribba, E., and Kroon, A. M., *Biochim. Biophys. Acta, 246,* 111 (1971).
32. Smith, A. E., and Marcker, K. A., *J. Mol. Biol., 38,* 241 (1968).
33. Galper, J. G., and Darnell, J. E., *Biochem. Biophys. Res. Commun., 34,* 205 (1969); *J. Mol. Biol., 57,* 363 (1971). end of tape
34. Bianchetti, R., Lucchini, G., and Santirana, M. L., *Biochem. Biophys. Res. Commun., 42,* 97 (1971).
35. Halbreich, A., and Rabinowitz, M., *Proc. Natl. Acad. Sci. U.S.A., 68,* 294 (1971).
36. Smith, A. E., and Marcker, K. A., *Nature, 226,* 607 (1970); Brown, J. C., and Smith, A. E., *Nature 226,* 610 (1970).
37. Wilson, D. B., and Dintzis, H. M., *Proc. Natl. Acad. Sci. U.S.A., 66,* 1282 (1970).
38. Marcus, A., Weeks, D. G., Leis, J. P., and Keller, E. B., *Proc. Natl. Acad. Sci. U.S.A., 67,* 1681 (1970).
39. Tarragó, A., Monasterio, O., and Allende, J. E., *Biochem. Biophys. Res. Commun., 41,* 765 (1970); Monasterio, O., Tarragó, A., and Allende, J. E., *J. Biol. Chem., 246,* 1539 (1971).
40. Richter, D., Lipmann, F., Tarragó, A., and Allende, J. E., *Proc. Natl. Acad. Sci. U.S.A., 68,* 1805 (1971).
41. Mans, R., and Novelli, G. D., *Arch. Biochem. Biophys., 94,* 48 (1961).
42. Kuff, E. L., and Roberts, N. E., *J. Mol. Biol., 26,* 211 (1967); see also Zomzely, C. E., Roberts, S., Brown, D. M., and Provost, C., *J. Mol. Biol., 20,* 455 (1966).
43. Henson, C. P., Weber, C. N., and Mahler, H. R., *Biochemistry, 7,* 4431 (1968).
44. Schweyen, R., and Kaudewitz, R., *Biochem. Biophys. Res. Commun., 38,* 728 (1970).
45. Kellerman, G. M., Griffiths, D. E., Hansby, J. E., Lamb, A. J., and Linnane, A. W., in Boardman, N. K., Linnane, A. W., and Smillie, R. M. (eds.), *Autonomy and Biogenesis of Mitochondria and Chloroplasts,* American Elsevier, New York (1971), p. 346.
46. Mahler, H. R., Perlman, P., and Mehrotra, B., in Boardman, N. K., Linnane, A. W., and Smillie, R. M. (eds.), *Autonomy and Biogenesis of Mitochondria and Chloroplasts,* American Elsevier, New York (1971), p. 492.
47. Neupert, W., Massinger, P., and Pfaller, A., in Boardman, N. K., Linnane, A. W., and Smillie, R. M. (eds.), *Autonomy and Biogenesis of Mitochondria and Chloroplasts,* American Elsevier, New York (1971), p. 328.
48. Hawley, E. S., and Greenawalt, J. W., *J. Biol. Chem., 245,* 3574 (1970).
49. Henson, C. P., Perlman, P., Weber, C. N., and Mahler, H. R., *Biochemistry, 7,* 4431 (1968).
50. Mahler, H. R., and Perlman, P. S., *Biochemistry, 10,* 2979 (1971).
51. Neupert, W., and Ludwig, G. D., *Europ. J. Biochem., 19,* 523 (1971).

52. Fish, W. W., Reynolds, J. A., and Tanford, C., *J. Biol. Chem., 245,* 5166 (1970); Trayer, H. R., Nozaki, Y., Reynolds, J. A., and Tanford, C., *J. Biol. Chem., 246,* 4485 (1971).
53. Mahler, H. R., Mackler, B., Slonimski, P. P., and Grandchamp, S., *Biochemistry, 3,* 677 (1964); Mahler, H. R., Neiss, G., Slonimski, P. P., and Mackler, B., *Biochemistry, 3,* 893 (1964).
54. Mackler, B., Douglas, H. C., Will, S., Hawthrone, D. C., and Mahler, H. R., *Biochemistry, 4,* 2016 (1965).
55. Mahler, H. R., Tewari, K. K., and Jayaraman, J., in Mills, A. K. (ed.), *Aspects of Yeast Metabolism* (Dublin Symposium, September 1965). Blackwell, Oxford (1967), p. 247.
56. Kraml, J., and Mahler, H. R., *Immunochemistry, 4,* 213 (1967).
57. Mehrotra, B. D., and Mahler, H. R., *Arch. Biochem. Biophys., 128,* 685 (1968).
58. Mahler, H. R., in Chance, B. (ed.), *Probes of Structure and Function of Macromolecules and Membranes,* Vol. 1, Academic Press, New York (1971), p. 411.
59. Perlman, P. S., and Mahler, H. R., *Arch. Biochem. Biophys., 136,* 245 (1970).
60. Perlman, P. S., and Mahler, H. R., *J. Bioenergetics, 1,* 113 (1970).
61. Mahler, H. R., Mehrotra, B. D., and Perlman, P. S., *Prog. Mol. Subcellular Biol., 2,* 274 (1971).
62. Schatz, G., *J. Biol. Chem., 243,* 2192 (1968).
63. Tzagoloff, A., *J. Biol. Chem., 244,* 5006 (1969); *245,* 1545 (1970); *246,* 3050 (1971); and in press.
64. Bernardi, G., Carnevali, F., Nicolaeff, A., Piperno, G., and Tecce, C., *J. Mol. Biol., 37,* 493 (1968).
65. Goldring, E. S., Grossman, L. I., Krupnick, D., Cryer, D. R., and Marmur, J., *J. Mol. Biol., 52,* 323 (1970); Goldring, E. S., Grossman, L. I., and Marmur, J., *J. Bacteriol., 107,* 377 (1971).
66. Nagley, P., and Linnane, A. W., *Biochem. Biophys. Res. Commun., 39,* 989 (1970).
67. South, D. J., and Mahler, H. R., *Nature, 218,* 1226 (1968).
68. Fukuhara, H., and Kujawa, C., *Biochem. Biophys. Res. Commun., 41,* 1002 (1970).
69. Kellerman, G. M., Biggs, D. A., and Linnane, A. W., *J. Cell Biol., 42,* 378 (1969).
70. Perlman, P.S., and Mahler, H. R., *Nature New Biology, 231,* 12 (1971).
71. Tuppy, H., and Birkmayer, C. D., *Europ. J. Biochem., 8,* 237 (1969).
72. Chen, W. L., and Charalampous, F. C., *J. Biol. Chem., 244,* 2767 (1969).
73. Shakespeare, P., and Mahler, H. R., *J. Biol. Chem., 246,* 7649 (1971).
74. Weiss, H., Sebald, W., and Bucher, T., *Europ. J. Biochem., 22,* 19 (1971).
75. Birkmayer, G. D., *Europ. J. Biochem., 21,* 258 (1971).
76. Swanson, R. F., *Nature, 231,* 31 (1971).
77. Attardi, B., and Attardi, G., *Proc. Natl. Acad. Sci. U.S.A., 58,* 1051 (1967); *61,* 261 (1968).
78. Gordon, G. N., and Sinsheimer, R. L., *Biochim. Biophys. Acta, 149,* 476 (1967).
79. Weisldgel, P. O., and Butow, R. A., *J. Biol. Chem., 246,* 5113 (1971).
80. Thomas, D. Y., and Williamson, D. H., *Nature New Biol., 233,* 196 (1971).
81. Yang, S., and Criddle, R. S., *Biochemistry, 9,* 3063 (1970).
82. Swank, R. T., Shier, G. I., and Munckres, K. D., *Biochemistry, 10,* 3924 (1971).

DISCUSSION

W. Colli (São Paulo, Brazil): Has someone looked to see if the mitochondrial RNA polymerase is coded for by a mitochondrial or a nuclear gene?

H. R. Mahler (Bloomington, U.S.A.): In all likelihood, although some controls still remain to be done, data from Wintersberger's, Criddle's, and our own laboratory suggest that since mitochondrial RNA polymerase is present in DNA-minus mutants (DNA-minus mutants being mutants that contain a mitochondrial DNA with a base composition of 96% adenine plus thymine and hence probably nonfunctional for coding purposes) it is specified by extramitochondrial genes. It is not present, Criddle has shown, in some DNA-zero mutants, but that is not surprising if DNA itself provides one of the anchoring points for the enzyme inside the mitochondria. Tentatively, the extramitochondrial specification also holds true certainly for one type of DNA polymerase activity that has been studied, since DNA-minus mutants replicate their DNA.

R. P. Perry (Philadelphia, U.S.A.): There have been some reports from Penman's laboratory and also from Chi and Suyama that the mitochondrial ribosomes have an unusually low buoyant density, indicating a higher than average protein/RNA ratio. Do you have any data along these lines?

H. R. Mahler: I have no data on these particular lines. These reports are both from work with animal mitochondria.

R. P. Perry: No, Chi and Suyama worked with yeast.

H. R. Mahler: Are you sure? No, I do not think so. That was with some protozoan. (Actually, *Tetrahymena.*)

A. S. Spirin (Moscow, USSR): Could you tell me what magnesium concentration you use in the experiments with cosedimentation of *E. coli* ribosomes, cytoplasmic ribosomes, and mitochondrial ribosomes?

H. R. Mahler: The magnesium concentration was 10 mM.

A. S. Spirin: And the monovalent ion concentration?

H. R. Mahler: The monovalent cation concentration was 100 mM NH$_4^+$, 10 mM tris.

A. S. Spirin: Did you try to fix ribosomes with formaldehyde before the sedimentation run?

H. R. Mahler: We have not done that yet, but it is on the list.

A. S. Spirin: And the buoyant density determination?

H. R. Mahler: That is the same thing that Dr. Perry asked. That is on the list. Dr. Spirin, we have been trying to be sure that we are dealing with a homogeneous population of uncontaminated ribosomes before undertaking any physical studies. I think now we are in a position to do so.

M. Burgos (Mendoza, Argentina): Is there any evidence for the synthesis or the presence of a contractile protein in the mitochondria?

H. R. Mahler: We have not done any work along these lines. We have followed the literature with a great deal of interest, and I think the current position would be that although mitochondria are capable of extrusion of water very, very actively, the presence of a myosin or actomyosin protein in mitochondria has not been substantiated.

R. Brentani (São Paulo, Brazil): If I understood correctly, the synthesis of DPN-cytochrome *c* reductase, while outside the mitochondria, was still inhibited by antimycin A.

H. R. Mahler: No, I refer to the NAD-cytochrome *c* reductase or succinate-cytochrone *c* reductase as the antimycin A-sensitive component. In answer to your question, the evidence concerning the extramitochondrial synthesis is completely unambiguous for both these entities. There is no question whatsoever that the whole respiratory chain prior to cytochrome *c* is not made by the mitochondria. I am not talking about the energy transduction mechanism now, but I am talking about the respiratory chain in the stricter sense.

P. P. Cohen (Madison, U.S.A.): Have you looked at the EM of these cells for any evidence of a structure in which transport of the extramitochondrial proteins might be insured to the mitochondria? We have proposed such a system in animal mitochondria, and if there is to be a significant and efficient production and utilization there must be a specific transport channel into these mitochondria.

H. R. Mahler: I could not agree more. We have looked very hard, but there are other groups more competent in electron microscopy than we are. There is no question that under appropriate conditions, particularly under conditions of maximal mitochondriogenesis or mitochondrial differentiation, as for instance during release from catabolite repression, you see structures that if you wish to be optimistic you could call "endoplasmic reticulum analogues" which practically envelope the mitochondria. This was done mainly by Schmitt in Belgium, and it is a fact that there exists a class of membrane-bound extramitochondrial ribosomes that is almost impossible to eliminate unless you use rather drastic methods. These two lines of evidence indicate to me that inquiries in that direction will definitely be fruitful in the future. Yes, there has to be a channel, there has to be a fairly direct communication. Let me give you one item of information that is pertinent to this. During release from catabolite repression, there is no way of establishing the transit time of pulse-labeled proteins synthesized in the cytoplasm into the inner membrane proteins of the mitochondria. In other words, the shortest time at which you can shear cells and break them open by mechanical means, to use them to purify mitochondria in the presence of inhibitors to stop any further protein synthesis, is 30 sec. In 30 sec, you already have cycloheximide-sensitive label entering the inner mitochondrial membrane. So not only does there have to be a channel of communication, it has to be an exceedingly efficient channel.

S. S. de Favelukes (Buenos Aires, Argentina): Can fusidic acid be used to differentiate mitochondrial protein synthesis *in vitro* from bacterial contamination?

H. R. Mahler: Yes, on the basis of Küntzel's results, very definitely. This is for *Neurospora*, but it has not been checked for yeast or for animal mitochondria. It is no problem in *Neurospora*.

F. L. Sacerdote (Mendoza, Argentina): I would like to ask you if this rather unfortunate situation that you have just described, of it being very difficult to get rid of elements of endoplasmic reticulum wrapping mitochondria, is restricted in your opinion to yeast or would you extrapolate that this difficulty also exists for animal cells?

H. R. Mahler: Well, as Dr. Cohen indicated, there is plenty of cytological evidence of intimate association of ER, particularly with the outer membrane; there are quite striking similarities in membrane composition and so forth. However, I am not competent to answer the particular question that you asked. My organism is *Saccharomyces cerevisiae*.

E. Bustamante Donayre (Lima, Peru): What is the percentage of component polypeptides in mitochondrial proteins synthesized by mitochondrial ribosomes, having methionine as the amino terminal residue, especially in the inner membrane?

H. R. Mahler: That is not an easy question to answer, because even among the inner mitochondrial membrane proteins, only a very small percentage, on the order of somewhere between 10-20% is contributed by the intramitochondrial system. Even if one found that only a very small fraction was initiated with methionine, the possibility of the removal of methionine by aminopeptidase has not encouraged investigations of this sort. I think now it will become definitely worthwhile to subfractionate mitochondria to obtain fractions that other lines indicate as being at least in large part provided by the mitochondrial system, and then look for methionine and even formylmethionine. There was a strange report last year, in the *Biochem Quickies*, that has probably gone unnoticed, that in honey bee mitochondria there appears to be formylmethionine persistent in the mature organelle.

A. O. M. Stoppani (Buenos Aires, Argentina): Does the aggregation state of yeast cytochrome oxidase have any effect on the catalytic properties of the enzyme?

H. R. Mahler: I cannot say much about the state of aggregation when cytochrome oxidase is still partly integrated into the inner mitochondrial membrane. Obviously, some of the characteristic features that allow one to assign certain aspects of the oxidase to a and the others to a_3, such as differential reduction or formation of carbon monoxide and cyanide complexes and so forth, are different for the membrane-bound and the solubilized enzyme, but that is true of the heart muscle enzyme, also. However, one can obtain the yeast enzyme in both an unaggregated and an aggregated form. One can obtain it in three forms: as a 100,000 molecular weight monomer; on standing, this is converted to a 200,000 molecular weight dimer which then has properties virtually indistinguishable from the heart muscle enzyme as ordinarily isolated. Stotz recently monomerized the heart muscle enzyme by exposure to alkali, and ours is somewhat similar to that one in its monomeric form. By omitting detergent, in particular during the isolation of the enzyme, one can also obtain the enzyme in a more highly aggregated form. All these three forms have the same catalytic constant.

A. O. M. Stoppani: The second question may have been in the mind of the previous discussant, and it is if you could make a comment about the mechanisms concerning the simultaneous and orderly operation of the mitochondrial and extramitochondrial protein synthetic systems.

H. R. Mahler: Obviously, very tight coordination between the two systems exists. We have looked very, very hard, particularly for the passage of signals. Because operationally it is somewhat easier, we have been interested in the passage of signals from the mitochondrion into the cytoplasm to set levels of certain cytoplasmic enzymes. This can be done rather neatly during release from catabolite repression and then the simultaneous use of various site-specific inhibitors of mitochondrial translation or transcription or mitochondrial functions such as antimycin A. We have been completely unsuccessful in demonstrating the passage of any such signals. That does not mean that such signals may not exist, but so far the application of techniques that have been quite successful in delineating the contribution of the two systems inside the mitochondria have been spectacularly unsuccessful in defining any mitochondrial contributions in the regulation of the extramitochondrial space. Nevertheless, I firmly believe that such things do exist, and the converse, also.

39

Stimulation of the Synthesis of Inner Mitochondrial Membrane Proteins in Rat Liver by Cuprizone

Néstor F. González-Cadavid, Flor Herrera, Alba Guevara, and Aíxa Viera

Departamento de Biología Celular
Facultad de Ciencias
Universidad Central de Venezuela
Caracas, Venezuela

During the past 5 years, an increasing body of evidence has confirmed earlier suggestions favoring the autonomy of the mitochondrial protein synthesizing machinery based on the ability of isolated organelles to incorporate amino acids into protein (1-3). Rather paradoxically, the discovery of mitochondrial DNA, RNA, polymerases, ribosomes, tRNA, etc., was concomitant with a progressive decrease in what was considered to be the degree of autonomy of mitochondrial replication. The initial evaluation of the very restricted information content of mitochondrial DNA (4) and the demonstration that cytochrome c is coded by the nuclear genome (5) was soon followed by proof of the synthesis of this mitochondrial protein by cytoplasmic ribosomes (6,7). Other proteins, such as those of mitochondrial ribosomes (8,9), outer membrane proteins (10), cytochrome oxidase (11,12), cytochrome b (12), and ATPase (13), were later shown to be synthesized outside the organelle. A recent assessment of the amount of protein synthesized by endogenous mitochondrial activity (14) implies that 90% of the mitochondrial proteins are, in fact, manufactured by 80S ribosomes.

Apparently, the organelle is only able to synthesize some large insoluble proteins (11) and perhaps peptides (15).

This situation poses several important questions; the question of particular interest to us is whether or not there is any functional specialization of cytoplasmic ribosomes for the synthesis of mitochondrial proteins. In other words, does this process take place in a section of the ribosomal population, or can it occur in virtually all the functionally active polysomes? If the first alternative is correct, is this restriction absolute or is there only a degree of topological segregation so that mitochondrial proteins are synthesized near the site of synthesis of other kinds of proteins? A first query in this direction concerns the role of free and membrane-bound polysomes in the synthesis of mitochondrial proteins, since there are conflicting views on this subject (16-18).

The clarification of this point would be a step forward in the study of the mechanisms that control the formation of mitochondrial proteins outside the organelle, particularly the possibility that signals of mitochondrial origin intervene in this regulation (e.g., transfer to the cytoplasm of mRNA or tRNA elaborated in the organelle).

A feasible approach to these problems is the use of drugs that preferentially inhibit or stimulate the synthesis of mitochondrial proteins in order to disturb the normal balance of formation of different kinds of cell proteins. In this way, one could expect to recognize those polysomes within the whole ribosomal population which are actively making mitochondrial proteins, since on a suitable fractionation they might be identified by a larger variation in their synthesizing ability. Similarly, the proteins which are more affected by the drugs are likely to be those which would be later exported to the mitochondria.

The first step is to demonstrate a clear-cut effect which justifies the use of a particular drug as a tool for our purpose. This is somewhat difficult, because a less drastic change is expected in the metabolic balance of cells in higher organisms as compared to lower eukaryotes such as yeast or fungi. Furthermore, if one considers that the mitochondria have about 30% of the total protein of the cell (19), and one assumes similar rates of synthesis for the average mitochondrial and nonmitochondrial protein, one would expect that a 50% change in the specific radioactivity of mitochondrial proteins would result from only a 20% variation in the overall protein-synthesizing abilitiy of the cytoplasmic ribosomes.

In principle, there are several inhibitors of mitochondrial protein synthesis which could be used for this purpose: chloramphenicol, oxytetracycline, erythromycin, and carbomycin are the most well known (20,21). Inhibitors of mitochondrial transcription, such as ethidium bromide and euflavine, can also be considered in this context (21).

Administration of chloramphenicol to partially hepatectomized rats for long periods results in the appearance of functionally defective liver mitochondria

(22). This effect is reversible and seems to be related to a small but significant inhibition in the specific radioactivity of the microsomal membrane (23) and in the *in vitro* protein-synthesizing ability of the isolated microsomal fraction (24). The stimulators of mitochondrial protein synthesis, with the possible exception of thyroid hormones (25,26), have been less studied in this respect. An amino-azo dye, 2-Me-DAB (27), atromid (28), and cuprizone (29) are all potential tools which require first a clarification of the degree of specificity of their effect as on mitochondrial *vs.* nonmitochondrial protein synthesis.

Another approach is to assess *in vitro* synthesis of specific mitochondrial proteins by different polysomal fractions. This is of course limited by the availability of a subcellular system that is able to carry out the net synthesis, or

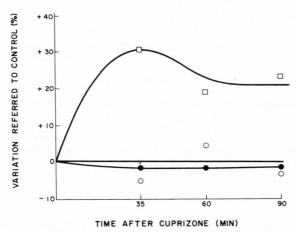

TIME AFTER CUPRIZONE (MIN)

Fig. 1. *Stimulation of the synthesis of mitochondrial proteins by cuprizone* in vivo. Male Sprague-Dawley rats (150 ± 10 g) were injected intraperitoneally with 2 ml of 0.15 *M* NaCl with or without 100 μg/ml of cuprizone. At various times, 5 μc of ^{14}C amino acids (54 *mc/m*Atom C) were given through the tail vein. The rats were killed 30 min later, and subcellular fractionation of the liver was carried out as previously described (22), except that the preparation of the mitochondrial fraction involved rehomogenization and washings of the nuclear pellet (30) followed by purification by the procedure of Sottocasa *et al.* (31). The radioactivity was determined on glass fiber discs (32) by liquid scintillation counting, and protein was estimated by the method of Lowry *et al.* (33). All values are averages of two separate experiments. □, Mitochondrial fraction (control value 207 dpm/mg); ○, microsomal fraction (control value 1036 dpm/mg); ●, homogenate (control value 428 dpm/mg).

Table I. Preferential Stimulation by Cuprizone of the
in vitro Synthesis of Mitochondrial Proteins in Liver Slices[a]

| | Protein specific radioactivity | | | |
| | No cycloheximide | | With cycloheximide | |
	Control value (dpm/mg)	Cuprizone/ control ratio	Control value (dpm/mg)	Cuprizone/ control ratio
Homogenate	3360	1.05	270	0.95
Mitochondria	1615	1.27	300	1.40
Microsomal fraction	10500	0.84	600	0.99

[a] Slices from 4 g of liver were washed for 20 min in 30 ml of Peters and Anfinsen medium (34), supplemented with 20 mM glucose, in 250 ml erlenmeyer flasks gassed with O_2-CO_2 (95-5%), at 37°, and then incubated for 30 min under the same conditions with fresh medium with or without 20 μg/ml of cuprizone. A mixture of ^{14}C amino acids was added to 0.5 μc/ml final concentration, and the incubation proceeded for 60 min. Mitochondria were obtained from an aliquot as described in Fig. 1. In another experiment, slices from 1 g of liver were incubated in a similar procedure, except that the final volume was 9 ml, the ^{14}C amino acid concentration was 1.1 μc/ml, and cychoheximide (0.5 mg/ml) was present in the incubation medium. Mitochondria were prepared directly by the procedure of Sottocasa *et al.* (31).

at least the elongation, of a well-characterized and homogeneous mitochondrial protein. The only case reported is the synthesis of cytochrome *c* by the isolated microsomal fraction of regenerating liver (30); however, the activity obtained is not entirely satisfactory for our purpose.

In the present work, we have restricted our interest to the study of the effect of cuprizone (bis-cyclohexanone oxaldihydrazone), a drug which induces the production of giant mitochondria in the liver of mice (29), on the synthesis of mitochondrial proteins both inside and outside the organelle. Our results, in combination with those obtained on the synthesis *in vitro* of cytochrome *c*, suggest that membrane-bound polysomes are the sites of the formation of the mitochondrial proteins.

RESULTS AND CONCLUSIONS

Our first aim was to decide if cuprizone preferentially enhances the synthesis of mitochondrial proteins or if it exerts a nonspecific effect. Secondly, can the stimulation be achieved by a single dose rather than by the rather long treatment necessary for the appearance of giant mitochondria? Figure 1 shows that the injection of 200 μg of cuprizone followed 5 min later by ^{14}C-leucine increased the specific radioactivity of the mitochondrial proteins when the rats were killed after a 30 min incubation period. The average radioactivity of the rest of the cell proteins was nearly unaffected. The effect apparently lasts for at least 90 min after injection, but at a lower level.

In order to investigate whether cuprizone acts directly on the hepatocyte, we incubated liver slices with 20 μg/ml of the drug, either by itself or in the presence of 0.5 mg/ml of cycloheximide to suppress microsomal protein synthesis. Table I shows that in both cases there is 30-40% stimulation of the synthesis of mitochondrial proteins, suggesting a direct effect of cuprizone on the mitochondrial protein-synthesizing machinery. A subfractionation performed with the same material demonstrated a preferential effect on the formation of mitochondrial inner membrane proteins (Table II). Higher doses of cuprizone (50 μg/ml) were slightly inhibitory.

Since the long-term effect of cuprizone *in vivo* is the induction of enlarged mitochondria, we wanted to look at the short-term effects of the drug on protein synthesis *in vitro*. The mitochondria, obtained from incubated liver slices by applying two different procedures of isolation, were fractionated by sedi-

Table II. Preferential Stimulation by Cuprizone of the *in vitro* Synthesis of Mitochondrial Membrane Proteins in Liver Slices[a]

| | Protein specific radioactivity | | | |
| | No cycloheximide | | With cycloheximide | |
	Control value (dpm/mg)	Cuprizone/ control ratio	Control value (dpm/mg)	Cuprizone/ control ratio
Matrix proteins	1740	1.17	368	0.93
Outer membrane proteins	2100	1.15	83	1.40
Inner membrane proteins	1360	1.40	369	1.58
Cytochrome oxidase	1070	1.45	–	–

[a] Mitochondria from the experiments described in Table I were subfractionated in the same way, applying the procedure of Sottocasa *et al.* (31). Purified cytochrome oxidase was prepared from the remainder of the "crude" mitochondrial fraction from the experiment without cycloheximide, as described by Jacobs *et al.* (35) but including several steps of fractionation with $(NH_4)_2SO_4$.

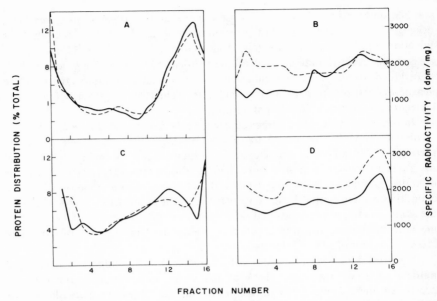

Fig. 2. Effect of cuprizone on the distribution and specific radioactivity of the mitochon-drial population fractionated by sedimentation velocity through a sucrose gradient. (A,B) Slices from 1 g of liver were incubated as described in Table I, except that the final concentration of radioactivity was 0.44 μc/ml. Mitochondria were prepared directly by the procedure of Sottocasa *et al.* (31) and layered onto 4.8 ml of a 0.5-1.0 *M* linear sucrose gradient with 0.5 ml of a 2.2 *M* sucrose cushion. Centrifugation was performed in the SW25.1 rotor at 3700 × g for 20 min, operating without the brake. Fractions of 0.36 ml were collected and used for protein and radioactivity determinations. A, protein distribu-tion; B, specific radioactivity; solid line, control; dashed line, cuprizone. (C, D) The experiment is similar to that depicted in A and B, except that the preparation of the mitochondrial fraction involved rehomogenization and washings of the nuclear pellet (30) and sedimentation and washings of the mitochondria at 8000 × g for 10 min. C, protein distribution; D, specific radioactivity, solid line, control; dashed line, curpizone.

mentation velocity through a continuous linear gradient from 0.5 *M* to 1.0 *M* sucrose. No significant difference was observed in the distribution of protein between the control and cuprizone-treated rats (Fig. 2A, C). A uniform enhance-ment of the specific radioactivity throughout the gradient was obtained with a mitochondrial preparation representative of the total population (Fig. 2D). However, when the fractionation was done by a procedure yielding a preparation artificially enriched in light or smaller mitochondria, the stimulation was evident only in the bottom layers, which contain the larger organelles (Fig. 2B). A similar although more complex situation occurred in the fractionation of mito-chondria prepared from slices incubated with the drug and with cycloheximide or emetine (Fig. 3A, B).

The stimulation, however, is not completely uniform. Figure 4A shows a polyacrylamide gel electropherogram of a mixture of inner membrane proteins from a control incubated with ^{14}C-leucine and a cuprizone-treated sample incubated with ^{3}H-leucine. It is apparent that there are three bands with a higher ^{3}H/^{14}C ratio than the rest; this does not seem to be related to the rate of synthesis, which suggests that there was a preferential enhancement of the formation of some proteins. A similar result was obtained with intact mitochondria from the lower zone of the gradient (Fig. 4B).

It is important to try to correlate the stimulation of the synthesis with changes in the protein-synthesizing ability of the cytoplasmic ribosomes. If one simply looks at the specific radioactivity of the microsomal fraction, there does not seem to be any significant variation either *in vivo* (Fig. 1) or *in vitro* in liver slices (Table I). However, this fraction was obtained from a 300,000 × g supernatant, and it lacks the heavier membrane-bound polysomes. Another possible explanation is that the free and membrane-bound polysomes exhibit opposite behavior, and changes in their labeling are mutually counteracted. Since the polyribosome profile is disarranged after incubation of liver slices, we decided to examine these questions with an *in vivo* experiment.

We gave ^{14}C amino acids *in vivo*, obtained a postmitochondrial supernatant at 120,000 × g, and separated free and bound ribosomes through a two-layer gradient. The cuprizone-treated rats showed a 20% average stimulation in the specific radioactivity of the membrane-bound polysomes and no change in the free polysomes (Tabe III). A similar degree of stimulation was observed in the protein-synthesizing ability of the bound polysomes when incubated *in vitro* with ^{14}C amino acids (Table IV). Free polysomes and detergent-treated poly-

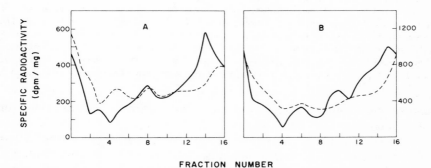

Fig. 3. Effect of cuprizone in vitro *on the endogenous protein-synthesizing ability of different mitochondrial populations.* (A) The experiment was performed as in Fig. 2A, B, except that the final concentration of radioactivity was 1.1 μc/ml and both incubation mixtures contained cycloheximide (0.5 mg/ml). (B) Similar to A, except that emetine (0.1 mg/ml) was substituted for cycloheximide.

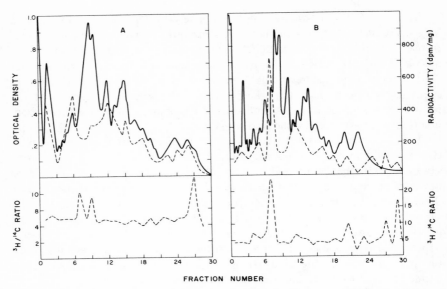

Fig. 4. *Preferential stimulation by cuprizone of the* in vitro *synthesis of certain kinds of mitochondrial proteins.* (A) Slices from 1 g of liver were incubated as described in Table I (without cycloheximide) except that the control had 2.2 μc/ml of L- U-^{14}C-leucine (330 μc/μmole) and the cuprizone had 22.2 μc/ml of L- G-^{3}H-leucine (250 μc/μmole). The mitochondrial inner membrane was prepared from a mixture of both samples applying the procedure of Sottocasa *et al.* (31). Polyacrylamide gel electrophoresis was carried out in duplicate in a 10% acrylamide, 1% SDS, 0.1 *M* phosphate, (*p*H 7.2) system (36), in 0.6 by 6.5 cm gels at 5 ma/gel for 5 hr. One sample (100 μg protein) was fixed and stained with Amido Black, and the other was cut in slices, treated with 0.1 ml of H_2O_2 at 50° for 6 hr, left for 18 hr at room temperature, and counted with 10 ml of a Triton X100-toluene scintillator (37). Solid line, densitometric tracing at 610 nm; dashed line, radioactivity of the cuprizone (^{3}H); dashed line (lower pattern), ^{3}H/^{14}C ratio of the cuprizone. (B) The experiment was similar to that of A except that the radioactivity was 2.2 μc/ml of ^{14}C-leucine and 11.1 μc/ml of L-4,5-^{3}H-leucine (3000 μc/μmole). Mitochondria were fractionated by sedimentation velocity as in Fig. 2A, B, and the bottom half of the gradient was pooled. Electrophoresis was done as in A, with the mitochondria sedimented at 2,000 × *g* for 10 min. Symbols as in A.

somes were slighly inhibited, suggesting a requirement of the membrane for stimulation.

This effect might be related to a decrease of the smaller polysomes in favor of the formation of the heavier ones (Fig. 5), which are more active in protein synthesis (39). In another experiment (results not shown here), no changes were observed in the incorporation of ^{14}C-uridine into the RNA associated with polysomes; it is likely, therefore, that the stimulation of protein synthesis by cuprizone is due to an effect at the level of translation. The increased activity was apparent particularly in the case of several protein classes separated by acrylamide electrophoresis (Fig. 6), some of which (e.g., No. 11) had the same mobility as those mitochondrial bands in Fig. 4 whose synthesis was more affected by the drug.

Table III. Stimulation by Cuprizone of *in vitro* Protein
Synthesis by Membrane-Bound Polysomes[a]

	RNA/protein ratio		Specific radioactivity	
	Control	Cuprizone	Control (dpm/mg RNA)	Cuprizone/ control ratio
Free polysomes	0.74	0.74	710	0.99
Bound polysomes	0.23	0.27	4250	1.21

[a] Each of two rats was treated as in Fig. 1. After 30 min, 5 μc of ^{14}C amino acid mixture was given intravenously. The rats were killed 30 min later, and free and bound polysomes were prepared according to the technique of Webb *et al.* (38) as modified by Ragnotti *et al.* (18), but using 2.0 M sucrose as bottom layer. Values are averages of four separate experiments.

Table IV. *In vivo* Stimulation by Cuprizone of the *in
vitro* Protein-Synthesizing Ability of Membrane-Bound
Polysomes[a]

	Specific radioactivity	
	Control (dpm/mg RNA)	Cuprizone/ control ratio
Free polysomes	15,820	0.86
Bound polysomes	11,400	1.22
Detergent-treated polysomes	14,750	0.93

[a] Each of two rats was treated as in Fig. 1. After 30 min the rats were killed, and free, bound, and detergent-treated polysomes were prepared as described in Table III. Incubations were performed for 30 min at 37° in a total volume of 0.5 ml containing ribosomal RNA (0.1-0.2 mg/ml), pH 5 fraction (p.5 mg protein/ml), ^{14}C amino acid mixture (0.25 μc/ml), Mg^{2+} (6 nM), K^+ (15 mM), sucrose (90 mM), Tris-Cl, pH 7.8 (20 mM0, phosphokinase (50 μg/ml), PEP (10 mM), ATP (2 mM), and GTP (0.25 mM). Values are averages of three separate experiments.

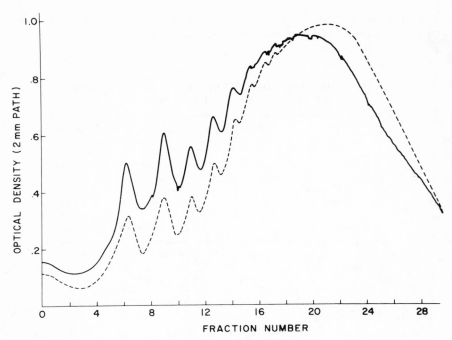

Fig. 5. Shift of the polyribosomal profile toward the region of larger polysomes by the effect of cuprizone in vivo. *Each of two rats was treated as in Fig. 1. After 30 min, the rats were killed and cytoplasmic polysomes were prepared as described in Table III. The pellet was dissolved in 1.0 ml of medium A (50 mM Tris-Cl, pH 7.8, 25 mM KCl, 5 mM MgSO$_4$) and layered onto a 15-50% linear sucrose gradient in medium A (18). After centrifugation for 3 hr at 25,000 rpm in the SW25.1 rotor operating without the brake, the gradient was pumped from the bottom at 1 ml/min through a 2 mm flow cell cuvette. A duplicate experiment gave essentially the same pattern.*

Perhaps the best proof supporting this indirect evidence in favor of the synthesis of mitochondrial proteins on membrane-bound polysomes was obtained with a different approach. Basically, it consisted of finding the polysome fraction that is able to carry out the synthesis of cytochrome *c in vitro*. The results appearing in Table V (González-Cadavid and González, unpublished data) show that the membrane-bound polysomes were around 15 times more active than the free polysomes in incorporating ^{14}C amino acids into cytochrome *c*. Similarly, the membrane seems to be necessary, since detergent-treated ribosomes were five times less active than the bound polysomes.

The main objective of the work so far presented was to discuss a strategy for the identification of the cytoplasmic polysomes engaged in the synthesis of mitochondrial proteins by using drugs which specifically or preferentially act on this process. We selected as an example the application of cuprizone, and although it induces some significant changes, it cannot be considered an ideal tool since the degree of stimulation is small and occasionally variable, perhaps due to its copper-chelating ability. But we hope that by applying this approach with other drugs it will be possible to select those compounds which elicit a

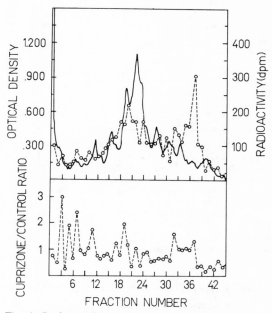

Fig. 6. *Preferential stimulation by cuprizone* in vivo *of the* in vitro *synthesis of certain kinds of proteins by membrane-bound polysomes.* The experiment was done as in Table IV, except that total volume was 2 ml and contained 100 μc of ^{3}H-leucine (3000 μc/μmole). Samples were precipitated with trichloroacetic acid and treated as in ref. 36. Polyacrylamide electrophoresis was carried out in 0.6 by 10 cm gels (100 μg protein) and 1.0 by 10 cm gels (300 μg protein) at 6 ma/cm^2 for 16 hr. Both gels contained ethylene diacrylate and glycerol. The first sample was fixed, stained, and used for densitometry, and the other was cut into slices and dissolved in H_2O_2-NH_3 (99:1) at 37° for 24 hr. After 12 hr standing at 0°, the vials were counted as in Fig. 4. Solid line, densitometric tracing at 610 nm; dashed line, radioactivity of the cuprizone, (lower pattern), cuprizone/control ratio.

Table V. *In vitro* **Synthesis of Cytochrome** *c* **by Membrane-Bound Polysomes**[a]

Experiment	Total protein (dpm/mg RNA)	Cytochrome c (dpm/mg RNA)	Cytochrome c/ protein ($\times 10^{-3}$)
I. ^{14}C amino acids (8 μc/ml)			
Detergent-treated polysomes	49,800	38	0.8
Bound polysomes	29,000	195	6.7
II. ^{3}H-leucine (6 μc/ml)[b]			
Detergent-treated polysomes	121,900	90	0.7
Free polysomes	76,600	26	0.3
Bound polysomes	71,000	390	5.5

[a] Free, bound, and detergent-treated polysomes were prepared from the livers of three rats as described in Table III. Incubations were performed at 37° for 30 min in 2.5 ml of medium containing ribosomal RNA (1-3 mg/ml), ATP (2 mM), PEP (10 mM), GTP (0.25 mM), phosphokinase (50 μg/ml), acetylglycine (2.5 mM), cytochrome c (0.1 mg), hemin (8 μM), Cleland's reagent (1 mM), cell sap (4 mg protein/ml), and the radioactive precursors. When labeled leucine was used, it was supplemented with an amino acid mixture (0.5 mM each). Cytochrome c was extracted, purified, estimated, and counted as previously described (32). Results are taken from unpublished data of González-Cadavid and González.
[b] Average of two separate experiments.

more definite response. This would allow a preliminary screening of the polysomal fractions before moving to such complex experiments as the *in vitro* synthesis of specific mitochondrial proteins. Of course, the main problem remains: how can one achieve a suitable fractionation of the polysomes that might correlate with their segregation by functional specialization? The use of antibodies against mitochondrial proteins, similar to what has been done with albumin (4), is a very interesting possibility and is under current investigation in our laboratory. We think that the application of drugs along these lines can play an important role in the clarification of the interrelationship between mitochondrial biogenesis and the cytoplasmic machinery for protein synthesis.

ACKNOWLEDGMENTS

This work was supported by grant DF-S1-063 from the Consejo Nacional de Investigaciones Científicas y Tecnológicas. F. H. is a recipient of a research fellowship from the same institution.

SUMMARY

Electron microscopic studies have shown that cuprizone, a copper-chelating agent, induces the formation of giant mitochondria in the liver of mice which have been fed the drug for several days. In the present work, we investigated the mechanism of a short-term cuprizone effect. The incorporation of ^{14}C amino acids into mitochondrial proteins in rat liver *in vivo* was stimulated by the drug. A similar effect was observed *in vitro* in incubations of liver slices, in both the presence and the absence of cychoheximide or emetine. The higher increase in specific radioactivity was in the total inner membrane proteins and in certain specific proteins known to be made outside the organelle, such as cytochrome oxidase. Polyacrylamide gel electrophoresis was used to show differential stimulation in some of the protein bands.

These changes were accompanied *in vivo* by a higher specific radioactivity in the membrane-bound polysomes and a slight shift of the polyribosomal profile toward the region of larger aggregates. Isolated bound polysomes from cuprizone-treated rats also showed a higher protein-synthesizing ability *in vitro*. These results suggest that the cytoplasmic synthesis of mitochondrial proteins takes place on membrane-bound polyribosomes. Further support for this assumption comes from experiments which showed that ^{14}C amino acid incorporation into cytochrome *c* occurs mainly in this class of ribosomes.

RESUMEN

Estudios de microscopía electrónica han demostrado que la cuprizona, un agente quelante, induce la formación de mitocondrias gigantes en el hígado de ratones que han sido alimentados con la droga por varios dias. En el presente trabajo hemos investigado el mecanismo del efecto a corto plazo de la cuprizona. La incorporación de amino-ácidos- ^{14}C en las proteínas mitocondriales en el hígado de rata *in vivo* es estimulada por la droga. Un efecto similar se observó *in vitro* en incubaciones de cortes de hígado en la presencia o ausencia de cicloheximida o emetina. El mayor aumento en la radioctividad específica fue totales en las proteínas de la membrana interna, y en ciertas proteínas específicas las cuales se sabe son sintetizadas fuera del organito a electroforesis en gels de poliacrilamida permitió demostrar la estimulación diferencial de algunas de las bandas de proteínas.

Estos cambios son acompañados, *in vivo,* por una mayor radioactividad específica alta en los polisomas asociados a membranas, y un pequeño desplazamiento del patrón poliribosomal hacia la region de agregados más grandes. Los polisomas asociados, obtenidos de ratas tratadas con cuprizona demostraron además una mayor capacidad para sintetizar proteínas *in vitro*. Estos resultados sugieren que la síntesis citoplasmica de proteínas mitocondriales se lleva a cabo en polisomas asociados a membranas. Un mayor respaldo de esta idea proviene de experimentos que demostraron que la incorporación de aminoácidos- ^{14}C en citocromo *c* ocurre principalmente en esta clase de ribosomas.

REFERENCES

1. Roodyn, D. B., and Wilkie, D., *The Biogenesis of Mitochondria,* Methuen & Co., Ltd., London (1968).
2. Ashwell, M., and Works, T. S., *Ann. Rev. Biochem., 39,* 251 (1970).
3. Rabinowitz, M., and Swift, H., *Physiol. Rev., 50,* 376 (1970).

4. Sinclair, J. H., and Stevens, B. J., *Proc. Natl. Acad. Sci. U.S.A., 56,* 508 (1966).
5. Sherman, F., Stewart, J. W., Margoliash, E., Parker, J., and Campbell, W., *Proc. Natl. Acad. Sci. U.S.A., 55,* 1498 (1966).
6. González-Cadavid, N. F., and Campbell, P. N., *Biochem. J., 105,* 443 (1967).
7. González-Cadavid, N. F., Bravo, M., and Campbell, P. N., *Biochem. J., 107,* 523 (1968).
8. Kuntzel, H., *Nature, 222,* 142 (1969).
9. Davey, P. J., Yu, R., and Linnane, A. W., *Biochem. Biophys. Res. Commun., 36,* 30 (1969).
10. Neupert, W., and Ludwig, G. D., *Europ. J. Biochem., 19,* 523 (1971).
11. Beattie, D. S., Patton, G. M., and Stuchell, R. N., *J. Biol. Chem., 245,* 2177 (1970).
12. Krymkiewicz, N., and González-Cadavid, N. F., *Biochem. J., 116,* 269 (1970).
13. Tzagoloff, A., *J. Biol. Chem., 246,* 3050 (1971).
14. Hawley, E. S., and Greenawalt, J. W., *J. Biol. Chem., 245,* 3574 (1970).
15. Kadenbach, B., *Biochem. Biophys. Res. Commun., 44,* 724 (1971).
16. Campbell, P. N., *FEBS Letters, 7,* 1 (1970).
17. Andrews, T. M., and Tata, J. R., *Biochem. J., 121,* 683 (1971).
18. Ragnotti, G., Lawford, G. R., and Campbell, P. N., *Biochem. J., 112,* 139 (1969).
19. Baudhuin, P., and Berthet, J., *J. Cell Biol., 35,* 631 (1967).
20. Davey, P. J., Haslam, J. M., and Linnane, A. W., *Arch. Biochem. Biophys., 136,* 54 (1970).
21. Kroon, A. M., and De Vries, H., in Boardman, N. K., Linnane, A. W., and Smillie, R. M. (eds.), *Autonomy and Biogenesis of Mitochondria and Chloroplasts,* American Elsevier, New York (1971), p. 318.
22. González-Cadavid, N. F., Avila Bello, E. M., and Ramírez, J. L., *Biochem. J., 118,* 577 (1970).
23. González-Cadavid, N. F., and Ramírez, J. L., submitted for publication (1972).
24. González-Cadavid, N. F., and Ramírez, J. L., *Acta Cientif. Venezol., 22,* R-23 (1971).
25. Gross, N. J., *J. Cell Biol., 48,* 29 (1971).
26. Roodyn, D. B., Freeman, K. B., and Tata, J. R., *Biochem. J., 94,* 628 (1965).
27. Lafontaine, J. G., and Allard, C., *J. Cell Biol., 22,* 143 (1964).
28. Ramakrishna Kurup, C. K., Aithal, H. N., and Ramasarma, T., *Biochem. J., 116,* 773 (1970).
29. Suzuki, K., *Science, 163,* 81 (1969).
30. González-Cadavid, N. F., and Campbell, P. N., *Biochem. J., 105,* 427 (1967).
31. Sottocasa, G. L., Kuylenstierna, B., Ernster, L., and Bergstrand, A., *Methods Enzymol., 10,* 448 (1967).
32. González-Cadavid, N. F., Ortega, J. P., and González, M., *Biochem. J., 124,* 685 (1971).
33. Lowry, O. H., Rosebrough, N. J., Farr, A. L., and Randall, R. J., *J. Biol. Chem., 193,* 265 (1951).
34. Peters, T., and Anfinsen, C. S., *J. Biol. Chem., 186,* 805 (1950).
35. Jacobs, E. E., Kirkpatrick, F. H., Andrews, E. C., Cunningham, W., and Crane, F. L., *Biochem. Biophys. Res. Commun., 25,* 96 (1966).
36. Shapiro, A. L., Viñuela, E., and Maizel, J. V., *Biochem. Biophys. Res. Commun., 28,* 815 (1967).
37. Patterson M. S., and Greene, R. C., *Anal. Chem., 37,* 854 (1965).
38. Webb, T. E., Blobel, G., and Potter, V. R., *Cancer Res., 24,* 1229 (1964).
39. Noll, H., Staehelin, T., and Wettstein, F. O., *Nature, 198,* 632 (1963).
40. Sottocasa, G. L., Kuglenstierna, B., Ernster, L., and Bergstrand, A., *J. Cell Biol., 32,* 415 (1967).

DISCUSSION

F. L. Sacerdote (Mendoza, Argentina): You stated that you used a slice technique, whereas from some of your data it would appear that you had employed homogenates.

N. F. González-Cadavid (Caracas, Venezuela): No, actually when I say homogenates, I mean after incubation. I homogenized and I looked at the radioactivity of the total protein.

F. L. Sacerdote: May I ask you which technique for separation of the mitochondrial components you have used: osmotic shock or sonication?

N. F. González-Cadavid: We used a very well-known technique of Sottocasa *et al.* (40). It is a procedure where you disrupt the mitochondria in three stages. The first stage is swelling in a very hypotonic medium, then you shrink them, with ATP in the presence of magnesium, and then you apply ultrasonics followed by the separation of the fractions through a discontinuous gradient.

R. Brentani (Sao Paulo, Brazil): Have you studied whether or not there are differences between the size of the compartments of free and bound ribosomes when you feed this drug to the animals? Is there a shift of free ribosomes toward the membranes?

N. F. González-Cadavid: We looked at that, but we did not observe any change in this sense. I do not believe too much in those changes unless they are really very marked, because the recovery of free and bound polysomes in the case of liver is somewhat variable.

R. Brentani: It has been shown by Campbell in *in vitro* studies that, for instance, DPN-cytochrome *c* reductase can be synthesized equally well by free and bound ribosomes, which is somewhat different than what you have shown for cytochrome *c*. I wonder if you would care to comment on this discrepancy.

N. F. González-Cadavid: There is not actually a discrepancy, because there are two different enzyme locations. In the case of TPNH-cytochrome *c* reductase, the enzyme studied by Campbell and colleagues (18) is a microsomal membrane constituent, whereas cytochrome *c* is a mitochondrial one. There might be a slight discrepancy from the point of view of the general implications, because one extreme interpretation for our findings would be that membrane-associated proteins are made exclusively on membrane-bound polysomes. But in fact we studied only cytochrome *c*, and I do not know whether that holds true for other proteins.

40

Hormonal Effects
on Mitochondrial Protein Synthesis

S. S. de Favelukes,
M. Schwarcz de Tarlovsky,
C. D. Bedetti, and A. O. M. Stoppani

Instituto de Química Biológica
Facultad de Medicina
Universidad de Buenos Aires
Buenos Aires, Argentina

Isolated mitochondria from widely different biological sources are capable of synthesizing protein *in vitro* (1,2). Extensive studies have proved that the mitochondrial synthesizing apparatus resembles the better-known cytoplasmic and bacterial systems, especially the latter one.

The assessment of the biological significance of *in vitro* protein synthesis by isolated mitochondria has met with difficulties. For example: (a) Mitochondrial DNA, due to its low amount, can code for only a few proteins (3,4). In accord with this, it is found that the amount of protein synthesized *in vivo* and the amount of labeled amino acids incorporated *in vitro* are also low. *In vivo*, it represents only 10-15% of the mitochondrion's own proteins (5). (b) Labeled amino acids incorporated *in vitro* by mitochondria are located in the inner membrane, mostly in the fraction described as "structural protein" (6,7). This protein is not homogeneous and can be resolved into several components by polyacrylamide gel electrophoresis. Moreover, the "structural protein" apparently does not have an enzymatic function.

In contrast to the above summarized information stressing the limited extent of protein synthesis in mitochondria and the unknown functions of the protein synthesized in the organelle, there is evidence of an essential physiological role of the endogenously formed protein. Observations with yeast mitochondria are particularly relevant; e.g., induction of "petite" mutants by agents such as the acridines, under conditions that permit specific interaction of dye with mitochondrial DNA, prevents the synthesis of the inner membrane cytochromes a, a_3, b, and c_1 and the assembly of a competent respiratory chain (8).

It is currently accepted that a certain number of hormones exert some of their actions by controlling the intracellular level of key enzymes; one aspect of this control is the induction of specific proteins. Thyroid hormones, insulin, and estrogens are typical examples (9). Since mitochondria are normal constituents of tissues subject to endocrine control, it seems reasonable to postulate that normal growth and biosynthesis under the influence of endocrine factors will involve the biosynthesis in a coordinate manner of mitochondrial and extramitochondrial cell constituents. This hypothesis is fully supported by the following facts: (a) maturation and growth alike influence amino acid incorporation by isolated mitochondria from liver (10), brain (11), and skeletal muscle (12); (b) tissue regeneration, such as occurs after partial hepatectomy, enhances protein biosynthesis in liver mitochondria *in vitro;* (c) the same occurs after administration of thyroid hormones to thyroidectomized rats whose content of mitochondria is abnormally low.

Coordination between intra- and extramitochondrial protein synthesis aimed at producing new, normal mitochondria was shown by Tata and coworkers (13). They demonstrated that a single dose of thyroid hormones brought about an increase in the activity of a number of mitochondrial enzymes and simultaneously a parallel increase in the amino acid incorporating activity of the microsomal system. Shäfer and Nägel (14) also found remarkable alterations in the pattern of activity of several mitochondrial enzymes under the influence of these hormones. In our laboratory, a decrease in the activity of the mitochondrial enzyme hydroxybutyrate dehydrogenase (E.C. 1.1.1.30) was demonstrated by Roldan *et al.* (15) in diabetic dogs; the activity could be restored by insulin administration. Moreover, Boveris and Stoppani (16) found that with NAD-dependent substrates, steroids inhibit *in vitro* electron transport in the mitochondrial respiratory chain. On these grounds, it seemed of interest to investigate the possibility that this group of substances exerts an action on mitochondrial protein synthesis. As a complement to these studies, the action of testosterone both *in vitro* and *in vivo* was investigated. Insulin and testosterone seemed of particular interest, since both were reported to promote an increase in the activity of isolated muscle ribosomes. We decided to investigate whether or not there was a similar increase in the synthetic activity of muscle mitochondria.

This work is part of a more general program in which a study of mitochondrial synthetic activities and enzyme patterns in different hormonal situations will be undertaken.

EXPERIMENTAL METHODS

White male rats, weighing 150-180 g, were obtained from the Instituto de Fisiología de la Facultad de Medicina. Diabetes was induced by rapid intravenous injection of streptozotocin (17), dissolved in citrate buffer, pH 4.5, at a dose of 65 mg/kg; normal animals were administered the same volume of buffer. Alloxan, dissolved in saline, was administered at the same dose by the same route. The animals injected with the antibiotic were used 7 days later. Glycemias of all animals used were determined by the method of Nikkilä and Hyvärinen (18); the values obtained were 98 ± 14 mg % for normal rats and 318 ± 27 (± standard deviation) mg % for diabetic nonfasted rats.

Methods for the preparation of liver and muscle mitochondria, determinations of oxygen uptake, determination of the incorporation of amino acids into protein, and counting of the incorporated radioactivity have been described (12). Protein was determined by the biuret method in the presence of deoxycholate (19).

Incubation conditions for the incorporation of the radioactive amino acid by isolated mitochondria were as follows (the figures in parentheses correspond to the muscle mitochondria system): 100 mM sucrose, 1 mM EDTA, 20 mM Tris-HCl (pH 7.4), 12 mM MgSO$_4$ (8 mM), 16 mM phosphate, (pH 7.4), oxidizable substrate 10-10-5 mM malate-glutamate-malonate, 1 mM ADP, 50 μg of an amino acid mixture of composition similar to the liver cell sap (equimolar amino acid mixture for muscle mitochondria), 0.25 μc ^{14}C-leucine of specific activity 6.5 mc$_1$ mM and 3-4 mg (1 mg) mitochondrial protein. The final volume was 1 ml and the pH 7.4. The reaction mixture in 25 ml erlenmeyer flasks was shaken for 60 min in a water bath at 30°. Sterile conditions were maintained as completely as possible. All glassware was routinely sterilized; solutions employed in the isolation and incubation of mitochondria were sterilized by filtration in

Table I. Incorporation of ^{14}C-leucine by Skeletal
Muscle Mitochondria of Normal and Diabetic Rats[a]

Source of mitochondria	^{14}C-leucine incorporated (cpm/mg of protein)	Percent of normal
Normal	222 ± 46 (12)	—
Diabetic	107 ± 39 (12)	48

[a] Incubation conditions were as described in *Experimental Methods*. All determinations were done in triplicate. Figures in parentheses correspond to the number of animals.

Table II. Action of Streptozotocin in Decreasing Protein Synthesis
at Different Times After Its Administration[a]

Source of mitochondria	Time after streptozotocin (days)	Glycemia (mg/100 ml)	^{14}C-leucine incorporated (cpm/mg of protein)	Percent of normal
Normal	—	100	196	—
Diabetic	2	300	126	64
Diabetic	4	360	71	36
Diabetic	6	320	118	60
Diabetic	8	280	122	62
Diabetic	38	290	112	57

[a] Conditions were as in Table I. Mean from two experiments.

Table III. Oxygen Uptake and Respiratory Control Ratios of
Muscle Mitochondria from Normal and Diabetic Rats[a]

Source of mitochondria	Oxygen uptake (n at g oxygen/min/mg of protein)	Respiratory control ratio
Normal	278 ± 54 (6)	5.9
Diabetic	248 ± 39 (6)	6.4

[a] Conditions were as in Table I.

adequate Millipore filter units using 0.22 μ filter discs. Direct counting of colonies of the incubation mixture on agar plates enriched with normal horse serum showed that contamination was between 10 and 10^3 colonies/ml, well below the limits established as safe by Kroon et al. (20).

RESULTS

Skeletal muscle mitochondria from diabetic rats incorporated ^{14}C-leucine into proteins half as effectively as did mitochondria from normal animals. The results can be seen in Table I.

The action of streptozotocin in decreasing mitochondrial protein synthesis was already present at 48 hr, at which time the diabetogenic action was also present (Table II).

Similar results were seen with alloxan 48-96 hr after its administration.

Incorporations were carried out in a system supported by ATP produced by oxidizable substrate and ADP through participation of the mitochondrial respiratory chain and phosphorylation apparatus. It was important to ascertain that the decrease in protein synthesis was not a secondary effect due to an impairment of energy-yielding mechanisms. Accordingly, oxygen uptakes and respiratory control ratios of normal and diabetic mitochondria were measured; no difference was observed (Table III). Decrease of the synthetic activity was thus not related to a concomitant decrease in the energy supply.

Diabetic mitochondria can be partially restored to near normal by administration of insulin. Table IV shows the results at 48 hr after the administration of 10 units of insulin. We have employed crystalline insulin for times up to 12 hr and protamine zinc insulin for longer periods. The effect was studied at times

Table IV. Restoration of Synthetic Activity of Diabetic Muscle Mitochondria by Insulin[a]

Source of mitochondria	^{14}C-leucine incorporated (cpm/mg of protein)	Percent of normal
Normal	222 ± 46 (12)	—
Diabetic	107 ± 39 (12)	48[b]
Diabetic + insulin	155 ± 60 (15)	70[c]

[a] Insulin was administered 48 hr before the experiment; the dose was 10 units protamine zinc insulin, subcutaneous injection. Conditions were as in Table I.
[b] $P < 0.001$.
[c] $P < 0.05$ (between b and c).

Table V. Effect of Starvation on Mitochondrial Protein Synthesis by Skeletal Muscle Mitochondria[a]

Source of mitochondria	^{14}C-leucine incorporated (cpm/mg of protein)	Percent of normal
Normal	216 ± 42 (3)	—
Starved 4 days	90 ± 4 (3)	42

[a] Conditions were as in Table I.

Table VI. Effect of Starvation on Protein Synthesis
by Diabetic Mitochondria[a]

Source of mitochondria	^{14}C-leucine incorporated (cpm/mg of protein)	Percent of normal
Normal	213 ±27 (6)	—
Diabetic (starved 48 hr)	57 ± 9 (6)	27

[a] Conditions were as in Table I.

between 15 min and 72 hr. Results showed a rather broad scattering, with a high percentage of restoration being present in most cases, though not all, at 48 hr. The overall restoration effect at 48 hr was 70%, with a significance of $p < 0.05$. When added *in vitro* to the incubation mixture, insulin was without effect on incorporation either by normal or by diabetic mitochondria.

Since starvation is known to produce some metabolic disturbances that resemble those present in diabetes, our next step was to investigate the effect of starvation of normal animals on mitochondrial protein synthesis. The results were as follows (Table V). The effect was only partially reversed by refeeding for 2 days, but reversion was total if insulin was given at the beginning of the administration of food.

It was of interest at this point to study the effect of starvation on mitochondrial protein synthesis in diabetic rats. As can be seen in Table VI, a dramatic decrease in the incorporation took place. This means a decrease of about 70% in incorporation; although this larger effect would make these animals better "reagents" for further experimentation, side effects such as extreme weakness precluded their use in our present studies with inhibitors. It was interesting, however, to try to obtain a clear-cut effect of insulin action in these animals. The results of such experiments are shown in Fig. 1. It can be seen that the maximal effect is obtained at 48 hr after the administration of insulin.

Since it is likely that different lots of animals show somewhat different time responses, if the time of observation of the effect is not optimal this would tend to make the average response lower.

At this point, the question arose whether the action of insulin is mediated by RNA or protein synthesis. In an attempt to ascertain this, we tried to block either RNA or protein synthesis by use of specific inhibitors. We have tried actinomycin D, ethidium bromide, cycloheximide, and chloramphenicol. Experimental design proved difficult because during the long period required for insulin to exert its action, toxic side effects of the drugs took place. This was reflected in the low incorporations obtained with mitochondria from normal animals injected with the inhibitors. We plan to pursue these studies using other inhibitors of lower toxicities.

In a preliminary screening of hormonal effects on mitochondrial protein synthesis, we also studied the action of steroid hormones *in vitro* on the incorporation of amino acids by isolated rat liver and skeletal muscle mitochondria. As was previously shown by Boveris and Stoppani (16), there is a steroid-sensitive site, located in the flavoprotein area of the mitochondrial respiratory chain. If steroids were included in the incubation mixture employed to study

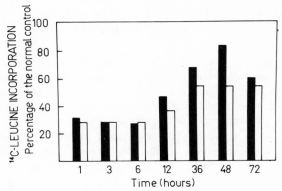

Fig. 1. Action of insulin administered in vivo *on protein synthesis by skeletal muscle mitochondria of fasted diabetic rats.* Black bars: diabetic rats, fasted, insulin treated; during insulin treatment, food was given *ad libitum.* White bars: control animals, fasted diabetic animals; food was administered during the same period as with insulin-treated rats.

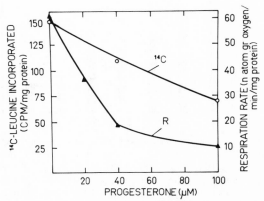

Fig. 2. Action of progesterone on protein synthesis and oxygen uptake by isolated liver mitochondria.

mitochondrial protein synthesis, a depression of the incorporation took place which was related to the inhibition of respiration. Results of a typical experiment can be seen in Fig. 2, which shows the results obtained with different concentrations of progesterone. This result was general with all steroids tested and NAD-dependent substrates. With succinate as substrate, inhibition of the incorporation was observed only at much higher concentration of the steroid, and this point should be remembered. In the presence of ATP and an ATP-generating system, there was no inhibition of the incorporation between 2 and 200 μM progesterone. Fig. 3 shows the results obtained with different steroids. It can be seen that the inhibition of incorporation is always less than the inhibition of respiration.

Similar experiments were also done with muscle mitochondria, especially in the presence of anabolic steroids, such as testosterone, but in no case was a change of the amount of mitochondrial protein synthesis obtained. We also performed these experiments with muscle mitochondria of immature rats, as well as with castrated animals, either immature or adult. As the respiration in muscle mitochondria was inhibited, sometimes to a considerable degree, we concluded that the discrepancy in the response of liver and skeletal muscle mitochondrial protein synthesis toward steroids could perhaps be explained on the basis of the much higher respiratory activity of the latter. That is, respiration could be inhibited to a considerable degree in muscle mitochondria, but still permit a production of sufficient ATP to support mitochondrial protein synthesis.

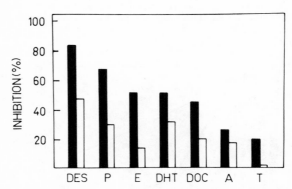

Fig. 3. Relationship between inhibition of respiration and inhibition of incorporation in liver mitochondria in the presence of different steroids. Black bars: inhibition of respiration. White bars: inhibition of incorporation. DES, diethylstilbestrol; PR, progesterone 17 β:17 β-estradiol; DHT, dihydrotestosterone; DOC, deoxycorticosterone acetate; A, androsterone; T, testosterone.

Breuer and Florini (21) showed a correlation between the anabolic action of testosterone and its capacity to enhance cell-free protein-synthesizing ability of skeletal muscle ribosomes from immature castrated rats. We tried similar conditions of testosterone administration to immature castrated rats to see if muscle mitochondria responded in a similar way, but could find no stimulation of protein synthesis by isolated mitochondria. We also found no stimulation using adult rats given different anabolic doses of testosterone after different castration periods.

Contrary to our results with insulin, there seems to be no relation between behavior *in vitro* of isolated ribosomes and isolated mitochondria under similar hormonal conditions.

CONCLUSIONS

The results presented above show that in the diabetic state a remarkable decrease in the protein synthetic ability of isolated rat skeletal muscle mitochondria takes place. This reduction can be partially reversed by administration of insulin 48 hr prior to sacrifice.

This would suggest that the synthesis of the proteins of the inner membrane, which are known to be synthesized by isolated mitochondria, is influenced by insulin. The importance of this influence can be considered in terms of control of the synthesis of a set of mitochondrial proteins which, as suggested by several authors (2,22,23), might have a regulatory role in the assembly of the mitochondrion.

Analyses of our own results, together with those found in the literature, suggest that different types of interrelationships seem to exist between the protein-synthesizing activities of the cytoplasmic and mitochondrial systems isolated from hormone-treated animals:

(a) Diabetes decreased and insulin restored the ability of muscle ribosomes to incorporate amino acids (24). This effect has also been found by us in the mitochondrial system, although kinetics of the insulin effect were different.

(b) Thyroidectomy and the administration of thyroid hormones produced similar changes in the synthetic activities of the microsomal and mitochondrial systems (25).

Insulin in diabetic animals (a) and thyroid hormones in thyroidectomized rats (b) show quite different time-effect relationships. In (a), Wool *et al.* (24) found that the activity of ribosomes was restored by the administration of 0.1 units of insulin in only 5 min, while the effect we have seen in mitochondria takes 36-48 hr to develop and requires 10 units of insulin. In (b), both mitochondrial and ribosomal systems are coordinated in time, with no lag in any of the systems.

Breuer and Florini (21) described an action of testosterone on the muscle ribosomal system of immature rats for which we have not found a counterpart at the mitochondrial level. Of course, the possibility cannot be completely discarded that our conditions do not permit us to detect changes in the mitochondrial system, even though we explored this under widely different experimental conditions.

Since there seem to be similarities in the cytoplasmic and mitochondrial protein-synthesizing systems, as far as the inclusion of ribosomes, messenger RNAs, transfer RNAs, and enzymes participating in the process are concerned, the difference between the responses of these systems to the hormones studied can be found in one of the following points of control.

In the case of insulin, Wool and coworkers interpret their results as being the consequence of the synthesis, under the action of insulin, of a factor they call "translation factor," which makes the ribosomes more able to translate messenger RNA. In our case, in view of the great differences in behavior toward insulin of the mitochondrial system, it can be expected that the mechanism would differ in many respects, possibly involving other points of control.

The fact that total reversal is not always seen with insulin could be the result of either the fact that we are not always observing the action of insulin at its optimal time or the hypothetical occurrence of irreversible damage to the mitochondria in the diabetic state.

In the case of thyroid hormones, the same mechanism of control could be operating synchronously at the mitochondrial and ribosomal levels.

As far as testosterone is concerned, action at the level of RNA synthesis to enhance the cytoplasmic synthesis of proteins, with no concerted action at the mitochondrial level, was considered by Breuer and Florini.

All the previous considerations lead to the conclusion that insulin and thyroid hormones, but not testosterone, *in vivo* may stimulate modifications of certain components of the mitochondrion which are present in the isolated organelles and are responsible for their increased synthetic ability *in vitro*.

ACKNOWLEDGMENTS

This study was aided by grants from the Consejo Nacional de Investigaciones Científicas y Técnicas and the Instituto de Farmacología, Secretaría de Salud Pública de la Nación Argentina. M. S. T. and A. O. M. S. are members of the Investigator Career, Consejo Nacional de Investigaciones Científicas y Técnicas. We are greatly indebted to Upjohn International, Inc., Kalamazoo, Michigan, U.S.A., for their generous gift of streptozotocin.

SUMMARY

A study of the effects of insulin, which is known to exert a profound effect on the muscle ribosomal system, has been undertaken. A considerable decrease of amino acid incorporation took place in mitochondria isolated from skeletal muscle of diabetic rats. This decrease was not due to impairment of the energy production by mitochondria, since oxygen uptake and respiratory control ratios were similar for mitochondria isolated from normal or from diabetic animals. Diabetic mitochondria showed a 52% decrease in their ability to incorporate amino acids *in vitro*. Diabetes was induced by the administration of streptozotocin. *In vitro,* the drug did not show any influence on the incorporation process. The decrease in incorporation could be partially reversed by administration of insulin *in vivo,* but restoration was achieved only after 48 hr. Starvation of normal animals for 4 days had a similar effect in decreasing protein synthesis. This effect could be reversed partially by refeeding for 2 days; recovery was complete if insulin was administered together with food. Starvation of diabetic rats was followed by a 70% decrease of the synthetic activity. The effect could again be reversed by refeeding plus insulin. The mechanism by which diabetes depresses and insulin restores the capacity of skeletal muscle mitochondria to synthesize proteins *in vitro* is being studied by the use of inhibitors of nucleic acid and protein synthesis.

The well-known anabolic action of testosterone in muscle prompted us to also study the effect of different steroids on mitochondrial protein synthesis. Preliminary experiments with steroids *in vitro* showed that protein synthesis by isolated liver mitochondria was decreased by those steroids which also inhibited mitochondrial respiration; the latter was shown to be the primary effect. The synthetic activity of muscle mitochondria either *in vivo* or *in vitro* was not affected by experimental changes in the level of testosterone, either by castration or by subsequent administration of physiological or anabolic doses of the hormone. These experiments show that muscle mitochondria are unresponsive to testosterone, at variance with its known stimulatory effect on the microsomal synthetic activity in muscle.

RESUMEN

Se llevó a cabo una investigación sobre el efecto de la insulina, que ejerce una acción profunda sobre el sistema citoplásmico del músculo. Se encontró una disminución considerable de la incorporación de aminoácidos en mitocondrias aisladas de músculo esquelético de ratas diabéticas. Esta disminución no era consecuencia de un impedimento en la producción de energía por las mitocondrias, ya que los consumos de oxígeno y controles respiratorios de las mitocondrias aisladas de animales normales y diabéticos eran semejantes. Las mitocondrias diabéticas exhibían una disminución de un 52% en su capacidad para incorporar aminoácidos *in vitro*. La diabetes se indujo por administración de streptozotocina; dicha droga *in vitro* no tenía acción sobre el proceso de incorporación. La disminución de la incorporación podría revertirse por administración de insulina *in vivo* pero la reversión tarda 48 horas en producirse. El ayuno de los animales durante cuatro días disminuye en forma semejante la síntesis de proteínas. El efecto puede ser parcialmente revertido por dos días de alimentación. La reversión era completa si se administraba insulina conjuntamente con la comida. El ayuno de ratas diabéticas condujo a un 70% de disminución de la actividad sintética. El efecto pudo ser también revertido por comida e insulina. Se está estudiando mediante el uso de inhibidores el mecanismo por el cual la diabetes disminuye y la insulina restablece la capacidad de las mitocondrias de músculo esquelético para sintetizar proteínas *in vitro*.

La conocida acción anabólica de la testosterona nos impulsó a estudiar también el efecto de diversos esteroides sobre la síntesis de proteína mitocondrial. Experimentos preliminares empleando esteroides *in vitro* demostraron que la síntesis de proteínas por mitocondrias aisladas de hígado era disminuida por aquellos esteroides que inhibián también la respiración mitocondrial; se demostró que este último era el efecto primario. La actividad sintética de mitocondrias de músculo, ya sea *in vivo* o *in vitro* no era afectada por cambios experimentales en los niveles de testosterona, producidos por castración o por la administración subsiguiente de dosis fisiológicas o anabólicas de la hormona. Estos experimentos demuestran que las mitocondrias de músculo no responden a la testosterona, en contraposición con el efecto que ésta ejerce sobre la actividad sintética en microsomas de músculo.

REFERENCES

1. Pullman, M. E., and Schatz, G., *Ann. Rev. Biochem., 36* (Part II), 539 (1967).
2. Schatz, G., in Racker, E. (ed.), *Membranes of Mitochondria and Chloroplasts,* Van Nostrand and Reinhold Co., New York (1970), p. 251.
3. Borst, P., and Kroon, A. M., *Internat. Rev. Cytol., 26,* 107 (1969).
4. Nass, M. M. K., *Science, 165,* 25 (1969).
5. Davey, P. J., Yu, R., and Linnane, A. W., *Biochem. Biophys. Res. Commun., 36,* 30 (1969).
6. Beattie, D. S., Basford, R. E., and Koritz, S. B., *Biochemistry, 6,* 3099 (1967).
7. Criddle, R. S., Bock, R. M., Green, D. E., and Tisdale, H., *Biochemistry, 1,* 827 (1962).
8. Kellerman, G. M., Biggs, D. R., and Linnane, A. W., *J. Cell Biol., 42,* 378 (1969).
9. Manchester, K. L., in Munro, H. N. (ed.), *Mammalian Protein Metabolism,* Academic Press, New York (1970), p. 229.
10. Roodyn, D. B., *Biochem. J., 97,* 782 (1965).
11. Klee, C. B., and Sokoloff, L., *Proc. Natl. Acad. Sci. U.S.A., 53,* 1014 (1965).
12. Favelukes, S. L. S. de, Schwarcz de Tarlovsky, M., and Stoppani, A. O. M., *Acta Physiol. Latinoam., 21,* 30 (1971).
13. Tata, J. R., in Tager, J. M., Papa, S., Quagliarello, E., and Slater, E. C. (eds.), *Regulation of Metabolic Processes in Mitochondria,* Elsevier Publishing Co., Amsterdam (1966), p. 489.
14. Shäfer, G., and Nägel, L., *Biochim. Biophys. Acta, 162,* 617 (1968).
15. Roldan, A. G., Del Castillo, E. J., Boveris, A., Garaza Pereira, A., and Stoppani, A. O. M., *Proc. Soc. Exptl. Biol. Med., 137,* 791 (1971).
16. Boveris, A., and Stoppani, A. O. M., *Arch. Biochem. Biophys., 141,* 641 (1970).
17. Junod, A., Lambert, A. E., Orci, L., Pictet, R., Gonet, A. E., and Renold, A. E., *Proc. Soc. Exptl. Biol. Med., 126,* 201 (1967).
18. Nikkilä, A. E., and Hyvärinen, A., *Clin. Chim. Acta, 7,* 140 (1962).
19. Jacobs, E. E., Jacob, M., Sanadi, D. R., and Bradley, L. B., *J. Biol. Chem., 223,* 147 (1956).
20. Kroon, A. M., Saccone, C., and Botman, M. J., *Biochim. Biophys. Acta, 142,* 552 (1967).
21. Breuer, C. B., and Florini, J. R., *Biochemistry, 4,* 1544 (1965).
22. Mahler, H. R., Perlman, P., Henson, C., and Weber, C., *Biochem. Biophys. Res. Commun., 31,* 3 (1968).
23. Ashwell, M. A., and Work, T. S., *Biochem. Biophys. Res. Commun., 32,* 1006 (1968).
24. Wool, I. G., Stirewalt, W. S., Kurihara, K., Low, R. B., Bailey, P., and Oyer, D., *Recent Progr. Hormone Res., 24,* 139 (1968).
25. Roodyn, D. B., Freeman, K. B., and Tata, J. R., *Biochem. J., 94,* 628 (1965).

DISCUSSION

P. P. Cohen (Madison, U.S.A.): I wish to offer a few comments which do not bear directly on the present paper but stem from the inquiry that was made earlier about the relationship between mitochondrial and extramitochondrial systems. In recent years, investigators have been dedicated to preparing highly purified mitochondria, and this has been laudable. However, one ought to reflect on the possibility that studies with less purified mitochondrial preparations might have considerable interest with respect to the regulation of protein synthesis and intracellular transport. We have a manuscript in press (*J. Biol. Chem.*) which demonstrates the operation of a concerted mechanism involving two mitochondrial enzymes and three extramitochondrial enzymes. These five enzymes are involved in urea biosynthesis. This biosynthetic pathway responds to the hormone thyroxine with a concerted response. The increase in activity of the mitochondrial enzymes follows right along with that of the extramitochondrial enzymes. Therefore, there must be regulatory factors which are operating to insure a relationship between what is going on in the nucleus, the cytoplasm, the ribosomes, and the mitochondria. Thus it is important that investigators studying regulated processes such as protein synthesis in mitochondria recognize that extramitochondrial factors are involved in the regulation of mitochondrial systems.

H. R. Mahler (Bloomington, U.S.A.): A comment on Dr. Cohen's comment and then a question to Dr. Favelukes. Of course, we are quite aware of this. We have actually gone further than that, we used the cell as our unit rather than impure mitochondria. Let me comment that when the signal is passed, whatever the signal may be, to lead to release from catabolite repression, there is complete coordinate synthesis of glutamate dehydrogenase (which in yeast is a completely extramitochondrial enzyme), malic dehydrogenase (which is extramitochondrial and matrix), and succinic dehydrogenase (which is mitochondrial in the membrane); this is quite analogous to what you have observed in your urea cycle enzymes, and that is on a cellular basis. Now the question, Dr. Favelukes, is the following: will you entertain a model for insulin action which would postulate that the primary action is extramitochondrial, that it leads to the synthesis of a component which is slowly integrated into the mitochondria and which then exerts the mitochondrial effects that you have observed such as the long lag and the partial restoration?

S. S. de Favelukes (Buenos Aires, Argentina): That could be one explanation; another possible explanation is the synthesis of some intramitochondrial component such as ribosomal RNA. That would have a long lag, too.

H. R. Mahler: Not in the systems that I am familiar with. I think this is true even of the animal mitochondria, at least Kroon believes very strongly that the transcription and translation are very tightly coupled.

K. L. Manchester (Kingston, Jamaica): If I could just comment on Dr. Mahler's comment, surely in the diabetic you might well expect that the amount of RNA in the mitochondria might well be down, the same as with total RNA in the tissue, and its restoration would take time, many hours, not just a few minutes. I think this was the point.

F. L. Sacerdote (Mendoza, Argentina): I would like to ask, not specifically with respect to the last speaker but with respect to the three mitochondrion papers which have been given this morning, whether anyone could speculate a bit. Since the contribution of the mitochondrion to protein synthesis, even perhaps to the synthesis of its own proteins, is apparently a small percentage of the protein of a cell, why do mitochondria synthesize protein at all?

S. S. de Favelukes: One reason to study this is that if insulin regulates the synthesis of the proteins of the inner membrane—we are aware of the limitations but we are supposing that the *in vitro* protein synthesis represents in some way the *in vivo* protein synthesis of the endogenous mitochondrial synthesizing system—if this protein synthesized by the mitochondria has a regulating or control action, it will be important to study this. Many people speculate that protein synthesized by the mitochondrion exerts a regulatory action on the cytoplasmic system for the synthesis of mitochondrial protein.

A. F. De Nicola (Buenos Aires, Argentina): Since you did not have any definite effect of testosterone on mitochondrial protein synthesis in muscle, what about the effect of testosterone in specific target organs such as the prostate, or estrogens in the uterus, or DOC or aldosterone in the kidney?

S. S. de Favelukes: Williams-Ashman has demonstrated that it has an action.

A. F. De Nicola: On mitochondrial protein synthesis?

S. S. de Favelukes: Not *in vitro*: testosterone administered *in vivo* to castrated animals acts to increase the capacity of prostate mitochondria for *in vitro* protein synthesis.

K. L. Manchester: With respect to one of the last questions, I think this is a good point. Could we ask Dr. Mahler to speculate wildly: what is the point of mitochondrial protein synthesis as it stands, because it is so small a proportion?

H. R. Mahler: We stuck our necks out on that, Dr. Manchester, in several recent publications and have asserted strongly that the function of the polypeptides specified by the mitochondrial genome and translated by the mitochondrial system of protein synthesis is in all likelihood a regulatory function. The recent identification of possibly a partial synthesis of cytochrome oxidase or cytochrome oxidase peptides and a peptide involved in the anchoring of the F1 ATPase to the membrane (unpublished observations of our own and others) tends to indicate that perhaps the polypeptides in question are not themselves part of the catalytic center of the molecule, but are involved in regulating the integration of those proteins into the membrane. It is already known from a number of studies that, based on some early work by Reilly and Sherman and some recent work by Dr. Peré in Dr. Slonimski's laboratory, cytochrome oxidase itself in turn exerts a regulatory function on the biosynthesis as well as the regulation of other mitochondrial enzymes. So one can entertain the picture of a cascade of regulatory events starting with an integrating polypeptide, responsible for the elaboration and the integration of a mitochondrial catalytic entity, itself specified externally, which then regulates mitochondrial biosynthesis and function, which in turn regulates certain key metabolic events in the cell as a whole. I would say that at the present moment this is the model that I would tend to test.

P. P. Cohen: I would like to add another point which Dr. Mahler did not refer to, probably in the interest of brevity. As you know, the mitochondrion is considered to be a vestigial organelle. It has been suggested that plastids in plant cells and mitochondria in animal cells have an evolutionary symbiotic origin. In the course of evolution, the eukaryotic cell has not only exploited the properties of plastids and mitochondria to carry out the production of ATP, etc., but also has utilized them to sequester certain systems to provide additional mechanisms for regulation of cell functions.

H. R. Mahler: Just to complete this particular discussion, I think it is very important to re-emphasize the additional functions of mitochondria, and this sequestration of essential cellular functions and cellular regulatory events inside the mitochondria is one of them. Once again, I think many of us have lost sight, because of the obvious implication of mitochondria in energy formation and transduction, of the additional essential functions the mitochondria fulfill. The particular example I would like to mention here is the mitochondria in the DNA-zero mutants, which have absolutely no respiration whatsoever, no oxidative phosphorylation whatsoever, but a complete retention of mitochondria, an essential retention of mitochondrial topography and topology, and perpetuation of mitochondria even in the complete absence of the mitochondrial genetic apparatus.

Index